# MEDICAL INSTRUMENTATION

## Application and Design

# MEDICAL INSTRUMENTATION

## Application and Design

FOURTH EDITION

**John G. Webster, Editor**

Contributing Authors

**John W. Clark, Jr.**
Rice University

**Michael R. Neuman**
Michigan Technological University

**Walter H. Olson**
Medtronic, Inc.

**Robert A. Peura**
Worcester Polytechnic Institute

**Frank P. Primiano, Jr.**
Consultant

**Melvin P. Siedband**
University of Wisconsin-Madison

**John G. Webster**
University of Wisconsin-Madison

**Lawrence A. Wheeler**
Nutritional Computing Concepts

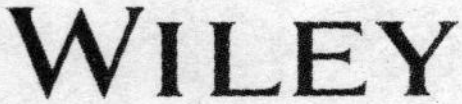

**Medical Instrumentation:** Application and Design
*Fourth Edition*

Authorized reprint by Wiley India Pvt. Ltd., 4435-36/7, Ansari Road, Daryaganj, New Delhi – 110002.



Cover Image: Getty Images



**Reprint:** 2016

**Printed at:** Raj Kamal Press, Delhi

ISBN: 978-81-265-5379-2

# PREFACE

*Medical Instrumentation*: Application and Design, Fourth Edition, is written for a senior to graduate-level course in biomedical engineering. It describes the principles, applications, and design of the medical instruments most commonly used in hospitals. Because equipment changes with time, we have stressed fundamental principles of operation and general types of equipment, avoiding detailed descriptions and photographs of specific models. Furthermore, because biomedical engineering is an interdisciplinary field requiring good communication with health-care personnel, we have provided some applications for each type of instrument. However, to keep the book to a reasonable length, we have omitted much of the physiology.

Most of those who use this text have had an introductory course in chemistry, are familiar with mathematics through differential equations, have a strong background in physics, and have taken courses in electric circuits and electronics. However, readers without this background will gain much from the descriptive material and should find this text a valuable reference. In addition, we recommend reading background material from an inexpensive physiology text, such as W. F. Ganong's *Review of Medical Physiology*, 22nd edition (New York: McGraw-Hill, 2005).

## EMPHASIS ON DESIGN

Throughout the book, we emphasize design. A scientist or engineer who has some background in electronics and instrumentation will glean enough information, in many of the areas we address, to be able to design medical instruments. This ability should be especially valuable in those situations—so frequently encountered—where special instruments that are not commercially available are required.

## PEDAGOGY

The book provides 300 homework problems, located at the end of each chapter, plus 64 in-text worked examples. Problems are designed to cover a wide variety of applications ranging from analysis of the waves of the electrocardiogram to circuit design of biopotential amplifiers and identification of electric safety hazards.

## REFERENCES

Rather than giving an exhaustive list of references, we have provided a list of review articles and books that can serve as a point of departure for further study on any given topic.

## ORGANIZATION

Each chapter has been carefully reviewed and updated for the fourth edition, and many new examples and references are included.

Chapter 1 covers general concepts that are applicable to all instrumentation systems, including on the commercial development of medical instruments, on biostatistics, and on the regulation of medical devices. Chapter 2 describes basic sensors, and Chapter 3 presents the design of amplifiers for them. Chapters 4 through 6 deal with biopotentials, tracing the topic from the origin of biopotentials, through electrodes, to the special amplifier design required.

Chapters 7 and 8 cover the measurement of cardiovascular dynamics—pressure, sound, flow, and volume of blood. Chapter 9 presents the measurement of respiratory dynamics—pressure, flow, and concentration of gases.

Chapter 10 describes the developing field of biosensors: sensors that measure chemical concentrations within the body via catheters or implants. Chapter 11 describes that area in the hospital where the greatest number of measurements is made, the clinical laboratory. Chapter 12 starts with general concepts of medical imaging and shows their applications to x-ray techniques, magnetic resonance imaging, positron emission tomography, and Doppler ultrasonic images.

Chapter 13 deals with devices used in therapy, such as the pacemaker, defibrillator, cochlear prosthesis, transcutaneous electrical nerve stimulation, implantable automatic defibrillators, the total artificial heart, lithotripsy, infant radiant warmers, drug infusion pumps, and anesthesia machines. Chapter 14 presents a guide both to electric safety in the hospital and to minimization of hazards.

We have used the recommended International System of Units (SI) throughout this book. In the case of units of pressure, we have presented both the commonly used millimeters of mercury and its SI unit, the pascal. To help the reader follow the trend toward employing SI units, the Appendix provides the most common conversion factors. The Appendix also provides a number of physical constants used in the book and a list of abbreviations.

A Solutions Manual containing complete solutions to all problems is available free to adopters of this text.

## ACKNOWLEDGMENTS

We would like to thank the reviewers of previous editions.

*First Edition Reviewers*
David Arnett, *Pennsylvania State University*
Robert B. Northrup, *University of Connecticut (Storrs)*
Kenneth C. Mylrea, *University of Arizona*
Curran S. Swift, *Iowa State University*

*Second Edition Reviewers*
Jonathan Newell, *Rensselaer Polytechnic Institute*
Robert B. Northrup, *University of Connecticut (Storrs)*

*Third Edition Reviewers*
Noel Thompson, *Stanford University*
W. Ed Hammond, *Duke University*
Robert B. Northrup, *University of Connecticut*
Richard Jendrucko, *University of Tennessee, Knoxville*

*Fourth Edition Reviewers*
Paul J. Benkeser, *Georgia Institute of Technology*
Lawrence V. Hmurcik, *University of Bridgeport*
Art Koblasz, *Georgia Institute of Technology*
Anant Madabhushi, *Rutgers University*
Andrew Mason, Michigan State University
Ken Meissner, *Texas A&M University*
Peter Molnar, *Clemson University*
Homer Nazeran, *The University of Texas at El Paso*
John A. Pearce, *The University of Texas at Austin*
Nadine Barrie Smith, *The Pennsylvania State University*

The authors welcome your suggestions for improvement of subsequent printings and editions.

*John G. Webster*

# LIST OF SYMBOLS

This list gives single-letter symbols for quantities, without subscripts or modifiers. Symbols for physical constants are given in Appendix A.1, multi-letter symbols in Appendix A.4, and chemical symbols in Appendix A.5.

| Symbol | Quantity | Introduced in Section |
|---|---|---|
| $a$ | Absorptivity | 10.3 |
| $a$ | Activity | 5.2 |
| $a$ | Coefficient | 1.10 |
| $\mathbf{a}$ | Lead vector | 6.2 |
| $A$ | Absorbance | 10.3 |
| $A$ | Area | 2.2 |
| $A$ | Coefficient | 1.9 |
| $A$ | Gain | 3.1 |
| $A$ | Percent | 1.7 |
| $b$ | Coefficient | 1.9 |
| $b$ | Intercept | 1.9 |
| $B$ | Coefficient | 1.10 |
| $B$ | Percent | 1.9 |
| $B$ | Viscous friction | 1.10 |
| $\mathbf{B}$ | Magnetic flux density | 8.3 |
| $c$ | Coefficient | 7.13 |
| $c$ | Specific heat | 8.1 |
| $c$ | Velocity of sound | 8.4 |
| $C$ | Capacitance | 1.10 |
| $C$ | Compliance | 7.3 |
| $C$ | Concentration | 10.3 |
| $C$ | Contrast | 12.1 |
| $d$ | Derivative | 1.10 |
| $d$ | Diameter | 1.10 |
| $d$ | Distance | 4.1 |
| $D$ | Density | 12.4 |
| $D$ | Detector responsivity | 2.17 |

(*Continued*)

| Symbol | Quantity | Introduced in Section |
|---|---|---|
| $D$ | $d/dt$ | 1.10 |
| $D$ | Diameter | 5.8 |
| $D$ | Diffusing capacity | 9.8 |
| $D$ | Distance | 4.4 |
| $E$ | emf | 2.7 |
| $E$ | Energy | 2.13 |
| $E$ | Exposure | 12.4 |
| $E$ | Irradiance | 2.17 |
| $E$ | Modulus of elasticity | 7.3 |
| $f$ | Force | 2.6 |
| $f$ | Frequency | 1.10 |
| $f$ | Function | 4.2 |
| $F$ | Filter transmission | 2.17 |
| $F$ | Flow | 7.3 |
| $F$ | Force | 2.2 |
| $F$ | Fraction | 12.1 |
| $F$ | Molar fraction | 9.3 |
| $g$ | Conductance/area | 4.1 |
| $G$ | Conductance | 2.9 |
| $G$ | Form factor | 2.4 |
| $G$ | Gage factor | 2.2 |
| $G$ | Gain | 1.7 |
| $h$ | Height | 7.13 |
| $H$ | Feedback gain | 1.7 |
| $i$ | Current | 2.6 |
| $I$ | Current | 3.7 |
| $I$ | Intensity | 10.3 |
| $j$ | $+(-1)^{1/2}$ | 1.10 |
| $J$ | Number of standard deviations | 12.1 |
| $k$ | Constant | 6.7 |
| $k$ | Piezoelectric constant | 2.6 |
| $K$ | Constant | 1.10 |
| $K$ | Number | 12.1 |
| $K$ | Sensitivity | 1.10 |
| $K$ | Solubility product | 5.3 |
| $K$ | Spring constant | 1.10 |
| $L$ | Inductance | 2.4 |
| $L$ | Inertance | 7.3 |
| $L$ | Length | 2.2 |
| $L$ | Line-source response | 12.10 |
| $m$ | Average number | 12.1 |
| $m$ | Mass | 7.3 |
| $m$ | Slope | 1.9 |
| $M$ | Mass | 1.10 |
| $M$ | Measured values | 12.2 |
| $\overline{M}$ | Modulation | 12.1 |
| $\mathbf{M}$ | Cardiac vector | 6.2 |
| $n$ | Number | 1.8 |

| Symbol | Quantity | Introduced in Section |
|---|---|---|
| $n$ | Refractive index | 2.14 |
| $N$ | Noise equivalent bandwidth | 12.3 |
| $N$ | Number | 5.3 |
| $N$ | Turns ratio | 3.13 |
| $p$ | Change in pressure | 9.1 |
| $p$ | Probability | 12.1 |
| $P$ | Power | 1.9 |
| $P$ | Pressure | 7.3 |
| $P$ | Projection | 12.8 |
| $q$ | Charge | 2.6 |
| $q$ | Rate of heat | 8.1 |
| $q$ | Change in volume flow | 9.1 |
| $Q$ | Heat content | 8.2 |
| $Q$ | Volume flow | 9.1 |
| $r$ | Correlation coefficient | 1.8 |
| $r$ | Radius | 7.3 |
| $r$ | Resistance/length | 4.2 |
| $R$ | Range | 8.4 |
| $R$ | Ratio | 10.3 |
| $R$ | Resistance | 1.10 |
| $S$ | Standard deviation | 1.8 |
| $S$ | Modulation transfer function | 12.2 |
| $S$ | Saturation | 10.1 |
| $S$ | Slew rate | 3.11 |
| $S$ | Source output | 2.17 |
| $t$ | Thickness | 5.8 |
| $t$ | Time | 1.10 |
| $T$ | Interval | 1.10 |
| $T$ | Temperature | 2.8 |
| $T$ | Transmittance | 11.1 |
| $u$ | Velocity | 4.2 |
| $u$ | Work function | 12.6 |
| $U$ | Molar uptake | 9.1 |
| $v$ | Voltage | 1.10 |
| $v$ | Change in volume | 9.1 |
| $V$ | Voltage | 1.10 |
| $V$ | Volume | 2.2 |
| $W$ | Power | 2.10 |
| $W$ | Weight | 10.3 |
| $W$ | Weighting factor | 12.8 |
| $x$ | Constant | 10.3 |
| $x$ | Distance | 2.4 |
| $x$ | Input | 1.7 |
| $X$ | Chemical species | 9.1 |
| $X$ | Effort variable | 1.9 |
| $X$ | Value | 1.8 |
| $y$ | Constant | 10.3 |

(*Continued*)

| Symbol | Quantity | Introduced in Section |
|---|---|---|
| $y$ | Output | 1.7 |
| $Y$ | Admittance | 1.9 |
| $Y$ | Flow variable | 1.9 |
| $Y$ | Value | 1.8 |
| $z$ | Distance | 4.1 |
| $Z$ | Atomic number | 12.6 |
| $Z$ | Impedance | 1.9 |

## Greek Letters

| Symbol | Quantity | Introduced in Section |
|---|---|---|
| $\alpha$ | Polytropic constant | 9.5 |
| $\alpha$ | Thermistor coefficient | 2.9 |
| $\alpha$ | Thermoelectric sensitivity | 2.8 |
| $\beta$ | Thermistor constant | 2.9 |
| $\Delta$ | Deviation | 10.3 |
| $\varepsilon$ | Emissivity | 2.10 |
| $\varepsilon$ | Dielectric constant | 2.5 |
| $\zeta$ | Damping ratio | 1.10 |
| $\eta$ | Viscosity | 7.3 |
| $\theta$ | Angle | 2.14 |
| $\Lambda$ | Logarithmic decrement | 1.10 |
| $\lambda$ | Wavelength | 2.10 |
| $\mu$ | Attenuation coefficient | 12.8 |
| $\mu$ | Mobility | 5.2 |
| $\mu$ | Permeability | 2.4 |
| $\mu$ | Poisson's ratio | 2.2 |
| $\rho$ | Density | 7.3 |
| $\rho$ | Mole density | 9.1 |
| $\rho$ | Resistivity | 2.2 |
| $\sigma$ | Conductance | 13.4 |
| $\sigma$ | Conductivity/distance | 4.7 |
| $\sigma^2$ | Variance | 12.1 |
| $\tau$ | Time constant | 1.10 |
| $\phi$ | Number of photons | 12.6 |
| $\phi$ | Phase shift | 1.10 |
| $\phi$ | Divergence | 8.4 |
| $\Phi$ | Potential | 4.6 |
| $\omega$ | Frequency | 1.10 |

# CONTENTS

# 5 BIOPOTENTIAL ELECTRODES 189

**Michael R. Neuman**



# 6 BIOPOTENTIAL AMPLIFIERS 241

**Michael R. Neuman**

# 7 BLOOD PRESSURE AND SOUND 293

**Robert A. Peura**



# 8 MEASUREMENT OF FLOW AND VOLUME OF BLOOD 338

**John G. Webster**

# 14 ELECTRICAL SAFETY 638

**Walter H. Olson**



# APPENDIX 676



# INDEX 683

# 1

# BASIC CONCEPTS OF MEDICAL INSTRUMENTATION

Walter H. Olson

The invention, prototype design, product development, clinical testing, regulatory approval, manufacturing, marketing, and sale of a new medical instrument add up to a complex, expensive, and lengthy process. Very few new ideas survive the practical requirements, human barriers, and inevitable setbacks of this arduous process. Usually there is one person who is the "champion" of a truly new medical instrument or device. This person—who is not necessarily the inventor—must have a clear vision of the final new product and exactly how it will be used. Most importantly, this person must have the commitment and persistence to overcome unexpected technical problems, convince the naysayers, and cope with the bureaucratic apparatus that is genuinely needed to protect patients.

One of five inventors' stories from *New Medical Devices: Invention, Development and Use* (Eckelman, 1988) is reprinted here to illustrate this process. The automated biochemical analyzer uses spectrophotometric methods in a continuous-flow system to measure the amount of many clinically important substances in blood or urine samples (Section 11.2).

***Development of Technicon's Auto Analyzer***

*Edwin C. Whitehead*

*In 1950 Alan Moritz, chairman of the department of pathology at Case Western Reserve University and an old friend of mine, wrote to tell me about Leonard Skeggs, a young man in his department who had developed an instrument that Technicon might be interested in. I was out of my New York office on a prolonged trip, and my father, cofounder with me of Technicon Corporation, opened the letter. He wrote to Dr. Moritz saying that Technicon was always interested in new developments and enclosed a four-page confidential disclosure form. Not surprisingly, Dr. Moritz thought that Technicon was not really interested in Skeggs's instrument, and my father dismissed the matter as routine.*

*Three years later Ray Roesch, Technicon's only salesman at the time, was visiting Joseph Kahn at the Cleveland Veterans Administration Hospital. Dr. Kahn asked Ray why Technicon had turned down Skeggs's invention. Ray responded that he had never heard of it and asked, "What invention?" Kahn replied, "A machine to automate chemical analysis." When Ray called me and asked why I had turned Skeggs's idea down, I said I had not heard of it either. When he told me that Skeggs's idea was to automate clinical chemistry, my reaction was, "Wow! Let's look at it and make sure Skeggs doesn't get away."*

*That weekend, Ray Roesch loaded some laboratory equipment in his station wagon and drove Leonard Skeggs and his wife Jean to New York. At Technicon, Skeggs set up a simple device consisting of a peristaltic pump to draw the specimen sample and reagent streams through the system, a continuous dialyzer to remove protein molecules that might interfere with the specimen-reagent reaction, and a spectrophotometer equipped with a flow cell to monitor the reaction. This device demonstrated the validity of the idea, and we promptly entered negotiations with Skeggs for a license to patent the Auto Analyzer. We agreed on an initial payment of $6,000 and royalties of 3 percent after a certain number of units had been sold.*

*After Technicon "turned-down" the project in 1950, Skeggs had made arrangements first with the Heinecke Instrument Co. and then the Harshaw Chemical Co. to sell his device. Both companies erroneously assumed that the instrument was a finished product. However, neither company had been able to sell a single instrument from 1950 until 1953. This was not surprising, because Skeggs's original instrument required an expensive development process to make it rugged and reliable, and to modify the original, manual chemical assays. Technicon spent 3 years refining the simple model developed by Skeggs into a commercially viable continuous-flow analyzer.*

*A number of problems unique to the Auto Analyzer had to be overcome. Because the analyzer pumps a continuous-flow stream of reagents interrupted by specimen samples, one basic problem was the interaction between specimen samples. This problem was alleviated by introducing air bubbles as physical barriers between samples. However, specimen carryover in continuous-flow analyzers remains sensitive to the formation and size of bubbles, the inside diameter of the tubing through which fluids flow, the pattern of peristaltic pumping action, and other factors.*

*Development of the Auto Analyzer was financed internally at Technicon. In 1953 Technicon had ongoing business of less than $10 million per year: automatic tissue processors and slide filing cabinets for histology laboratories, automatic fraction collectors for chromatography, and portable respirators for polio patients. Until it went public in 1969, Technicon had neither borrowed money nor sold equity. Thus, Technicon's patent on Skegg's original invention was central to the development of the Auto Analyzer. Without patent protection, Technicon could never have afforded to pursue the expensive development of this device.*

*Early in the instrument's development, I recognized that traditional marketing techniques suitable for most laboratory instruments would not work for something as revolutionary as the Auto Analyzer. At that time, laboratory instruments were usually sold by catalog salesmen or by mail from specification sheets listing instrument specifications, price, and perhaps product benefits. In contrast, we decided that Technicon had to market the Auto Analyzer as a complete system—instrument, reagents, and instruction.*

*Technicon's marketing strategy has been to promote the Auto Analyzer at professional meetings and through scientific papers and journal articles. Technicon employs only direct salesmen. The company has never used agents or distributors, except in countries where the market is too small to support direct sales.*

*To introduce technology as radical as the Auto Analyzer into conservative clinical laboratories, Technicon decided to perform clinical evaluations. Although unusual at that time, such evaluations have since become commonplace. An important condition of the clinical evaluations was Technicon's insistence that the laboratory conducting the evaluation call a meeting of its local professional society to announce the results. Such meetings generally resulted in an enthusiastic endorsement of the Auto Analyzer by the laboratory director. I believe this technique had much to do with the rapid market acceptance of the Auto Analyzer.*

*Other unusual marketing strategies employed by Technicon to promote the Auto Analyzer included symposia and training courses. Technicon sponsored about 25 symposia on techniques in automated analytical chemistry. The symposia were generally 3-day affairs, attracting between 1,000 and 4,500 scientists, and were held in most of the major countries of the world including the United States.*

*Because we realized that market acceptance of the Auto Analyzer could be irreparably damaged by incompetent users, Technicon set up a broad-scale training program. We insisted that purchasers of Auto Analyzers come to our training centers located around the world for a 1-week course of instruction. I estimate that we have trained about 50,000 people to use Auto Analyzers.*

*Introduction of Technicon's continuous-flow Auto Analyzer in 1957 profoundly changed the character of the clinical laboratory, allowing a hundredfold increase in the number of laboratory tests performed over a 10-year period. When we began to develop the Auto Analyzer in 1953, I estimated a potential market of 250 units. Currently, more than 50,000 Auto Analyzer Channels are estimated to be in use around the world.*

*In reviewing the 35-year history of the Auto Analyzer, I have come to the conclusion that several factors significantly influenced our success. First, the Auto Analyzer allowed both an enormous improvement in the quality of laboratory test results and an enormous reduction in the cost of doing chemical analysis. Second, physicians began to realize that accurate laboratory data are useful in diagnosis. Last, reimbursement policies increased the availability of health care.*

(Reprinted with permission from *New Medical Devices, Invention, Development and Use,* (c) 1988 by the National Academy of Sciences. Published by National Academy Press, Washington, D.C.)

This success story demonstrates that important new ideas rarely flow smoothly to widespread clinical use. There are probably 100 untold failure stories for each success story! New inventions usually are made by the wrong person with the wrong contacts and experience, in the wrong place at the wrong time. It is important to understand the difference between a crude feasibility prototype and a well-developed, reliable, manufacturable product. Patents are important to protect ideas during the development process and to provide incentives for making the financial investments needed. Many devices have failed because they were too hard to use, reliability and ruggedness were inadequate, marketing was misdirected, user education was lacking, or service was poor and/or slow.

An evolutionary product is a new model of an existing product that adds new features, improves the technology, and reduces the cost of production. A revolutionary new product either solves a totally new problem or uses a new principle or concept to solve an old problem in a better way that displaces old methods. A medical instrument that improves screening, diagnosis, or monitoring may not add value by improving patient outcome unless improvements in the application of therapy occur as a result of using the medical instrument.

## 1.1 TERMINOLOGY OF MEDICINE AND MEDICAL DEVICES

Most biomedical engineers learn the physical sciences first in the context of traditional engineering, physics, or chemistry. When they become interested in medicine, they usually take at least a basic course in physiology, which does not describe disease or pathologic terminology. The book *Medical Terminology: An Illustrated Guide* (Cohen, 2004) is recommended. It emphasizes the Latin and Greek roots in a workbook format (with answers) that includes clinical case studies, flash cards, and simple, clear illustrations. An unabridged medical dictionary such as *Dorland's Illustrated Medical Dictionary*, 30th ed. (Dorland, 2003), is often useful. Physicians frequently use abbreviations and acronyms that are difficult to look up, and ambiguity or errors result. Six references on medical abbreviations are given (Cohen, 2004; Davis, 2001; Firkin and Whitworth, 1996; Haber, 1988; Hamilton and Guides, 1988; Heister, 1989). Medical eponyms are widely used to describe diseases and syndromes by the name of the person who first identified them. Refer to *Dictionary of Medical Eponyms* (Firkin and Whitworth, 1996).

The name used to describe a medical instrument or device should be informative, consistent, and brief. The annual *Health Devices Sourcebook*

(Anonymous, 2007) is a directory of U.S. and Canadian medical device products, trade names, manufacturers, and related services. This book uses internationally accepted nomenclature and a numerical coding system for over 5000 product categories. The *Product Development Directory* (1996) lists all specific medical products by the FDA standard product category name since enactment of the Medical Devices Amendments in April 1976. The *Encyclopedia of Medical Devices and Instrumentation* (Webster, 2006) has many detailed descriptions. But beware of borrowing medical terminology to describe technical aspects of devices or instruments. Confounding ambiguities can result.

Recent information on medical instrumentation can be found by searching World Wide Web servers such as www.google.com or www.uspto.gov, Library Online Catalogs, and journal electronic databases such as Engineering Village, Science Citation Index, and PubMed.

## 1.2 GENERALIZED MEDICAL INSTRUMENTATION SYSTEM

Every instrumentation system has at least some of the functional components shown in Figure 1.1. The primary flow of information is from left to right. Elements and relationships depicted by dashed lines are not essential. The major difference between this system of medical instrumentation and

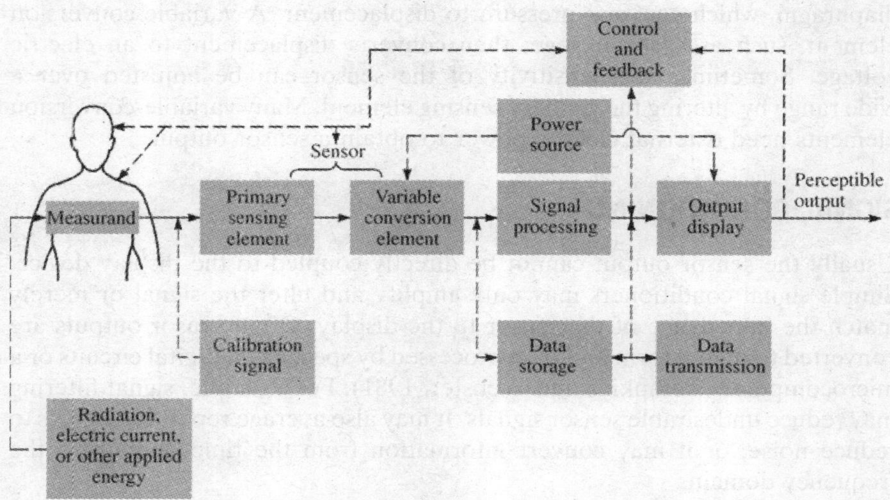


**Figure 1.1 Generalized instrumentation system** The sensor converts energy or information from the measurand to another form (usually electric). This signal is then processed and displayed so that humans can perceive the information. Elements and connections shown by dashed lines are optional for some applications.

conventional instrumentation systems is that the source of the signals is living tissue or energy applied to living tissue.

## MEASURAND

The physical quantity, property, or condition that the system measures is called the *measurand*. The accessibility of the measurand is important because it may be internal (blood pressure), it may be on the body surface (electrocardiogram potential), it may emanate from the body (infrared radiation), or it may be derived from a tissue sample (such as blood or a biopsy) that is removed from the body. Most medically important measurands can be grouped in the following categories: biopotential, pressure, flow, dimensions (imaging), displacement (velocity, acceleration, and force), impedance, temperature, and chemical concentrations. The measurand may be localized to a specific organ or anatomical structure.

## SENSOR

Generally, the term *transducer* is defined as a device that converts one form of energy to another. A sensor converts a physical measurand to an electric output. The sensor should respond only to the form of energy present in the measurand, to the exclusion of all others. The sensor should interface with the living system in a way that minimizes the energy extracted, while being minimally invasive. Many sensors have a primary sensing element such as a diaphragm, which converts pressure to displacement. A variable-conversion element, such as a strain gage, then converts displacement to an electric voltage. Sometimes the sensitivity of the sensor can be adjusted over a wide range by altering the primary sensing element. Many variable-conversion elements need external electric power to obtain a sensor output.

## SIGNAL CONDITIONING

Usually the sensor output cannot be directly coupled to the display device. Simple signal conditioners may only amplify and filter the signal or merely match the impedance of the sensor to the display. Often sensor outputs are converted to digital form and then processed by specialized digital circuits or a microcomputer (Tompkins and Webster, 1981). For example, signal filtering may reduce undesirable sensor signals. It may also average repetitive signals to reduce noise, or it may convert information from the time domain to the frequency domain.

## OUTPUT DISPLAY

The results of the measurement process must be displayed in a form that the human operator can perceive. The best form for the display may be numerical or graphical, discrete or continuous, permanent or temporary—depending on the particular measurand and how the operator will use the information. Although most displays rely on our visual sense, some information (Doppler ultrasonic signals, for example) is best perceived by other senses (here, the auditory sense). User controls and the output display should conform to the *Human Factors Engineering Guidelines and Preferred Practices for the Design of Medical Devices* (AAMI, 1993).

### AUXILIARY ELEMENTS

A calibration signal with the properties of the measurand should be applied to the sensor input or as early in the signal-processing chain as possible. Many forms of control and feedback may be required to elicit the measurand, to adjust the sensor and signal conditioner, and to direct the flow of output for display, storage, or transmission. Control and feedback may be automatic or manual. Data may be stored briefly to meet the requirements of signal conditioning or to enable the operator to examine data that precede alarm conditions. Alternatively, data may be stored before signal conditioning, so that different processing schemes can be utilized. Conventional principles of communications can often be used to transmit data to remote displays at nurses' stations, medical centers, or medical data-processing facilities.

## 1.3 ALTERNATIVE OPERATIONAL MODES

### DIRECT-INDIRECT MODES

Often the desired measurand can be interfaced directly to a sensor because the measurand is readily accessible or because acceptable invasive procedures are available. When the desired measurand is not accessible, we can use either another measurand that bears a known relation to the desired one or some form of energy or material that interacts with the desired measurand to generate a new measurand that is accessible. Examples include cardiac output (volume of blood pumped per minute by the heart), determined from measurements of respiration and blood gas concentration or from dye dilution; morphology of internal organs, determined from x-ray shadows; and pulmonary volumes, determined from variations in thoracic impedance plethysmography.

### SAMPLING AND CONTINUOUS MODES

Some measurands—such as body temperature and ion concentrations—change so slowly that they may be sampled infrequently. Other quantities—such as the electrocardiogram and respiratory gas flow—may require continuous monitoring. The frequency content of the measurand, the objective of the measurement, the condition of the patient, and the potential liability of the physician all influence how often medical data are acquired. Many data that are collected may go unused.

## GENERATING AND MODULATING SENSORS

Generating sensors produce their signal output from energy taken directly from the measurand, whereas modulating sensors use the measurand to alter the flow of energy from an external source in a way that affects the output of the sensor. For example, a photovoltaic cell is a generating sensor because it provides an output voltage related to its irradiation, without any additional external energy source. However, a photoconductive cell is a modulating sensor; to measure its change in resistance with irradiation, we must apply external energy to the sensor.

## ANALOG AND DIGITAL MODES

Signals that carry measurement information are either *analog*, meaning continuous and able to take on any value within the dynamic range, or *digital*, meaning discrete and able to take on only a finite number of different values. Most currently available sensors operate in the analog mode, although some inherently digital measuring devices have been developed. Increased use of digital signal processing has required concurrent use of analog-to-digital and digital-to-analog converters to interface computers with analog sensors and analog display devices. Researchers have developed indirect digital sensors that use analog primary sensing elements and digital variable-conversion elements (optical shaft encoders). Also quasi-digital sensors, such as quartz-crystal thermometers, give outputs with variable frequency, pulse rate, or pulse duration that are easily converted to digital signals.

The advantages of the digital mode of operation include greater accuracy, repeatability, reliability, and immunity to noise. Furthermore, periodic calibration is usually not required. Digital numerical displays are replacing many analog meter movements because of their greater accuracy and readability. Many clinicians, however, prefer analog displays when they are determining whether a physiological variable is within certain limits and when they are looking at a parameter that can change quickly, such as beat-to-beat heart rate. In the latter case, digital displays often change numbers so quickly that they are very difficult and annoying to observe.

## REAL-TIME AND DELAYED-TIME MODES

Of course sensors must acquire signals in real time as the signals actually occur. The output of the measurement system may not display the result immediately, however, because some types of signal processing, such as averaging and transformations, need considerable input before any results can be produced. Often such short delays are acceptable unless urgent feedback and control tasks depend on the output. In the case of some measurements, such as cell cultures, several days may be required before an output is obtained.

## 1.4 MEDICAL MEASUREMENT CONSTRAINTS

The medical instrumentation described throughout this book is designed to measure various medical and physiological parameters. The principal measurement and frequency ranges for each parameter are major factors that affect the design of all the instrument components shown in Figure 1.1. To get a brief overview of typical medical parameter magnitude and frequency ranges, refer to Table 1.1. Shown here are approximate ranges that are intended to include normal and abnormal values. Most of the parameter measurement ranges are quite low compared with nonmedical parameters. Note, for example, that most voltages are in the microvolt range and that pressures are low (about 100 mm Hg = 1.93 psi = 13.3 kPa). Also note that all the signals listed are in the audio-frequency range or below and that many signals contain direct current (dc) and very low frequencies. These general properties of medical parameters limit the practical choices available to designers for all aspects of instrument design.

Many crucial variables in living systems are inaccessible because the proper measurand–sensor interface cannot be obtained without damaging the system. Unlike many complex physical systems, a biological system is of such a nature that it is not possible to turn it off and remove parts of it during the measurement procedure. Even if interference from other physiological systems can be avoided, the physical size of many sensors prohibits the formation of a proper interface. Either such inaccessible variables must be measured indirectly, or corrections must be applied to data that are affected by the measurement process. The cardiac output is an important measurement that is obviously quite inaccessible.

Variables measured from the human body or from animals are seldom deterministic. Most measured quantities vary with time, even when all controllable factors are fixed. Many medical measurements vary widely among normal patients, even when conditions are similar. This inherent *variability* has been documented at the molecular and organ levels, and even for the whole body. Many internal anatomical variations accompany the obvious external differences among patients. Large tolerances on physiological measurements are partly the result of interactions among many physiological systems. Many feedback loops exist among physiological systems, and many of the interrelationships are poorly understood. It is seldom feasible to control or neutralize the effects of these other systems on the measured variable. The most common method of coping with this variability is to assume empirical statistical and probabilistic distribution functions. Single measurements are then compared with these *norms* (see Section 1.8).

**Table 1.1 Medical and Physiological Parameters**

| Parameter or Measuring Technique | Principal Measurement Range of Parameter | Signal Frequency Range, Hz | Standard Sensor or Method |
|---|---|---|---|
| Ballistocardiography (BCG) | 0–7 mg | dc–40 | Accelerometer, strain gage |
| | 0–100 μm | dc–40 | Displacement linear variable differential transformer (LVDT) |
| Bladder pressure | 1–100 cm $H_2O$ | dc–10 | Strain-gage manometer |
| Blood flow | 1–300 ml/s | dc–20 | Flowmeter (electromagnetic or ultrasonic) |
| Blood pressure, arterial | | | |
| Direct | 10–400 mm Hg | dc–50 | Strain-gage manometer |
| Indirect | 25–400 mm Hg | dc–60 | Cuff, auscultation |
| Blood pressure, venous | 0–50 mm Hg | dc–50 | Strain gage |
| Blood gases | | | |
| $P_{O_2}$ | 30–100 mm Hg | dc–2 | Specific electrode, volumetric or manometric |
| $P_{CO_2}$ | 40–100 mm Hg | dc–2 | Specific electrode, volumetric or manometric |
| $P_{N_2}$ | 1–3 mm Hg | dc–2 | Specific electrode, volumetric or manometric |
| $P_{CO}$ | 0.1–0.4 mm Hg | dc–2 | Specific electrode, volumetric or manometric |
| Blood pH | 6.8–7.8 pH units | dc–2 | Specific electrode |
| Cardiac output | 4–25 liter/min | dc–20 | Dye dilution, Fick |
| Electrocardiography (ECG) | 0.5–4 mV | 0.01–250 | Skin electrodes |
| Electroencephalography (EEG) | 5–300 μV | dc–150 | Scalp electrodes |
| (Electrocorticography and brain depth) | 10–5000 μV | dc–150 | Brain-surface or depth electrodes |
| Electrogastrography (EGG) | 10–1000 μV | dc–1 | Skin-surface electrodes |
| | 0.5–80 mV | dc–1 | Stomach-surface electrodes |
| Electromyography (EMG) | 0.1–5 mV | dc–10,000 | Needle electrodes |
| Eye potentials | | | |
| Electro-oculogram (EOG) | 50–3500 μV | dc–50 | Contact electrodes |
| Electroretinogram (ERG) | 0–900 μV | dc–50 | Contact electrodes |
| Galvanic skin response (GSR) | 1–500 kΩ | 0.01–1 | Skin electrodes |
| Gastric pH | 3–13 pH units | dc–1 | pH electrode; antimony electrode |

**Table 1.1** *(Continued)*

| Parameter or Measuring Technique | Principal Measurement Range of Parameter | Signal Frequency Range, Hz | Standard Sensor or Method |
|---|---|---|---|
| Gastrointestinal pressure | 0–100 cm $H_2O$ | dc–10 | Strain-gage manometer |
| Gastrointestinal forces | 1–50 g | dc–1 | Displacement system, LVDT |
| Nerve potentials | 0.01–3 mV | dc–10,000 | Surface or needle electrodes |
| Phonocardiography | Dynamic range 80 dB, threshold about 100 μPa | 5–2000 | Microphone |
| Plethysmography (volume change) | Varies with organ measured | dc–30 | Displacement chamber or impedance change |
| Circulatory | 0–30 ml | dc–30 | Displacement chamber or impedance change |
| Respiratory functions Pneumotachography (flow rate) | 0–600 liter/min | dc–40 | Pneumotachograph head and differential pressure |
| Respiratory rate | 2–50 breaths/min | 0.1–10 | Strain gage on chest, impedance, nasal thermistor |
| Tidal volume | 50–1000 ml/breath | 0.1–10 | Above methods |
| Temperature of body | 32–40 °C 90–104 °F | dc–0.1 | Themistor, thermocouple |

SOURCE: Revised from *Medical Engineering*. C. D. Ray (ed.). Copyright © 1974 by Year Book Medical Publishers, Inc., Chicago. Used by permission.

Nearly all biomedical measurements depend either on some form of energy being applied to the living tissue or on some energy being applied as an incidental consequence of sensor operation. X-ray and ultrasonic imaging techniques and electromagnetic or Doppler ultrasonic blood flowmeters depend on externally applied energy interacting with living tissue. Safe levels of these various types of energy are difficult to establish, because many mechanisms of tissue damage are not well understood. A fetus is particularly vulnerable during the early stages of development. The heating of tissue is one effect that must be limited, because even reversible physiological changes can affect measurements. Damage to tissue at the molecular level has been demonstrated in some instances at surprisingly low energy levels.

Operation of instruments in the medical environment imposes important additional constraints. Equipment must be reliable, easy to operate, and capable of withstanding physical abuse and exposure to corrosive chemicals. Electronic equipment must be designed to minimize electric-shock hazards (Chapter 14). The safety of patients and medical personnel must be considered in all phases of the design and testing of instruments. The Medical Device Amendments of 1976 and the Safe Medical Devices Act of 1990 amend the

Federal Food, Drug, and Cosmetics Act to provide for the safety and effectiveness of medical devices intended for human use (Section 1.13).

## 1.5 CLASSIFICATIONS OF BIOMEDICAL INSTRUMENTS

The study of biomedical instruments can be approached from at least four viewpoints. Techniques of biomedical measurement can be grouped according to the *quantity that is sensed*, such as pressure, flow, or temperature. One advantage of this classification is that it makes different methods for measuring any quantity easy to compare.

A second classification scheme uses the *principle of transduction*, such as resistive, inductive, capacitive, ultrasonic, or electrochemical. Different applications of each principle can be used to strengthen understanding of each concept; also, new applications may be readily apparent.

Measurement techniques can be studied separately for each *organ system*, such as the cardiovascular, pulmonary, nervous, and endocrine systems. This approach isolates all important measurements for specialists who need to know only about a specific area, but it results in considerable overlap of quantities sensed and principles of transduction.

Finally, biomedical instruments can be classified according to the *clinical medicine specialties*, such as pediatrics, obstetrics, cardiology, or radiology. This approach is valuable for medical personnel who are interested in specialized instruments. Of course, certain measurements—such as blood pressure—are important to many different medical specialties.

## 1.6 INTERFERING AND MODIFYING INPUTS

*Desired inputs* are the measurands that the instrument is designed to isolate. *Interfering inputs* are quantities that inadvertently affect the instrument as a consequence of the principles used to acquire and process the desired inputs. If spatial or temporal isolation of the measurand is incomplete, the interfering input can even be the same quantity as the desired input. *Modifying inputs* are undesired quantities that indirectly affect the output by altering the performance of the instrument itself. Modifying inputs can affect processing of either desired or interfering inputs. Some undesirable quantities can act as both a modifying input and an interfering input.

A typical electrocardiographic recording system, shown in Figure 1.2, will serve to illustrate these concepts. The desired input is the electrocardiographic voltage $v_{ecg}$ that appears between the two electrodes on the body surface. One interfering input is 60 Hz noise voltage induced in the shaded loop by environmental alternating current (ac) magnetic fields. The desired and the interfering voltages are in series, so both components appear at the input to the

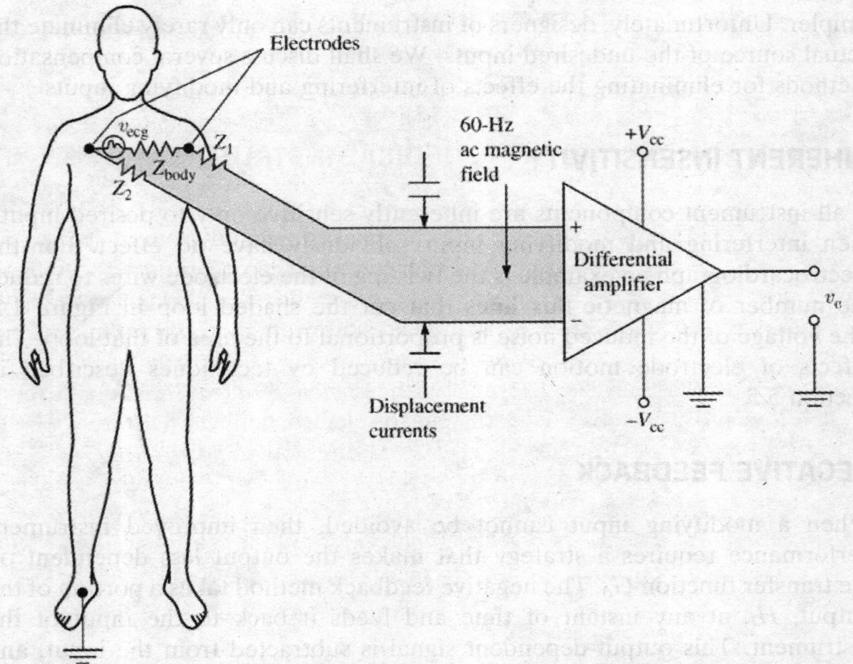


**Figure 1.2 Simplified electrocardiographic recording system** Two possible interfering inputs are stray magnetic fields and capacitively coupled noise. Orientation of patient cables and changes in electrode–skin impedance are two possible modifying inputs. $Z_1$ and $Z_2$ represent the electrode–skin interface impedances.

differential amplifier. Also, the difference between the capacitively coupled displacement currents flowing through each electrode and the body to ground causes an interfering voltage to appear across $Z_{body}$ between the two electrodes and two interfering voltages across $Z_1$ and $Z_2$, the electrode impedances.

An example of a modifying input is the orientation of the patient cables. If the plane of the cables is parallel to the ac magnetic field, magnetically introduced interference is zero. If the plane of the cables is perpendicular to the ac magnetic field, magnetically introduced interference is maximal.

## 1.7 COMPENSATION TECHNIQUES

The effects of most interfering and modifying inputs can be reduced or eliminated either by altering the design of essential instrument components or by adding new components designed to offset the undesired inputs. The former alternative is preferred when it is feasible, because the result is usually simpler. Unfortunately, designers of instruments can only rarely eliminate the actual source of the undesired inputs. We shall discuss several compensation methods for eliminating the effects of interfering and modifying inputs.

## INHERENT INSENSITIVITY

If all instrument components are inherently sensitive only to desired inputs, then interfering and modifying inputs obviously have no effect. For the electrocardiograph an example is the twisting of the electrode wires to reduce the number of magnetic flux lines that cut the shaded loop in Figure 1.2. The voltage of the induced noise is proportional to the area of that loop. The effects of electrode motion can be reduced by techniques described in Section 5.5.

## NEGATIVE FEEDBACK

When a modifying input cannot be avoided, then improved instrument performance requires a strategy that makes the output less dependent on the transfer function $G_d$. The negative feedback method takes a portion of the output, $H_f$, at any instant of time and feeds it back to the input of the instrument. This output-dependent signal is subtracted from the input, and the difference becomes the effective system input. For input $x_d$ and output $y$, we can write

$$(x_d - H_f y)G_d = y \tag{1.1}$$

$$x_d G_d = y(1 + H_f G_d) \tag{1.2}$$

$$y = \frac{G_d}{1 + H_f G_d} x_d \tag{1.3}$$

$G_d$ usually includes amplification, so $H_f G_d \gg 1$ and $y \cong (1/H_f)(x_d)$. This well-known relationship shows that only the feedback element, $H_f$, determines the output for a given input. Of course, this strategy fails if $H_f$ is also affected by modifying inputs. Usually the feedback device carries less power, so it is more accurate and linear. Less input-signal power is also needed for this feedback scheme, so less loading occurs. The major disadvantage of using this feedback principle is that dynamic instability leading to oscillations can occur, particularly if $G_d$ contains time delays. The study of feedback systems is a well-developed discipline that cannot be pursued further here (Kuo and Golnaraghi, 2003).

## SIGNAL FILTERING

A filter separates signals according to their frequencies. Most filters accomplish this by attenuating the part of the signal that is in one or more frequency bands. A more general definition for a *filter* is "a device or program that separates data, signals, or material in accordance with specified criteria" (IEEE, 1997).

Filters may be inserted at the instrument input, at some point within the instrument, or at the output of the instrument. In fact, the limitations of people's senses may be used to filter unwanted signal components coming from display devices. An example is the utilization of flicker fusion for rapidly changing images from a real-time ultrasonic scanner.

Input filtering blocks interfering and modifying inputs but does not alter the desired input. Filter elements may be distinct devices that block or pass all inputs, or they may be embodied in a single device that selectively blocks only undesired inputs. Many designers do not use input filters that are electric circuits but use instead mechanical, pneumatic, thermal, or electromagnetic principles to block out undesired environmental inputs. For example, instruments are often shock-mounted to filter vibrations that affect sensitive instrument components. Electromagnetic shielding is often used to block interfering electric and magnetic fields, such as those indicated in Figure 1.2.

Electronic filters are often incorporated at some intermediate stage within the instrument. To facilitate filtering based on differences in frequency, mixers and modulators are used to shift desired and/or undesired signals to another frequency range where filtering is more effective. Digital computers are used to filter signals on the basis of template-matching techniques and various time-domain signal properties. These filters may even have time- or signal-dependent criteria for isolating the desired signal.

Output filtering is possible, though it is usually more difficult because desired and undesired output signals are superimposed. The selectivity needed may be easier to achieve with higher-level output signals.

## OPPOSING INPUTS

When interfering and/or modifying inputs cannot be filtered, additional interfering inputs can be used to cancel undesired output components. These extra intentional inputs may be the same as those to be canceled. In general, the unavoidable and the added opposing inputs can be quite different, as long as the two output components are equal so that cancellation results. The two outputs must cancel despite variations in all the unavoidable interfering inputs and variations in the desired inputs. The actual cancellation of undesired output components can be implemented either before or after the desired and undesired outputs are combined. Indeed, either the intentional or the unavoidable interfering input signal might be processed by $G_d$. The method of opposing inputs can also be used to cancel the effects of modifying inputs.

Automatic real-time corrections are implied for the method of opposing inputs just described. Actually, output corrections are often calculated manually or by computer methods and applied after data are collected. This requires quantitative knowledge of the interfering and/or modifying input at the time of the measurement and also of how these inputs affect the output. This method is usually cumbersome, loses real-time information, and is often used only for rather static interfering inputs, such as temperature and atmospheric pressure.

An example of using the opposing-input method is to intentionally induce a voltage from the same 60 Hz magnetic field present in Figure 1.2 to be amplified and inverted until cancellation of the 60 Hz interference in the output is achieved. An obvious disadvantage of this method is that the amplifier gain has to be adjusted whenever the geometry of the shaded loop in Figure 1.2 changes. In electronic circuits that must operate over a wide temperature range, *thermistors* (temperature-dependent resistors) are often used to counteract unavoidable temperature-dependent changes in characteristics of active circuit elements, such as transistors and integrated circuits.

## 1.8 BIOSTATISTICS

The application of statistics to medical data is used to design experiments and clinical studies; to summarize, explore, analyze, and present data; to draw inferences from data by estimation or hypothesis testing; to evaluate diagnostic procedures; and to assist clinical decision making (Dawson-Saunders and Trapp, 2004).

Medical research studies can be *observational studies*, wherein characteristics of one or more groups of patients are observed and recorded, or *experimental intervention studies*, wherein the effect of a medical procedure or treatment is investigated. The simplest observational studies are *case-series* studies that describe some characteristics of a group. These studies are without control subjects, in order only to identify questions for further research. *Case-control* observational studies use individuals selected because they have (or do not have) some outcome or disease and then look backward to find possible causes or risk factors. *Cross-sectional* observational studies analyze characteristics of patients at one particular time to determine the status of a disease or condition. *Cohort* observational studies prospectively ask whether a particular characteristic is a precursor or risk factor for an outcome or disease. Experimental clinical trials are *controlled* if the outcome for patients administered a drug, device, or procedure is compared to the outcome for patients given a placebo or another accepted treatment. The trials are *uncontrolled* if there is no such comparison. *Concurrent controls* are best, because patients are selected in the same way and for the same time period. *Double-blind* study with *randomized* selection of patients to treatment options is preferred, because this design minimizes investigator and patient bias. Medical outcome studies show cost-effective improvements in patient health are increasingly required prior to adoption and reimbursement for new medical technologies (Anonymous, 2001).

Quantitative data are measured on a continuous or discrete *numerical scale* with some precision. Qualitative data values that fit into categories are measured on *nominal scales* that show the names of the categories. An *ordinal scale* is used when the categories exhibit an inherent order. Descriptive statistics are useful to summarize data and their attributes. *Distributions* of empirical or theoretical data reflect the values of a variable or characteristic and the frequency of occurrence of those values.

Measures of the middle, or central tendency, include the well-known *mean*, which is the sum of observed values divided by the number of observations. The mean, found as follows,

$$\overline{X} = \frac{\sum X_i}{n} \tag{1.4}$$

works best as the measure of central tendency for symmetric distributions. The *median* is the value for which half the observations are smaller and half are larger; it is used for skewed numerical data or ordinal data. The *mode* is the observation that occurs most frequently; it is used for bimodal distributions. The *geometric mean* (GM) is the $n$th root of the product of the observations:

$$\text{GM} = \sqrt[n]{X_1 X_2 X_3 \cdots X_n} \tag{1.5}$$

It is used with data on a logarithmic scale.

Measures of spread or dispersion of data describe the variation in the observations. The *range*, which is the difference between the largest and smallest observations, is used to emphasize extreme values. The *standard deviation* is a measure of the spread of data about the mean. It is computed as follows:

$$s = \sqrt{\frac{\sum (X_i - \overline{X})^2}{n-1}} \tag{1.6}$$

It is used with the mean for symmetric distributions of numerical data. Regardless of the type of symmetric distribution, at least 75% of the values always lie between $\overline{X} - 2s$ and $\overline{X} + 2s$. The *coefficient of variation* (CV) is calculated as follows:

$$\text{CV} = \left(\frac{s}{\overline{X}}\right)(100\%) \tag{1.7}$$

It standardizes the variation, making it possible to compare two numerical distributions that are measured on different scales. A *percentile* gives the percentage of a distribution that is less than or equal to the percentile number; it may be used with the median for ordinal data or skewed numerical data. The *interquartile range* is the difference between the 25th and 75th percentiles, so it describes the central 50% of a distribution with any shape. The *standard error of the mean* (SEM) (i.e., standard deviation of the mean), $s_{\overline{X}} = s/\sqrt{n-1}$, expresses the variability to be expected among the *means* in future samples, whereas the *standard deviation* describes the variability to be expected among *individuals* in future samples.

**EXAMPLE 1.1** Your samples from a population are 1, 1, 3, 5, 5. Estimate the mean $\overline{X}$, the standard deviation $s$, and the standard deviation of the mean $s_{\overline{X}}$.

**ANSWER** Mean $\overline{X}$ = (sum of values)/(number of values) $= (1 + 1 + 3 + 5 + 5)/5 = 3$ standard deviation $s = \{[(1-3)^2 + (1-3)^2 + (3-3)^2 + (5-3)^2 + (5-3)^2]/(5-1)\}^{1/2} = (16/4)^{1/2} = 2$ standard deviation of mean $s_{\overline{X}} = s/\sqrt{n-1} = 2/\sqrt{5-1} = 1$.

Often we need to study relationships between two numerical characteristics. The *correlation coefficient r* is a measure of the relationship between numerical variables $X$ and $Y$ for paired observations.

$$r = \frac{\sum(X_i - \overline{X})(Y_i - \overline{Y})}{\sqrt{\sum(X_i - \overline{X})^2}\sqrt{\sum(Y_i - \overline{Y})^2}} \tag{1.8}$$

The correlation coefficient ranges from $-1$ for a negative linear relationship to $+1$ for a positive linear relationship; 0 indicates that there is no linear relationship between $X$ and $Y$. The correlation coefficient is independent of the units employed to measure the variables, which can be different. Like the standard deviation, the correlation coefficient is strongly influenced by outlying values. Because the correlation coefficient measures only a straight-line relationship, it may be small for a strong curvilinear relationship. Of course, a high correlation does *not* imply a cause-and-effect relationship between the variables.

Estimation and hypothesis testing are two ways to make an inference about a value in a population of subjects from a set of observations drawn from a sample of such subjects. In estimation, *confidence intervals* are calculated for a statistic such as the mean. The confidence intervals indicate that a percentage—say 95%—of such confidence intervals contain the true value of the population mean. The confidence intervals indicate the degree of confidence we can have that they contain the true mean. Hypothesis testing reveals whether the sample gives enough evidence for us to reject the *null hypothesis*, which is usually cast as a statement that expresses the opposite of what we think is true. A *P-value* is the probability of obtaining, if the null hypothesis is true, a result that is at least as extreme as the one observed. The *P*-value indicates how often the observed difference would occur by chance alone if, indeed, nothing but chance were affecting the outcome. Recent trends favor using estimation and confidence intervals rather than hypothesis testing.

Methods for measuring the accuracy of a diagnostic procedure use three pieces of information. The *sensitivity* [TP/(TP + FN)] of a test is the probability of its yielding true positive (TP) results in patients who actually have the disease. A test with high sensitivity has a low *false-negative* (FN) rate. The *specificity* [TN/(TN + FP)]of a test is the probability of its yielding negative results in patients who do not have the disease. A test with high specificity has a low *false-positive* (FP) rate; it does not give a false positive (FP) result in many patients who do not have the disease. The third piece of information is the *prior probability*, or prevalence [(TP + FN)/(TN + TP + FN + FP)] of the condition prior to the test (all diseased persons divided by all persons). There are several methods for revising the probability that a patient has a condition on the basis of the results of a diagnostic test. Taking into consideration the results of a diagnostic procedure is only one part of the complex clinical decision-making process. Decision tree analysis and other forms of decision analysis that include economic implications are also used in an effort to make optimal decisions (Webster, 2004).

## 1.9 GENERALIZED STATIC CHARACTERISTICS

To enable purchasers to compare commercially available instruments and evaluate new instrument designs, quantitative criteria for the performance of instruments are needed. These criteria must clearly specify how well an instrument measures the desired input and how much the output depends on interfering and modifying inputs. Characteristics of instrument performance are usually subdivided into two classes on the basis of the frequency of the input signals.

*Static characteristics* describe the performance of instruments for dc or very low frequency inputs. The properties of the output for a wide range of constant inputs demonstrate the quality of the measurement, including nonlinear and statistical effects. Some sensors and instruments, such as piezoelectric devices, respond only to time-varying inputs and have no static characteristics.

*Dynamic characteristics* require the use of differential and/or integral equations to describe the quality of the measurements. Although dynamic characteristics usually depend on static characteristics, the nonlinearities and statistical variability are usually ignored for dynamic inputs, because the differential equations become difficult to solve. Complete characteristics are approximated by the sum of static and dynamic characteristics. This necessary oversimplification is frequently responsible for differences between real and ideal instrument performance.

### ACCURACY

The *accuracy* of a single measured quantity is the difference between the true value and the measured value divided by the true value. This ratio is usually expressed as a percent. Because the true value is seldom available, the accepted true value or reference value should be traceable to the National Institute of Standards and Technology.

The accuracy usually varies over the normal range of the quantity measured, usually decreases as the full-scale value of the quantity decreases on a multirange instrument, and also often varies with the frequency of desired, interfering, and modifying inputs. Accuracy is a measure of the total error without regard to the type or source of the error. The possibility that the measurement is low and that it is high are assumed to be equal. The accuracy can be expressed as percent of reading, percent of full scale, $\pm$ number of digits for digital readouts, or $\pm 1/2$ the smallest division on an analog scale. Often the accuracy is expressed as a sum of these, for example, on a digital device, $\pm 0.01\%$ of reading $\pm 0.015\%$ of full-scale $\pm 1$ digit. If accuracy is expressed simply as a percentage, full scale is usually assumed. Some instrument manufacturers specify accuracy only for a limited period of time.

## PRECISION

The *precision* of a measurement expresses the number of distinguishable alternatives from which a given result is selected. For example, a meter that displays a reading of 2.434 V is more precise than one that displays a reading of 2.43 V. High-precision measurements do not imply high accuracy, however, because precision makes no comparison to the true value.

## RESOLUTION

The smallest incremental quantity that can be measured with certainty is the *resolution*. If the measured quantity starts from zero, the term *threshold* is synonymous with *resolution*. Resolution expresses the degree to which nearly equal values of a quantity can be discriminated.

## REPRODUCIBILITY

The ability of an instrument to give the same output for equal inputs applied over some period of time is called *reproducibility* or *repeatability*. Reproducibility does not imply accuracy. For example, a broken digital clock with an AM or PM indicator gives very reproducible values that are accurate only once a day.

## STATISTICAL CONTROL

The accuracy of an instrument is not meaningful unless all factors, such as the environment and the method of use, are considered. Statistical control ensures that random variations in measured quantities that result from all factors that influence the measurement process are tolerable. Any systematic errors or bias can be removed by calibration and correction factors, but random variations pose a more difficult problem. The measurand and/or the instrument may introduce statistical variations that make outputs unreproducible. If the cause of this variability cannot be eliminated, then statistical analysis must be used to determine the error variation. Making multiple measurements and averaging the results can improve the estimate of the true value.

## STATIC SENSITIVITY

A static calibration is performed by holding all inputs (desired, interfering, and modifying) constant except one. This one input is varied incrementally over the normal operating range, resulting in a range of incremental outputs. The static sensitivity of an instrument or system is the ratio of the incremental output quantity to the incremental input quantity. This ratio is the static component of $G_{\mathrm{d}}$ for desired inputs within the range of the incremental inputs. The incremental slope can be obtained from either the secant between two adjacent points or the tangent to one point on the calibration curve. The static sensitivity may be constant for only part of the normal operating range of the instrument, as shown in Figure 1.3(a). For input–output data that indicate a straight-line calibration curve, the slope $m$ and intercept $b$ for the line with the minimal sum of the squared differences between data points and the line are given by the following equations:

$$m = \frac{n\sum x_{\mathrm{d}}y - (\sum x_{\mathrm{d}})(\sum y)}{n\sum x_{\mathrm{d}}^2 - (\sum x_{\mathrm{d}})^2} \tag{1.9}$$

$$b = \frac{(\sum y)(\sum x_{\mathrm{d}}^2) - (\sum x_{\mathrm{d}}y)(\sum x_{\mathrm{d}})}{n\sum x_{\mathrm{d}}^2 - (\sum x_{\mathrm{d}})^2} \tag{1.10}$$

$$y = mx_{\mathrm{d}} + b \tag{1.11}$$

where $n$ is the total number of points and each sum is for all $n$ points. The static sensitivity for modulating sensors is usually given per volt of excitation, because the output voltage is proportional to the excitation voltage. For example, the static sensitivity for a blood-pressure sensor containing a strain-gage bridge might be $50\ \mu\mathrm{V}\cdot\mathrm{V}^{-1}\ \mathrm{mm\ Hg}^{-1}$.

## ZERO DRIFT

Interfering and/or modifying inputs can affect the static calibration curve shown in Figure 1.3(a) in several ways. Zero drift has occurred when all output values increase or decrease by the same absolute amount. The slope of the sensitivity curve is unchanged, but the output-axis intercept increases or decreases as shown in Figure 1.3(b). The following factors can cause zero drift: manufacturing misalignment, variations in ambient temperature, hysteresis, vibration, shock, and sensitivity to forces from undesired directions. A change in the dc-offset voltage at the electrodes in the electrocardiograph example in Figure 1.2 is an example of zero drift. Slow changes in the dc-offset voltage do not cause a

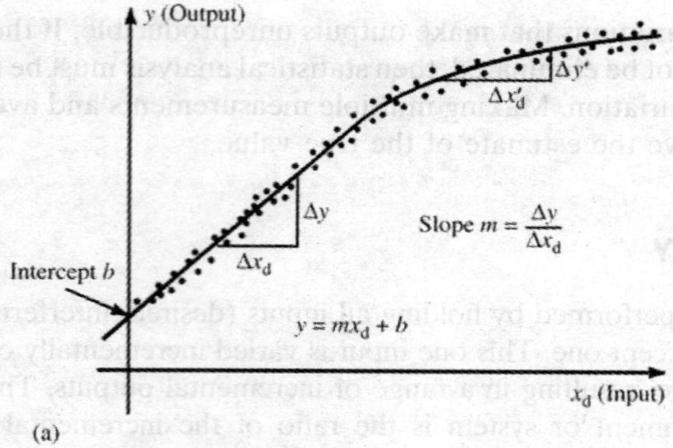


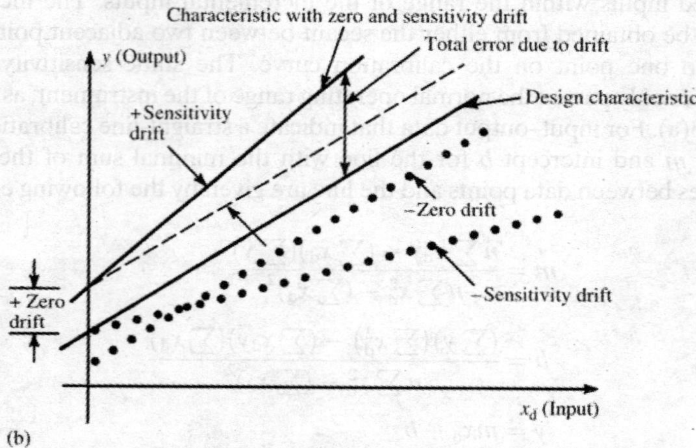


**Figure 1.3** (a) Static-sensitivity curve that relates desired input $x_d$ to output $y$. Static sensitivity may be constant for only a limited range of inputs. (b) Static sensitivity: zero drift and sensitivity drift. Dotted lines indicate that zero drift and sensitivity drift can be negative. [Part (b) modified from *Measurement Systems: Application and Design*, E. O. Doebelin. Copyright © 1990 by McGraw-Hill, Inc. Used with permission of McGraw-Hill Book Co.]

problem, because the ECG amplifier is ac-coupled. Fast changes due to motion of the subject do cause low-frequency artifact to appear at the output.

## SENSITIVITY DRIFT

When the slope of the calibration curve changes as a result of an interfering and/or modifying input, a drift in sensitivity results. Sensitivity drift causes error that is proportional to the magnitude of the input. The slope of the calibration curve can either increase or decrease, as indicated in Figure 1.3(b). Sensitivity drift can result from manufacturing tolerances, variations in power supply, nonlinearities, and changes in ambient temperature and pressure. Variations in the electrocardiograph-amplifier voltage gain as a result of fluctuations in dc power-supply voltage or change in temperature are examples of sensitivity drift.

## LINEARITY

A system or element is linear if it has properties such that if $y_1$ is the response to $x_1$ and $y_2$ is the response to $x_2$, then $y_1 + y_2$ is the response to $x_1 + x_2$, and $Ky_1$ is the response to $Kx_1$. These two requirements for system linearity are restated in Figure 1.4(a).

They are clearly satisfied for an instrument with a calibration curve that is a straight line.

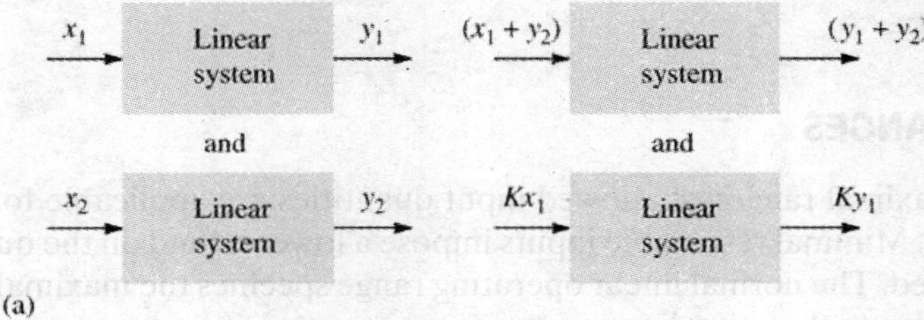


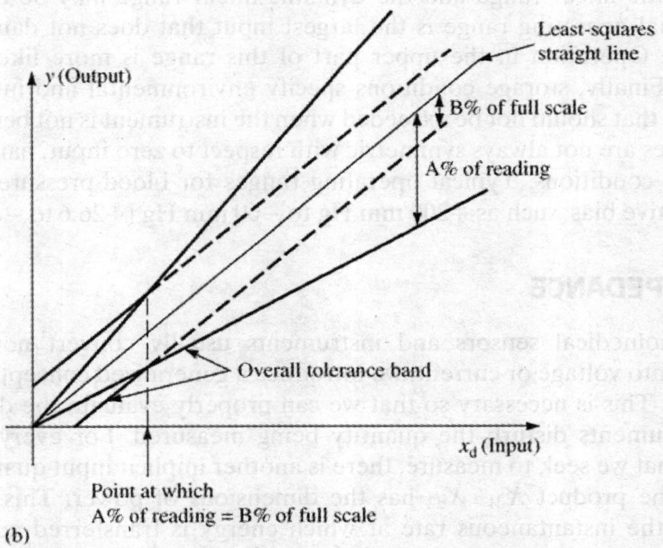


**Figure 1.4** (a) Basic definition of linearity for a system or element. The same linear system or element is shown four times for different inputs. (b) A graphical illustration of independent nonlinearity equals ±A% of the reading, or ±B% of full scale, whichever is greater (that is, whichever permits the larger error). [Part (b) modified from *Measurement Systems: Application and Design*, E. O. Doebelin. Copyright © 1990 by McGraw-Hill, Inc. Used with permission of McGraw-Hill Book Co.]

Keep in mind, however, that high accuracy does not necessarily imply linearity. In practice, no instrument has a perfect linear response, so a measure of deviation from linearity is needed. *Independent nonlinearity* expresses the maximal deviation of points from the least-squares fitted line as either $\pm A\%$ of the reading or $\pm B\%$ of full scale, whichever is greater (that is, whichever permits the larger error). This linearity specification is shown in Figure 1.4(b). For up-scale readings, the percent-of-reading figure is desirable because most errors are proportional to the reading. For small readings near zero, however, percentage of full scale is more realistic because it is not feasible to test for small percent-of-reading deviations near zero. All data points must fall inside the "funnel" shown in Figure 1.4(b). For most instruments that are essentially linear, if other sources of error are minimal, the accuracy is equal to the nonlinearity.

## INPUT RANGES

Several maximal ranges of allowed input quantities are applicable for various conditions. Minimal resolvable inputs impose a lower bound on the quantity to be measured. The normal linear operating range specifies the maximal or near-maximal inputs that give linear outputs.

The static linear range and the dynamic linear range may be different. The maximal operating range is the largest input that does not damage the instrument. Operation in the upper part of this range is more likely to be nonlinear. Finally, storage conditions specify environmental and interfering input limits that should not be exceeded when the instrument is not being used. These ranges are not always symmetric with respect to zero input, particularly for storage conditions. Typical operating ranges for blood-pressure sensors have a positive bias, such as +200 mm Hg to −60 mm Hg (+26.6 to −8.0 kPa).

## INPUT IMPEDANCE

Because biomedical sensors and instruments usually convert nonelectric quantities into voltage or current, we introduce a generalized concept of input impedance. This is necessary so that we can properly evaluate the degree to which instruments disturb the quantity being measured. For every desired input $X_{d1}$ that we seek to measure, there is another implicit input quantity $X_{d2}$ such that the product $X_{d1} \cdot X_{d2}$ has the dimensions of power. This product represents the instantaneous rate at which energy is transferred across the tissue–sensor interface. The generalized input impedance $Z_x$ is the ratio of the phasor equivalent of a steady-state sinusoidal *effort* input variable (voltage, force, pressure) to the phasor equivalent of a steady-state sinusoidal *flow* input variable (current, velocity, flow).

$$Z_x = \frac{X_{d1}}{X_{d2}} = \frac{\text{effort variable}}{\text{flow variable}} \tag{1.12}$$

The power $P$ is the time rate of energy transfer from the measurement medium.

$$P = X_{d1}X_{d2} = \frac{X_{d1}^2}{Z_x} = Z_x X_{d2}^2 \quad (1.13)$$

To minimize $P$, when measuring effort variables $X_{d1}$, we should make the generalized input impedance as large as possible. This is usually achieved by minimizing the flow variable. However, most instruments function by measuring minute values of the flow variable, so the flow variable cannot be reduced to zero. On the other hand, when we are measuring flow variables $X_{d2}$, small input impedance is needed to minimize $P$. The loading caused by measuring devices depends on the magnitude of the input impedance $|Z_x|$ compared with the magnitude of the source impedance $|Z_s|$ for the desired input. Unfortunately, biological source impedances are usually unknown, variable, and difficult to measure and control. Thus the instrument designer must usually focus on maximizing the input impedance $Z_x$ for effort-variable measurement. When the measurand is a flow variable instead of an effort variable, it is more convenient to use the admittance $Y_x = 1/Z_x$ than the impedance.

## 1.10 GENERALIZED DYNAMIC CHARACTERISTICS

Only a few medical measurements, such as body temperature, are constant or slowly varying quantities. Most medical instruments must process signals that are functions of time. It is this time-varying property of medical signals that requires us to consider dynamic instrument characteristics. Differential or integral equations are required to relate dynamic inputs to dynamic outputs for continuous systems. Fortunately, many engineering instruments can be described by ordinary linear differential equations with constant coefficients. The input $x(t)$ is related to the output $y(t)$ according to the following equation:

$$a_n \frac{d^n y}{dt^n} + \cdots + a_1 \frac{dy}{dt} + a_0 y(t) = b_m \frac{d^m x}{dt^m} + \cdots + b_1 \frac{dx}{dt} + b_0 x(t) \quad (1.14)$$

where the constants $a_i (i = 0, 1, \ldots, n)$ and $b_j (j = 0, 1, \ldots, m)$ depend on the physical and electric parameters of the system. By introducing the differential operator $D^k \equiv d^k()/dt^k$, we can write this equation as

$$(a_n D^n + \cdots + a_1 D + a_0) y(t) = (b_m D^m + \cdots + b_1 D + b_0) x(t) \quad (1.15)$$

Readers familiar with Laplace transforms may recognize that $D$ can be replaced by the Laplace parameter s to obtain the equation relating the transforms $Y(s)$ and $X(s)$. This is a *linear* differential equation, because the linear properties stated in Figure 1.4(a) are assumed and the coefficients

$a_i$ and $b_j$ are not functions of time or the input $x(t)$. The equation is *ordinary*, because there is only one independent variable $y$. Essentially such properties mean that the instrument's methods of acquiring and analyzing the signals do not change as a function of time or the quantity of input. For example, an autoranging instrument may violate these conditions.

Most practical instruments are described by differential equations of zero, first, or second order; thus $n = 0, 1, 2$, and derivatives of the input are usually absent, so $m = 0$.

The input $x(t)$ can be classified as transient, periodic, or random. No general restrictions are placed on $x(t)$, although, for particular applications, bounds on amplitude and frequency content are usually assumed. Solutions for the differential equation depend on the input classifications. The step function is the most common transient input for instrumentation. Sinusoids are the most common periodic function to use because, through the Fourier-series expansion, any periodic function can be approximated by a sum of sinusoids. Band-limited white noise (uniform-power spectral content) is a common random input because one can test instrument performance for all frequencies in a particular bandwidth.

## TRANSFER FUNCTIONS

The transfer function for a linear instrument or system expresses the relationship between the input signal and the output signal mathematically. If the transfer function is known, the output can be predicted for any input. The *operational transfer function is the ratio* $y(D)/x(D)$ as a function of the differential operator $D$.

$$\frac{y(D)}{x(D)} = \frac{b_m D^m + \cdots + b_1 D + b_0}{a_n D^n + \cdots + a_1 D + a_0} \tag{1.16}$$

This form of the transfer function is particularly useful for transient inputs. For linear systems, the output for transient inputs, which occur only once and do not repeat, is usually expressed directly as a function of time, $y(t)$, which is the solution to the differential equation.

The *frequency transfer function* for a linear system is obtained by substituting $j\omega$ for $D$ in (1.16).

$$\frac{Y(j\omega)}{X(j\omega)} = \frac{b_m(j\omega)^m + \cdots b_1(j\omega) + b_0}{a_n(j\omega)^n + \cdots a_1(j\omega) + a_0} \tag{1.17}$$

where $j = +\sqrt{-1}$ and $\omega$ is the angular frequency in radians per second. The input is usually given as $x(t) = A_x \sin(\omega t)$, and all transients are assumed to have died out. The output $y(t)$ is a sinusoid with the same frequency, but the amplitude and phase depend on $\omega$; that is, $y(t) = B(\omega)\sin[\omega t + \phi(\omega)]$. The frequency transfer function is a complex quantity having a magnitude that is the ratio of the magnitude of the output to the magnitude of the input and a phase angle $\phi$ that is the phase of the output $y(t)$ minus the phase of the input $x(t)$. The phase angle for most instruments is negative. We do not usually express the output of the system as $y(t)$ for each frequency, because we know that it is just a sinusoid with a particular magnitude and phase. Instead, the amplitude ratio and the phase angle are given separately as functions of frequency.

The dynamic characteristics of instruments are illustrated below by examples of zero-, first-, and second-order linear instruments for step and sinusoidal inputs.

## ZERO-ORDER INSTRUMENT

The simplest nontrivial form of the differential equation results when all the $a$'s and $b$'s are zero except $a_0$ and $b_0$.

$$a_0 y(t) = b_0 x(t) \tag{1.18}$$

This is an algebraic equation, so

$$\frac{y(D)}{x(D)} = \frac{Y(j\omega)}{X(j\omega)} = \frac{b_0}{a_0} = K = \text{static sensitivity} \tag{1.19}$$

where the single constant $K$ replaces the two constants $a_0$ and $b_0$. This zero-order instrument has ideal dynamic performance, because the output is proportional to the input for all frequencies and there is no amplitude or phase distortion.

A linear potentiometer is a good example of a zero-order instrument. Figure 1.5 shows that if the potentiometer has pure uniform resistance, then the output voltage $y(t)$ is directly proportional to the input displacement $x(t)$, with no time delay for any frequency of input. In practice, at high frequencies, some parasitic capacitance and inductance might cause slight distortion. Also, low-resistance circuits connected to the output can load this simple zero-order instrument.

## FIRST-ORDER INSTRUMENT

If the instrument contains a single energy-storage element, then a first-order derivative of $y(t)$ is required in the differential equation.

$$a_1 \frac{dy(t)}{dt} + a_0 y(t) = b_0 x(t) \tag{1.20}$$

This equation can be written in terms of the differential operator $D$ as

$$(\tau D + 1) y(t) = K x(t) \tag{1.21}$$

where $K = b_0/a_0 =$ static sensitivity, and $\tau = a_1/a_0 =$ time constant.

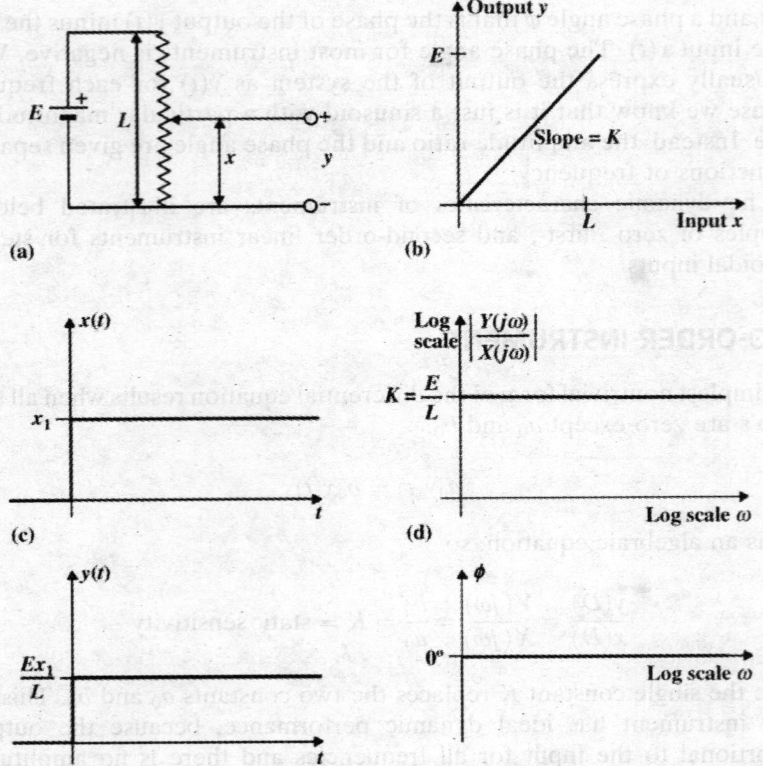


**Figure 1.5** (a) A linear potentiometer, an example of a zero-order system. (b) Linear static characteristic for this system. (c) Step response is proportional to input. (d) Sinusoidal frequency response is constant with zero phase shift.

Exponential functions offer solutions to this equation when appropriate constants are chosen. The operational transfer function is

$$\frac{y(D)}{x(D)} = \frac{K}{1 + \tau D} \tag{1.22}$$

and the frequency transfer function is

$$\frac{Y(j\omega)}{X(j\omega)} = \frac{K}{1 + j\omega\tau} = \frac{K}{\sqrt{1 + \omega^2\tau^2}} \underline{/\phi = \arctan\ (-\omega\tau/1)} \tag{1.23}$$

The *RC* low-pass filter circuit shown in Figure 1.6(a) is an example of a first-order instrument. The input is the voltage $x(t)$, and the output is the voltage $y(t)$ across the capacitor. The first-order differential equation for this

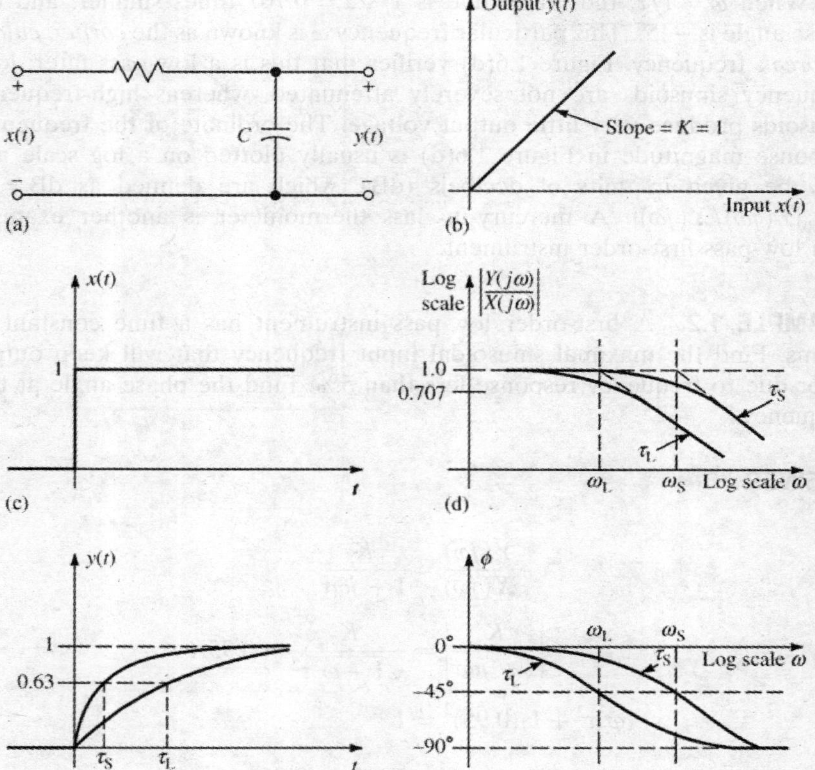


**Figure 1.6** (a) A low-pass $RC$ filter, an example of a first-order instrument. (b) Static sensitivity for constant inputs. (c) Step response for large time constants ($\tau_L$) and small time constants ($\tau_S$). (d) Sinusoidal frequency response for large and small time constants.

circuit is $RC[dy(t)/dt] + y(t) = Kx(t)$. The static-sensitivity curve given in Figure 1.6(b) shows that static outputs are equal to static inputs. This is verified by the differential equation because, for static conditions, $dy/dt = 0$. The step response in Figure 1.6(c) is exponential with a time constant $\tau = RC$.

$$y(t) = K(1 - e^{-t/\tau}) \tag{1.24}$$

The smaller the time constant, the faster the output approaches the input. For sinusoids, (1.23) and Figure 1.6(d) show that the magnitude of the output decreases as frequency increases. For larger time constants, this decrease occurs at lower frequency.

When $\omega = 1/\tau$, the magnitude is $1/\sqrt{2} = 0.707$ times smaller, and the phase angle is $-45°$. This particular frequency $\omega$ is known as the *corner, cutoff*, or *break* frequency. Figure 1.6(d) verifies that this is a low-pass filter; low-frequency sinusoids are not severely attenuated, whereas high-frequency sinusoids produce very little output voltage. The ordinate of the frequency-response magnitude in Figure 1.6(d) is usually plotted on a log scale and may be given in units of decibels (dB), which are defined as dB $= 20 \log_{10}|Y(j\omega)/X(j\omega)|$. A mercury-in-glass thermometer is another example of a low-pass first-order instrument.

**EXAMPLE 1.2** A first-order low-pass instrument has a time constant of 20 ms. Find the maximal sinusoidal input frequency that will keep output error due to frequency response less than 5%. Find the phase angle at this frequency.

**ANSWER**

$$\frac{Y(j\omega)}{X(j\omega)} = \frac{K}{1 + j\omega\tau}$$

$$\left|\frac{K}{1 + j\omega\tau}\right| = \frac{K}{\sqrt{1 + \omega^2\tau^2}} = 0.95K$$

$$(\omega^2\tau^2 + 1)(0.95)^2 = 1$$

$$\omega^2 = \frac{1 - (0.95)^2}{(0.95)^2(20 \times 10^{-3})^2}$$

$$\omega = 16.4 \text{ rad/s}$$

$$f = \frac{\omega}{2\pi} = 2.62 \text{ Hz}$$

$$\phi = \tan^{-1}\left(\frac{-\omega\tau}{1}\right) = -18.2°$$

If $R$ and $C$ in Figure 1.6(a) are interchanged, the circuit becomes another first-order instrument known as a *high-pass filter*. The static characteristic is zero for all values of input, and the step response jumps immediately to the step voltage but decays exponentially toward zero as time increases. Thus $y(t) = Ke^{-t/\tau}$. Low-frequency sinusoids are severely attenuated, whereas high-frequency sinusoids are little attenuated. The sinusoidal transfer function is $Y(j\omega)/X(j\omega) = j\omega\tau/(1 + j\omega\tau)$.

**EXAMPLE 1.3** From a 2 kV source in series with a 20 kΩ resistor, calculate the time required to charge a 100 μF defibrillator capacitor to 1.9 kV

**ANSWER** Circuit is shown in Figure 1.6(a). Use (1.24) $v_C = V - Ve^{-\frac{t}{RC}}$

$$1900\,\text{V} = 2000\,\text{V} - 2000\,\text{V} \cdot e^{-\frac{t}{(20{,}000\Omega)(100\times10^{-6}\,\text{F})}}$$

$$-100\,\text{V} = -2000\,\text{V} \cdot e^{-\frac{t}{(20{,}000\Omega)(100\times10^{-6}\,\text{F})}}$$

$$0.05 = e^{-\frac{t}{(20{,}000\Omega)(100\times10^{-6}\,\text{F})}}$$

$$\ln 0.05 = -\frac{t}{2\,\Omega \cdot \text{F}}$$

$$t = 5.99\,\text{s}$$

## SECOND-ORDER INSTRUMENT

An instrument is second order if a second-order differential equation is required to describe its dynamic response.

$$a_2 \frac{d^2y(t)}{dt^2} + a_1 \frac{dy(t)}{dt} + a_0 y(t) - b_0 x(t) \tag{1.25}$$

Many medical instruments are second order or higher, and low pass. Furthermore, many higher-order instruments can be approximated by second-order characteristics if some simplifying assumptions can be made. The four constants in (1.25) can be reduced to three new ones that have physical significance:

$$\left[\frac{D^2}{\omega_n^2} + \frac{2\zeta D}{\omega_n} + 1\right] y(t) = Kx(t) \tag{1.26}$$

where

$$K = \frac{b_0}{a_0} = \text{static sensitivity, output units divided by input units}$$

$$\omega_n = \sqrt{\frac{a_0}{a_2}} = \text{undamped natural frequency, rad/s}$$

$$\zeta = \frac{a_1}{2\sqrt{a_0 a_1}} = \text{damping ratio, dimensionless}$$

Again exponential functions offer solutions to this equation, although the exact form of the solution varies as the damping ratio becomes greater than, equal to, or less than unity. The operational transfer function is

$$\frac{y(D)}{x(D)} = \frac{K}{\dfrac{D^2}{\omega_n^2} + \dfrac{2\zeta D}{\omega_n} + 1} \tag{1.27}$$

and the frequency transfer function is

$$\frac{Y(j\omega)}{X(j\omega)} = \frac{K}{(j\omega/\omega_n)^2 + (2\zeta j\omega/\omega_n) + 1}$$
$$= \frac{K}{\sqrt{[1-(\omega/\omega_0)^2]^2 + 4\zeta^2\omega^2/\omega_n^2}} \Big/ \phi = \arctan\frac{2\zeta}{\omega/\omega_n - \omega_n/\omega} \quad (1.28)$$

A mechanical force-measuring instrument illustrates the properties of a second-order instrument (Doebelin, 1990). Mass, spring, and viscous-damping elements oppose the applied input force $x(t)$, and the output is the resulting displacement $y(t)$ of the movable mass attached to the spring [Figure 1.7(a)]. If the natural frequency of the spring is much greater than the frequency components in the input, the dynamic effect of the spring can be included by adding one-third of the spring's mass to the mass of the moving elements to obtain the equivalent total mass $M$.

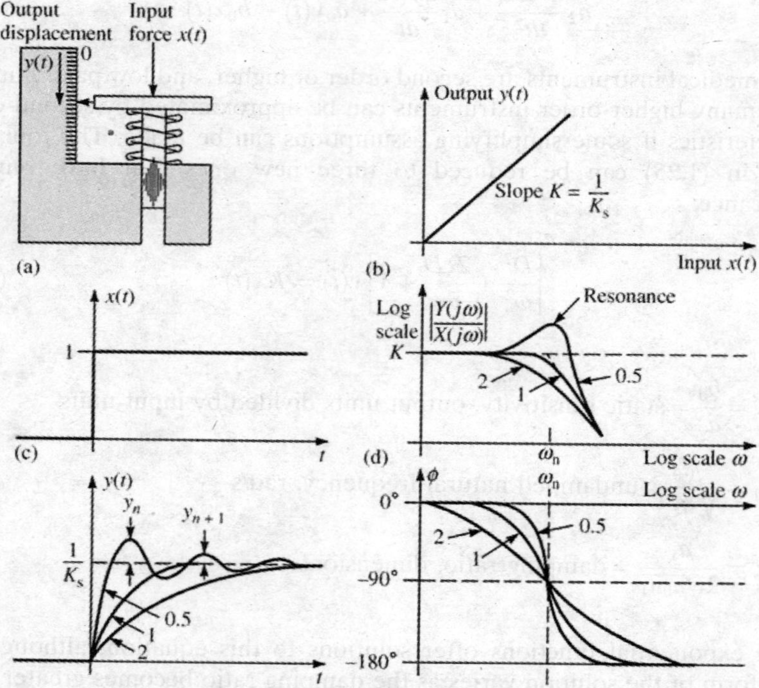


**Figure 1.7** (a) Force-measuring spring scale, an example of a second-order instrument. (b) Static sensitivity. (c) Step response for overdamped case $\zeta = 2$, critically damped case $\zeta = 1$, underdamped case $\zeta = 0.5$. (d) Sinusoidal steady-state frequency response, $\zeta = 2$, $\zeta = 1$, $\zeta = 0.5$. [Part (a) modified from *Measurement Systems: Application and Design*, E. O. Doebelin. Copyright © 1990 by McGraw-Hill, Inc. Used with permission of McGraw-Hill Book Co.]

Hooke's law for linear springs is assumed, so the spring constant is $K_s$. Dry friction is neglected and perfect viscous friction is assumed, with constant $B$.

To eliminate gravitational force from the equation, we adjust the scale until $y = 0$ when $x = 0$. Then the sum of the forces equals the product of mass and acceleration.

$$x(t) - B\frac{dy(t)}{dt} - K_s y(t) = M\frac{d^2y(t)}{dt^2} \tag{1.29}$$

This equation has the same form as (1.26) when the static sensitivity, undamped natural frequency, and damping ratio are defined in terms of $K_s$, $B$, and $M$, as follows:

$$K = \frac{1}{K_s} \tag{1.30}$$

$$\omega_n = \sqrt{K_s/M} \tag{1.31}$$

$$\zeta = \frac{B}{2\sqrt{K_m M}} \tag{1.32}$$

The static response is $y(t) = Kx(t)$, as shown in Figure 1.7(b). The step response can have three forms, depending on the damping ratio. For a unit-step input, these three forms are

Overdamped, $\zeta > 1$:

$$y(t) = -\frac{\zeta + \sqrt{\zeta^2 - 1}}{2\sqrt{\zeta^2 - 1}} K e^{\left(-\zeta + \sqrt{\zeta^2 - 1}\right)\omega_n t} + \frac{\zeta - \sqrt{\zeta^2 - 1}}{2\sqrt{\zeta^2 - 1}} K e^{\left(-\zeta - \sqrt{\zeta^2 - 1}\right)\omega_n t} + K \tag{1.33}$$

Critically damped, $\zeta = 1$:

$$y(t) = -(1 + \omega_n t) K e^{-\omega_n t} + K \tag{1.34}$$

Underdamped, $\zeta < 1$:

$$y(t) = -\frac{e^{-\zeta\omega_n t}}{\sqrt{1 - \zeta^2}} K \sin\left(\sqrt{1 - \zeta^2}\,\omega_n t + \phi\right) + K$$
$$\phi = \arcsin\sqrt{1 - \zeta^2} \tag{1.35}$$

Examples of these three step responses are represented in Figure 1.7(c). Only for damping ratios less than unity does the step response overshoot the final value. Equation (1.35) shows that the frequency of the oscillations in the underdamped response in Figure 1.7(c) is the damped natural frequency $\omega_d = \omega_n\sqrt{1-\zeta^2}$. A practical compromise between rapid rise time and minimal overshoot is a damping ratio of about 0.7.

**EXAMPLE 1.4** For underdamped second-order instruments, find the damping ratio $\zeta$ from the step response.

**ANSWER** To obtain the maximums for the underdamped response, we take the derivative of (1.35) and set it to zero. For $\zeta < 0.3$ we approximate positive maximums when the sine argument equals $3\pi/2$, $7\pi/2$, and so forth. This occurs at

$$t_n = \frac{3\pi/2 - \phi}{\omega_n\sqrt{1-\zeta^2}} \quad \text{and} \quad t_{n+1} = \frac{7\pi/2 - \phi}{\omega_n\sqrt{1-\zeta^2}} \tag{1.36}$$

The ratio of the first positive overshoot $y_n$ to the second positive overshoot $y_{n+1}$ [Figure 1.7(c)] is

$$\frac{y_n}{y_{n+1}} = \frac{\dfrac{K}{\sqrt{1-\zeta^2}}\exp\left(-\zeta\omega_n\dfrac{(3\pi/2-\phi)}{\omega_n\sqrt{1-\zeta^2}}\right)}{\dfrac{K}{\sqrt{1-\zeta^2}}\exp\left(-\zeta\omega_n\dfrac{(7\pi/2-\phi)}{\omega_n\sqrt{1-\zeta^2}}\right)}$$

$$= \exp\frac{2\pi\zeta}{\sqrt{1-\zeta^2}}$$

$$\ln\frac{y_n}{y_{n+1}} = \Lambda = \frac{2\pi\zeta}{\sqrt{1-\zeta^2}} \tag{1.37}$$

where $\Lambda$ is defined as *logarithmic decrement*. Solving for $\zeta$ yields

$$\zeta = \frac{\Lambda}{\sqrt{4\pi^2 + \Lambda^2}} \tag{1.38}$$

For sinusoidal steady-state responses, the frequency transfer function (1.28) and Figure 1.7(d) show that low-pass frequency responses result. The rate of decline in the amplitude frequency response is twice the rate of that decline for first-order instruments. Note that resonance phenomena can occur if the damping ratio is too small. Also note that the output phase lag can be as much as 180°, whereas for single-order instruments, the maximal phase lag is 90°.

## TIME DELAY

Instrument elements that give an output that is exactly the same as the input, except that it is delayed in time by $\tau_d$, are defined as *time-delay elements*. The mathematical expression for these elements is

$$y(t) = K_x(t - \tau_d), \quad t > \tau_d \tag{1.39}$$

These elements may also be called analog delay lines, transport lags, or dead times. Although first-order and second-order instruments have negative phase angles that imply time delays, the phase angle varies with frequency, so the delay is not constant for all frequencies. For time delays, the static characteristic is the constant $K$, the step response is specified by (1.39), and the sinusoidal frequency response for magnitude and phase is

$$\frac{Y(j\omega)}{X(j\omega)} = Ke^{-j\omega\tau_d} \tag{1.40}$$

Time delays are present in transmission lines (electric, mechanical, hydraulic blood vessels, and pneumatic respiratory tubing), magnetic tape recorders, and some digital signal-processing schemes. Usually these time delays are to be avoided, especially in instruments or systems that involve feedback, because undesired oscillations may result.

If the instrument is used strictly for measurement and is not part of a feedback-control system, then some time delay is usually acceptable. The transfer function for undistorted signal reproduction with time delay becomes $Y(j\omega)/X(j\omega) = K\underline{/-\omega\tau_d}$. Our previous study of time-delay elements shows that the output magnitude is $K$ times the input magnitude for all frequencies and that the phase lag increases linearly with frequency.

The transfer-function requirements concern the *overall* instrument transfer function. The overall transfer function of linear elements connected in series is the product of the transfer functions for the individual elements. Many combinations of nonlinear elements can produce the overall linear transfer function required. Various forms of modulation and demodulation are used, and unavoidable sensor nonlinearities can sometimes be compensated for by other instrument elements.

## 1.11 DESIGN CRITERIA

As shown, many factors affect the design of biomedical instruments. The factors that impose constraints on the design are of course different for each type of instrument. However, some of the general requirements can be categorized as signal, environmental, medical, and economic factors.

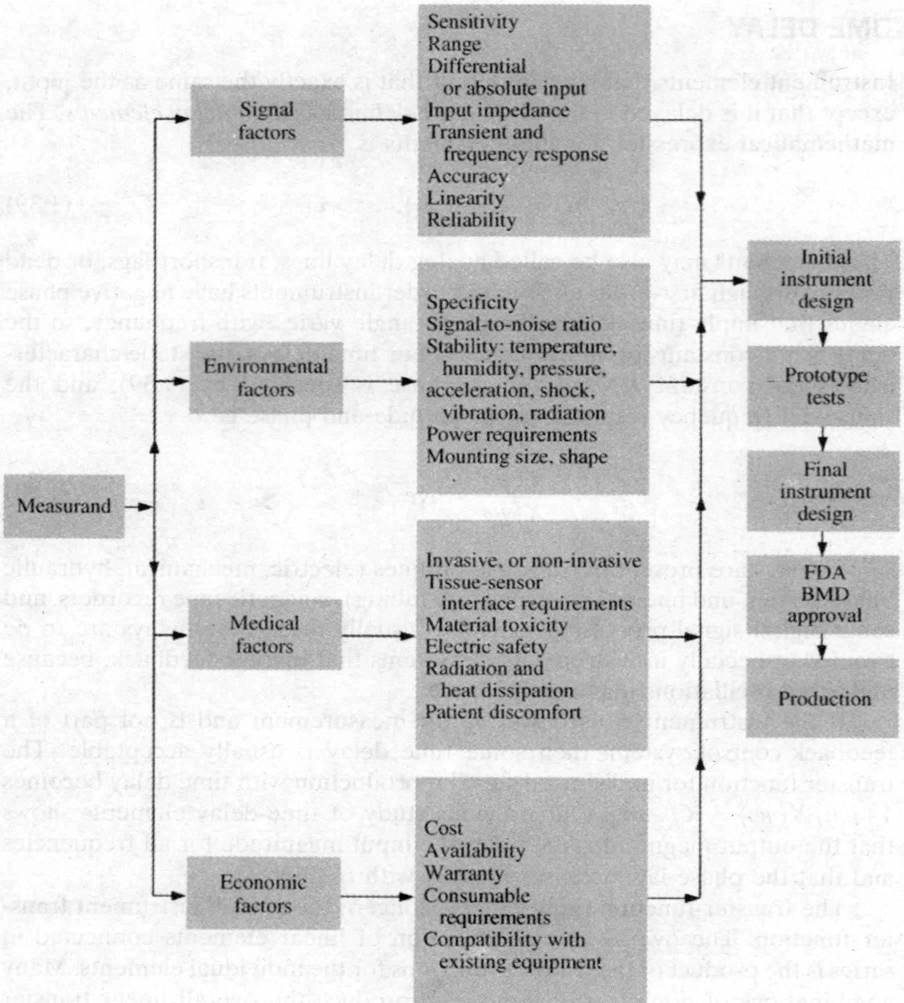


**Figure 1.8 Design process for medical instruments** Choice and design of instruments are affected by signal factors and also by environmental, medical, and economic factors. (Revised from *Transducers for Biomedical Measurements: Application and Design*, R. S. C. Cobbold. Copyright © 1974, John Wiley and Sons, Inc. Used by permission of John Wiley and Sons, Inc.)

Figure 1.8 shows how these factors are incorporated into the initial design and development of an instrument.

Note that the type of sensor selected usually determines the signal-processing equipment needed, so an instrument specification includes more than just what type of sensor to use. To obtain a final design, some compromises in specifications are usually required. Actual tests on a prototype are always needed before final design decisions can be made. Changes in performance and interaction of the elements in a complex instrument often dictate design modifications. Good designs are frequently the result of many compromises throughout the development of the instrument. In Chapter 2, we shall examine basic methods of sensing biomedical quantities to ensure that many sensor design alternatives are considered (King and Fries, 2009).

## 1.12 COMMERCIAL MEDICAL INSTRUMENTATION DEVELOPMENT PROCESS

A commercial medical instrument project has many phases, and the size of the team needed grows as the project progresses. Ideas often come from people working where health care is delivered, because clinical needs are most evident there. Physicians, nurses, clinical engineers, and sales personnel are therefore good sources of ideas. Industry engineers and marketing personnel should spend time in hospitals observing how their products are actually being used (and misused). Unsolicited inventions are often presented to industry. Most companies have one or more people who are responsible for evaluating new ideas, so it is very important for those who want to propose a new idea to be in contact with a person who can understand the idea and who has the authority to proceed with a detailed evaluation. A simple, signed nondisclosure agreement is adequate (but essential) to protect patent rights when detailed ideas are discussed.

At this early stage even the best ideas are crudely defined, and they are often not appreciated until at least a preliminary *feasibility analysis* is done. The feasibility analysis and written *product description* should consider the medical need for the product, its technical feasibility, and how well it fits with the company's current or planned product lines and sales methods. Determining medical feasibility entails examining the clinical need for the product, including patient indications, number of patients, clinical specialty, and exactly how, why, and by whom the device will be utilized. Marketing research and analysis can be useful for evolutionary products but are not reliable for revolutionary products, especially when a change in medical practice is required. Technical feasibility analysis should include a description of the core technologies needed, suitability of existing or readily modifiable components, breakthroughs or inventions required, systems analysis, and preliminary cost estimates. A functional prototype that includes the sensor, primary signal processing elements, and other new or unique components should be built and tested on animals and humans as early as possible. The manufacturing feasibility analysis should be done early, when major alternative technologies can still be selected. A brief business plan should assess financial aspects, personnel requirements, competition, patents, standards, manufacturing requirements, sales and service requirements, and the time schedule for the project. Experience has shown that abbreviating the feasibility phase or adding features after this phase usually causes disasters later. A detailed feasibility review should be required at the end of this phase. If the results are not clearly favorable, the project should be abandoned or the feasibility phase should be continued.

After a favorable feasibility review is complete, a detailed *product specification* must be written to describe all the product features. Included should be numerical values for performance, many internal testing requirements, user interface requirements, environmental testing requirements, and even the size, weight, and color of the instrument. The product specification should say everything about "what" is required but nothing about "how" it is to be achieved. This gives design engineers important flexibility. The product specification is used by design and development engineers, test equipment design engineers, quality assurance engineers, and manufacturing engineers throughout the product life cycle. The product specification remains a confidential document in most companies; only the main external performance specifications appear in user technical manuals and promotional materials.

Design and development uses the product specification to make a manufacturable prototype. For most instruments, functions must be partitioned into hardware and software before detailed design can begin. Circuit diagrams, detailed software requirements, and mechanical designs are made by means of computer-aided-design (CAD) tools that allow such detailed simulations of functional operation that there is little need for "breadboard" prototypes. Design reviews focus on systems issues and problems that the company may encounter in meeting the product specification. True prototypes that are very similar to the final product are thus developed much earlier and can be used by test, design assurance, and manufacturing engineers. These prototypes are also tested on animals or human subjects to verify expected operation and performance at a few clinical testing centers. Data from these *clinical feasibility trials* (including repeated observations of users) should be studied closely, because design flaws that cause user frustration or errors must be discovered at this critical stage. A final *design review* should include test results for all specifications, clinical results including subjective user feedback, an assessment of manufacturability, and more detailed cost estimates.

Production engineers must be involved throughout the design and development process to avoid a redesign for manufacturability. Special production equipment usually has a long lead time. Many fixtures and automatic tests must be designed. All final documents that describe how the product is made must be released by the design and development engineers. Any changes made after the final design review must be authorized via an *engineering change order* (ECO). Small production runs are usually needed to discover problems and improve efficiency. Most medical instruments and devices are not produced in high volume, as consumer products are, so full automation of production is not cost-effective. Even after full production begins, some ECOs may be needed to correct problems that occur in the field. Any failures of medical devices must be documented, along with the corrective action taken.

Throughout the product life cycle, which includes the period after the product is no longer offered for sale, technical support for user questions and problems must be provided. Successful companies must be committed to repairing or replacing their products throughout the entire expected lifetime of the product.

## 1.13 REGULATION OF MEDICAL DEVICES

In 1976 the United States Congress passed what are known as the **Medical Device Amendments** (Public Law 94-295) to the Federal Food, Drug, and Cosmetics Act that dates back to the 1930s. In the Safe Medical Devices Act of 1990, further amendments were made (Pacela, 1991). The primary purpose was to ensure the safety and efficacy of new medical devices prior to marketing of the device. The law's definition of the term *medical device* is "any item promoted for a medical purpose that does not rely on chemical action to achieve its intended effect" (Kessler *et al.*, 1987). Medical devices were classified in two ways. First, the division of such devices into Class I, II, and III was based on the principle that devices that pose greater potential hazards should be subject to more regulatory requirements. Second, seven categories were established: preamendment, postamendment, substantially equivalent, implant, custom, investigational, and transitional (Enderle *et al.*, 2005).

The seven categories into which medical devices are divided are described in Table 1.2, which also includes classification rules and examples. Software used in medical devices has become an area of increasing concern; several serious accidents have been traced to software bugs (Murfitt, 1990). Increased requirements for maintaining traceability of devices to the ultimate customer, postmarketing surveillance for life-sustaining and life-supporting implants, and hospital reporting requirements for adverse incidents were added to the law in 1990.

***Class I general controls.*** Manufacturers are required to perform registration, premarketing notification, record keeping, labeling, reporting of adverse experiences, and good manufacturing practices. These controls apply to all three classes.

***Class II performance standards.*** These standards were to be defined by the federal government, but the complexity of procedures called for in the amendments and the enormity of the task have resulted in little progress having been made toward defining the 800 standards needed. The result has been overreliance on the postamendment "substantial equivalence" known as the 510(k) process.

***Class III premarketing approval.*** Such approval is required for devices used in supporting or sustaining human life and preventing impairment of human health. The FDA has extensively regulated these devices by requiring manufacturers to prove their safety and effectiveness prior to market release.

**Table 1.2 FDA Medical Device Categories**

| Category | Description | Classification Rules | Examples |
|---|---|---|---|
| Preamendment devices (or old devices) | Devices on the market before May 28, 1976, when the Medical Device Amendments were enacted. | Devices are assigned to 1 of 3 classes. A presumption exists that preamendment devices should be placed in Class I unless their safety and effectiveness cannot be ensured without the greater regulation afforded by Classes II and III. A manufacturer may petition the FDA for reclassification. | Analog electrocardiography machine; electrohydraulic lithotriptor; contraceptive intrauterine device and accessories; infant radiant warmer; contraceptive tubal occlusion device; automated heparin analyzer; automated differential cell counter; automated blood-cell separator; transabdominal aminoscope. |
| Postamendment devices (or new devices) | Devices put on the market after May 28, 1976. | Unless shown to be substantially equivalent to a device that was on the market before the amendments took effect, these devices are automatically placed in Class III. A manufacturer may petition the FDA for reclassification. | Magnetic resonance imager; extracorporeal shock-wave lithotriptor; absorbable sponge; YAG laser; AIDS-antibody test kit; hydrophilic contact lenses; percutaneous catheter for transluminal coronary angioplasty; implantable defibrillator; bone-growth stimulator; alpha-fetoprotein RIA kit; hepatitis B-antibody detection kit. |
| Substantially equivalent devices | Postamendment devices that are substantially equivalent to preamendment devices. | Devices are assigned to the same class as their preamendment counterparts and subject to the same requirements. If and when the FDA requires testing and approval of preamendment devices, their substantially equivalent counterparts will also be subject to testing and approval. | Digital electrocardiography machines; YAG lasers for certain uses; tampons; ELISA diagnostic kits; devices used to test for drug abuse. |

**Table 1.2** *(Continued)*

| Category | Description | Classification Rules | Examples |
|---|---|---|---|
| Implanted devices | Devices that are inserted into a surgically formed or natural body cavity and intended to remain there for $\geq$ 30 days. | Devices are assumed to require placement in Class III unless a less-regulated class will ensure safety and effectiveness. | Phrenic-nerve stimulator; pacemaker pulse generator; intracardiac patch; vena cava clamp. |
| Custom devices | Devices not generally available to other licensed practitioners and not available in finished form. Product must be specifically designed for a particular patient and may not be offered for general commercial distribution. | Devices are exempt from premarketing testing and performance standards but are subject to general controls. | Dentures; orthopedic shoes. |
| Investigational devices | Unapproved devices undergoing clinical investigation under the authority of an Investigational Device Exemption. | Devices are exempt if an Investigational Device Exemption has been granted. | Artificial heart; ultrasonic hyperthermia equipment; DNA probes; laser angioplasty devices; positron emission tomography machines. |
| Transitional devices | Devices that were regulated as drugs before enactment of the statute but are now defined as medical devices. | Devices are automatically assigned to Class III but may be reclassified in Class I or II. | Antibiotic susceptibility disks; bone heterografts; gonorrhea diagnostic products; injectable silicone; intraocular lenses; surgical sutures; soft contact lenses. |

SOURCE: Reprinted with permission from *The New England Journal of Medicine* 317(6), 357–366, 1987.

## PROBLEMS

**1.1** Find the independent nonlinearity, as defined in Figure 1.4(b), for the following set of inputs and outputs from a nearly linear system. Instrument was designed for an output equal to twice the input. Full scale is 20.

| Inputs | 0.50 | 1.50 | 2.00 | 5.00 | 10.00 |
|---|---|---|---|---|---|
| Outputs | 0.90 | 3.05 | 4.00 | 9.90 | 20.50 |

**1.2** Find the correlation coefficient $r$ for the set of five inputs and outputs given in Problem 1.1.

**1.3** Derive the operational transfer function and the sinusoidal transfer function for an *RC* high-pass filter. Plot the step response and the complete frequency response (magnitude and phase).

**1.4** A first-order low-pass instrument must measure hummingbird wing displacements (assume sinusoidal) with frequency content up to 100 Hz with an amplitude inaccuracy of less than 5%. What is the maximal allowable time constant for the instrument? What is the phase angle at 50 Hz and at 100 Hz?

**1.5** A mercury thermometer has a cylindrical capillary tube with an internal diameter of 0.2 mm. If the volume of the thermometer and that of the bulb are not affected by temperature, what volume must the bulb have if a sensitivity of 2 mm/°C is to be obtained? Assume operation near 24 °C. Assume that the stem volume is negligible compared with the bulb internal volume. Differential expansion coefficient of Hg $= 1.82 \times 10^{-4}$ ml/(ml · °C).

**1.6** For the spring scale shown in Figure 1.7(a), find the transfer function when the mass is negligible.

**1.7** Find the time constant from the following differential equation, given that $x$ is the input, $y$ is the output, and $a$ through $h$ are constants.

$$a\frac{dy}{dt} + bx + c + hy = e\frac{dy}{dt} + fx + g$$

**1.8** A low-pass first-order instrument has a time constant of 20 ms. Find the frequency, in hertz, of the input at which the output will be 93% of the dc output. Find the phase angle at this frequency.

**1.9** A second-order instrument has a damping ratio of 0.4 and an undamped natural frequency of 85 Hz. Sketch the step response, and give numerical values for the amplitude and time of the first two positive maxima. Assume that the input goes from 0 to 1 and that the static sensitivity is 10.

**1.10** Consider an underdamped second-order system with step response as shown in Figure 1.7(c). A different way to define logarithmic decrement is

$$\Gamma = \ln \frac{y_n}{y_{n+1}}$$

Here $n$ refers not to the number of positive peaks shown in Figure 1.7(c) but to both positive and negative peaks. That is, $n$ increases by 1 for each half cycle. Derive an equation for the damping ratio $\zeta$ in terms of this different definition of logarithmic decrement.

## REFERENCES


Anonymous, *Designers Handbook: Medical Electronics. A Resource and Buyers Guide for Medical Electronics Engineering and Design*, 3rd ed. Santa Monica, CA: Canon Communications, Inc., 1994.

Anonymous, *Health Devices Sourcebook*. Plymouth Meeting, PA: ECRI, 2007.

Anonymous, *Human Factors Engineering Guidelines and Preferred Practices for the Design of Medical Devices*, 2nd ed. Arlington, VA: ANSI/AAMI HE48, 1993.

Anonymous, *Medical Outcomes and Guidelines Sourcebook*. New York, NY: Faulkner and Gray, Inc., 2001.

Anonymous, *Product Development Directory*. Montvale, NJ: Medical Economics Co., 1996.

Bronzino, J. D. (ed.), *The Biomedical Engineering Handbook*, 3rd ed. Boca Raton, FL: CRC Press, 2006.

Brush, L. C., *The Guide to Biomedical Standards*, 21st ed. Brea, CA: Quest Publishing Co., 1999.

Cobbold, R. S. C., *Transducers for Biomedical Measurements: Principles and Applications*. New York: Wiley, 1974.

Cohen, B. J., *Medical Terminology: An Illustrated Guide*, 4th ed. Philadelphia: Lippincott, 2004.

Cromwell, L., F. J. Weibell, and E. A. Pfeiffer, *Biomedical Instrumentation and Measurements*, 2nd ed. Englewood Cliffs, NJ: Prentice-Hall, 1980.

Davis, N. M., *Medical Abbreviations: 15,000 Conveniences at the Expense of Communication and Safety*, 10th ed. Huntington Valley, PA: Neil M. Davis Associates, 2001.

Dawson-Saunders, B., and R. G. Trapp, *Basic and Clinical Biostatistics*. 4th ed. Norwalk, CT: Appleton & Lange, 2004.

Doebelin, E. O., *Measurement Systems: Application and Design*, 4th ed. New York: McGraw-Hill, 1990.

Dorland, N. W. (ed.), *Dorland's Illustrated Medical Dictionary*, 30th ed. Philadelphia: Saunders, 2003.

Ekelman, K. B., *New Medical Devices: Invention, Development, and Use*. Washington, DC: National Academy Press, 1988.

Enderle, J. D., S. M. Blanchard, and J. D. Bronzino, *Introduction to Biomedical Engineering*, 2nd ed., San Diego: Academic, 2005.

Firkin, B. G., and J. A. Whitworth, *Dictionary of Medical Eponyms*, 2nd ed. Park Ridge, NJ: Parthenon, 1996.

Geddes, L. A., and L. E. Baker, *Principles of Applied Biomedical Instrumentation*, 3rd ed. New York: Wiley, 1989.

Haber, K., *Common Abbreviations in Clinical Medicine*. New York: Raven Press, 1988.

Hamilton, B., and B. Guides, *Medical Acronyms, Symbols and Abbreviations*, 2nd ed. New York: Neal-Schuman, 1988.

Heister, R., *Dictionary of Abbreviations in Medical Sciences*. New York: Springer, 1989.

Institute of Electrical and Electronics Engineers (IEEE), *IEEE Standard Dictionary of Electrical and Electronic Terms*, 6th ed. Piscataway, NJ: Institute of Electrical and Electronics Engineers, 1997.

Jacobson, B., and J. G. Webster, *Medicine and Clinical Engineering*. Englewood Cliffs, NJ: Prentice-Hall, 1977.

Kessler, D. A., "The federal regulation of medical devices." *N. Engl. J. Med.*, 1987, 317(6), 357–366.

King, P. H., and R. C. Fries, *Design of Biomedical Devices and Systems*, 2nd ed. Boca Raton, FL: CRC Press, 2009.

Kuo, B., and F. Golnaraghi, *Automatic Control Systems*, 8th ed. New York: Wiley, 2003.

Murfitt, R. R., "United States government regulation of medical device software: A review." *J. Med. Eng. Technol.*, 1990, 14(3), 111–113.

Pacela, A. F. (ed.), "Safe medical devices law: Sweeping changes for hospitals and the standards industry," *Biomed. Safety and Stand.* Special Supplement No. 12, February 1991.

Rabbitt, J. T., and P. A. Bergh, *The ISO 9000 Book*, 2nd ed. White Plains, NY: Quality Resources, 1994.

Ray, C. D. (ed.), *Medical Engineering*. Chicago: Year Book, 1974.

Scott, D., and J. G. Webster, "Development phases for medical devices." *Med. Instrum.*, 1986, 20(1), 48–52.

Stanaszek, M. J., *The Inverted Medical Dictionary*, 2nd ed. Lancaster, PA: Technomic Publishing Co., 1991.

Tompkins, W. J., and J. G. Webster (eds.), *Design of Microcomputer-Based Medical Instrumentation*. Englewood Cliffs, NJ: Prentice-Hall, 1981.

Webster, J. G. (ed.), *Bioinstrumentation*. Hoboken NJ: Wiley, 2004.

Webster, J. G. (ed.), *Encyclopedia of Medical Devices and Instrumentation*, 2nd ed. Vols. 1-6. New York: Wiley, 2006.

Webster, J. G., and A. M. Cook (eds.), *Clinical Engineering: Principles and Practices*. Englewood Cliffs, NJ: Prentice-Hall, 1979.

# 2

# BASIC SENSORS AND PRINCIPLES

Robert A. Peura and John G. Webster

This chapter deals with basic mechanisms and principles of the sensors used in a number of medical instruments. A *transducer* is a device that converts energy from one form to another. A *sensor* converts a physical parameter to an electric output. An *actuator* converts an electric signal to a physical output. An electric output from the sensor is normally desirable because of the advantages it gives in further signal processing (Pallas-Areny and Webster, 2001). As we shall see in this chapter, there are many methods used to convert physiological events to electric signals. Dimensional changes may be measured by variations in resistance, inductance, capacitance, and piezoelectric effect. Thermistors and thermocouples are employed to measure body temperatures. Electromagnetic-radiation sensors include thermal and photon detectors. In our discussion of the design of medical instruments in the following chapters, we shall use the principles described in this chapter (Togawa *et al.*, 1997).

## 2.1 DISPLACEMENT MEASUREMENTS

The physician and biomedical researcher are interested in measuring the size, shape, and position of the organs and tissues of the body. Variations in these parameters are important in discriminating normal from abnormal function. Displacement sensors can be used in both direct and indirect systems of measurement. Direct measurements of displacement are used to determine the change in diameter of blood vessels and the changes in volume and shape of cardiac chambers.

Indirect measurements of displacement are used to quantify movements of liquids through heart valves. An example is the movement of a microphone diaphragm that detects the movement of the heart indirectly and the resulting heart murmurs.

Here we will describe the following types of displacement-sensitive measurement methods: resistive, inductive, capacitive, and piezoelectric (Nyce, 2004).

## 2.2 RESISTIVE SENSORS

### POTENTIOMETERS

Figure 2.1 shows three types of potentiometric devices for measuring displacement. The potentiometer shown in Figure 2.1(a) measures translational displacements from 2 to 500 mm. Rotational displacements ranging from 10° to more than 50° are detected as shown in Figure 2.1(b) and (c). The resistance elements (composed of wire-wound, carbon-film, metal-film, conducting-plastic, or ceramic material) may be excited by either dc or ac voltages. These potentiometers produce a linear output (within 0.01% of full scale) as a function of displacement, provided that the potentiometer is not electrically loaded.

The resolution of these potentiometers is a function of the construction. It is possible to achieve a continuous stepless conversion of resistance for low-resistance values up to 10 Ω by utilizing a straight piece of wire. For greater variations in resistance, from several ohms to several megohms, the resistance wire is wound on a mandrel or card. The variation in resistance is thereby not continuous, but rather stepwise, because the wiper moves from one turn of wire to the next. The fundamental limitation of the resolution is a function of the wire spacing, which may be as small as 20 μm. The frictional and inertial components of these potentiometers should be low in order to minimize dynamic distortion of the system.

### STRAIN GAGES

When a fine wire (25 μm) is strained within its elastic limit, the wire's resistance changes because of changes in the diameter, length, and resistivity. The resulting strain gages may be used to measure extremely small displacements, on the order of nanometers. The following derivation shows how each of these parameters influences the resistance change. The basic equation for the

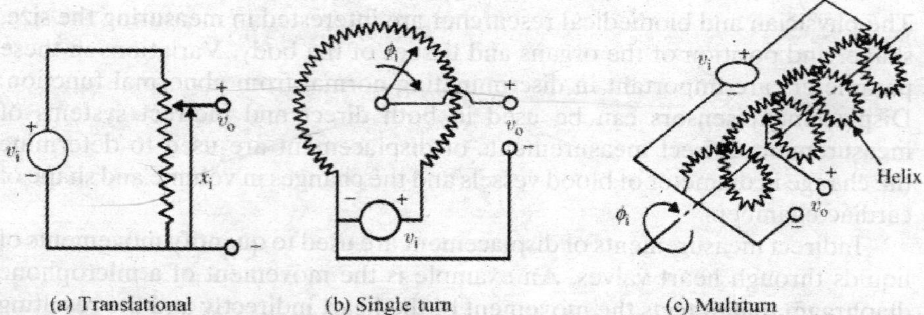


**Figure 2.1 Three types of potentiometric devices for measuring displacements** (a) Translational. (b) Single-turn, (c) Multiturn. (From *Measurement Systems: Application and Design*, by E. O. Doebelin. Copyright © 1990 by McGraw-Hill, Inc. Used with permission of McGraw-Hill Book Co.)

resistance $R$ of a wire with resistivity $\rho$ (ohm·meter), length $L$ (meters), and cross-sectional area $A$ (meter squared) is given by

$$R = \frac{\rho L}{A} \tag{2.1}$$

The differential change in $R$ is found by taking the differential

$$dR = \frac{\rho dL}{A} - \rho A^{-2} L\,dA + L\frac{d\rho}{A} \tag{2.2}$$

We shall modify this expression so that it represents finite changes in the parameters and is also a function of standard mechanical coefficients. Thus dividing members of (2.2) by corresponding members of (2.1) and introducing incremental values, we get

$$\frac{\Delta R}{R} = \frac{\Delta L}{L} - \frac{\Delta A}{A} + \frac{\Delta\rho}{\rho} \tag{2.3}$$

Poisson's ratio $\mu$. relates the change in diameter $\Delta D$ to the change in length: $\Delta D/D = -\mu\,\Delta L/L$. Substituting this into the center term of (2.3) yields

$$\frac{\Delta R}{R} = \underbrace{(1+2\mu)\frac{\Delta L}{L}}_{\substack{\text{Dimensional}\\ \text{effect}}} + \underbrace{\frac{\Delta\rho}{\rho}}_{\substack{\text{Piezoresistive}\\ \text{effect}}} \tag{2.4}$$

Note that the change in resistance is a function of changes in dimension—length ($\Delta L/L$) and area ($2\mu\,\Delta L/L$)—plus the change in resistivity due to strain-induced changes in the lattice structure of the material, $\Delta\rho/\rho$. The gage factor $G$, found by dividing (2.4) by $\Delta L/L$, is useful in comparing various strain-gage materials.

$$G = \frac{\Delta R/R}{\Delta L/L} = (1+2\mu) + \frac{\Delta\rho/\rho}{\Delta L/L} \tag{2.5}$$

Table 2.1 gives the gage factors and temperature coefficient of resistivity of various strain-gage materials. Note that the gage factor for semiconductor materials is approximately 50 to 70 times that of the metals.

Also note that the gage factor for metals is primarily a function of dimensional effects. For most metals, $\mu = 0.3$ and thus $G$ is at least 1.6, whereas for semiconductors, the piezoresistive effect is dominant. The desirable feature of higher gage factors for semiconductor devices is offset by their greater resistivity–temperature coefficient.

Designs for instruments that use semiconductor materials must incorporate temperature compensation.

Strain gages can be classified as either unbonded or bonded. An unbonded strain-gage unit is shown in Figure 2.2(a). The four sets of strain-sensitive wires

**Table 2.1 Properties of Strain-Gage Materials**

| Material | Composition (%) | Gage Factor | Temperature Coefficient of Resistivity $(^\circ C^{-1}\text{–}10^{-5})$ |
|---|---|---|---|
| Constantan (advance) | $Ni_{45}$, $Cu_{55}$ | 2.1 | ±2 |
| Isoelastic | $Ni_{36}$, $Cr_8$ $(Mn, Si, Mo)_4$ $Fe_{52}$ | 3.52 to 3.6 | +17 |
| Karma | $Ni_{74}$, $Cr_{20}$, $Fe_3$ $Cu_3$ | 2.1 | +2 |
| Manganin | $Cu_{84}$, $Mn_{12}$, $Ni_4$ | 0.3 to 0.47 | ±2 |
| Alloy 479 | $Pt_{92}$, $W_8$ | 3.6 to 4.4 | +24 |
| Nickel | Pure | −12 to −20 | 670 |
| Nichrome V | $Ni_{80}$, $Cr_{20}$ | 2.1 to 2.63 | 10 |
| Silicon | (*p* type) | 100 to 170 | 70 to 700 |
| Silicon | (*n* type) | −100 to −140 | 70 to 700 |
| Germanium | (*p* type) | 102 | |
| Germanium | (*n* type) | −150 | |

SOURCE: From R. S. C. Cobbold, *Transducers for Biomedical Measurements*, 1974, John Wiley & Sons, Inc.. Used with permission of John Wiley & Sons, Inc., New York.

are connected to form a Wheatstone bridge, as shown in Figure 2.2(b). These wires are mounted under stress between the frame and the movable armature such that preload is greater than any expected external compressive load. This is necessary to avoid putting the wires in compression. This type of sensor may be used for converting blood pressure to diaphragm movement, to resistance change, then to an electric signal.

A bonded strain-gage element, consisting of a metallic wire, etched foil, vacuum-deposited film, or semiconductor bar, is cemented to the strained surface. Figure 2.3 shows typical bonded strain gages. The deviation from linearity is approximately 1%. One method of temperature compensation for the natural temperature sensitivity of bonded strain gages involves using a second strain gage as a dummy element that is also exposed to the temperature variation, but not to strain. When possible, the four-arm bridge shown in Figure 2.2 should be used, because it not only provides temperature compensation but also yields four times greater output if all four arms contain active gages. Four bonded metal strain gages can be used on cantilever beams to measure bite force in dental research (Dechow, 2006).

Strain-gage technology advanced in the 1960s with the introduction of the semiconductor strain-gage element, which has the advantage of having a high gage factor, as shown in Table 2.1. However, it is more temperature sensitive and inherently more nonlinear than metal strain gages because the piezoresistive effect varies with strain. Semiconductor elements can be used as

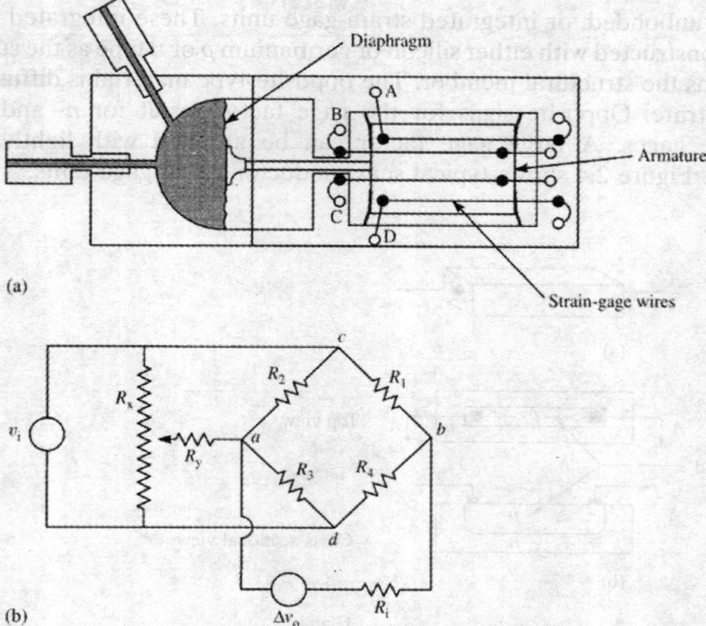


**Figure 2.2** (a) Unbonded strain-gage pressure sensor. The diaphragm is directly coupled by an armature to an unbonded strain-gage system. With increasing pressure, the strain on gage pair B and C is increased, while that on gage pair A and D is decreased. (b) Wheatstone bridge with four active elements: $R_1 = \text{B}$, $R_2 = \text{A}$, $R_3 = \text{D}$, and $R_4 = \text{C}$ when the unbonded strain gage is connected for translational motion. Resistor $R_y$ and potentiometer $R_x$ are used to initially balance the bridge, $v_i$ is the applied voltage, and $\Delta v_o$ is the output voltage on a voltmeter or similar device with an internal resistance of $R_i$.

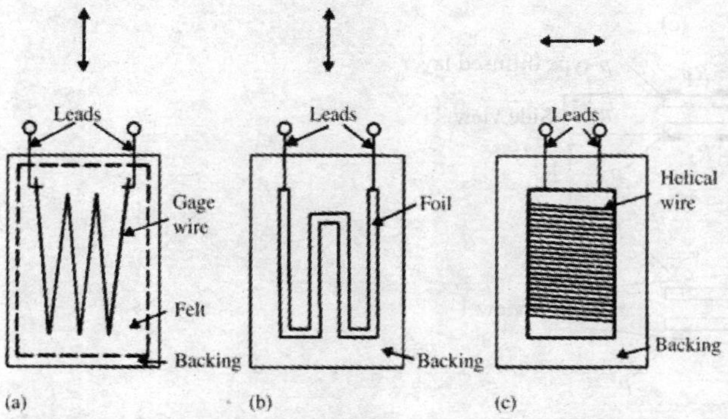


**Figure 2.3 Typical bonded strain-gage units** (a) resistance-wire type, (b) foil type, (c) helical-wire type. Arrows above units show direction of maximal sensitivity to strain. [Parts (a) and (b) are modified from *Instrumentation in Scientific Research*, K. S. Lion. Copyright © 1959 by McGraw-Hill, Inc. Used with permission of McGraw-Hill Book Co.]

bonded, unbonded, or integrated strain-gage units. These integrated devices can be constructed with either silicon or germanium *p* or *n* type as the substrate that forms the structural member. The opposite-type material is diffused into the substrate. Opposite signs for the gage factor result for *n*- and *p*-type substrate gages. A large gage factor can be attained with lightly doped material. Figure 2.4 shows typical semiconductor strain-gage units.

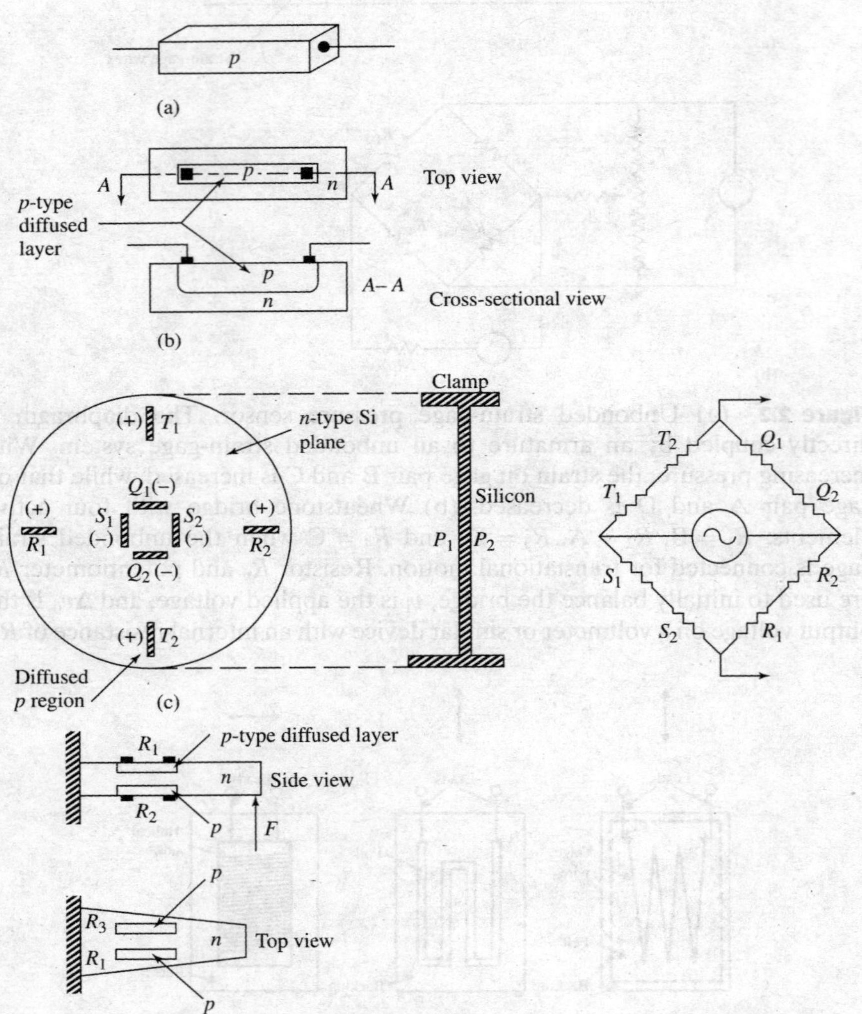


**Figure 2.4 Typical semiconductor strain-gage units** (a) unbonded, uniformly doped, (b) diffused *p*-type gage, (c) integrated pressure sensor, (d) integrated cantilever-beam force sensor. (From *Transducers for Medical Measurements: Application and Design*, R. S. C. Cobbold. Copyright © 1974, John Wiley & Sons, Inc. Reprinted by permission of John Wiley & Sons, Inc.)

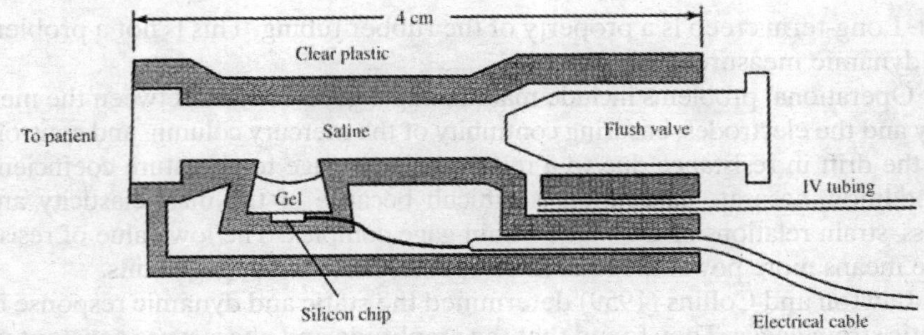


**Figure 2.5 Isolation in a disposable blood-pressure sensor** Disposable blood-pressure sensors are made of clear plastic so air bubbles are easily seen. Saline flows from an intravenous (IV) bag through the clear IV tubing and the sensor to the patient. This flushes blood out of the tip of the indwelling catheter to prevent clotting. A lever can open or close the flush valve. The silicon chip has a silicon diaphragm with a four-resistor Wheatstone bridge diffused into it. Its electrical connections are protected from the saline by a compliant silicone elastomer gel, which also provides electrical isolation. This prevents electric shock from the sensor to the patient and prevents destructive currents during defibrillation from the patient to the silicon chip.

The integrated-type sensor has an advantage in that a pressure sensor can be fabricated by using a silicon substrate for the structural member of the diaphragm. The gages are diffused directly onto the diaphragm. When pressure is applied to the diaphragm, a radial stress component occurs at the edge. The sign of this component is opposite to that of the tangential stress component near the center. The placement of the eight diffused strain-gage units shown in Figure 2.4(c) gives high sensitivity and good temperature compensation (Cobbold, 1974). Figure 2.5 shows a disposable blood-pressure sensor that uses an integrated silicon chip. Silicon strain-gage pressure sensors can be placed on the tip of a catheter and inserted directly into the blood, resulting in more accurate measurements and faster response times (Korites, 1987).

Elastic-resistance strain gages are extensively used in biomedical applications, especially in cardiovascular and respiratory dimensional and plethysmographic (volume-measuring) determinations. These systems normally consist of a narrow silicone-rubber tube [0.5 mm inner diameter (ID), 2 mm outer diameter (OD)] from 3 to 25 cm long and filled with mercury or with an electrolyte or conductive paste. The ends of the tube are sealed with electrodes (amalgamated copper, silver, or platinum). As the tube stretches, the diameter of the tube decreases and the length increases, causing the resistance to increase. The resistance per unit length of typical gages is approximately 0.02 to 2 Ω/cm. These units measure much higher displacements than other gages.

The elastic strain gage is linear within 1% for 10% of maximal extension. As the extension is increased to 30% of maximum, the nonlinearity reaches 4% of full scale. The initial nonlinearity (dead band) is ascribed to slackness of the unit. Long-term creep is a property of the rubber tubing. This is not a problem for dynamic measurements.

Operational problems include maintaining a good contact between the mercury and the electrodes, ensuring continuity of the mercury column, and controlling the drift in resistance due to a relatively large gage temperature coefficient. In addition, accurate calibration is difficult because of the mass-elasticity and stress–strain relations of the tissue–strain-gage complex. The low value of resistance means more power is required to operate these strain-gage units.

Lawton and Collins (1959) determined the static and dynamic response of elastic strain gages. They found that the amplitude and phase were constant up to 10 Hz. Significant distortion occurred for frequencies greater than 30 Hz. Cobbold (1974) indicated that a problem not fully appreciated is that the gage does not distend fully during pulsations when diameter of the vessel is being measured. The mass of the gage and its finite mechanical resistance can cause it to dig into the vessel wall as the vessel expands, so it can give a reading several times lower than that measured using ultrasonic or cineangiographic methods.

Hokanson *et al.* (1975) described an electrically calibrated mercury-in-rubber strain gage. Lead-wire errors are common with these devices because of the low resistance of the strain gage. In Hokanson's design, the problem was eliminated by effectively placing the strain gage at the corners of the measurement bridge. A constant-current source causes an output that is linear for large changes in gage resistance. Figure 2.6 shows the device and its output when applied to the human calf.

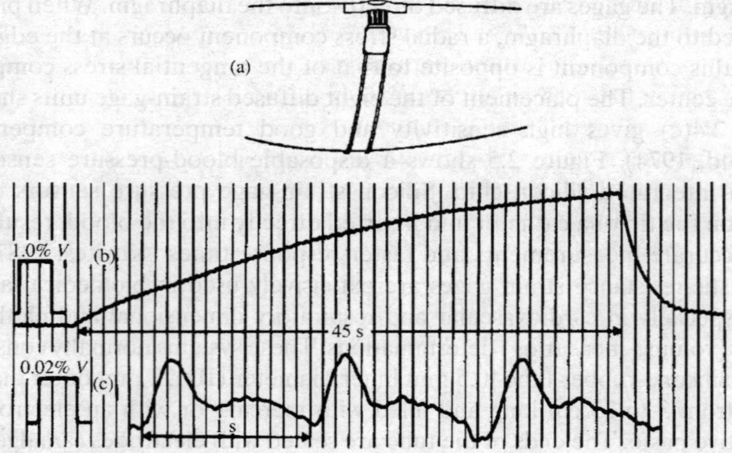


**Figure 2.6 Mercury-in-rubber strain-gage plethysmography** (a) Four-lead gage applied to human calf, (b) Bridge output for venous-occlusion plethysmography. (c) Bridge output for arterial-pulse plethysmography. [Part (a) is based on D. E. Hokanson, D. S. Sumner, and D. E. Strandness, Jr., "An electrically calibrated plethysmograph for direct measurement of limb blood flow." 1975, BME-22, 25–29; used with permission of *IEEE Trans. Biomed. Eng.*, 1975, New York.]

## 2.3 BRIDGE CIRCUITS

The Wheatstone bridge circuit is ideal for measuring small changes in resistance. Figure 2.2(b) shows a Wheatstone bridge with an applied dc voltage of $v_i$ and a readout meter $\Delta v_o$ with internal resistance $R_i$. It can be shown by the voltage-divider approach that $\Delta v_o$ is zero—that is, the bridge is balanced—when $R_1/R_2 = R_4/R_3$.

Resistance-type sensors may be connected in one or more arms of a bridge circuit. The variation in resistance can be detected by measuring $\Delta v_o$ with a differential amplifier feeding an analog-to-digital converter (ADC), which feeds a computer.

Assume that all values of resistance of the bridge are initially equal to $R_0$ and that $R_0 \ll R_i$. An increase in resistance, $\Delta R$, of all resistances still results in a balanced bridge. However, if $R_1$ and $R_3$ increase by $\Delta R$, and $R_2$ and $R_4$ decrease by $\Delta R$, then

$$\Delta v_o = \frac{\Delta R}{R_0} v_i \tag{2.6}$$

Because of the symmetry a similar expression results if $R_2$ and $R_4$ increase by $\Delta R$ and $R_1$ and $R_3$ decrease by $\Delta R$. Note that (2.6), for the four-active-arm bridge, shows that $\Delta v_o$ is linearly related to $\Delta R$. A nonlinearity in $\Delta R/R_0$ is present even when $R_0/R_i = 0$.

It is common practice to incorporate a balancing scheme in the bridge circuit [see Figure 2.2(b)]. Resistor $R_y$ and potentiometer $R_x$ are used to change the initial resistance of one or more arms. This arrangement brings the bridge into balance so that zero voltage output results from "zero" (or *base-level*) input of the measured parameter.

To minimize loading effects, $R_x$ is approximately 10 times the resistance of the bridge leg, and $R_y$ limits the maximal adjustment. Strain-gage applications normally use a value of $R_y = 25$ times the resistance of the bridge leg. Alternating-current (ac) balancing circuits are more complicated because a reactive as well as a resistive imbalance must be compensated.

## 2.4 INDUCTIVE SENSORS

An inductance $L$ can be used to measure displacement by varying any three of the coil parameters:

$$L = n^2 G \mu \tag{2.7}$$

where

$n$ = number of turns of coil

$G$ = geometric form factor

$\mu$ = effective permeability of the medium

Each of these parameters can be changed by mechanical means.

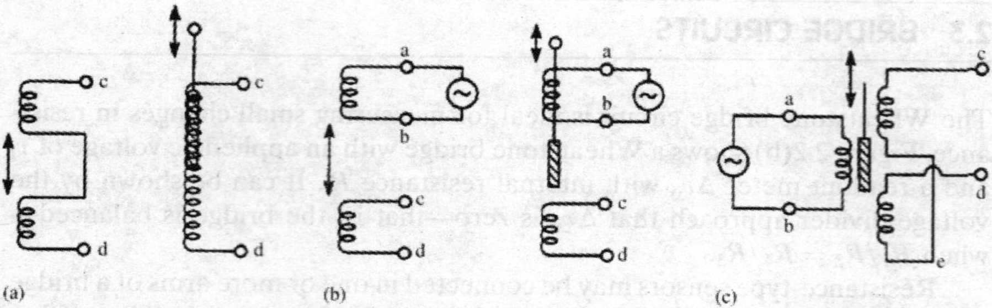


**Figure 2.7 Inductive displacement sensors** (a) self-inductance, (b) mutual inductance, (c) differential transformer.

Figure 2.7 shows (a) self-inductance, (b) mutual-inductance, and (c) differential transformer types of inductive displacement sensors. It is usually possible to convert a mutual-inductance system into a self-inductance system by series of parallel connections of the coils. Note in Figure 2.7 that the mutual-inductance device (b) becomes a self-inductance device (a) when terminals *b–c* are connected.

An inductive sensor has an advantage in not being affected by the dielectric properties of its environment. However, it may be affected by external magnetic fields due to the proximity of magnetic materials.

The variable-inductance method employing a single displaceable core is shown in Figure 2.7(a). This device works on the principle that alterations in the self-inductance of a coil may be produced by changing the geometric form factor or the movement of a magnetic core within the coil. The change in inductance for this device is not linearly related to displacement. The fact that these devices have low power requirements and produce large variations in inductance makes them attractive for radiotelemetry applications.

The mutual-inductance sensor employs two separate coils and uses the variation in their mutual magnetic coupling to measure displacement [Figure 2.7(b)]. Cobbold (1974) describes the application of these devices in measuring cardiac dimensions, monitoring infant respiration, and ascertaining arterial diameters.

Van Citters (1966) provides a good description of applications of mutual inductance transformers in measuring changes in dimension of internal organs (kidney, major blood vessels, and left ventricle). The induced voltage in the secondary coil is a function of the geometry of the coils (separation and axial alignment), the number of primary and secondary turns, and the frequency and amplitude of the excitation voltage. The induced voltage in the secondary coil is a nonlinear function of the separation of the coils. In order to maximize the output signal, a frequency is selected that causes the secondary coil (tuned circuit) to be in resonance. The output voltage is detected with standard demodulator and amplifier circuits.

The linear variable differential transformer (LVDT) is widely used in physiological research and clinical medicine to measure pressure, displacement, and force (Kesavan and Reddy, 2006). As shown in Figure 2.7(c), the LVDT is composed of a primary coil (terminals a–b) and two secondary coils (c–e and d–e) connected in series. The coupling between these two coils is changed by the motion of a high-permeability alloy slug between them. The two secondary coils are connected in opposition in order to achieve a wider region of linearity.

The primary coil is sinusoidally excited, with a frequency between 60 Hz and 20 kHz. The alternating magnetic field induces nearly equal voltages $v_{ce}$ and $v_{de}$ in the secondary coils. The output voltage $v_{cd} = v_{ce} - v_{de}$. When the slug is symmetrically placed, the two secondary voltages are equal and the output signal is zero.

Linear variable differential transformer characteristics include linearity over a large range, a change of phase by 180° when the core passes through the center position, and saturation on the ends. Specifications of commercially available LVDTs include sensitivities on the order of 0.5 to 2 mV for a displacement of 0.01 mm/V of primary voltage, full-scale displacement of 0.1 to 250 mm, and linearity of ±0.25%. Sensitivity for LVDTs is much higher than that for strain gages.

A disadvantage of the LVDT is that it requires more complex signal-processing instrumentation. Figure 2.8 shows that essentially the same

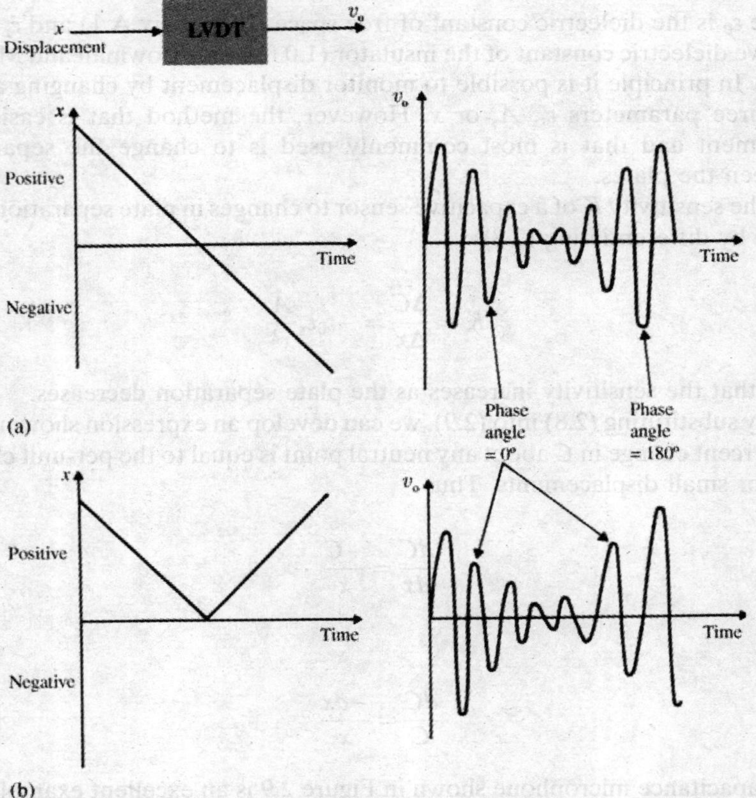


**Figure 2.8** (a) As $x$ moves through the null position, the phase changes 180°, while the magnitude of $v_o$ is proportional to the magnitude of $x$. (b) An ordinary rectifier demodulator cannot distinguish between (a) and (b), so a phase-sensitive demodulator is required.

magnitude of output voltage results from two very different input displacements. The direction of displacement may be determined by using the fact that there is a 180° phase shift when the core passes through the null position. A phase-sensitive demodulator is used to determine the direction of displacement. Figure 3.17 shows a ring-demodulator system that could be used with the LVDT.

## 2.5 CAPACITIVE SENSORS

The capacitance between two parallel plates of area $A$ separated by distance $x$ is

$$C = \varepsilon_0 \varepsilon_r \frac{A}{x} \tag{2.8}$$

where $\varepsilon_0$ is the dielectric constant of free space (Appendix A.1) and $\varepsilon_r$ is the relative dielectric constant of the insulator (1.0 for air) (Bowman and Meindl, 1988). In principle it is possible to monitor displacement by changing any of the three parameters $\varepsilon_r$, $A$, or $x$. However, the method that is easiest to implement and that is most commonly used is to change the separation between the plates.

The sensitivity $K$ of a capacitive sensor to changes in plate separation $\Delta x$ is found by differentiating (2.8).

$$K = \frac{\Delta C}{\Delta x} = -\varepsilon_0 \varepsilon_r \frac{A}{x^2} \tag{2.9}$$

Note that the sensitivity increases as the plate separation decreases.

By substituting (2.8) into (2.9), we can develop an expression showing that the percent change in $C$ about any neutral point is equal to the per-unit change in $x$ for small displacements. Thus

$$\frac{dC}{dx} = \frac{-C}{x} \tag{2.10}$$

or

$$\frac{dC}{C} = \frac{-dx}{x} \tag{2.11}$$

The capacitance microphone shown in Figure 2.9 is an excellent example of a relatively simple method for detecting variation in capacitance (Doebelin, 1990; Cobbold, 1974). This is a dc-excited circuit, so no current flows when the capacitor is stationary (with separation $x_0$), and thus $v_1 = E$. A change in

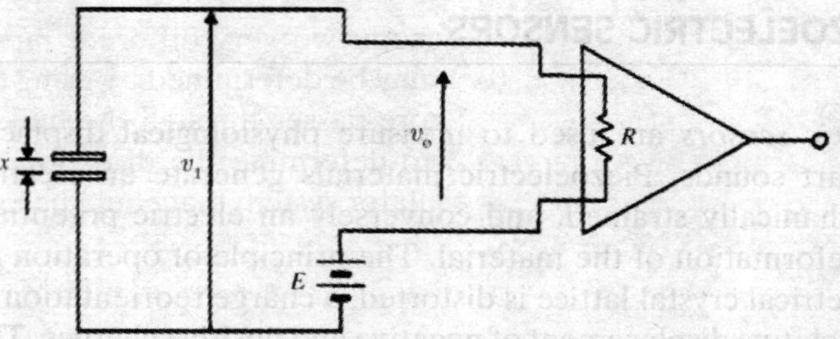


**Figure 2.9** Capacitance sensor for measuring dynamic displacement changes.

position $\Delta x = x_1 - x_0$ produces a voltage $v_o = v_1 - E$. The output voltage $V_o$ is related to $x_1$ by

$$\frac{V_o(j\omega)}{X_1(j\omega)} = \frac{(E/x_0)\, j\omega\tau}{j\omega\tau + 1} \tag{2.12}$$

where $\tau = RC = R\varepsilon_0\varepsilon_r A/x_0$.

Typically, $R$ is 1 MΩ or higher, and thus the readout device must have a high (10 MΩ or higher) input impedance.

For $\omega\tau \gg 1$, $V_0(j\omega)/X_1(j\omega) \cong E/x_0$, which is a constant. However, the response drops off for low frequencies, and it is zero when $\omega = 0$. Thus (2.12) describes a high-pass filter. This frequency response is quite adequate for a microphone that does not measure sound pressures at frequencies below 20 Hz. However, it is inadequate for measuring most physiological variables because of their low-frequency components.

Compliant plastics of different dielectric constants may be placed between foil layers to form a capacitive mat to be placed on a bed. Patient movement generates charge, which is amplified and filtered to display respiratory movements from the lungs and ballistographic movements from the heart (Alihanka *et al*, 1982).

A capacitance sensor can be fabricated from layers of mica insulators sandwiched between corrugated metal layers. Applied pressure flattens the corrugations and moves the metallic plates closer to each other, thus increasing the capacitance. The sensor is not damaged by large overloads, because flattening of the corrugations does not cause the metal to yield. The sensor measures the pressure between the foot and the shoe (Patel *et al.*, 1989). Tsoukalas *et al.* (2006) describe micromachined silicon capacitive sensors and their electronic interfaces.

**EXAMPLE 2.1** For a 1 cm$^2$ capacitance sensor, $R$ is 100 MΩ. Calculate $x$, the plate spacing required to pass sound frequencies above 20 Hz.

**ANSWER** From the corner frequency, $C = 1/2\pi fR = 1/(2\pi 20 \times 10^8) =$ 80 pF From (2.8) we can calculate $x$ given the value of $C$.

$$x = \frac{\varepsilon_0\varepsilon_r A}{C} = \frac{(8.854 \times 10^{-12})(1 \times 10^{-4})}{80 \times 10^{-12}} = 1.11 \times 10^5 \text{ m} = 11.1\ \mu\text{m}$$

## 2.6 PIEZOELECTRIC SENSORS

*Piezoelectric sensors* are used to measure physiological displacements and record heart sounds. Piezoelectric materials generate an electric potential when mechanically strained, and conversely an electric potential can cause physical deformation of the material. The principle of operation is that when an asymmetrical crystal lattice is distorted, a charge reorientation takes place, causing a relative displacement of negative and positive charges. The displaced internal charges induce surface charges of opposite polarity on opposite sides of the crystal. Surface charge can be determined by measuring the difference in voltage between electrodes attached to the surfaces.

Initially, we assume infinite leakage resistance. Then, the total induced charge $q$ is directly proportional to the applied force $f$.

$$q = kf \tag{2.13}$$

where $k$ is the piezoelectric constant, C/N. The change in voltage can be found by assuming that the system acts like a parallel-plate capacitor where the voltage $v$ across the capacitor is charge $q$ divided by capacitance $C$. Then, by substitution of (2.8), we get

$$v = \frac{kf}{C} = \frac{kfx}{\varepsilon_0 \varepsilon_r A} \tag{2.14}$$

Tables of piezoelectric constants are given in the literature (Lion, 1959; and Cobbold, 1974).

Typical values for $k$ are 2.3 pC/N for quartz and 140 pC/N for barium titanate. For a piezoelectric sensor of 1 $cm^2$ area and 1 mm thickness with an applied force due to a 10 g weight, the output voltage $v$ is 0.23 mV and 14 mV for the quartz and barium titanate crystals, respectively.

There are various modes of operation of piezoelectric sensors, depending on the material and the crystallographic orientation of the plate (Lion, 1959). These modes include the thickness or longitudinal compression, transversal compression, thickness-shear action, and face-shear action.

Also available are piezoelectric polymeric films, such as polyvinylidene fluoride (PVDF) (Hennig, 1988; Webster, 1988). These films are very thin, lightweight and pliant, and they can be cut easily and adapted to uneven surfaces. The low mechanical quality factor does not permit resonance applications, but it permits acoustical broadband applications for microphones and loudspeakers.

Piezoelectric materials have a high but finite resistance. As a consequence, if a static deflection $x$ is applied, the charge leaks through the leakage resistor (on the order of 100 G$\Omega$). It is obviously quite important that the input impedance of the external voltage-measuring device be an order of magnitude higher than that of the piezoelectric sensor. It would be helpful to look at the

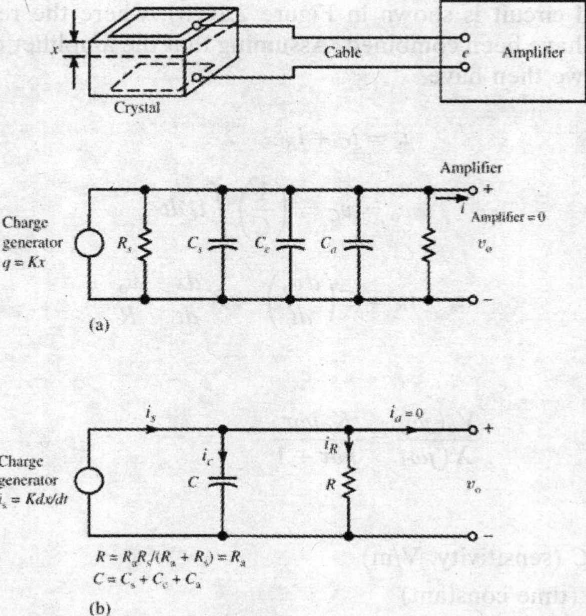


**Figure 2.10** (a) Equivalent circuit of piezoelectric sensor, where $R_s$ = sensor leakage resistance, $C_s$ = sensor capacitance, $C_c$ = cable capacitance, $C_a$ = amplifier input capacitance, $R_a$ = amplifier input resistance, and $q$ = charge generator. (b) Modified equivalent circuit with current generator replacing charge generator. (From *Measurement Systems: Application and Design*, by E. O. Doebelin. Copyright © 1990 by McGraw-Hill, Inc. Used with permission of McGraw-Hill Book Co.)

equivalent circuit for the piezoelectric sensor [Figure 2.10(a)] in order to quantify its dynamic-response characteristics.

This circuit has a charge generator $q$ defined by

$$q = Kx \tag{2.15}$$

where where

$K$ = proportionality constant, C/m
$x$ = deflection

The circuit may be simplified by converting the charge generator to a current generator, $i_s$.

$$i_s = \frac{dq}{dt} = K\frac{dx}{dt} \tag{2.16}$$

The modified circuit is shown in Figure 2.10(b), where the resistances and capacitances have been combined. Assuming that the amplifier does not draw any current, we then have

$$i_s = i_C + i_R \tag{2.17}$$

$$v_o = v_C = \left(\frac{1}{C}\right)\int i_C dt \tag{2.18}$$

$$i_s - i_R = C\left(\frac{dv_o}{dt}\right) = K\frac{dx}{dt} - \frac{v_o}{R} \tag{2.19}$$

or

$$\frac{V_o(j\omega)}{X(j\omega)} = \frac{K_s j\omega\tau}{j\omega\tau + 1} \tag{2.20}$$

where

$K_s = K/C$ (sensitivity, V/m)
$\tau = RC$ (time constant)

**EXAMPLE 2.2** A piezoelectric sensor has $C = 500$ pF. The sensor leakage resistance is 10 GΩ. The amplifier input impedance is 5 MΩ. What is the low-corner frequency?

**ANSWER** We may use the modified equivalent circuit of the piezoelectric sensor given in Figure 2.10(b) for this calculation.

$$f_c = 1/(2\pi RC) = 1/[2\pi(5 \times 10^6)(500 \times 10^{-12})] = 64 \text{ Hz}$$

Note that by increasing the input impedance of the amplifier by a factor of 100, we can lower the low-corner frequency to 0.64 Hz.

**EXAMPLE 2.3** For a piezoelectric sensor plus cable that has 1 nF capacitance, design a *voltage amplifier* (not a charge amplifier) by using only *one* noninverting amplifier that has a gain of 10. It should handle a charge of 1 μC generated by the carotid pulse without saturation. It should not drift into saturation because of bias currents. It should have a frequency response from 0.05 to 100 Hz. Add the minimal number of extra components to achieve the design specifications.

**ANSWER** Calculate the voltage from $V = Q/C = 1\,\mu\text{C}/1\,\text{nF} = 1\,\text{kV}$. Because this is too high, add a shunt capacitor $C_s = 1\,\mu\text{F}$ to achieve 1.0 V. Allow for a gain of 10. To achieve low-corner frequency, add shunt

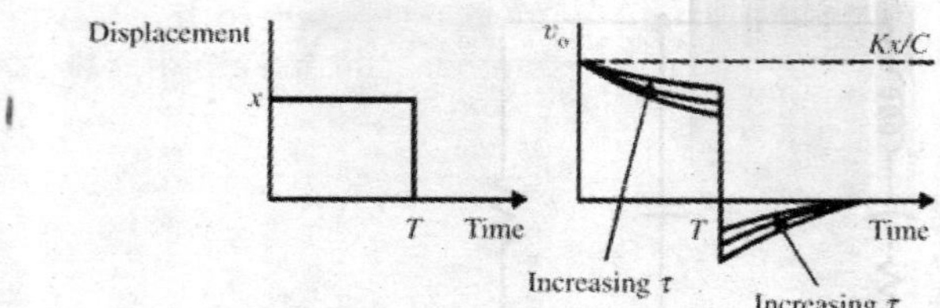


**Figure 2.11 Sensor response to a step displacement** (From Doebelin, E. O. 1990. *Measurement Systems: Application and Design*, New York: McGraw-Hill.)

$R_s = 1/2\pi f_c C = 1/2\pi(0.05)(1\,\mu F) = 3.2\,M\Omega$. To achieve gain of +10 in a noninverting amplifier, select $R_f = 10\,k\Omega$ and $R_i = 11.1\,k\Omega$. To achieve high-corner frequency, $C_f = 1/2\pi f_c R_f = 1/2\pi(100)(10\,k\Omega) = 160\,nF$.

Figure 2.11 shows the voltage-output response of a piezoelectric sensor to a step displacement $x$. The output decays exponentially because of the finite internal resistance of the piezoelectric material. At time equal to $T$ the force is released, and a displacement restoration results that is equal to and opposite of the original displacement. This causes a sudden decrease in voltage of magnitude $Kx/C$, with a resulting undershoot equal to the decay prior to the release of the displacement. The decay and undershoot can be minimized by increasing the time constant, $\tau = RC$. The simplest approach to increasing $\tau$ is to add a parallel capacitor. However, doing so reduces the sensitivity in the midband frequencies according to (2.20).

Another approach to improving the low-frequency response is to use the charge amplifier described in Section 3.8.

Because of its mechanical resonance, the high-frequency equivalent circuit for a piezoelectric sensor is complex. This effect can be represented by adding a series *RLC* circuit in parallel with the sensor capacitance and leakage resistance. Figure 2.12 shows the high-frequency equivalent circuit and its frequency response. Note that in some applications—for example, in the case of crystal filters—the mechanical resonance is useful for accurate frequency control.

Piezoelectric sensors are used quite extensively in cardiology for external (body-surface) and internal (intracardiac) phonocardiography. They are also used in the detection of Korotkoff sounds in blood-pressure measurements (Chapter 7). Additional applications of piezoelectric sensors involve their use in measurements of physiological accelerations. A piezoelectric sensor and circuit can measure the acceleration due to human movements and provide an estimate of energy expenditure (Servais *et al.*, 1984). Section 8.4 describes ultrasonic blood-flow meters in which the piezoelectric element operating at mechanical resonance emits and senses high-frequency sounds. Li and Su (2006) describe piezoelectric sensors as sensitive mass sensors to detect and measure a broad variety of biomedical analytes in both gas and liquid phases based on the adsorption and/or desorption of target analyte(s) on the sensor surface.

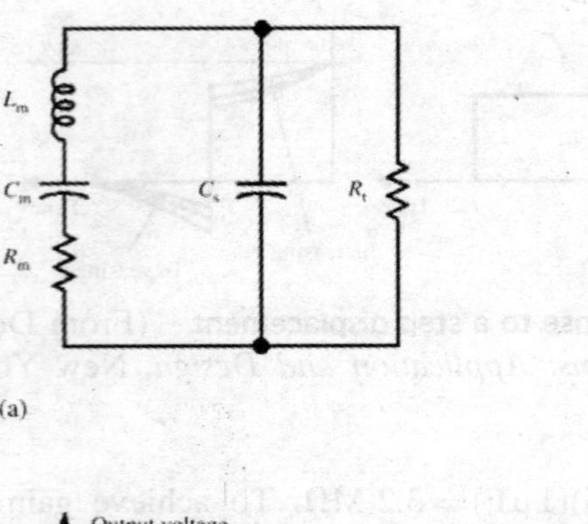


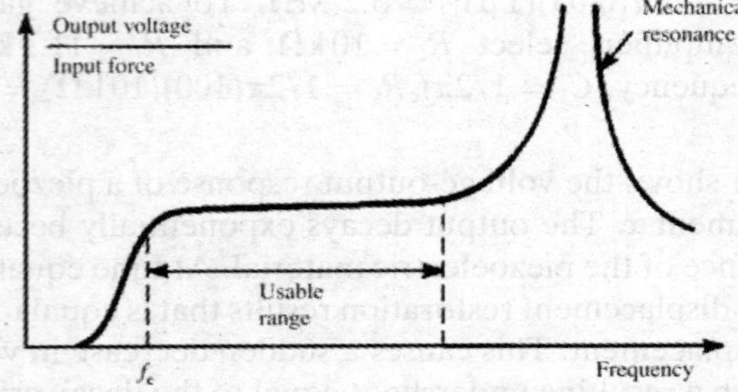


**Figure 2.12** (a) High-frequency circuit model for piezoelectric sensor. $R_s$ is the sensor leakage resistance and $C_s$ is the capacitance. $L_m$, $C_m$, and $R_m$ represent the mechanical system, (b) Piezoelectric sensor frequency response. (From *Transducers for Biomedical Measurements: Principles and Applications*, by R. S. C. Cobbold. Copyright (c) 1974, John Wiley and Sons, Inc. Reprinted by permission of John Wiley and Sons, Inc.)

## 2.7 TEMPERATURE MEASUREMENTS

A patient's body temperature gives the physician important information about the physiological state of the individual. External body temperature is one of many parameters used to evaluate patients in shock, because the reduced blood pressure of a person in circulatory shock results in low blood flow to the periphery. A drop in the big-toe temperature is a good early clinical warning of shock. Infections, on the other hand, are usually reflected by an increase in body temperature, with a hot, flushed skin and loss of fluids. Increased ventilation, perspiration, and blood flow to the skin result when high fevers destroy temperature-sensitive enzymes and proteins. Anesthesia decreases body temperature by depressing the thermal regulatory center. In fact, physicians routinely induce hypothermia in surgical cases in which they wish to decrease a patient's metabolic processes and blood circulation.

In pediatrics, special heated incubators are used for stabilizing the body temperature of infants. Accurate monitoring of temperature and regulatory control systems are used to maintain a desirable ambient temperature for the infant.

In the study of arthritis, physicians have shown that temperatures of joints are closely correlated with the amount of local inflammation. The increased blood flow due to arthritis and chronic inflammation can be detected by thermal measurements.

The specific site of body-temperature recording must be selected carefully so that it truly reflects the patient's temperature. Also, environmental changes and artifacts can cause misleading readings. For example, the skin and oral-mucosa temperature of a patient seldom reflects true body-core temperature.

The following types of thermally sensitive methods of measurement will be described here: thermocouples, thermistors, and radiation and fiber-optic detectors (Samaras, 2006). The voltage across a *p–n* junction changes about 2 mV/°C so temperature sensors that use this principle are available (Togawa, 2006).

## 2.8 THERMOCOUPLES

*Thermoelectric thermometry* is based on the discovery of Seebeck in 1821. He observed that an *electromotive force* (emf) exists across a junction of two dissimilar metals. This phenomenon is due to the sum of two independent effects. The first effect, discovered by Peltier, is an emf due solely to the contact of two unlike metals and the junction temperature. The net Peltier emf is roughly proportional to the difference between the temperatures of the two junctions. The second effect, credited to Thomson (Lord Kelvin), is an emf due to the temperature gradients along each single conductor. The net Thomson emf is proportional to the difference between the squares of the absolute junction temperatures ($T_1$ and $T_2$). The magnitudes of the Peltier and Thomson emfs can be derived from thermodynamic principles (Anonymous, 1974), and either may predominate, depending on the metals chosen.

Knowledge of these two effects is not generally useful in practical applications, so empirical calibration data are usually curve fitted with a power series expansion that yields the Seebeck voltage,

$$E = aT + \frac{1}{2}bT^2 + \cdots \tag{2.21}$$

where $T$ is in degrees Celsius and the reference junction is maintained at 0 °C.

Figure 2.13(a) is a thermocouple circuit with two dissimilar metals, $A$ and $B$, at two different temperatures, $T_1$, and $T_2$. The net emf at terminals $c$–$d$ is a function of the difference between the temperatures at the two junctions and the properties of the two metals. In the practical situation, one junction is held at a constant known temperature (by an ice bath or controlled oven) for a reference in order to determine the desired or unknown temperature.

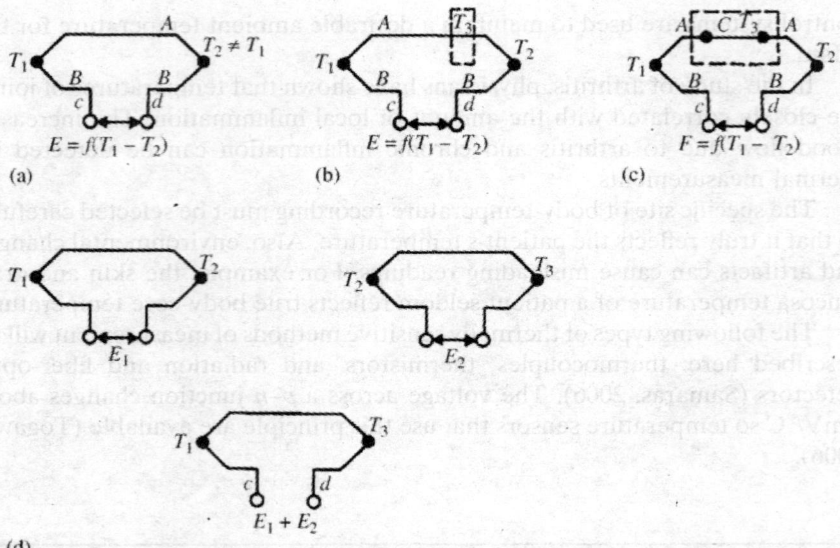


**Figure 2.13** **Thermocouple circuits** (a) Peltier emf, (b) law of homogeneous circuits, (c) law of intermediate metals, (d) law of intermediate temperatures.

An understanding of the three empirical thermocouple laws leads to using them properly. The first law, *homogeneous circuits*, states that in a circuit composed of a single homogeneous metal, one cannot maintain an electric current by the application of heat alone. In Figure 2.13(b), the net emf at *c–d* is the same as in Figure 2.13(a), regardless of the fact that a temperature distribution ($T_3$) exists along one of the wires ($A$).

The second law, *intermediate metals*, states that the net emf in a circuit consisting of an interconnection of a number of unlike metals, maintained at the same temperature, is zero. The practical implication of this principle is that lead wires may be attached to the thermocouple without affecting the accuracy of the measured emf, provided that the newly formed junctions are at the same temperature [Figure 2.13(c)].

The third law, successive or *intermediate temperatures*, is illustrated in Figure 2.13(d), where emf $E_1$ is generated when two dissimilar metals have junctions at temperatures $T_1$ and $T_2$ and emf $E_2$ results for temperatures $T_2$ and $T_3$. It follows that an emf $E_1 + E_2$ results at *c–d* when the junctions are at temperatures $T_1$ and $T_3$. This principle makes it possible for calibration curves derived for a given reference-junction temperature to be used to determine the calibration curves for another reference temperature.

The *thermoelectric sensitivity* $\alpha$ (also called the *thermoelectric power* or the *Seebeck coefficient*) is found by differentiating (2.21) with respect to $T$. Then

$$\alpha = \frac{dE}{dT} = a + bT + \cdots \tag{2.22}$$

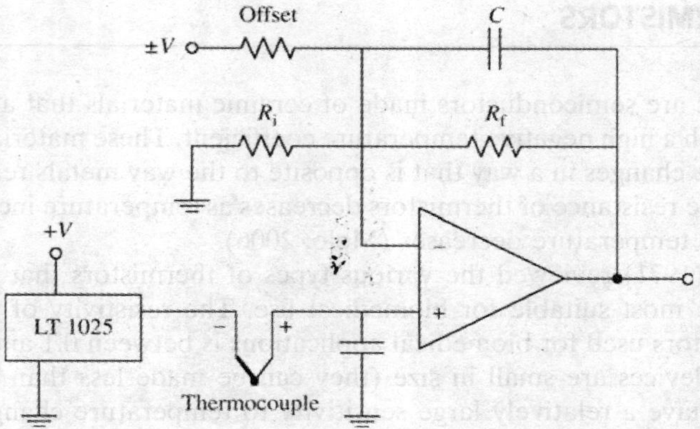


**Figure 2.14** The LT1025 electronic cold junction and the hot junction of the thermocouple yield a voltage that is amplified by an inverting amplifier.

Note that $\alpha$ is not a constant but varies (usually increases) with temperature. The sensitivities of common thermocouples range from 6.5 to 80 μV/°C at 20 °C, with accuracies from ¼% to 1%.

For accurate readings, the reference junction should be kept in a triple-point-of-water device the temperature of which is $0.01 \pm 0.0005$ °C (Doebelin, 1990). Normally the accuracy of a properly constructed ice bath, 0.05 °C with a reproducibility of 0.001 °C is all that is necessary. Temperature-controlled ovens can maintain a reference temperature to within ±0.4 °C. Figure 2.14 shows that modern thermocouple signal conditioners contain an electronic cold junction (Tompkins and Webster, 1988; Sheingold, 1980).

Increased sensitivity may be achieved by connecting a number of thermocouples in series, all of them measuring the same temperature and using the same reference junction. An arrangement of multiple-junction thermocouples is referred to as a *thermopile*. Parallel combinations may be used to measure average temperature.

It is easy to obtain a direct readout of the thermocouple voltage using a digital voltmeter. Chart recordings may be secured by using a self-balancing potentiometer system. The linearity of this latter device is dependent only on the thermocouple and potentiometer; it is independent of the other circuitry.

Thermocouples have the following advantages: fast response time (time constant as small as 1 ms), small size (down to 12 μm diameter), ease of fabrication, and long-term stability. Their disadvantages are small output voltage, low sensitivity, and the need for a reference temperature.

Numerous examples of the use of thermocouples in biomedical research are given in the literature (Wren, 2006). Thermocouples can be made small in size, so they can be inserted into catheters and hypodermic needles.

## 2.9 THERMISTORS

Thermistors are semiconductors made of ceramic materials that are thermal resistors with a high negative temperature coefficient. These materials react to temperature changes in a way that is opposite to the way metals react to such changes. The resistance of thermistors decreases as temperature increases and increases as temperature decreases (Melo, 2006).

Sapoff (1971) reviewed the various types of thermistors that have been found to be most suitable for biomedical use. The resistivity of thermistor semiconductors used for biomedical applications is between 0.1 and 100 Ω·m.

These devices are small in size (they can be made less than 0.5 mm in diameter), have a relatively large sensitivity to temperature changes (−3 to −5%/°C), and have excellent long-term stability characteristics (±0.2% of nominal resistance value per year).

Figure 2.15(a) shows a typical family of resistance-versus-temperature characteristics of thermistors. These properties are measured for the

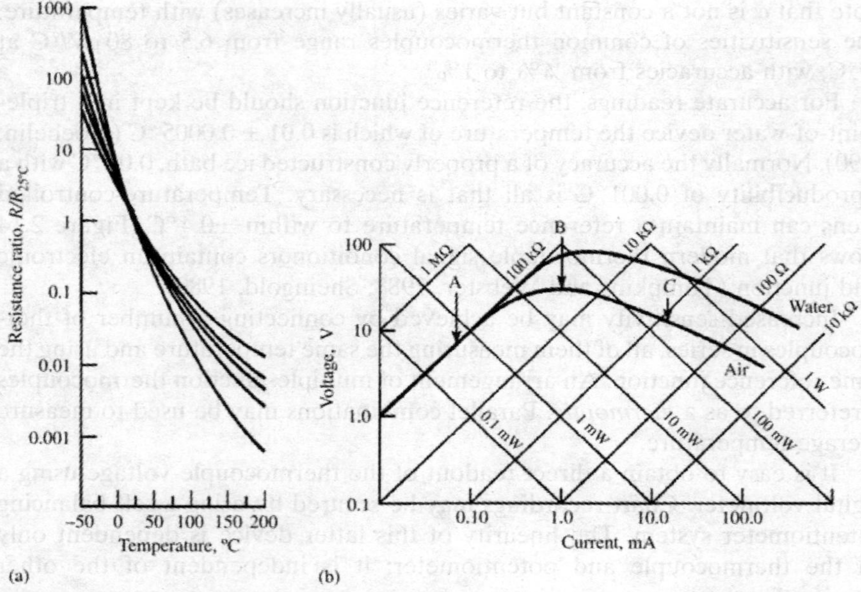


**Figure 2.15** (a) Typical thermistor zero-power resistance ratio–temperature characteristics for various materials. (b) Thermistor voltage-versus-current characteristic for a thermistor in air and water. The diagonal lines with a positive slope give linear resistance values and show the degree of thermistor linearity at low currents. The intersection of the thermistor curves and the diagonal lines with negative slope give the device power dissipation. Point *A* is the maximal current value for no appreciable self-heat. Point *B* is the peak voltage. Point *C* is the maximal safe continuous current in air. [Part (b) is from *Thermistor Manual*, EMC-6, © 1974, Fenwal Electronics, Framingham, MA. Used by permission.]

thermistor operated at a very small amount of power such that there is negligible self-heating. This resistance is commonly referred to as *zero-power resistance*. The empirical relationship between the thermistor resistance $R_t$ and absolute temperature $T$ in kelvin (K) (the SI unit *kelvin* does not use a degree sign) is

$$R_t = R_0 e^{[\beta(T_0 - T)/TT_0]} \tag{2.23}$$

where

$\beta$ = material constant for thermistor, K

$T_0$ = standard reference temperature, K

The value of $\beta$ increases slightly with temperature. However, this does not present a problem over the limited temperature spans for biomedical work (10 °C to 20 °C). $\beta$, also known as the characteristic temperature, is in the range of 2500 to 5000 K. It is usually about 4000 K.

The temperature coefficient $\alpha$ can be found by differentiating (2.23) with respect to $T$ and dividing by $R_t$. Thus

$$\alpha = \frac{1}{R_t}\frac{dR_1}{dT} = -\frac{\beta}{T^2}(\%/\mathrm{K}) \tag{2.24}$$

Note from (2.24) that $\alpha$ is a nonlinear function of temperature. This nonlinearity is also reflected in Figure 2.15(a).

The voltage-versus-current characteristics of thermistors, as shown in Figure 2.15(b), are linear up to the point at which self-heating becomes a problem. When there is large self-heating, the thermistor voltage drop decreases as the current increases. This portion of the curve displays a negative-resistance characteristic.

In the linear portion, Ohm's law applies and the current is directly proportional to the applied voltage. The temperature of the thermistor is that of its surroundings. However, at higher currents a point is reached, because of increased current flow, at which the heat generated in the thermistor raises the temperature of the thermistor above ambient. At the peak of the $v$–$i$ characteristic, the incremental resistance is zero, and for higher currents a negative-resistance relationship occurs. Operations in this region render the device vulnerable to thermal destruction.

Figure 2.15(b) shows the difference in the self-heat regions for a thermistor in water and air due to the differences in thermal resistance of air and water. The principle of variation in thermal resistance can be used to measure blood velocity, as described in Section 8.5.

**EXAMPLE 2.4** Sketch typical thermistor $v$–$i$ characteristics with and without a heat sink. Explain why there is a difference.

**ANSWER** Figure 2.15(b) shows typical thermistor $v$–$i$ characteristics in water and air. For low currents Ohm's law applies, and the current is directly proportional to the applied voltage in both cases. The thermistor temperature is close to ambient. The system with water can reach higher current levels and still remain in a linear portion of the $v$–$i$ curve since the water keeps the thermistor close to ambient temperature. Eventually the thermistor-water combination will self-heat and a negative-resistance relationship will result. In the same manner, the heat sink keeps the thermistor temperature close to ambient at higher current levels and yields characteristics similar to Figure 2.15(b).

**EXAMPLE 2.5** For a thermistor assume self-heating $< 0.1\,^{\circ}\mathrm{C}$, voltage $= 5\,\mathrm{V}$, dissipation coefficient (DC) $= 2.0\,\mathrm{mW}/^{\circ}\mathrm{C}$. Calculate minimum thermistor resistance.

**ANSWER**

$$\Delta T = \frac{P}{\mathrm{D.C.}} = \frac{V^2/R}{\mathrm{D.C.}}$$

$$R = \frac{V^2}{\Delta T(\mathrm{D.C.})} = \frac{5^2}{0.1\,^{\circ}\mathrm{C}(0.002\,\mathrm{W}/^{\circ}\mathrm{C})} = 125,000\ \Omega$$

Choose next larger available size $= 500,000\,\Omega$

The current–time characteristics of a thermistor are important in any dynamic analysis of the system. When a step change in voltage is applied to a series circuit consisting of a resistor and a thermistor, a current flows. The time delay for the current to reach its maximal value is a function of the voltage applied, the mass of the thermistor, and the value of the series-circuit resistance. Time delays from milliseconds to several minutes are possible with thermistor circuits. Similar time delays occur when the temperature surrounding the thermistor is changed in a step fashion.

Various circuit schemes for linearizing the resistance-versus-temperature characteristics of thermistors have been proposed (Cobbold, 1974; Doebelin, 1990). Modern instruments use microcomputers to correct for nonlinearities, rather than the former circuit schemes.

The circuitry used for thermistor readout is essentially the same as for conductive sensors, and many of the same techniques apply. Bridge circuits give high sensitivity and good accuracy. The bridge circuit shown in Figure 2.2(b) could be used with $R_3 = R_t$ and $R_4 =$ the thermistor resistance at the midscale value.

Very small differences in temperature can be found using a differential-temperature bridge. It is often necessary to measure such minute differences in biological work. An example is the need to determine the temperature difference between two organs or between multiple sites in the same organ.

A dc differential bridge can achieve a linearity of better than 1% of full-scale output when bead thermistors matched to within ±1% of each other at 25 °C are used. The dc stability of this bridge is not normally a problem, because the output voltage of the bridge—even for temperature differences of 0.01%—is larger than the dc drift of good integrated-circuit operational amplifiers (Cobbold, 1974).

Operational-amplifier circuits may be used to measure the current in a thermistor as a function of temperature. In essence, this circuit applies a constant voltage to the thermistor and monitors its current with a current-to-voltage converter.

Various shapes of thermistors are available: beads, chips, rods, and washers (Sapoff, 1971). The glass-encapsulated bead thermistor is the one most commonly used in biomedical applications. The glass coating protects the sensing element from the hostile environment of the body without significantly affecting the thermal response time of the system. The small size of these thermistors makes possible their placement at the tip of catheters or hypodermic needles. The thermodilution-catheter system discussed in Section 8.2 employs a four-lumen catheter with a thermistor located near the catheter tip.

An additional application of thermistors is in the clinical measurement of oral temperature. Thermistor probes with disposable sheaths are presently used, but these exhibit a first-order step response as shown in Figure 1.6(c). To yield the oral temperature prior to stabilization, a fixed correction of about 1 °C is added to the probe temperature when the rate of change of probe temperature decreases below 0.1 °C/s.

A problem with thermistor neonatal skin surface temperature-monitoring instruments is that the probes fall off. Thermal contact with the skin can be monitored by applying a 14 s pulse every 4.5 min and monitoring the resultant temperature rise (Re and Neuman, 1991).

## 2.10 RADIATION THERMOMETRY

The basis of *radiation thermometry* is that there is a known relationship between the surface temperature of an object and its radiant power. This principle makes it possible to measure the temperature of a body without physical contact with it. Medical thermography is a technique whereby the temperature distribution of the body is mapped with a sensitivity of a few tenths of a kelvin. It is based on the recognition that skin temperature can vary from place to place depending on the cellular or circulatory processes occurring at each location in the body. Thermography has been used for the early detection of breast cancer, but the method is controversial. It has also been used for determining the location and extent of arthritic disturbances, for gauging the depth of tissue destruction from frostbite and burns, and for detecting various peripheral circulatory disorders (venous thrombosis, carotid artery occlusions, and so forth) (Qi, 2006). Here we shall deal with the basic principles of thermal radiation and detector systems.

Every body that is above absolute zero radiates electromagnetic power, the amount being dependent on the body's temperature and physical properties. For objects at room temperature, the spectrum is predominantly in the far- and extreme-far-infrared regions.

A blackbody is an ideal thermal radiator; as such, it absorbs all incident radiation and emits the maximal possible thermal radiation. The radiation emitted from a body is given by Planck's law multiplied by emissivity $\varepsilon$. This expression relates the radiant flux per unit area per unit wavelength $W_\lambda$ at a wavelength $\lambda$ (μm) and is stated as

$$W_\lambda = \frac{\varepsilon C_1}{\lambda^5 (e^{C_2/\lambda T} - 1)} \quad (\text{W/cm}^2 \cdot \mu\text{m}) \tag{2.25}$$

where

$C_1 = 3.74 \times 100 \ (\text{W} \cdot \mu\text{m}^4/\text{cm}^2)$

$C_2 = 1.44 \times 10^4 \quad (\mu\text{m} \cdot \text{K})$

$T$ = blackbody temperature, K

$\varepsilon$ = emissivity, the extent by which a surface deviates from a blackbody ($\varepsilon = 1$)

Figure 2.16(a) shows a plot of (2.25), the spectral radiant emittance versus wavelength for a blackbody at 300 K.

Wien's displacement law gives the wavelength $\lambda_m$ for which $W_\lambda$ is a maximum. It can simply be found by differentiating (2.25) and setting this to zero.

$$\lambda_m = \frac{2898}{T} \quad (\mu\text{m}) \tag{2.26}$$

Figure 2.16(a) indicates $\lambda_m = 9.66\ \mu\text{m}$ ($T = 300$ K). Note from (2.25) that the maximal level of spectral emittance increases with $T$, and from (2.26) that $\lambda_m$ is inversely related to $T$.

The total radiant power $W_t$, can be found by integrating the area under the curve. This expression is known as the *Stefan–Boltzmann law*.

$$W_t = \varepsilon \sigma T^4 \quad (\text{W/cm}^2) \tag{2.27}$$

where $\sigma$ is the Stefan–Boltzmann constant (see Appendix).

It is of interest to examine how the percentage of total radiant power varies with wavelength for room-temperature objects. This parameter, plotted in Figure 2.14(a), is found by dividing $\int_0^\lambda W_\lambda d\lambda$ by the total radiant power $W_t$ (2.27). Note that approximately 80% of the total radiant power is found in the wavelength band from 4 to 25 μm.

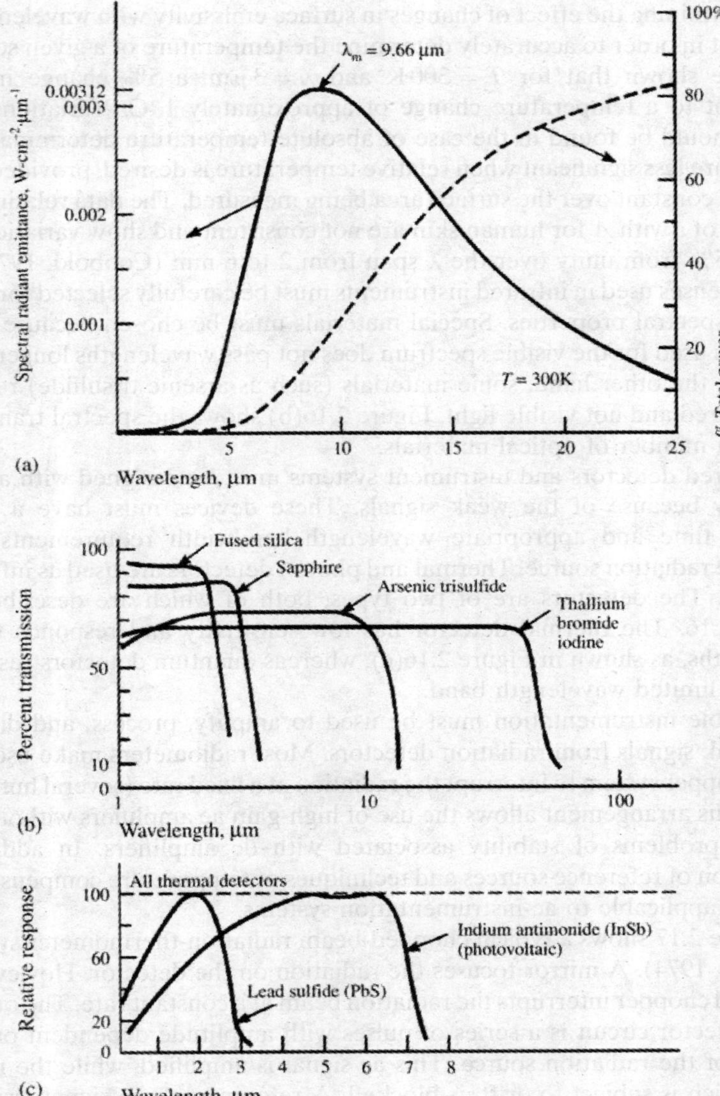


**Figure 2.16** (a) Spectral radiant emittance versus wavelength for a blackbody at 300 K on the left vertical axis; percentage of total energy on the right vertical axis. (b) Spectral transmission for a number of optical materials. (c) Spectral sensitivity of photon and thermal detectors. [Part (a) is from *Transducers for Biomedical Measurements: Principles and Applications*, R. S. C. Cobbold. Copyright © 1974, John Wiley & Sons, Inc. Reprinted by permission of John Wiley & Sons, Inc. Parts (b) and (c) are from *Measurement Systems: Application and Design*, E. O. Doebelin. Copyright © 1990 by McGraw-Hill, Inc. Used with permission of McGraw-Hill Book Co.]

Determining the effect of changes in surface emissivity with wavelength is important in order to accurately determine the temperature of a given source. It can be shown that for $T = 300\,\text{K}$ and $\lambda = 3\,\mu\text{m}$, a 5% change in $\varepsilon$ is equivalent to a temperature change of approximately $1\,^\circ\text{C}$. Variations in $\varepsilon$ with $A$ should be found in the case of absolute-temperature determinations, but they are less significant when relative temperature is desired, provided that $\varepsilon$ remains constant over the surface area being measured. The data relating the variation of $\varepsilon$ with $A$ for human skin are not consistent and show variations as large as 5% from unity over the $\lambda$ span from 2 to 6 mm (Cobbold, 1974).

The lenses used in infrared instruments must be carefully selected for their infrared spectral properties. Special materials must be chosen because standard glass used for the visible spectrum does not pass wavelengths longer than $2\,\mu\text{m}$. On the other hand, some materials (such as arsenic trisulfide) readily pass infrared and not visible light. Figure 2.16(b) shows the spectral transmission for a number of optical materials.

Infrared detectors and instrument systems must be designed with a high sensitivity because of the weak signals. These devices must have a short response time and appropriate wavelength–bandwidth requirements that match the radiation source. Thermal and photon detectors are used as infrared detectors. The detectors are of two types, both of which are described in Section 2.16. The thermal detector has low sensitivity and responds to all wavelengths, as shown in Figure 2.16(c), whereas quantum detectors respond only to a limited wavelength band.

Suitable instrumentation must be used to amplify, process, and display these weak signals from radiation detectors. Most radiometers make use of a beam-chopper system to interrupt the radiation at a fixed rate (several hundred hertz). This arrangement allows the use of high-gain ac amplifiers without the inherent problems of stability associated with dc amplifiers. In addition, comparison of reference sources and techniques of temperature compensation are more applicable to ac-instrumentation systems.

Figure 2.17 shows a typical chopped-beam radiation-thermometer system (Cobbold, 1974). A mirror focuses the radiation on the detector. However, a blackened chopper interrupts the radiation beam at a constant rate. The output of the detector circuit is a series of pulses with amplitude dependent on the strength of the radiation source. This ac signal is amplified, while the mean value, which is subject to drift, is blocked. A reference-phase signal, used to synchronize the phase-sensitive demodulator (Section 3.15), is generated in a special circuit consisting of a light source and detector. The signal is then filtered to provide a dc signal proportional to the target temperature. This signal can then be displayed or recorded. Infrared microscopes have also been designed using these techniques.

Figure 2.18 shows one application of radiation thermometry is an instrument that determines the internal or core body temperature of the human by measuring the magnitude of infrared radiation emitted from the tympanic membrane and surrounding ear canal. The tympanic membrane and hypothalamus are perfused by the same vasculature. The hypothalamus is the

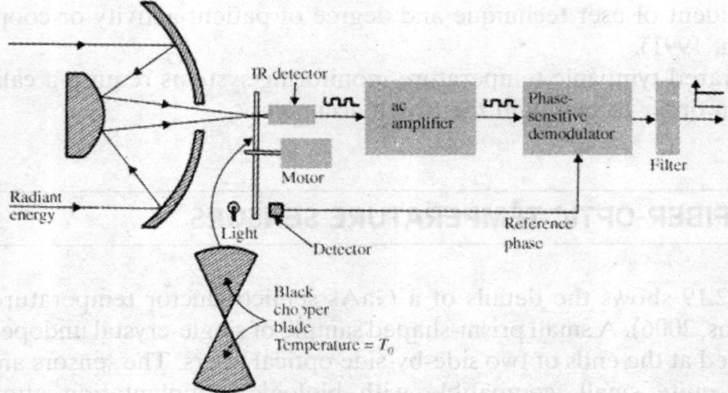


**Figure 2.17** Stationary chopped-beam radiation thermometer (From *Transducers for Biomedical Measurements: Principles and Applications,* by R. S. C. Cobbold. Copyright (c) 1974, John Wiley and Sons, Inc. Reprinted by permission of John Wiley and Sons, Inc.)

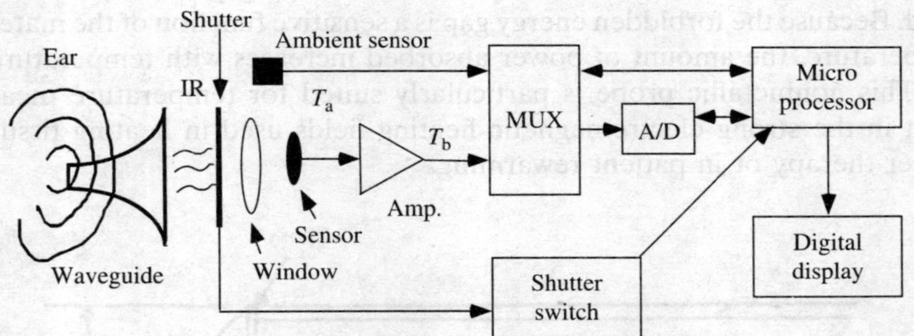


**Figure 2.18** The infrared thermometer opens a shutter to expose the sensor to radiation from the tympanic membrane. [From J. G. Webster (ed.), *Bioinstrumentation*, New York: John Wiley & Sons, 2004.]

body's main thermostat, which regulates the core body temperature. This approach has advantages over using mercury thermometers, thermocouples, or thermistors. The standard temperature-measuring techniques measure the temperature of the sensor, not that of the subject. The sensor must be in contact with the patient long enough for its temperature to become the same as, or close to, that of the subject whose temperature is being measured. However, the infrared thermometry device detects emitted energy that is proportional to the actual temperature of the subject. There is negligible thermal time constant for the pyroelectric sensor (Fraden, 1997). The infrared tympanic temperature-monitoring system has a response time in the order of 0.1 s and an accuracy of approximately 0.1 °C. A disposable sanitary probe cover is used to prevent cross-contamination from patient to patient. Ear thermometry offers several clinical benefits over taking sublingual (oral) or rectal measurements. Response is rapid, and readings can be obtained independent of user technique and degree of patient activity or cooperation (Fraden, 1991).

Infrared tympanic temperature-monitoring systems require a calibration target in order to maintain their high accuracy.

## 2.11 FIBER-OPTIC TEMPERATURE SENSORS

Figure 2.19 shows the details of a GaAs semiconductor temperature probe (Samaras, 2006). A small prism-shaped sample of single-crystal undoped GaAs is epoxied at the ends of two side-by-side optical fibers. The sensors and fibers can be quite small, compatible with biological implantation after being sheathed. One fiber transmits light from a light-emitting diode source to the sensor, where it is passed through the GaAs and collected by the other fiber for detection in the readout instrument. Some of the optical power traveling through the semiconductor is absorbed, by the process of raising valence-band electrons, across the forbidden energy gap into the conduction band. Because the forbidden energy gap is a sensitive function of the material's temperature, the amount of power absorbed increases with temperature.

This nonmetallic probe is particularly suited for temperature measurement in the strong electromagnetic heating fields used in heating tissue for cancer therapy or in patient rewarming.

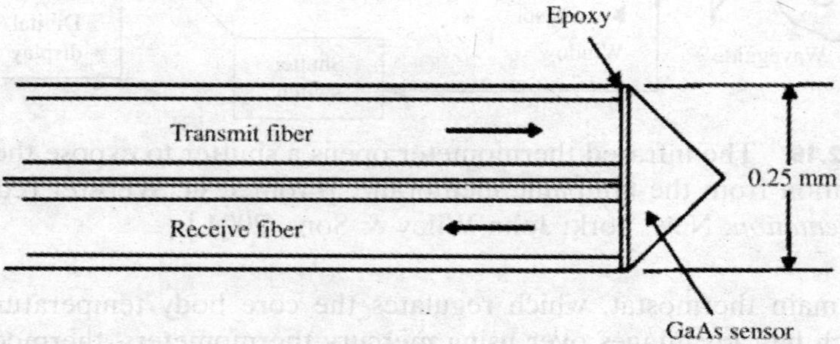


**Figure 2.19** Details of the fiber-sensor arrangement for the GaAs semiconductor temperature probe.

## 2.12 OPTICAL MEASUREMENTS

Optical systems are widely used in medical diagnosis. The most common use occurs in the clinical-chemistry lab, in which technicians analyze samples of blood and other tissues removed from the body. Optical instruments are also used during cardiac catheterization to measure the oxygen saturation of hemoglobin and to measure cardiac output.

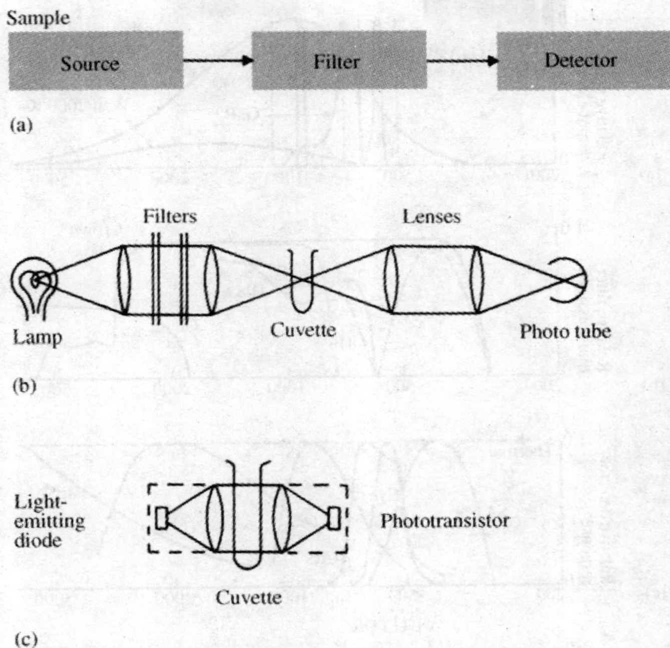


**Figure 2.20** (a) General block diagram of an optical instrument. (b) Highest efficiency is obtained by using an intense lamp and lenses to gather and focus the light on the sample in the cuvette, and a sensitive detector. (c) Solid-state lamps and detectors may simplify the system.

Figure 2.20(a) shows that the usual optical instrument has a source, filter, and detector. Figure 2.20(b) shows a common arrangement of components. Figure 2.20(c) shows that in some cases, the function of source, filter, sample, and detector may be accomplished by solid-state components.

The remainder of this chapter is divided into sections that deal with sources, geometrical optics, filters, detectors, and combinations thereof.

## 2.13 RADIATION SOURCES

### TUNGSTEN LAMPS

Incandescent tungsten-wire filament lamps are the most commonly used sources of radiation. Their radiant output varies with temperature and wavelength, as given by (2.25). For $\lambda < 1\ \mu m$, tungsten has an emissivity of about 0.4 and thus emits about 40% of what it would if the emissivity were 1.0. The relative-output spectrum shown in Figure 2.21(a) is only slightly altered. For higher temperatures, $\lambda_m$, the maximal wavelength of the radiant-output

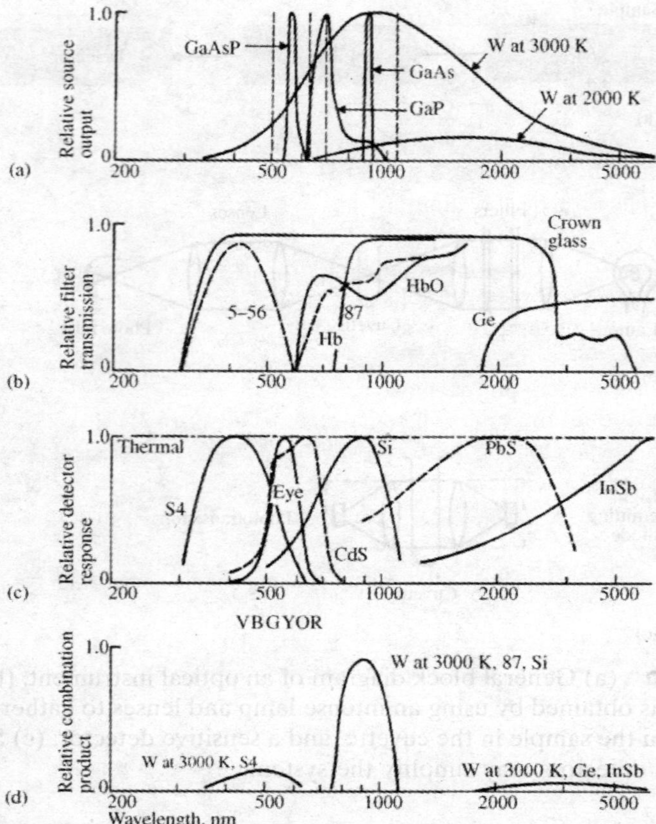


**Figure 2.21 Spectral characteristics of sources, filters, detectors, and combinations thereof** (a) Light sources: tungsten (W) at 3000 K has a broad spectral output. At 2000 K, output is lower at all wavelengths and peak output shifts to longer wavelengths. Light-emitting diodes yield a narrow spectral output with GaAs in the infrared, GaP in the red, and GaAsP in the green. Monochromatic outputs from common lasers are shown by dashed lines: Ar, 515 nm; HeNe, 633 nm; ruby, 693 nm; Nd, 1064 nm; $CO_2$ (not shown), 10,600 nm. (b) Filters: A Corning 5-56 glass filter passes a blue wavelength band. A Kodak 87 gelatin filter passes infrared and blocks visible wavelengths. Germanium lenses pass long wavelengths that cannot be passed by glass. Hemoglobin Hb and oxyhemoglobin HbO pass equally at 805 nm and have maximal difference at 660 nm. (c) Detectors: The S4 response is a typical phototube response. The eye has a relatively narrow response, with colors indicated by VBGYOR. CdS plus a filter has a response that closely matches that of the eye. Si *p–n* junctions are widely used. PbS is a sensitive infrared detector. InSb is useful in far infrared. *Note*: These are only relative responses. Peak responses of different detectors differ by $10^7$. (d) Combination: Indicated curves from (a), (b), and (c) are multiplied at each wavelength to yield (d), which shows how well source, filter, and detector are matched. (e) Photon energy: If it is less than 1 eV, it is too weak to cause current flow in Si *p–n* junctions.

curves, shifts to a shorter wavelength, as given by (2.26) and as shown in Figure 2.21(a).

Low temperatures, then, yield a reddish color (infrared lamps), whereas high temperatures yield a bluish color (photoflood lamps). The total radiation is given by (2.27). Hence the radiant output increases rapidly with temperature, as do the efficiency, the evaporation of tungsten, and the blackening of the glass bulb. The life of the filament is thus drastically shortened by higher temperatures.

Filaments are usually coiled to increase their emissivity and efficiency. For use in instruments, short linear coils may be arranged within a compact, nearly square area lying in a single plane. To produce a source of uniform radiant output over a substantial area, ribbon filaments may be used.

Tungsten–halogen lamps have iodine or bromine added to the gases normally used to fill the bulb. The small quartz bulbs operate at temperatures above 250 °C and usually require cooling by a blower. The halogen combines with tungsten at the wall. The resulting gas migrates back to the filament, where it decomposes and deposits tungsten on the filament. As a result, these lamps maintain more than 90% of their initial radiant output throughout their life. The radiant output of a conventional lamp, on the other hand, declines as much as 50% over its lifetime.

## ARC DISCHARGES

The fluorescent lamp is filled with a low-pressure Ar–Hg mixture. Electrons are accelerated and collide with the gas atoms, which are raised to an excited level. As a given atom's electron undergoes a transition from a higher level to a lower level, the atom emits a quantum of energy. The energy per quantum $E = hv = hc/\lambda$, where $h$ = Planck's constant, $v$ = frequency, $c$ = velocity of light, and $\lambda$ = wavelength.

Because the strongest transition of the mercury atom corresponds to about 5 eV, Figure 2.21(e) shows the resulting wavelength to be about 250 nm. A phosphor on the inside of the glass bulb absorbs this ultraviolet radiation and emits light of longer, visible wavelengths. The fluorescent lamp has low radiant output per unit area, so it is not used in optical instruments. However, it can be rapidly turned on and off in about 20 μs, so it is used in the *tachistoscope* (which presents brief stimuli to the eye) used in measurements of visual perception. Other low-pressure discharge lamps include the glow lamp (such as the neon lamp), the sodium-vapor lamp, and the laser.

High-pressure discharge lamps are more important for optical instruments because the arc is compact and the radiant output per unit area is high. The carbon arc has been in use for the longest time, but it has largely been replaced by the mercury lamp (bluish-green color), the sodium lamp (yellow color), and the xenon lamp (white color). These lamps usually have a clear quartz bulb with electrodes at both ends of the spherical bulb. The zirconium arc lamp provides an intense point source.

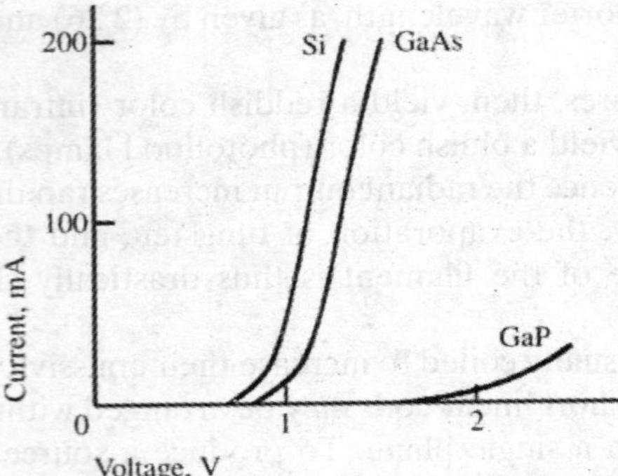


**Figure 2.22** Forward characteristics for *p–n* junctions. Ordinary silicon diodes have a band gap of 1.1 eV and are inefficient radiators in the near-infrared range. GaAs has a band gap of 1.44 eV and radiates at 900 nm. GaP has a band gap of 2.26 eV and radiates at 700 nm.

## LIGHT-EMITTING DIODES (LEDS)

Light-emitting diodes are *p–n* junction devices that are optimized for radiant output. The ordinary silicon *p–n* junction characteristic shown in Figure 2.22 emits radiant power when a current (typically 20 mA) passes in the forward direction. Spontaneous recombination of injected hole and electron pairs results in the emission of radiation. Because the silicon band gap is 1.1 eV, the wavelength is at about 1100 nm. The silicon device is not efficient. However, GaAs has a slightly higher band gap, as shown in Figure 2.22, and therefore radiates at 900 nm, as shown in Figure 2.21(a). Although the output is not visible, the efficiency is high and the GaAs device is widely used. It can be switched in less than 10 ns.

Figure 2.21(c) and Figure 2.21(e) show that, in order to produce visible light, the band gap of a *p–n* junction must exceed 1.9 eV. The GaP LED in Figure 2.22 has a band gap of 2.26 eV, requires a larger forward-bias voltage than silicon diodes, and is electroluminescent at 700 nm, as shown in Figure 2.21(a). It is an efficient visible LED and produces a bright red light. The GaAsP LEDs make use of a special phosphor that absorbs two photons at one wavelength and emits a single photon at a shorter wavelength. The GaAs is Si doped to emit radiation at 940 nm. Power at this wavelength is absorbed by the phosphor coating that emits green light at 540 nm, as shown in Figure 2.21(a). The decay time of the phosphor is about 1 ms.

Light-emitting diodes are compact, rugged, economical, and nearly monochromatic. They are widely used in a variety of medical, transportation, and industrial circuits. A variety of circuits are available for LEDs and photodetectors using either steady or modulated radiation.

## LASERS

*Laser* (light amplification by stimulated emission of radiation) action can occur in GaAs. The end faces that are perpendicular to the *p–n* junction are polished to serve as partial mirrors, thus forming a resonant optical cavity. The forward current pumps a large population of the molecules to an excited energy level. Radiation incident on the molecules causes the production of additional radiation that is identical in character. This phenomenon, known as *stimulated emission*, is produced by the feedback from the mirrors. Laser output is highly monochromatic, collimated (parallel), and phase coherent. However, *p–n* junction lasers are not widely used because they operate in the infrared and require current densities of $10^3$ A/cm$^2$ or more, thus necessitating pulsed (10–100 ns) operation rather than continuous wave (CW).

The most common laser is the He–Ne laser that operates at 633 nm in the red region, as shown in Figure 2.21(a). The laser is operated by a low-pressure arc similar to a neon sign and provides up to 100 mW. Partially reflective mirrors at each end provide the resonant optical cavity and laser action.

Argon lasers provide the highest continuous-power levels (1–15 W) in the visible part of the spectrum at 515 nm [Figure 2.21(a)]. This high-power output permits photocoagulation of blood vessels in the eyes of patients suffering from diabetic retinopathy.

$CO_2$ lasers provide 50–500 W of CW output power and are used for cutting plastics, rubber, and metals up to 1 cm thick.

Two solid-state lasers—both usually operated in the pulsed mode—are widely used. The lasers are pumped by firing a flash tube that is wound around them. The ruby laser has a moderate (1 mJ) output in the red region of the spectrum at 693 nm, as shown in Figure 2.21(a). The neodymium in yttrium aluminum garnet (Nd: YAG) laser has a high (2 W/mm$^2$) output in the infrared region at 1064 nm, as shown in Figure 2.21(a).

The most important medical use of the laser has been to mend tears in the retina. A typical photocoagulator uses a pulsed ruby laser with a controllable output. It is focused on a tear in the retina. The heat dissipated by the pulse forms a burn, which, on healing, develops scar tissue that mends the original tear. Section 13.10 provides further information on therapeutic applications of lasers.

Safety to the eye should be considered with respect to some light sources. It is safe to look at a 100 W frosted light bulb for long periods of time. However, looking at clear incandescent lamps, the sun, high-pressure arc sources, or lasers can cause burns on the retina. Protective eyewear worn by the physician to protect against lasers usually consists of a set of filters that attenuate at the specific wavelengths emitted by the laser but transmit as much visible radiation as possible.

## 2.14 GEOMETRICAL AND FIBER OPTICS

### GEOMETRICAL OPTICS

There are a number of geometric factors that modify the power transmitted between the source and the detector. In Figure 2.20(b), the most obvious optical elements are the lenses. The lamp emits radiation in all directions. The first lens should have as small an *f number* (ratio of focal length to diameter) as practical. Thus it collects the largest practical solid angle of radiation from the lamp. The first lens is usually placed one focal length away from the lamp, so that the resulting radiation is *collimated* (that is, the rays are parallel). Thus, for a point source, the second lens can be placed at any distance without losing any radiation. Also, some interference filters operate best in collimated rays.

The second lens focuses the radiation on a small area of sample in the cuvette. Because the radiation now diverges, third and fourth lenses are used to collect all the radiation and focus it on a detector. Some spectrophotometers [Figure 2.20(c)] transmit collimated radiation through the sample section. The lenses can be coated with a coating that is a quarter-wavelength thick to prevent reflective losses at air–glass surfaces. Full mirrors may be used to fold the optical path to produce a compact instrument. Half-silvered mirrors enable users to split the beam into two beams for analysis or to combine two beams for analysis by a single detector. Curved mirrors may function as lenses for wavelengths that are absorbed by normal glass lenses.

Scattered radiation must be prevented from reaching the detector. Internal support structures and mechanical components of optical instruments are internally painted flat black to prevent scattered radiation. Stops (apertures that pass only the desired beam size) may be placed at several locations along the instrument's optical axis to trap scattered radiation.

## FIBER OPTICS

Fiber optics are an efficient way of transmitting radiation from one point to another (Modell and Perelman, 2006). Transparent glass or plastic fiber with a refractive index $n_1$ is coated or surrounded by a second material of a lower refractive index $n_2$. By Snell's law,

$$n_2 \sin \theta_2 = n_1 \sin \theta_1 \tag{2.28}$$

where $\theta$ is the angle of incidence shown in Figure 2.23. Because $n_1 > n_2$, $\sin \theta_2 > \sin \theta_1$, so $\sin \theta_2 = 1.0$ for a value of $\theta_1$ that is less than 90°. For values of $\theta_1$ greater than this, $\sin\ \theta_2$ is greater than unity, which is impossible, and the ray is internally reflected. The critical angle for reflection ($\theta_{ic}$) is found by setting $\sin\ \theta_2 = 1.0$, which gives

$$\sin \theta_{ic} = \frac{n_2}{n_1} \tag{2.29}$$

A ray is internally reflected for all angles of incidence greater than $\theta_{ic}$. Because rays entering the end of a fiber are usually refracted from air ($n = 1.0$) into glass ($n = 1.62$ for one type), a larger cone of radiation ($\theta_3$) is accepted by a fiber than that indicated by calculations using $90° - \theta_{ic}$. Rays entering the end of the fiber at larger angles ($\theta_4$) are not transmitted down the fiber; they escape through the walls.

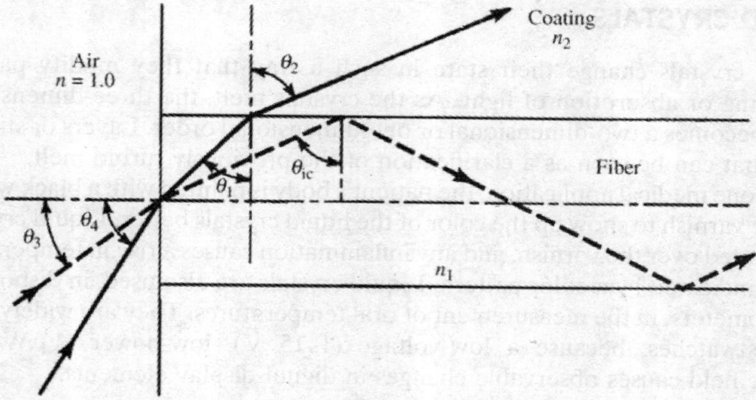


**Figure 2.23 Fiber optics** The solid line shows refraction of rays that escape through the wall of the fiber. The dashed line shows total internal reflection within a fiber.

Fiber-optic (FO) sensors are replacing some conventional sensors for measuring a variety of electrical, electronic, mechanical, pneumatic, and hydraulic variables (Sirohi and Kothiyal, 1991; Udd, 1991). They are chemically inert and have freedom from electromagnetic interference.

A 50 cm glass fiber exhibits a transmission exceeding 60% for wavelengths between 400 and 1200 nm. A 50 cm plastic fiber has a transmission exceeding 70% for wavelengths between 500 and 850 nm. Although a single fiber is useful for sampling incident radiation of a small area, most applications use flexible bundles of about 400 fibers. In *noncoherent bundles* (called *light guides*), the diameter of a fiber is typically 13 to 100 nm. There is no correlation between a fiber's spatial position at the input and at the output. These fibers are useful only for transmitting radiation. In one application, light is transmitted through the flexible bundle for viewing internal organs (Northrop, 2002). In a second application, an instrument that measures blood oxygen saturation within the vessels alternately transmits radiation at two wavelengths down one bundle (Chapter 10). The radiation is backscattered by the red-blood cells and returned to the instrument for analysis through a second bundle.

In *coherent-fiber bundles*, the fibers occupy the same relative position at both end faces. An image at one end is faithfully transmitted to the other end. The most important medical application of these fibers is in the *endoscope* (a tube for examining body cavities through natural openings) (Hooper, 2006). A typical endoscope is 1 m long and 1 cm in diameter and may be used for viewing the lining of the stomach, intestines, and so forth. A noncoherent bundle transmits light for illumination. A small lens focuses the image of the lining onto the end of a coherent bundle, which transmits the image in such a way that it may be viewed or photographed. External levers make it possible to steer the internal end of the optical-fiber device over a 360° range so that the examining physician can look at cavity walls and around corners.

### LIQUID CRYSTALS

Liquid crystals change their state in such a way that they modify passive scattering or absorption of light. As the crystals melt, the three-dimensional order becomes a two-dimensional or one-dimensional order. Layers or strands form that can be seen as a clarification of the previously turbid melt.

In one medical application, the patient's body is painted with a black water-soluble varnish to show up the color of the liquid crystals better. Liquid crystals are painted over the varnish, and any inflammation causes a rise in temperature that is indicated by a color pattern. Liquid crystals are also used, in disposable thermometers, in the measurement of oral temperatures. They are widely used in wristwatches, because a low-voltage (1–15 V), low-power (1 $\mu W/cm^2$) electric field causes observable changes in digital-display elements.

## 2.15 OPTICAL FILTERS

### FILTERS

Filters are frequently inserted in the optical system to control the distribution of radiant power or wavelength. To reduce radiant power only, neutral-density filters are used. When glass is partially silvered, most of the power is reflected, and the desired fraction of the power is transmitted. When carbon particles are suspended in plastic, most of the power is absorbed and the desired fraction of the power is transmitted. Two Polaroid filters may also be used to attenuate the light. Each filter transmits only that portion of the light that is in a particular state of polarization. As one is rotated with respect to the other, the optical transmission of the combination varies.

Color filters transmit certain wavelengths and reject others. Gelatin filters are the most common type of absorption filters. An organic dye is dissolved in an aqueous gelatin solution, and a thin film is dried on a glass substrate. An example shown in Figure 2.21(b) is the infrared Kodak 87 Wratten filter. Glass filters, made by combining additives with the glass itself in its molten state, are extensively used. They provide rather broad passbands, as illustrated by the blue Corning 5-56 filter shown in Figure 2.21(b).

*Interference filters* are formed by depositing a reflective stack of layers on both sides of a thicker spacer layer. This sandwich construction provides multiple reflection and interference effects that yield sharp-edge high, low, and bandpass filters with bandwidths from 0.5 to 200 nm. Interference filters are generally used with collimated radiation and cost more than those just mentioned. Interference coatings are used on dichroic mirrors (cold mirrors), which reflect visible radiation from projection lamps. The nonuseful infrared radiation is transmitted through the coating and mirror to the outside of the optical system. This reduces heat within the optical system without sacrificing the useful light.

*Diffraction gratings* are widely employed to produce a wavelength spectrum in the spectrometer. Plane gratings are formed by cutting thousands of closely spaced parallel grooves in a material. The grating is coated with aluminum, which reflects and disperses white light into a diffraction spectrum. A narrow slit selects a narrow band of wavelengths for use.

Although clear glass is not ordinarily thought of as a filter, Figure 2.21(b) shows that crown glass does not transmit below 300 nm. For instruments that operate in the ultraviolet, fused quartz (silica glass) is used. Most glasses do not transmit well above 2600 nm, so instrument makers use either curved mirrors for infrared instruments or lenses made of Ge, Si, $AsS_3$, $CaF_2$, or $Al_2O_3$.

Conway *et al.* (1984) describe an optical method for measuring the percentage of fat in the body. They found that fat has an absorption band at 930 and that water has an absorption band at 970 nm. From a single-beam rapid-scanning spectrophotometer, they conducted light to and reflected light from five sites on the body through a fiber-optic probe. The method successfully predicted percent body fat in 17 subjects ($r = 0.91$) when compared with the $D_2O$ dilution technique.

## 2.16 RADIATION SENSORS

Radiation sensors may be classified into two general categories: thermal sensors and quantum sensors (Mendelson, 2006).

### THERMAL SENSORS

The *thermal sensor* absorbs radiation and transforms it into heat, thus causing a rise in temperature in the sensors. Typical thermal sensors are the thermistor and the thermocouple. The sensitivity of such a sensor does not change with (is flat with) wavelength, and the sensor has slow response [Figure 2.21(c)]. Changes in output due to changes in ambient temperature cannot be distinguished from changes in output due to the source, so a windmill-shaped mechanical chopper is frequently used to interrupt the radiation from the source periodically.

The *pyroelectric sensor* (Fraden, 1997) absorbs radiation and converts it into heat. The resulting rise in temperature changes the polarization of the crystals, which produces a current proportional to the rate of change of temperature. As it is for the piezoelectric sensor, dc response is zero, so a chopper is required for dc measurements.

### QUANTUM SENSORS

*Quantum sensors* absorb energy from individual photons and use it to release electrons from the sensor material. Typical quantum sensors are the eye, the phototube, the photodiode, and photographic emulsion. Such sensors are sensitive over only a restricted band of wavelengths; most respond rapidly. Changes in ambient temperature cause only a second-order change in sensitivity of these sensors.

## PHOTOEMISSIVE SENSORS

*Photoemissive sensors*—an example is the *phototube*—have photocathodes coated with alkali metals. If the energy of the photons of the incoming radiation is sufficient to overcome the work function of the photocathode, the forces that bind electrons to the photocathode are overcome, and it emits electrons. Electrons are attracted to a more positive anode and form a current that is measured by an external circuit. Photon energies below 1 eV are not large enough to overcome the work function, so wavelengths longer than 1200 nm cannot be detected. Figure 2.21(c) shows the spectral response of the most common photocathode, the S4, which has lower sensitivity in the ultraviolet region because of absorption of radiation in the glass envelope.

The *photomultiplier* shown in Figure 2.24 is a phototube combined with an electron multiplier (Lion, 1975). Each accelerated electron hits the first dynode with enough energy to liberate several electrons by secondary emission. These electrons are accelerated to the second dynode, where the process is repeated, and so on. Time response is less than 10 ns. Photomultipliers are the most sensitive photodetectors. When they are cooled (to prevent electrons from being thermally generated), they can count individual photons. The eye is almost as sensitive; under the most favorable conditions, it can detect six photons arriving in a small area within 100 ms. Photodiodes have replaced photomultipliers in many applications.

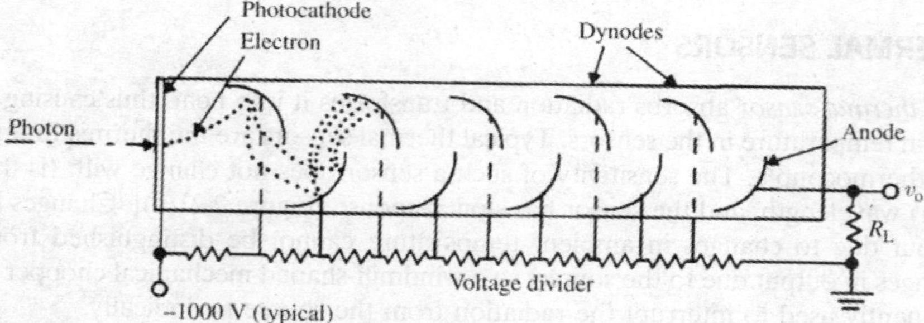


**Figure 2.24 Photomultiplier** An incoming photon strikes the photocathode and liberates an electron. This electron is accelerated toward the first dynode, which is 100 V more positive than the cathode. The impact liberates several electrons by secondary emission. They are accelerated toward the second dynode, which is 100 V more positive than the first dynode. This electron multiplication continues until it reaches the anode, where currents of about 1 μA flow through $R_L$.

## PHOTOCONDUCTIVE CELLS

*Photoresistors* are the simplest solid-state photoelectric sensors. A photosensitive crystalline material such as CdS or PbS [Figure 2.21(c)] is deposited on a ceramic substrate, and ohmic electrodes are attached. If a photon of the incoming radiation has sufficient energy to jump the band gap, hole–electron pairs are produced because the electron is raised from the valence band to the conduction band. The presence of the electrons in the conduction band and of the holes in the valence band increases the conductivity of the crystalline material so that the resistance decreases with input radiation. Photocurrent is linear at low levels of radiation but nonlinear at levels that are normally used. It is independent of the polarity of applied voltage. After a step increase or decrease of radiation, the photocurrent response rises and decays with a time constant of from 10 to 0.01 s, depending on whether the radiation is low or high.

## PHOTOJUNCTION SENSORS

Photojunction sensors are formed from *p–n* junctions and are usually made of silicon. If a photon has sufficient energy to jump the band gap, hole–electron pairs are produced that modify the junction characteristics, as shown in Figure 2.25. If the junction is reverse-biased, the reverse photocurrent flowing from the cathode to the anode increases linearly with an increase in radiation. The resulting photodiode responds in about 1 μs. In phototransistors, the base lead is not connected, and the resulting radiation-generated base current is multiplied by the current gain (beta) of the transistor to yield a large current from collector to emitter. The radiation–current characteristics have a nonlinearity of about 2% because beta varies with collector current. The response time is about 10 μs.

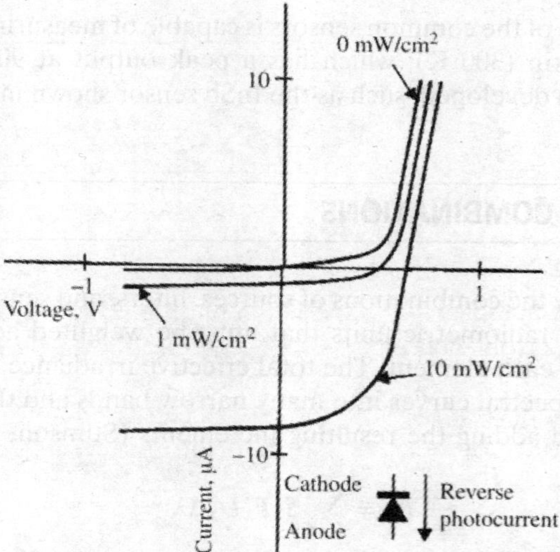


**Figure 2.25 Voltage–current characteristics of irradiated silicon *p–n* junction**
For 0 irradiance, both forward and reverse characteristics are normal. For 1 mW/cm$^2$, open-circuit voltage is 500 mV, and short-circuit current is 0.8 μA. For 10 mW/cm$^2$, open-circuit voltage is 600 mV, and short-circuit current is 8 μA.

Silicon *p–n* junctions are also manufactured as photo Darlington transistors, photo FETs, photo unijunction transistors, and photo silicon-controlled rectifiers (SCRs). Photon couplers are LED–photodiode combinations that are used for isolating electric circuits. For example, they are used for breaking ground loops and for preventing dangerous levels of current from leaking out of equipment and entering the heart of a patient (Section 14.9). Modern photojunction sensors have become so sensitive and with rapid response times so that in many applications they have replaced photomultipliers.

### PHOTOVOLTAIC SENSORS

The same silicon *p–n* junction can be used in the photovoltaic mode. Figure 2.25 shows that there is an open-circuit voltage when the junction receives radiation. The voltage rises logarithmically from 100 to 500 mV as the input radiation increases by a factor of 104. This is the principle of the solar cell that is used for direct conversion of the sun's radiation into electric power.

### SPECTRAL RESPONSE

All of the aforementioned silicon sensors have the spectral response shown in Figure 2.21(c). There is no response above 1100 nm because the energy of the photons is too low to permit them to jump the band gap. For wavelengths shorter than 900 nm, the response drops off because there are fewer, more-energetic photons per watt. Each photon generates only one hole–electron pair.

Because none of the common sensors is capable of measuring the radiation emitted by the skin (300 K), which has a peak output at 9000 nm, special sensors have been developed, such as the InSb sensor shown in Figure 2.21(c).

## 2.17 OPTICAL COMBINATIONS

In order to specify the combinations of sources, filters, and sensors, instrument designers require radiometric units that must be weighted according to the response curve of each element. The total effective irradiance, $E_e$, is found by breaking up the spectral curves into many narrow bands and then multiplying each together and adding the resulting increments (Stimson, 1974). Thus

$$E_e = \sum S_\lambda F_\lambda D_\lambda \Delta\lambda \tag{2.30}$$

where

$S_\lambda$ = relative source output
$F_\lambda$ = relative filter transmission
$D_\lambda$ = relative sensor responsivity

Figure 2.21(d) shows several results of this type of calculation. One of the examples shown is an efficient system capable of making measurements in the dark without stimulating the eye. Such a device can be used for tracking eye movements. It can be formed from a tungsten source, a Kodak 87 Wratten filter, and a silicon sensor. If GaAs provides enough output, it can replace both the tungsten source and the Kodak 87 Wratten filter (Borah, 2006).

## PROBLEMS

**2.1** For Figure P2.1, plot the ratio of the output voltage to the input voltage $v_o/v_i$ as a function of the displacement $x_i$ of a potentiometer with a total displacement $x_t$ for ranges of $R_m$, the input resistance of the meter. Show that the maximal error occurs in the neighborhood of $x_i/x_t = 0.67$. What is the value of this maximal error?

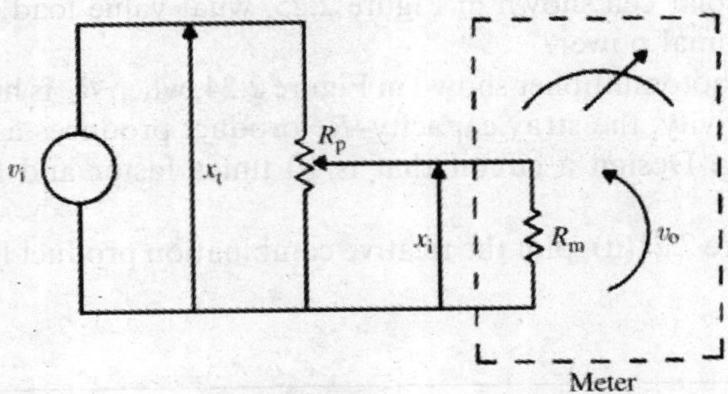


**Figure P2.1**

**2.2** The practical limitation for wire spacing in potentiometer construction is between 20 and 40 turns/mm. Find the resolution limitation for a translational and a rotational potentiometer. Propose a way to increase the resolution of a rotational potentiometer.

**2.3** Discuss some of the possible problems involved in elastic-resistance strain-gage sensors and their solutions.

**2.4** The electromotive force $E$ for a thermocouple is given by (2.21). Calculate and plot $E$ for conditions in which the reference source is at 0 °C and temperature varies from 0 °C to 50 °C. The thermocouple material is copper constantan with $a = 38.7\ \mu\text{V/°C}$ and $b = 0.082\ \mu\text{V/°C}^2$. How significant is the second term in your calculations? Note that these calculated curves are not exactly satisfied in the practical situation. Thus an experimental calibration must be measured over the range of interest.

**2.5** Using the results of Problem 2.4, calculate the sensitivity $\alpha$ at 37 °C for the copper–constantan thermocouple.

**2.6** Calculate the value of the thermistor temperature coefficient $\alpha$ for $T =$ 300 K and $b = 4000$ K.

**2.7** For the LVDT shown in Figure 2.6(c), sketch the voltages c–e, d–e, and c–d as the core is displaced through its normal range.

**2.8** For Example 2.1, what size shunting capacitor should be added to extend the low-corner frequency to 0.05 Hz, as is required to detect pulse waveforms? How is the sensitivity changed?

**2.9** Design a charge amplifier for a piezoelectric sensor that has 500 pF capacitance. It should pass frequencies from 0.05 to 100 Hz so that it can detect carotid pulses, and it should not drift into saturation.

**2.10** Sketch typical thermistor $v$–$i$ characteristics with and without a heat sink. Explain why there is a difference.

**2.11** Calculate and sketch a curve for the radiant output of the skin at 300 K at 2000, 5000, 10,000, and 20,000 nm.

**2.12** Sketch an optical system using curved mirrors instead of lenses that could replace the system shown in Figure 2.20(b).

**2.13** Sketch the circuit for a photo Darlington transistor, which is two cascaded emitter–follower transistors. Estimate its linearity and response time.

**2.14** For the solar cell shown in Figure 2.25, what value load resistor would receive the maximal power?

**2.15** For the photomultiplier shown in Figure 2.24, when $R_L$ is high enough for adequate sensitivity, the stray capacity–$R_L$ product produces a time constant that is too long. Design a circuit that is 10 times faster and has no loss in sensitivity.

**2.16** For Figure 2.21(d), plot the relative combination product for GaP, HbO, CdS.

## REFERENCES


Alihanka, J., K. Vaahtoranta, and S.-E Björkqvist, Apparatus in medicine for the monitoring and/or recording of the body movements of a person on a bed, for instance of a patient. United States Patent 4,320,766, 1982.

Anonymous, *Manual on the Use of Thermocouples in Temperature Measurement.* Publication 470A. Philadelphia: American Society for Testing and Materials, 1974.

Borah, J., "Eye movement, measurement techniques for." In J. G. Webster (ed.), *Encyclopedia of Medical Devices and Instrumentation*, 2nd ed. New York: Wiley, 2006, Vol. 3, pp. 263–286.

Bowman, L., and J. D. Meindl, "Capacitive sensors." In J. G. Webster (ed.), *Encyclopedia of Medical Devices and Instrumentation.* New York: Wiley, 1988, pp. 551–556.

Cobbold, R. S. C, *Transducers for Biomedical Measurements.* New York: John Wiley & Sons, Inc., 1974.

Conway, J. M., K. H. Norris, and C. E. Bodwell, "A new approach for the estimation of body composition: Infrared interactance." *Am. J. Clin. Nutr.*, 1984, 40, 1123–1130.

Dechow, P. C., and Q. Wang, "Strain gages." In J. G. Webster (ed.), *Encyclopedia of Medical Devices and Instrumentation.* 2nd ed. New York: Wiley, 2006, Vol. 6, pp. 282–290.

Doebelin, E. O., *Measurement Systems: Application and Design*, 4th ed. New York: McGraw-Hill, 1990.

Fraden, J., "Noncontact temperature measurements in medicine." In D. L. Wise (ed.), *Bioinstrumentation and Biosensors.* New York: Marcel Dekker, 1991, pp. 511–550.

Fraden, J., *Handbook of Modern Sensors: Physics, Designs, and Applications*. 2nd ed. Woodbury, NY: American Institute of Physics, 1997.

Geddes, L. A., and L. E. Baker, *Principles of Applied Biomedical Instrumentation*, 3rd ed. New York: Wiley, 1989.

Hennig, E. M., "Piezoelectric sensors." In J. G. Webster (ed.), *Encyclopedia of Medical Devices and Instrumentation*. New York: Wiley, 1988, pp. 2310–2319.

Hokanson, D. E., D. S. Sumner, and D. E. Strandness, Jr.. "An electrically calibrated plethysmograph for direct measurement of limb blood flow." *IEEE Trans. Biomed. Eng.*, 1975, BME-22, 25–29.

Hooper, B. A., "Endoscopes." In J. G. Webster (ed.), *Encyclopedia of Medical Devices and Instrumentation*, 2nd ed., New York: Wiley, 2006, Vol. 3, pp. 177–189.

Kesavan, S. K., and N. P. Reddy, "Linear variable differential transformers." In J. G. Webster (ed.), *Encyclopedia of Medical Devices and Instrumentation*. 2nd ed., New York: Wiley, 2006, Vol. 4, pp. 252–257.

Korites, B. J., *Microsensors*. Rockland, MA: Kern International, 1987.

Lawton, R. W., and C. C. Collins, "Calibration of an aortic circumference gauge." *J Appl. Physiol.*, 1959, 14, 465–467.

Li, Y., and X.-L. Su, "Piezoelectric sensors," in J. G. Webster (ed.), *Encyclopedia of Medical Devices and Instrumentation*, 2nd ed., New York: Wiley, 2006, Vol. 5, pp. 359–367.

Lion, K. S., *Elements of Electronic and Electrical Instrumentation*. New York: McGraw-Hill, 1975.

Lion, K. S., *Instrumentation in Scientific Research*. New York: McGraw-Hill, 1959.

Mendelson, Y., "Optical sensors." In J. G. Webster (ed.), *Encyclopedia of Medical Devices and Instrumentation*, 2nd ed. New York: Wiley, 2006, Vol. 5, pp. 160–175.

Melo, P. L., "Thermistors." In J. G. Webster (ed.), *Encyclopedia of Medical Devices and Instrumentation*, 2nd ed. New York: Wiley, 2006, Vol. 6, pp. 320–340.

Modell, M. D., and L. T. Perelman, "Fiber optics in medicine." In J. G. Webster (ed.), *Encyclopedia of Medical Devices and Instrumentation*, 2nd ed. New York: Wiley, 2006, Vol. 3, pp. 301–315.

Northrop, R. B., *Noninvasive Instrumentation and Measurement in Medical Diagnosis*. Boca Raton: CRC Press, 2002.

Nyce, D. S., *Linear Position Sensors Theory and Application*, Hoboken: Wiley, 2004.

Pallás-Areny, R., and J. G. Webster, *Sensors and Signal Conditioning*, 2nd ed. New York: Wiley, 2001.

Patel, A., M. Kothari, J. G. Webster, W. J. Tompkins, and J. J. Wertsch, "A capacitance pressure sensor using a phase-locked loop." *J. Rehabil. Res. Devel.*, 1989, 26(2), 55–62.

Qi, H., "Thermography" In J. G. Webster (ed.), *Encyclopedia of Medical Devices and Instrumentation*, 2nd ed. New York: Wiley, 2006, Vol. 6, pp. 346–355.

Re, T. J., and M. R. Neuman, "Thermal contact-sensing electronic thermometer." *Biomed. Instrum. Technol.*, 1991, 25, 54–59.

Samaras, T., "Thermometry." In J. G. Webster (ed.), *Encyclopedia of Medical Devices and Instrumentation*, 2nd. ed. New York: Wiley, 2006, Vol. 6, pp. 355–362.

Sapoff, M., *Thermistors for Biomedical Use*. Fifth Symposium on Temperature, Proceedings. Washington, DC: Instrument Society of America, 1971, 2109–2121.

Servais, S. B., J. G. Webster, and H. J. Monotoye, "Estimating human energy expenditure using an accelerometer device." *J. Clin. Eng.*, 1984, 9, 159–171.

Sheingold, D. H. (ed.), *Transducer Interfacing Handbook*. Norwood, MA: Analog Devices, Inc., 1980.

Sirohi, R. S., and M. P. Kothiyal, *Optical Components, Systems, and Measurement Techniques*. New York: Marcel Dekker, 1991.

Stimson, A., *Photometry and Radiometry for Engineers*. New York: Wiley, 1974.

Sydenham, P. H., N. H. Hancock, and R. Thorn, *Introduction to Measurement Science and Engineering*, New York; Wiley, 1992.

Togawa, T., "Integrated circuit temperature sensor." In J. G. Webster (ed.), *Encyclopedia of Medical Devices and Instrumentation* 2nd ed. New York: Wiley, 2006, Vol. 4, pp. 157–162.

Togawa, T., T. Tamura, and P. A. Oberg, *Biomedical Transducers and Instruments*. Boca Raton: CRC Press, 1997.

Tompkins, W. J., and J. G. Webster (eds.), *Interfacing Sensors to the IBM PC*. Englewood Cliffs, NJ: Prentice-Hall, 1988.

Tsoukalas, D., S. Chatzandrouroulis, and D. Goustouridis, "Capacitive microsensors for biomedical applications." In J. G. Webster (ed.), *Encyclopedia of Medical Devices and Instrumentation*, 2nd ed. New York: Wiley, 2006, Vol. 2, pp. 1–12.

Udd, E. (ed.), *Fiber Optic Sensors: An Introduction for Engineers and Scientists*. New York: Wiley, 1991.

vanCitters, R. L., "Mutual inductance transducers." In R. F. Rushmer (ed.), *Methods in Medical Research*. Vol. XI. Chicago: Year Book, 1966, 26–30.

Webster, J. G. (ed.), *Tactile Sensors for Robotics and Medicine*. New York: Wiley, 1988.

Wren, J., "Thermocouples." In J. G. Webster (ed.), *Encyclopedia of Medical Devices and Instrumentation*, 2nd ed. New York: Wiley, 2006, Vol. 6, pp. 340–346.

# 3

# AMPLIFIERS AND SIGNAL PROCESSING

John G. Webster

Most bioelectric signals are small and require amplification. Amplifiers are also used for interfacing sensors that sense body motions, temperature, and chemical concentrations. In addition to simple amplification, the amplifier may also modify the signal to produce frequency filtering or nonlinear effects. This chapter emphasizes the *operational amplifier* (op amp), which has revolutionized electronic circuit design. Most circuit design was formerly performed with discrete components, requiring laborious calculations, many components, and large expense. Now a 20-cent op amp, a few resistors, and knowledge of Ohm's law are all that is needed.

## 3.1 IDEAL OP AMPS

An *op amp* is a high-gain dc differential amplifier. It is normally used in circuits that have characteristics determined by external negative-feedback networks.

The best way to approach the design of a circuit that uses op amps is first to assume that the op amp is ideal. After the initial design, the circuit is checked to determine whether the nonideal characteristics of the op amp are important. If they are not, the design is complete; if they are, another design check is made, which may require additional components.

### IDEAL CHARACTERISTICS

Figure 3.1 shows the equivalent circuit for a nonideal op amp. It is a dc differential amplifier, which means that any differential voltage, $v_d = (v_2 - v_1)$, is multiplied by the very high gain $A$ to produce the output voltage $v_o$.

To simplify calculations, we assume the following characteristics for an ideal op amp:

**1.** $A = \infty$ (gain is infinity)
**2.** $v_o = 0$, when $v_1 = v_2$ (no offset voltage)

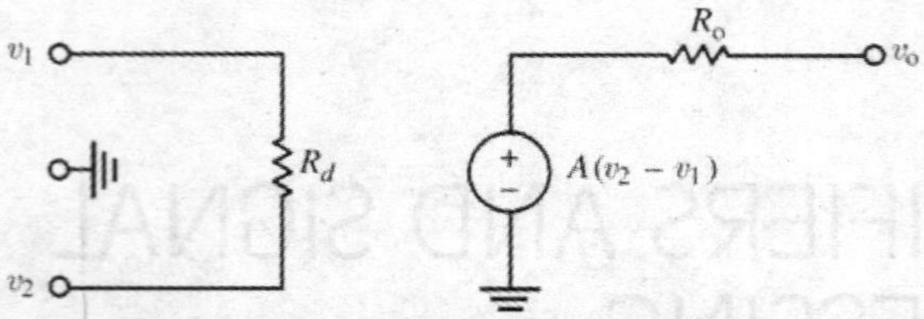


**Figure 3.1 Op-amp equivalent circuit** The two inputs are $v_1$ and $v_2$. A differential voltage between them causes current flow through the differential resistance $R_d$. The differential voltage is multiplied by $A$, the gain of the op amp, to generate the output-voltage source. Any current flowing to the output terminal $v_o$ must pass through the output resistance $R_o$.

3. $R_d = \infty$ (input impedance is infinity)
4. $R_o = 0$ (output impedance is zero)
5. Bandwidth $= \infty$ (no frequency-response limitations) and no phase shift

Later in the chapter we shall examine the effect on the circuit of characteristics that are not ideal.

Figure 3.2 shows the op-amp circuit symbol, which includes two differential input terminals and one output terminal. All these voltages are measured with respect to the ground shown. Power supplies, usually $\pm 15$ V, must be connected to terminals indicated on the manufacturer's specification sheet (Jung, 1986; Horowitz and Hill, 1989).

## TWO BASIC RULES

Throughout this chapter we shall use two basic rules (or input terminal restrictions) that are very helpful in designing op-amp circuits.

**RULE 1** *When the op-amp output is in its linear range, the two input terminals are at the same voltage.*

This is true because if the two input terminals were not at the same voltage, the differential input voltage would be multiplied by the infinite gain to yield an infinite output voltage. This is absurd; most op amps use a power supply of $\pm 15$ V, so $v_o$ is restricted to this range. Actually the op-amp specifications guarantee a

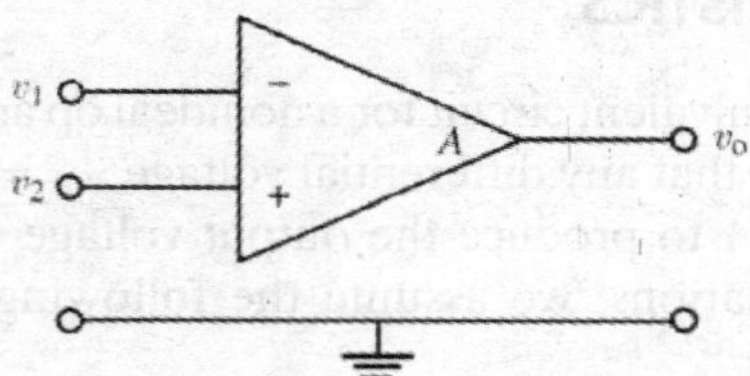


**Figure 3.2 Op-amp circuit symbol** A voltage at $v_1$, the inverting input, is greatly amplified and inverted to yield $v_o$. A voltage at $v_2$, the noninverting input, is greatly amplified to yield an in-phase output at $v_o$.

linear output range of only ±10 V, although some saturate at about ±13 V. A single supply is adequate with some op amps, such as the LM358 (Horowitz and Hill, 1989).

**RULE 2** *No current flows into either input terminal of the op amp.*

This is true because we assume that the input impedance is infinity, and no current flows into an infinite impedance. Even if the input impedance were finite, Rule 1 tells us that there is no voltage drop across $R_d$; so therefore, no current flows.

## 3.2 INVERTING AMPLIFIERS

### CIRCUIT

Figure 3.3(a) shows the basic inverting-amplifier circuit. It is widely used in instrumentation. Note that a portion of $v_o$ is fed back via $R_f$ to the negative input of the op amp. This provides the inverting amplifier with the many advantages associated with the use of negative feedback—increased bandwidth, lower output impedance, and so forth. If $v_o$ is ever fed back to the positive input of the op amp, examine the circuit carefully. Either there is a mistake, or the circuit is one of the rare ones in which a regenerative action is desired.

### EQUATION

Note that the positive input of the op amp is at 0 V. Therefore, by Rule 1, the negative input of the op amp is also at 0 V. Thus no matter what happens to the rest of the circuit, the negative input of the op amp remains at 0 V, a condition known as a *virtual ground.*

Because the right side of $R_i$, is at 0 V and the left side is $v_i$, by Ohm's law the current $i$ through $R_i$, is $i = v_i/R_i$. By Rule 2, no current can enter the op amp; therefore $i$ must also flow through $R_f$. This produces a voltage drop across $R_f$ of $iR_f$. Because the left end of $R_f$ is at 0 V, the right end must be

$$v_o = -iR_f = -v_i\frac{R_f}{R_i} \quad \text{or} \quad \frac{v_o}{v_i} = \frac{-R_f}{R_i} \tag{3.1}$$

Thus the circuit inverts, and the *inverting-amplifier* gain (not the op-amp gain) is given by the ratio of $R_f$ to $R_i$.

### LEVER ANALOGY

Figure 3.3(b) shows an easy way to visualize the circuit's behavior. A lever is formed with arm lengths proportional to resistance values. Because the

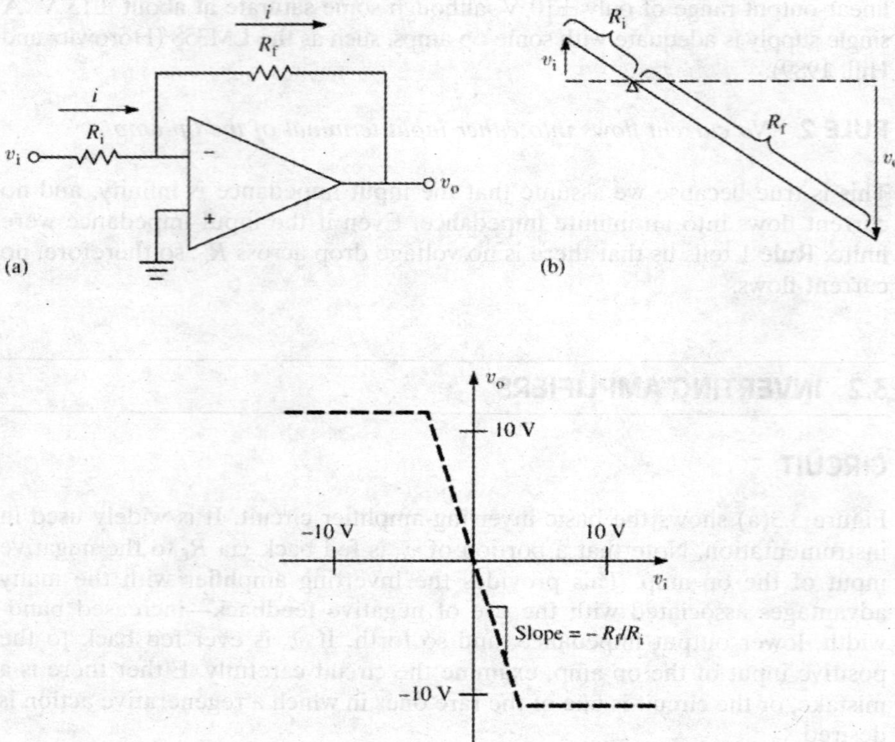


**Figure 3.3** (a) An inverting amplifier. Current flowing through the input resistor $R_i$ also flows through the feedback resistor $R_f$. (b) A lever with arm lengths proportional to resistance values enables the viewer to visualize the input–output characteristics easily. (c) The input–output plot shows a slope of $-R_f/R_i$ in the central portion, but the output saturates at about ±13 V.

negative input is at 0 V, the fulcrum is placed at 0 V, as shown. If $R_f$ is three times $R_i$, as shown, any variation of $v_i$ results in a three-times-bigger variation of $v_o$. The circuit in Figure 3.3(a) is a voltage-controlled current source (VCCS) for any load $R_f$ (Jung, 1986). The current $i$ through $R_f$ is $v_i/R_i$, so $v_i$ controls $i$. Current sources are useful in electrical impedance plethysmography for passing a fixed current through the body (Section 8.7).

## INPUT–OUTPUT CHARACTERISTIC

Figure 3.3(c) shows that the circuit is linear only over a limited range of $v_i$. When $v_o$ exceeds about ±13 V, it *saturates* (limits), and further increases in $v_i$ produce no change in the output. The linear swing of $v_o$ is about 4 V less than the difference in power-supply voltages. Although op amps usually have power-supply voltages set at ±15 V, reduced power-supply voltages may be used, with a corresponding reduction in the saturation voltages and the linear swing of $v_o$.

## SUMMING AMPLIFIER

The inverting amplifier may be extended to form a circuit that yields the weighted sum of several input voltages. Each input voltage $v_{i1}, v_{i2}, \ldots, v_{ik}$ is connected to the negative input of the op amp by an individual resistor the conductance of which $(1/R_{ik})$ is proportional to the desired weighting.

**EXAMPLE 3.1** The output of a biopotential preamplifier that measures the electro-oculogram (EOG) (Section 4.7) is an undesired dc voltage of ±5 V due to electrode half-cell potentials (Section 5.1), with a desired signal of ±1 V superimposed. Design a circuit that will balance the dc voltage to zero and provide a gain of −10 for the desired signal without saturating the op amp.

**ANSWER** Figure E3.1(a) shows the design. We assume that $v_b$, the balancing voltage available from the 5 kΩ potentiometer, is ±10 V. The undesired voltage at $v_i = 5$ V. For $v_o = 0$, the current through $R_f$ is zero. Therefore the sum of the currents through $R_i$ and $R_b$, is zero.

$$\frac{v_i}{R_i} + \frac{v_b}{R_b} = 0$$

$$R_b = \frac{-R_i v_b}{v_i} = \frac{-10^4(-10)}{5} = 2 \times 10^4\ \Omega$$

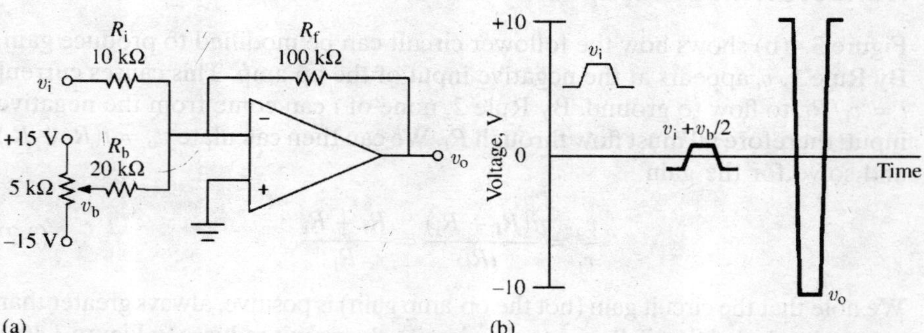


**Figure E3.1** (a) This circuit sums the input voltage $v_i$ plus one-half of the balancing voltage $v_b$. Thus the output voltage $v_o$ can be set to zero even when $v_i$ has a nonzero dc component, (b) The three waveforms show $v_i$, the input voltage; $(v_i + v_b/2)$, the balanced-out voltage; and $v_o$, the amplified output voltage. If $v_i$ were directly amplified, the op amp would saturate.

For a gain of −10, (3.1) requires $R_f/R_i, = 10$, or $R_f, = 100\,\text{k}\Omega$. The circuit equation is

$$v_o = -R_f\left(\frac{v_i}{R_i} + \frac{v_b}{R_b}\right)$$

$$v_o = -10^5\left(\frac{v_i}{10^4} + \frac{v_b}{2\times 10^4}\right)$$

$$v_o = -10\left(v_i + \frac{v_b}{2}\right)$$

The potentiometer can balance out any undesired voltage in the range ±5 V, as shown by Figure E3.1(b). Here we have selected resistors of 10 kΩ to 100 kΩ from the common resistors used in electronic circuits that have values between 10 Ω and 22 MΩ.

## 3.3 NONINVERTING AMPLIFIERS

### FOLLOWER

Figure 3.4(a) shows the circuit for a unity-gain follower. Because $v_i$ exists at the positive input of the op amp, by Rule 1 $v_i$ must also exist at the negative input. But $v_o$ is also connected to the negative input. Therefore $v_o = v_i$, or the output voltage follows the input voltage. At first glance it seems nothing is gained by using this circuit; the output is the same as the input. However, the circuit is very useful as a *buffer*, to prevent a high source resistance from being loaded down by a low-resistance load. By Rule 2, no current flows into the positive input, and therefore the source resistance in the external circuit is not loaded at all.

### NONINVERTING AMPLIFIER

Figure 3.4(b) shows how the follower circuit can be modified to produce gain. By Rule 1, $v_i$ appears at the negative input of the op amp. This causes current $i = v_i/R_i$, to flow to ground. By Rule 2, none of $i$ can come from the negative input; therefore all must flow through $R_f$. We can then calculate $v_o = i(R_f + R_i)$ and solve for the gain.

$$\frac{v_o}{v_i} = \frac{i(R_f + R_i)}{iR_i} = \frac{R_f + R_i}{R_i} \tag{3.2}$$

We note that the circuit gain (not the op-amp gain) is positive, always greater than or equal to 1; and that if $R_i = \infty$ (open circuit), the circuit reduces to Figure 3.4(a).

Figure 3.4(c) shows how a lever makes possible an easy visualization of the input–output characteristics. The fulcrum is placed at the left end, because $R_i$ is grounded at the left end. $v_i$ appears between the two resistors, so it provides an input at the central part of the diagram. $v_o$ travels through an output excursion determined by the lever arms.

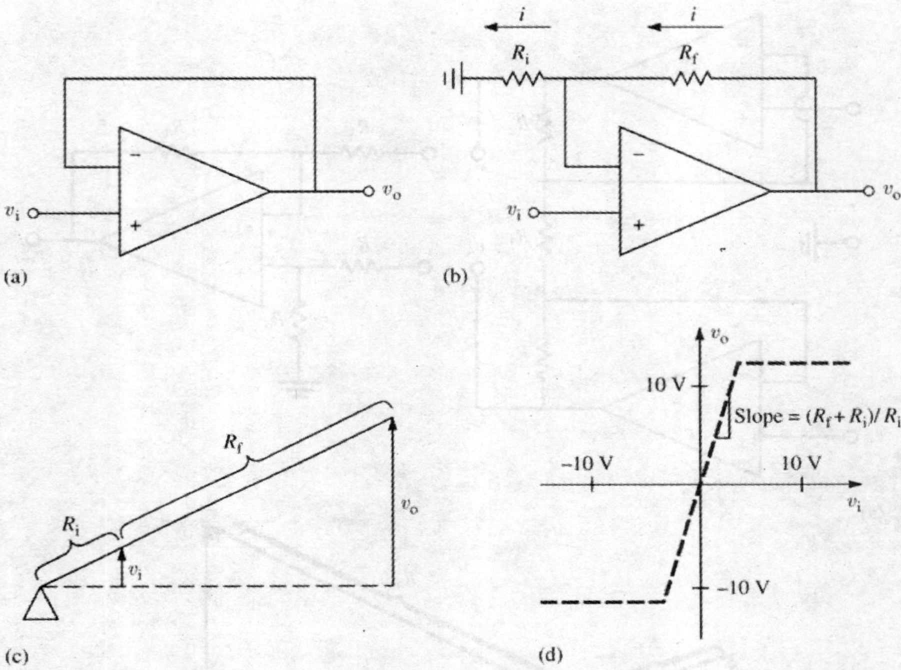


**Figure 3.4** (a) A follower, $v_o = v_i$. (b) A noninverting amplifier, $v_i$ appears across $R_i$, producing a current through $R_i$ that also flows through $R_f$. (c) A lever with arm lengths proportional to resistance values makes possible an easy visualization of input–output characteristics. (d) The input–output plot shows a positive slope of $(R_f + R_i)/R_i$ in the central portion, but the output saturates at about ±13 V.

Figure 3.4(d), the input–output characteristic, shows that a one-op-amp circuit can have a positive amplifier gain. Again saturation is evident.

## 3.4 DIFFERENTIAL AMPLIFIERS

### ONE-OP-AMP DIFFERENTIAL AMPLIFIER

The right side of Figure 3.5(a) shows a simple one-op-amp differential amplifier. Current flows from $v_4$ through $R_3$ and $R_4$ to ground. By Rule 2, no current flows into the positive input of the op amp. Hence $R_3$ and $R_4$, act as a simple voltage-divider attenuator, which is unaffected by having the op amp attached or by any other changes in the circuit. The voltages in this part of the circuit are visualized in Figure 3.5(b) by the single lever that is attached to the fulcrum (ground).

By Rule 1, whatever voltage appears at the positive input also appears at the negative input. Once this voltage is fixed, the top half of the circuit

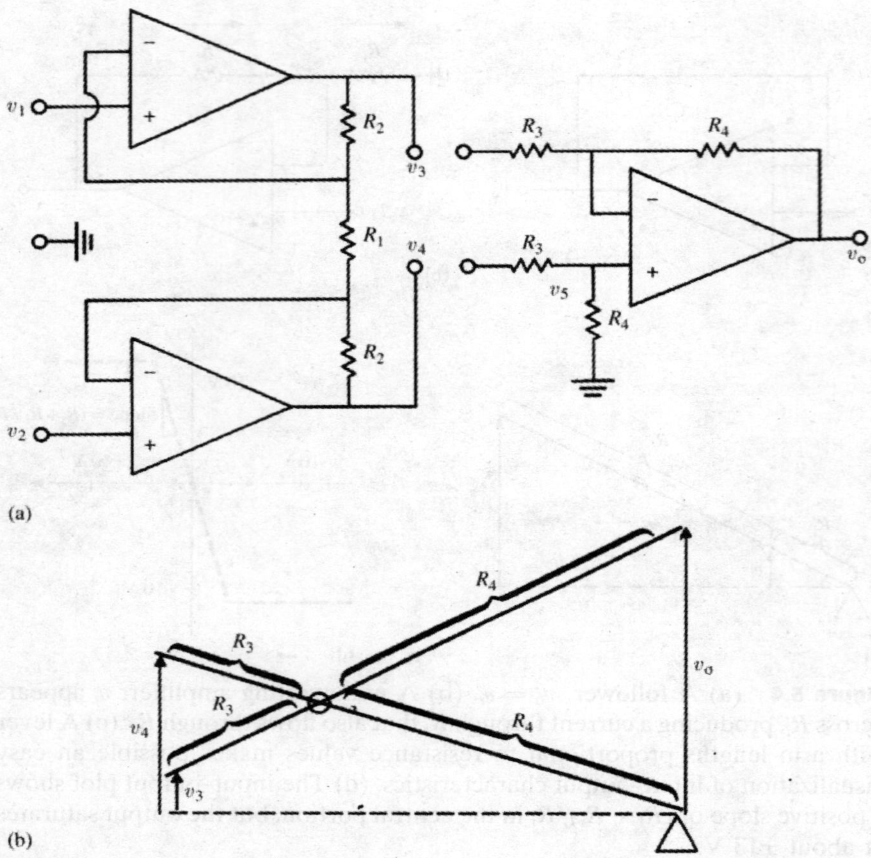


**Figure 3.5** (a) The right side shows a one-op-amp differential amplifier, but it has low input impedance. The left side shows how two additional op amps can provide high input impedance and gain. (b) For the one-op-amp differential amplifier, two levers with arm lengths proportional to resistance values make possible an easy visualization of input–output characteristics.

behaves like an inverting amplifier. For example, if $v_4$ is 0 V, the positive input of the op amp is 0 V and the $v_3$–$v_o$ circuit behaves exactly like an inverting amplifier. For other values of $v_4$, an inverting relation is obtained about some voltage intermediate between $v_4$ and 0 V. The relationship can be visualized in Figure 3.5(b) by noting that the two levers behave like a pair of scissors. The thumb and finger holes are $v_4$ and $v_3$, and the points are at $v_o$ and 0 V.

We solve for the gain by finding $v_5$.

$$v_5 = \frac{v_4 R_4}{R_3 + R_4} \tag{3.3}$$

Then, solving for the current in the top half, we get

$$i = \frac{v_3 - v_5}{R_3} = \frac{v_5 - v_o}{R_4} \tag{3.4}$$

Substituting (3.3) into (3.4) yields

$$v_o = \frac{(v_4 - v_3)R_4}{R_3} \tag{3.5}$$

This is the equation for a differential amplifier. If the two inputs are hooked together and driven by a common source, with respect to ground, then the *common-mode voltage* $v_c$ is $v_3 = v_4$. Equation (3.5) shows that the ideal output is 0. The differential amplifier-circuit (not op-amp) *common-mode gain* $G_c$ is 0. In Figure 3.5(b), imagine the scissors to be closed. No matter how the inputs are varied, $v_o = 0$.

If on the other hand $v_3 \neq v_4$, then the differential voltage $(v_4 - v_3)$ produces an amplifier-circuit (not op-amp) *differential gain* $G_d$ that from (3.5) is equal to $R_4/R_3$. This result can be visualized in Figure 3.5(b) by noting that as the scissors open, $v_o$ is geometrically related to $(v_4 - v_3)$ in the same ratio as the lever arms, $R_4/R_3$.

No differential amplifier perfectly rejects the common-mode voltage. To quantify this imperfection, we use the term *common-mode rejection ratio* (CMRR), which is defined as

$$\text{CMRR} = \frac{G_d}{G_c} \tag{3.6}$$

This factor may be lower than 100 for some oscilloscope differential amplifiers and higher than 10,000 for a high-quality biopotential amplifier.

**EXAMPLE 3.2** A blood-pressure sensor uses a four-active-arm Wheatstone strain gage bridge excited with 5 V dc. At full scale, each arm changes resistance by ±0.3%. Design an amplifier that will provide a full-scale output over the op amp's full range of linear operation. Use the minimal number of components.

**ANSWER** From (2.6), $\Delta v_o = v_i \Delta R/R = 5\,\text{V}(0.003) = 0.015\,\text{V}$. Gain = 20/0.015 = 1333. Assume $R = 120\ \Omega$. Then the Thevenin source impedance = 60 Ω. Use this to replace $R_3$ of Figure 3.5(a) right side. Then $R_4 = R_3(\text{gain}) = 60\ \Omega(1333) = 80\,\text{k}\Omega$.

## THREE-OP-AMP DIFFERENTIAL AMPLIFIER

The one-op-amp differential amplifier is quite satisfactory for low-resistance sources, such as strain-gage Wheatstone bridges (Section 2.3). But the input resistance is too low for high-resistance sources. Our first recourse is to add the simple follower shown in Figure 3.4(a) to each input. This provides the required buffering. Because this solution uses two additional op amps, we can also obtain gain from these buffering amplifiers by using a noninverting amplifier, as shown in Figure 3.4(b). However, this solution amplifies the common-mode voltage, as well as the differential voltage, so there is no improvement in CMRR.

A superior solution is achieved by hooking together the two $R_i$'s of the noninverting amplifiers and eliminating the connection to ground. The result is shown on the left side of Figure 3.5(a). To examine the effects of common-mode voltage, assume that $v_1 = v_2$. By Rule 1, $v_1$, appears at both negative inputs to the op amps. This places the same voltage at both ends of $R_1$. Hence current through $R_1$ is 0. By Rule 2, no current can flow from the op-amp inputs. Hence the current through both $R_2$'s is 0, so $v_1$ appears at both op-amp outputs and the $G_c$ is 1.

To examine the effects when $v_1 \neq v_2$, we note that $v_1 - v_2$ appears across $R_1$. This causes a current to flow through $R_1$ that also flows through the resistor string $R_2$, $R_1$, $R_2$. Hence the output voltage

$$v_3 - v_4 = i(R_2 + R_1 + R_2)$$

whereas the input voltage

$$v_1 - v_2 = iR_1$$

The differential gain is then

$$G_d = \frac{v_3 - v_4}{v_1 - v_2} = \frac{2R_2 + R_1}{R_1} \tag{3.7}$$

Since the $G_c$ is 1, the CMRR is equal to the $G_d$, which is usually much greater than 1. When the left and right halves of Figure 3.5(a) are combined, the resulting three-op-amp amplifier circuit is frequently called an *instrumentation amplifier.* It has high input impedance, a high CMRR, and a gain that can be changed by adjusting $R_1$. This circuit finds wide use in measuring biopotentials (Section 6.7), because it rejects the large 60 Hz common-mode voltage that exists on the body.

## 3.5 COMPARATORS

### SIMPLE

A comparator is a circuit that compares the input voltage with some reference voltage. The comparator's output flips from one saturation limit to the other, as the negative input of the op amp passes through 0 V. For $v_i$ greater than the comparison level, $v_o = -13$ V. For $v_i$ less than the comparison level,

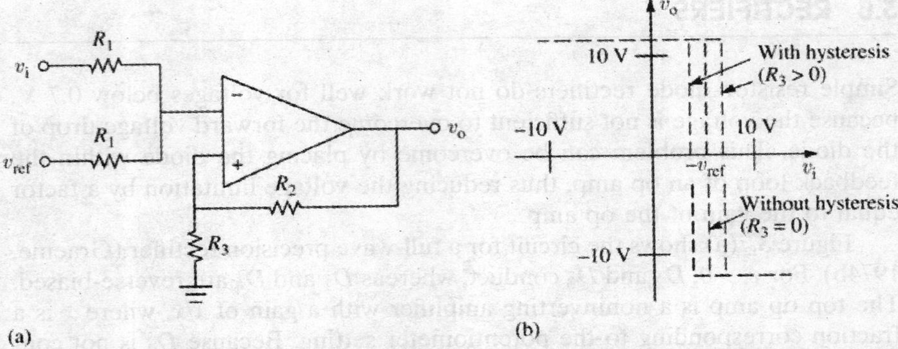


**Figure 3.6** (a) Comparator. When $R_3 = 0$, $v_o$ indicates whether $(v_I + v_{ref})$ is greater or less than 0 V. When $R_3$ is larger, the comparator has hysteresis, as shown in, (b) the input–output characteristic.

$v_o = +13$ V. Thus this circuit performs the same function as a *Schmitt trigger,* which detects an analog voltage level and yields a logic level output. The simplest comparator is the op amp itself, as shown in Figure 3.2. If a reference voltage is connected to the positive input and $v_i$ is connected to the negative input, the circuit is complete. The inputs may be interchanged to invert the output. The input circuit may be expanded by adding the two $R_1$ resistors shown in Figure 3.6(a). This provides a known input resistance for the circuit and minimizes overdriving the op-amp input. Figure 3.6(b) shows that the comparator flips when $v_i = -v_{ref}$. To avoid building a separate power supply for $v_{ref}$, we can connect $v_{ref}$ to the −15 V power supply and adjust the values of the input resistors so that the negative input of the op amp is at 0 V when $v_i$ is at the desired positive comparison level. When negative comparison levels are desired, $v_{ref}$ is connected to the +15 V power supply.

## WITH HYSTERESIS

For a simple comparator, if $v_i$ is at the comparison level and there is noise on $v_i$, then $v_o$ fluctuates wildly. To prevent this, we can add hysteresis to the comparator by adding $R_2$ and $R_3$, as shown in Figure 3.6(a). The effect of this positive feedback is illustrated by the input–output characteristics shown in Figure 3.6(b). To analyze this circuit, first assume that $v_{ref} = -5$ V and $v_i = +10$ V. Then, because the op amp inverts and saturates, $v_o = -13$ V. Divide $v_o$ by $R_2$ and $R_3$ so that the positive input is at, say, −1 V. As $v_i$ is lowered, the comparator does not flip until $v_i$ reaches +3 V, which makes the negative input equal to the positive input, −1 V. At this point, $v_o$ flips to +13 V, causing the positive input to change to +1 V. Noise on $v_i$ cannot cause $v_o$ to flip back, because the negative input must be raised to +1 V to cause the next flip. This requires $v_i$ to be raised to +7 V, at which level the circuit can flip back to its original state. From this example, we see that the width of the hysteresis is four times as great as the magnitude of the voltage across $R_3$. The width of the hysteresis loop can be varied by replacing $R_3$ by a potentiometer.

## 3.6 RECTIFIERS

Simple resistor–diode rectifiers do not work well for voltages below 0.7 V, because the voltage is not sufficient to overcome the forward voltage drop of the diode. This problem can be overcome by placing the diode within the feedback loop of an op amp, thus reducing the voltage limitation by a factor equal to the gain of the op amp.

Figure 3.7(a) shows the circuit for a full-wave precision rectifier (Graeme, 1974b). For $v_i > 0$, $D_2$ and $D_3$ conduct, whereas $D_1$ and $D_4$ are reverse-biased. The top op amp is a noninverting amplifier with a gain of $1/x$, where $x$ is a fraction corresponding to the potentiometer setting. Because $D_4$ is not conducting, the lower op amp does not contribute to the output.

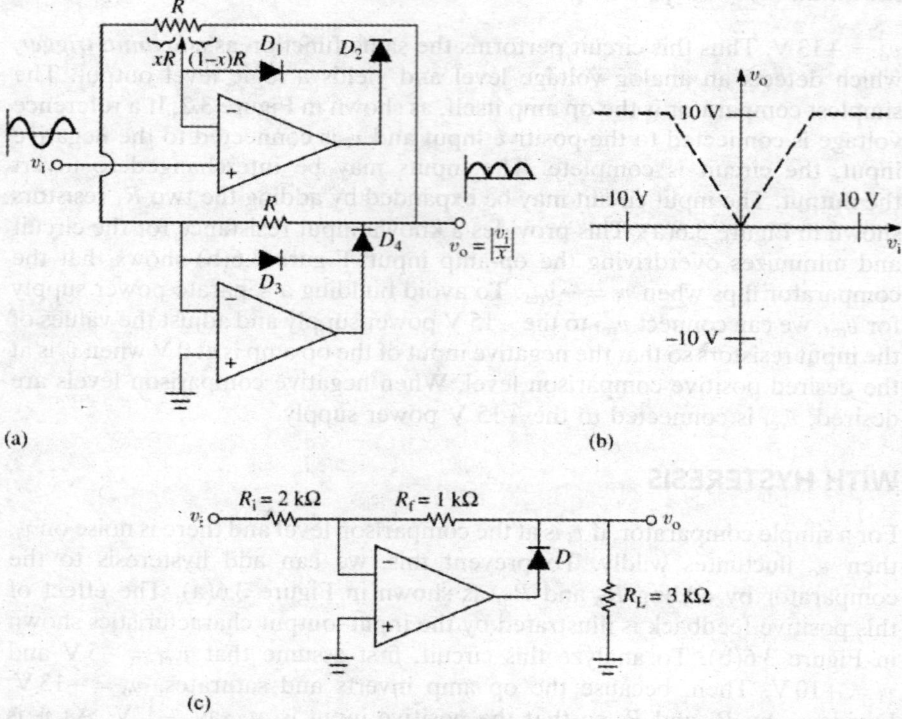


**Figure 3.7** (a) Full-wave precision rectifier. For $v_i > 0$, the noninverting amplifier at the top is active, making $v_o > 0$. For $v_i < 0$, the inverting amplifier at the bottom is active, making $v_o > 0$. Circuit gain may be adjusted with a single pot. (b) Input–output characteristics show saturation when $v_o > +13$ V. (Reprinted with permission from *Electronics* Magazine, copyright © December 12, 1974; Penton Publishing, Inc.) (c) One-op-amp full-wave rectifier. For $v_i < 0$, the circuit behaves like the inverting amplifier rectifier with a gain of +0.5. For $v_i > 0$, the op amp disconnects and the passive resistor chain yields a gain of +0.5.

For $v_i < 0$, $D_1$ and $D_4$ conduct, while $D_2$ and $D_3$ are reverse-biased. At the potentiometer wiper $v_i$ serves as the input to the lower op-amp inverting amplifier, which has a gain of $-1/x$. Because $D_2$ is not conducting, the upper op amp does not contribute to the output. And because the polarity of the gain switches with the polarity of $v_i$, $v_o = |v_i/x|$.

The advantage of this circuit over other full-wave rectifier circuits (Wait, 1975, p. 173) is that the gain can be varied with a single potentiometer and the input resistance is very high. If only a half-wave rectifier is needed, either the noninverting amplifier or the inverting amplifier can be used separately, thus requiring only one op amp. The perfect rectifier is frequently used with an integrator to quantify the amplitude of electromyographic signals (Section 6.8).

Figure 3.7(c) shows a one-op-amp full-wave rectifier (Tompkins and Webster, 1988). Unlike other full-wave rectifiers, it requires the load to remain constant, because the gain is a function of load.

## 3.7 LOGARITHMIC AMPLIFIERS

The logarithmic amplifier makes use of the nonlinear volt–ampere relation of the silicon planar transistor (Jung, 1986).

$$V_{BE} = 0.060 \log\left(\frac{I_C}{I_S}\right) \tag{3.8}$$

where

$V_{BE}$ = base – emitter voltage

$I_C$ = collector current

$I_S$ = reverse saturation current, $10^{-13}$ A at 27 °C

The transistor is placed in the *transdiode* configuration shown in Figure 3.8(a), in which $I_C = v_i/R_i$. Then the output $v_o = V_{BE}$ is logarithmically related to $v_i$ as given by (3.8) over the approximate range $10^{-7}\text{ A} < I_C < 10^{-2}\text{ A}$. The approximate range of $v_o$ is –0.36 to –0.66 V, so larger ranges of $v_o$ are sometimes obtained by the alternate switch position shown in Figure 3.8(a). The resistor network feeds back only a fraction of $v_o$ in order to boost $v_o$ and uses the same principle as that used in the noninverting amplifier. Figure 3.8(b) shows the input–output characteristics for each of these circuits.

Because semiconductors are temperature sensitive, accurate circuits require temperature compensation. Antilog (exponential) circuits are made by interchanging the resistor and semiconductor. These log and antilog circuits are used to multiply a variable, divide it, or raise it to a power; to compress large dynamic ranges into small ones; and to linearize the output of devices with logarithmic o exponential input-output relations. In the photometer

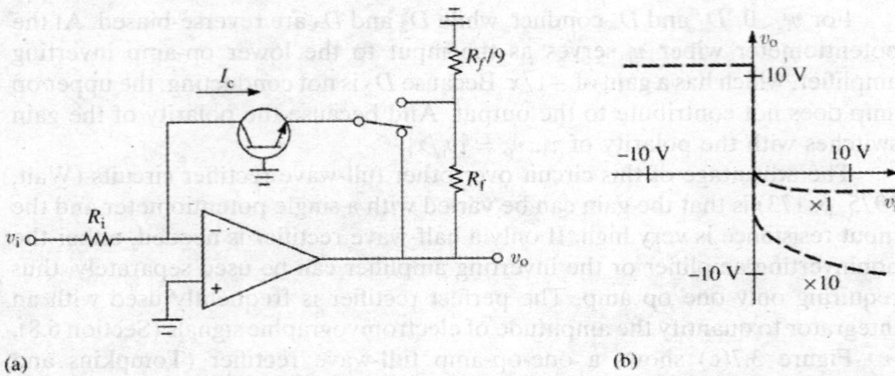


**Figure 3.8** (a) A logarithmic amplifier makes use of the fact that a transistor's $V_{BE}$ is related to the logarithm of its collector current. With the switch thrown in the alternate position, the circuit gain is increased by 10. (b) Input–output characteristics show that the logarithmic relation is obtained for only one polarity; ×1 and ×10 gains are indicated.

(Section 11.1), the logarithmic converter can be used to convert transmittance to absorbance.

## 3.8 INTEGRATORS

So far in this chapter, we have considered only circuits with a flat gain-versus-frequency characteristic. Now let us consider circuits that have a deliberate change in gain with frequency. The first such circuit is the *integrator*. Figure 3.9

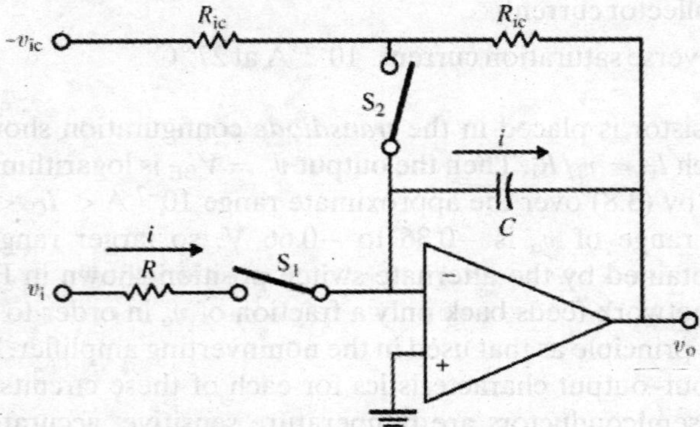


**Figure 3.9 A three-mode integrator** With $S_1$ open and $S_2$ closed, the dc circuit behaves as an inverting amplifier. Thus $v_o = v_{ic}$ and $v_o$ can be set to any desired initial condition. With $S_1$ closed and $S_2$ open, the circuit integrates. With both switches open, the circuit holds $v_o$ constant, making possible a leisurely readout.

shows the circuit for an *integrator,* which is obtained by closing switch $S_i$. The voltage across an initially uncharged capacitor is given by

$$v = \frac{1}{C}\int_0^{t_1} i dt \tag{3.9}$$

where $i$ is the current through $C$ and $t_1$ is the integration time. For the integrator, for $v_i$ positive, the input current $i = v_i/R$ flows through $C$ in a direction to cause $v_o$ to move in a negative direction. Thus

$$v_o = -\frac{1}{RC}\int_0^{t_1} v_i dt + v_{ic} \tag{3.10}$$

This shows that $v_o$ is equal to the negative integral of $v_i$, scaled by the factor 1/ $RC$ and added to $v_{ic}$, the voltage due to the initial condition. For $v_o = 0$ and $v_i =$ constant, $v_o = -v_i$ after an integration time equal to $RC$. Because any real integrator eventually drifts into saturation, a means must be provided to restore $v_o$ to any desired initial condition. If an initial condition of $v_o = 0\,\text{V}$ is desired, a simple switch to short out $C$ is sufficient. For more versatility, $S_1$ is opened and $S_2$ closed. This dc circuit then acts as an inverting amplifier, which makes $v_o = v_{ic}$. During integration, $S_1$ is closed and $S_2$ open. After the integration, both switches may be opened to hold the output at the final calculated value, thus permitting time for a readout. The circuit is useful for computing the area under a curve, as technicians do when they calculate cardiac output (Section 8.2).

The frequency response of an integrator is easily analyzed because the formula for the inverting amplifier gain (3.1) can be generalized to any input and feedback impedances. Thus for Figure 3.9, with $S_1$ closed,

$$\frac{V_o(j\omega)}{V_i(j\omega)} = \frac{Z_f}{Z_i} = -\frac{1/j\omega C}{R} = -\frac{1}{j\omega RC} = -\frac{1}{j\omega\tau} \tag{3.11}$$

where $\tau = RC$, $\omega = 2\pi f$, and $f =$ frequency. Equation (3.11) shows that the circuit gain decreases as $R$ increases, Figure 3.10 shows the frequency response, and (3.11) shows that the circuit gain is 1 when $\omega\tau = 1$.

**EXAMPLE 3.3** The output of the piezoelectric sensor shown in Figure 2.11(b) may be fed directly into the negative input of the integrator shown in Figure 3.9, as shown in Figure E3.2. Analyze the circuit of this charge amplifier and discuss its advantages.

**ANSWER** Because the FET-op-amp negative input is a virtual ground, $i_{sC} = i_{sR} = 0$. Hence long cables may be used without changing sensor sensitivity or

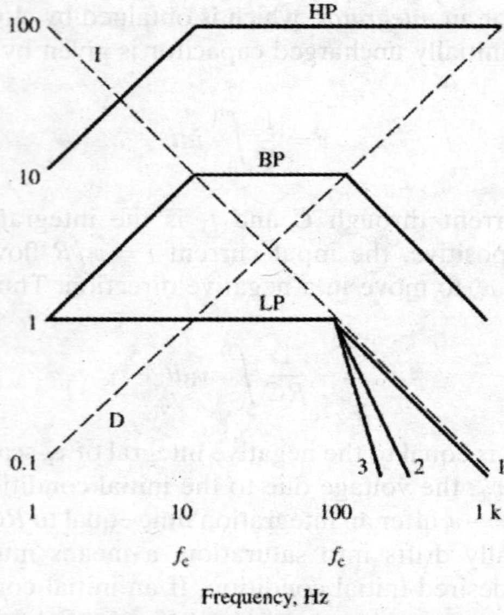


**Figure 3.10 Bode plot (gain versus frequency) for various filters** Integrator (I): differentiator (D); low pass (LP), 1, 2, 3 section (pole); high pass (HP); bandpass (BP). Corner frequencies $f_c$ for high-pass, low-pass, and bandpass filters.

time constant, as is the case with voltage amplifiers. From Figure E3.2, current generated by the sensor, $i_s = K\,dx/dt$, all flows into $C$, so, using (3.10), we find that $v_o$ is

$$v_o = -v - \frac{1}{C}\int_0^{t_1} \frac{Kdx}{dt}\,dt = -\frac{kX}{C}$$

which shows that $v_o$ is proportional to $x$, even down to dc. Like the integrator, the charge amplifier slowly drifts with time because of bias

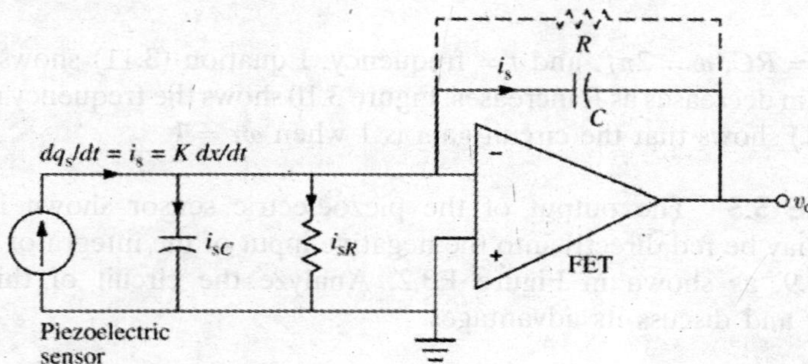


**Figure E3.2** The charge amplifier transfers charge generated from a piezoelectric sensor to the op-amp feedback capacitor $C$.

currents required by the op-amp input. A large feedback resistance $R$ must therefore be added to prevent saturation. This causes the circuit to behave as a high-pass filter, with a time constant $\tau = RC$. It then responds only to frequencies above $f_c = 1/(2\pi RC)$ and has no frequency-response improvement over the voltage amplifier. Common capacitor values are 10 pF to 1 μF.

## 3.9 DIFFERENTIATORS

Interchanging the integrator's $R$ and $C$ yields the differentiator shown in Figure 3.11. The current through a capacitor is given by

$$i = C\frac{dv}{dt} \tag{3.12}$$

If $dv_i/dt$ is positive, $i$ flows through $R$ in a direction such that it yields a negative $v_o$. Thus

$$v_o = -RC\frac{dv_i}{dt} \tag{3.13}$$

The frequency response of a differentiator is given by the ratio of feedback to input impedance.

$$\begin{aligned}\frac{V_o(j\omega)}{V_i(j\omega)} &= -\frac{Z_f}{Z_i} = -\frac{R}{1/j\omega C}\\ &= -j\omega RC = -j\omega\tau\end{aligned} \tag{3.14}$$

Equation (3.14) shows that the circuit gain increases as $f$ increases and that it is equal to unity when $\omega\tau = 1$. Figure 3.10 shows the frequency response.

Unless specific preventive steps are taken, the circuit tends to oscillate. The output also tends to be noisy, because the circuit emphasizes high frequencies. A differentiator followed by a comparator is useful for detecting

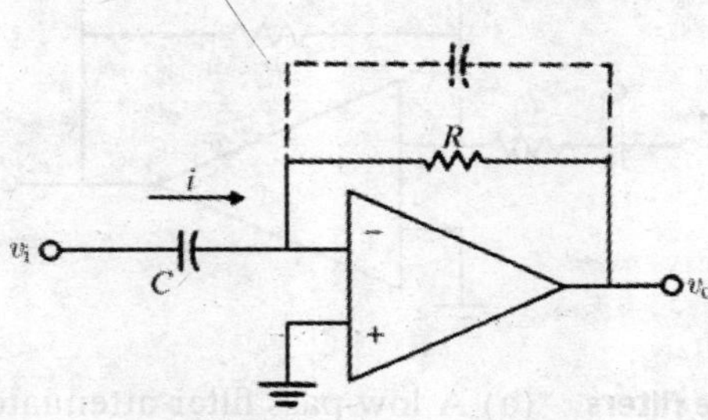


**Figure 3.11 A differentiator** The dashed lines indicate that a small capacitor must usually be added across the feedback resistor to prevent oscillation.

an event the slope of which exceeds a given value—for example, detection of the R wave in an electrocardiogram.

## 3.10 ACTIVE FILTERS

### LOW-PASS FILTER

Figure 1.9(a) shows a low-pass filter that is useful for attenuating high-frequency noise. A low-pass active filter can be obtained by using the one-op-amp circuit shown in Figure 3.12(a). The advantages of this circuit are that

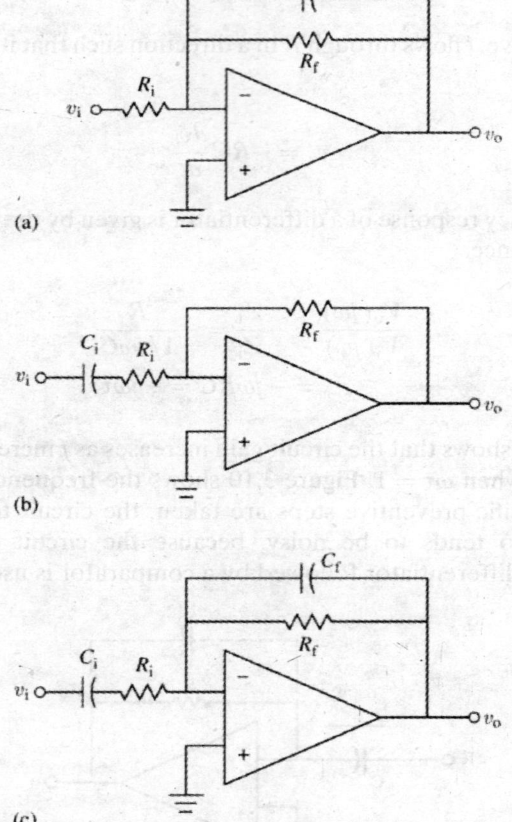


**Figure 3.12 Active filters** (a) A low-pass filter attenuates high frequencies. (b) A high-pass filter attenuates low frequencies and blocks dc. (c) A bandpass filter attenuates both low and high frequencies.

it is capable of gain and that it has a very low output impedance. The frequency response is given by the ratio of feedback to input impedance.

$$\frac{V_o(j\omega)}{V_i(j\omega)} = -\frac{Z_f}{Z_i} = -\frac{\dfrac{(R_f/j\omega C_f)}{[(1/j\omega C_f)+R_f]}}{R_i}$$

$$= \frac{R_f}{(1+j\omega R_f C_f)R_i} = \frac{R_f}{R_i}\frac{1}{1+j\omega\tau} \tag{3.15}$$

where $\tau = R_f C_f$. Note that (3.15) has the same form as (1.23). Figure 3.10 shows the frequency response, which is similar to that shown in Figure 1.8(d). For $\omega \ll 1/\tau$, the circuit behaves as an inverting amplifier (Figure 3.3), because the impedance of $C_f$ is large compared with $R_f$. For $\omega \gg 1/\tau$, the circuit behaves as an integrator (Figure 3.9), because $C_f$ is the dominant feedback impedance. The *corner frequency* $f_c$, which is defined by the intersection of the two asymptotes shown, is given by the relation $\omega\tau = 2\pi f_c \tau = 1$. When a designer wishes to limit the frequency of a wide-bandwideband amplifier, it is not necessary to add a separate stage, as shown in Figure 3.12(a), but only to add the correct size $C_f$ to the existing wide-band amplifier.

## HIGH-PASS FILTER

Figure 3.12(b) shows a one-op-amp high-pass filter. Such a circuit is useful for amplifying a small ac voltage that rides on top of a large dc voltage, because $C_i$, blocks the dc. The frequency-response equation is

$$\frac{V_o(j\omega)}{V_i(j\omega)} = -\frac{Z_f}{Z_i} = -\frac{R_f}{1/j\omega C_i + R_i}$$

$$= -\frac{j\omega R_f C_i}{1+j\omega C_i R_i} = -\frac{R_f}{R_i}\frac{j\omega\tau}{1+j\omega\tau} \tag{3.16}$$

where $\tau = R_i C_i$. Figure 3.10 shows the frequency response. For $\omega \ll 1/\tau$, the circuit behaves as a differentiator (Figure 3.11), because $C_i$: is the dominant input impedance. For $\omega \gg 1/\tau$, the circuit behaves as an inverting amplifier, because the impedance of $R_i$ is large compared with that of $C_i$. The corner frequency $f_c$, which is defined by the intersection of the two asymptotes shown, is given by the relation $\omega\tau = 2\pi f_c \tau = 1$.

## BANDPASS FILTER

A series combination of the low-pass filter and the high-pass filter results in a *bandpass filter*, which amplifies frequencies over a desired range and attenuates higher and lower frequencies. Figure 3.12(c) shows that the bandpass function can be achieved with a one-op-amp circuit. Figure 3.10 shows the frequency response. The corner frequencies are defined by the same relations as those for the low-pass and the high-pass filters. This circuit is useful for amplifying a certain band of frequencies, such as those required for recording heart sounds or the electrocardiogram.

## 3.11 FREQUENCY RESPONSE

Up until now, we have found it useful to consider the op amp as ideal. Now we shall examine the effects of several nonideal characteristics, starting with that of frequency response.

### OPEN-LOOP GAIN

Because the op amp requires very high gain, it has several stages. Each of these stages has stray or junction capacitance that limits its high-frequency response in the same way that a simple *RC* low-pass filter reduces high-frequency gain. At high frequencies, each stage has a −1 slope on a log–log plot of gain versus frequency, and each has a −90° phase shift. Thus a three-stage op amp, such as type 709, reaches a slope of −3, as shown by the dashed curve in Figure 3.13.

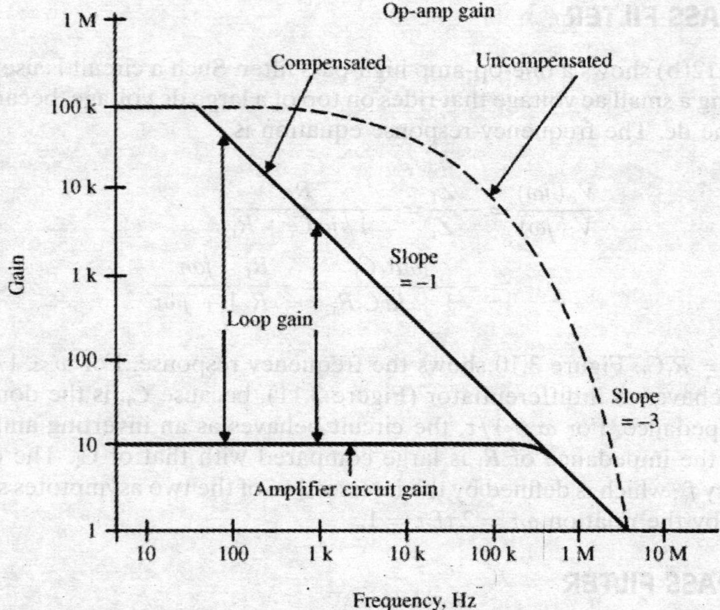


**Figure 3.13 Op-amp frequency characteristics** Early op amps (such as the 709) were uncompensated, had a gain greater than 1 when the phase shift was equal to −180°, and therefore oscillated unless compensation was added externally. A popular op amp, the 411, is compensated internally; so for a gain greater than 1, the phase shift is limited to −90°. When feedback resistors are added to build an amplifier circuit, the loop gain on this log–log plot is the difference between the op-amp gain and the amplifier–circuit gain.

The phase shift reaches −270°, which is quite satisfactory for a comparator, because feedback is not employed. For an amplifier, if the gain is greater than 1 when the phase shift is equal to −180° (the closed-loop condition for oscillation), there is undesirable oscillation.

## COMPENSATION

Adding an external capacitor to the terminals indicated on the specification sheet moves one of the *RC* filter corner frequencies to a very low frequency. This compensates the uncompensated op amp, resulting in a slope of −1 and a maximal phase shift of −90°. This is done with an internal capacitor in the 411, resulting in the solid curve shown in Figure 3.13. This op amp does not oscillate for any amplifier we have described. This op amp has very high dc gain, but the gain is progressively reduced at higher frequencies, until it is only 1 at 4 MHz.

## CLOSED-LOOP GAIN

It might appear that the op amp has very poor frequency response, because its gain is reduced for frequencies above 40 Hz. However, an amplifier circuit is never built using the op-amp open loop, so we shall therefore discuss only the circuit closed-loop response. For example, if we build an amplifier circuit with a gain of 10, as shown in Figure 3.13, the frequency response is flat up to 400 kHz and is reduced above that frequency only because the amplifier-circuit gain can never exceed the op-amp gain. We find this an advantage of using negative feedback, in that the frequency response is greatly extended.

## LOOP GAIN

The loop gain for an amplifier circuit is obtained by breaking the feedback loop at any point in the loop, injecting a signal, and measuring the gain around the loop. For example, in a unity-gain follower [Figure 3.4(a)] we break the feedback loop and then the injected signal enters the negative input, after which it is amplified by the op-amp gain. Therefore, the loop gain equals the op-amp gain. To measure loop gain in an inverting amplifier with a gain of −1 [Figure 3.3(a)], assume that the amplifier-circuit input is grounded. The injected signal is divided by 2 by the attenuator formed of $R_f$ and $R_i$, and is then amplified by the op-amp gain. Thus the loop gain is equal to (op-amp gain)/2.

Figure 3.13 shows the loop-gain concept for a noninverting amplifier. The amplifier-circuit gain is 10. On the log–log plot, the difference between the op-amp gain and the amplifier-circuit gain is the loop gain. At low frequencies, the loop gain is high and the closed-loop amplifier-circuit characteristics are determined by the feedback resistors. At high frequencies, the loop gain is low and the amplifier-circuit characteristics follow the op-amp characteristics. High loop gain is good for accuracy and stability, because the feedback resistors can be made much more stable than the op-amp characteristics.

## GAIN–BANDWIDTH PRODUCT

The gain–bandwidth product of the op amp is equal to the product of gain and bandwidth at a particular frequency. Thus in Figure 3.13 the unity-gain–bandwidth product is 4 MHz, a typical value for op amps. Note that along the entire curve with a slope of −1, the gain-bandwidth product is still constant, at 4 MHz. Thus, for any amplifier circuit, we can obtain its bandwidth by dividing the gain–bandwidth product by the amplifier-circuit gain. For higher-frequency applications, op amps such as the OP-37E are available with gain–bandwidth products of 60 MHz.

## SLEW RATE

Small-signal response follows the amplifier-circuit frequency response predicted by Figure 3.13. For large signals there is an additional limitation. When rapid changes in output are demanded, the capacitor added for compensation must be charged up from an internal source that has limited current capability $I_{max}$. The change in voltage across the capacitor is then limited, $dv/dt = I_{max}/C$, and $dv_o/dt$ is limited to a maximal slew rate (15 V/μs for the 411). If this slew rate $S_r$ is exceeded by a large-amplitude, high-frequency sine wave, distortion occurs. Thus there is a limitation on the sine-wave *full-power response*, or maximal frequency for rated output,

$$f_p = \frac{S_r}{2\pi V_{or}} \tag{3.17}$$

where $V_{or}$ is the rated output voltage (usually 10 V). If the slew rate is too slow for fast switching of a comparator, an uncompensated op amp can be used, because comparators do not contain the negative-feedback path that may cause oscillations.

# 3.12 OFFSET VOLTAGE

Another nonideal characteristic is that of offset voltage. The two op-amp inputs drive the bases of transistors, and the base-to-emitter voltage drop may be slightly different for each. Thus, so that we can obtain $v_o = 0$, the voltage $(v_1 - v_2)$ must be a few millivolts. This offset voltage is usually not important when $v_i$ is 1 to −10 V. But when $v_i$ is on the order of millivolts, as when amplifying the output from thermocouples or strain gages, the offset voltage must be considered.

## NULLING

The offset voltage may be reduced to zero by adding an external nulling pot to the terminals indicated on the specification sheet. Adjustment of this pot increases emitter current through one of the input transistors and lowers it through the other. This alters the base-to-emitter voltage of the two transistors until the offset voltage is reduced to zero.

## DRIFT

Even though the offset voltage may be set to 0 at 25 °C, it does not remain there if temperature is not constant. Temperature changes that affect the base-to-emitter voltages may be due to either environmental changes or to variations in the dissipation of power in the chip that result from fluctuating output voltage. The effects of temperature may be specified as a maximal offset voltage change in volts per degree Celsius or a maximal offset voltage change over a given temperature range, say −25 °C to +85 °C. If the drift of an inexpensive op amp is too high for a given application, tighter specifications (0.1 μV/°C) are available with temperature-controlled chips. An alternative technique modulates the dc as in chopper-stabilized and varactor op amps (Tobey *et al.*, 1971).

## NOISE

All semiconductor junctions generate noise, which limits the detection of small signals. Op amps have transistor input junctions, which generate both noise-voltage sources and noise-current sources. These can be modeled as shown in Figure 3.14. For low source impedances, only the noise voltage $v_n$ is important; it is large compared with the $i_nR$ drop caused by the current noise $i_n$. The noise is random, but the amplitude varies with frequency. For example, at low

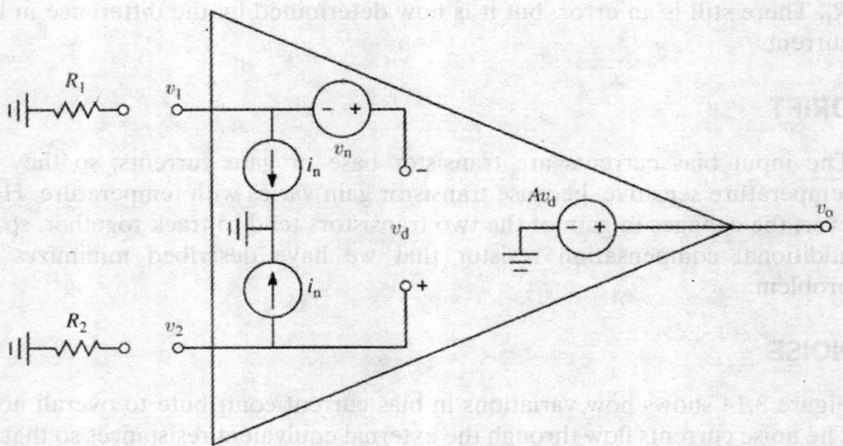


**Figure 3.14 Noise sources in an op amp** The noise-voltage source $v_n$ is in series with the input and cannot be reduced. The noise added by the noise-current sources in can be minimized by using small external resistances.

frequencies the noise power density varies as $1/f$ (flicker noise), so a large amount of noise is present at low frequencies. At the midfrequencies, the noise is lower and can be specified in root-mean-square (rms) units of $V \cdot Hz^{-1/2}$. In addition, some silicon planar-diffused bipolar integrated-circuit op amps exhibit bursts of noise, called *popcorn noise* (Wait *et al.*, 1975).

## 3.13 BIAS CURRENT

Because the two op-amp inputs drive transistors, base or gate current must flow all the time to keep the transistors turned on. This is called *bias current*, which for the 411 is about 200 pA. This bias current must flow through the feedback network. It causes errors proportional to feedback-element resistances. To minimize these errors, small feedback resistors, such as those with resistances of 10 kΩ, are normally used. Smaller values should be used only after a check to determine that the current flowing through the feedback resistor, plus the current flowing through all load resistors, does not exceed the op-amp output current rating (20 mA for the 411).

### DIFFERENTIAL BIAS CURRENT

The difference between the two input bias currents is much smaller than either of the bias currents alone. A degree of cancellation of the effects of bias current can be achieved by having each bias current flow through the same equivalent resistance. This is accomplished for the inverting amplifier and the noninverting amplifier by adding, in series with the positive input, a compensation resistor the value of which is equal to the parallel combination of $R_i$ and $R_f$. There still is an error, but it is now determined by the difference in bias current.

### DRIFT

The input bias currents are transistor base or gate currents, so they are temperature sensitive, because transistor gain varies with temperature. However, the changes in gain of the two transistors tend to track together, so the additional compensation resistor that we have described minimizes the problem.

### NOISE

Figure 3.14 shows how variations in bias current contribute to overall noise. The noise currents flow through the external equivalent resistances so that the total rms noise voltage is

$$v \cong \{[v_n^2 + (i_n R_1)^2 + (i_n R_2)^2 + 4\kappa T R_1 + 4\kappa T R_2]\mathrm{BW}\}^{1/2} \tag{3.18}$$

where

$R_1$ and $R_2$ = equivalent source resistances
$v_n$ = mean value of the rms noise voltage, in $V \cdot Hz^{-1/2}$, across the frequency range of interest
$i_n$ = mean value of the rms noise current, in $A \cdot Hz^{-1/2}$, across the frequency range of interest
$\kappa$ = Boltzmann's constant (Appendix)
T = temperature, K
BW = noise bandwidth, Hz

The specification sheet provides values of $v_n$ and $i_n$ (sometimes $v_n^2$ and $i_n^2$), thus making it possible to compare different op amps. If the source resistances are 10 kΩ, bipolar-transistor op amps yield the lowest noise. For larger source resistances, low-input-current amplifiers such as the field-effect transistor (FET) input stage are best because of their lower current noise. Ary (1977) presents design factors and performance specifications for a low-noise amplifier.

For ac amplifiers, the lowest noise is obtained by calculating the characteristic noise resistance $R_n = v_n/i_n$ and setting it equal to the equivalent source resistance $R_2$ (for the noninverting amplifier). This is accomplished by inserting a transformer with turns ratio 1 : $N$, where $N = (R_n/R_2)^{1/2}$, between the source and the op amp (Jung, 1986).

## 3.14 INPUT AND OUTPUT RESISTANCE

### INPUT RESISTANCE

The op-amp differential-input resistance $R_d$ is shown in Figures 3.1 and 3.15. For the FET-input 411, it is 1 TΩ, whereas for BJT-input op amps, it is about 2 MΩ, which is comparable to the value of some feedback resistors used. However, we shall see that its value is usually not important because of the benefits of feedback. Consider the follower shown in Figure 3.15. In order to calculate the amplifier-circuit input resistance $R_{ai}$, assume a change in input voltage $v_i$. Because this is a follower,

$$\Delta v_o = A\Delta v_d = A(\Delta v_i - \Delta v_o)$$

$$= \frac{A\Delta v_i}{A+1}$$

$$\Delta i_i = \frac{\Delta v_d}{R_d} = \frac{\Delta v_i - \Delta v_o}{R_d} = \frac{\Delta v_i}{(A+1)R_d}$$

$$R_{ai} = \frac{\Delta v_i}{\Delta i_i} = (A+1)R_d \cong AR_d \tag{3.19}$$

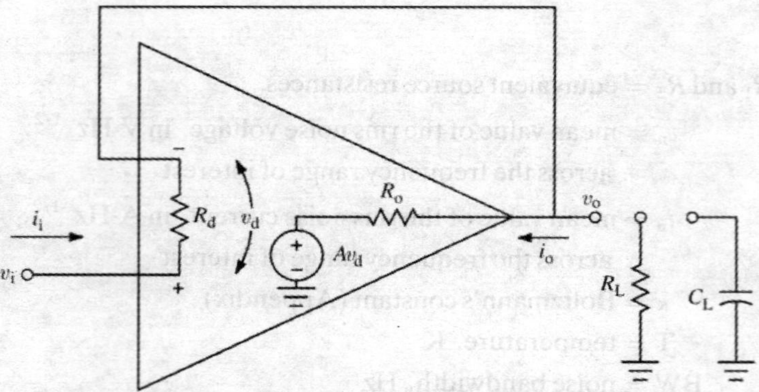


**Figure 3.15** The amplifier input impedance is much higher than the op-amp input impedance $R_d$. The amplifier output impedance is much smaller than the op-amp output impedance $R_o$.

Thus the amplifier-circuit input resistance $R_{ai}$ is about $(10^5) \times (2\ \text{M}\Omega) = 200\ \text{G}\Omega$. This value cannot be achieved in practice, because surface leakage paths in the op-amp socket lower it considerably. In general, all noninverting amplifiers have a very high input resistance, which is equal to $R_d$ times the loop gain. This is not to say that very large source resistances can be used, because the bias current usually causes much larger problems than the amplifier-circuit input impedance. For large source resistances, FET op amps such as the 411 are helpful.

The input resistance of an inverting amplifier is easy to determine. Because the negative input of the op amp is a virtual ground,

$$R_{ai} = \frac{\Delta v_i}{\Delta i_i} = R_i \tag{3.20}$$

Thus the amplifier-circuit input resistance $R_{ai}$ is equal to $R_i$, the input resistor. Because $R_i$ is usually a small value, the inverting amplifier has small input resistance.

## OUTPUT RESISTANCE

The op-amp output resistance $R_o$ is shown in Figures 3.1 and 3.15. It is about 40 Ω for the typical op amp, which may seem large for some applications. However, its value is usually not important because of the benefits of feedback. Consider the follower shown in Figure 3.15. In order to calculate the amplifier-circuit output resistance $R_{ao}$, assume that load resistor $R_L$ is attached to the output, causing a change in output current $\Delta i_o$. Because $i_o$ flows through $R_o$, there is an additional voltage drop $\Delta i_o R_o$.

$$-\Delta v_d = \Delta v_o = A\Delta v_d + \Delta i_o R_o = -A\Delta v_o + \Delta i_o R_o$$

$$(A+1)\Delta v_o = \Delta i_o R_o$$

$$R_{ao} = \frac{\Delta v_o}{\Delta i_o} = \frac{R_o}{A+1} \cong R_o/A \tag{3.21}$$

Thus the amplifier-circuit output resistance $R_{ao}$ is about $40/10^5 = 0.0004\ \Omega$, a value negligible in most circuits. In general, all noninverting and inverting amplifiers have an output resistance that is equal to $R_o$ divided by the loop gain. This is not to say that very small load resistances can be driven by the output. If $R_L$ shown in Figure 3.15 is smaller than 500 Ω, the op amp saturates internally, because the maximal current output for a typical op amp is 20 mA. This maximal current output must also be considered when driving large capacitances $C_L$ at a high slew rate. Then the output current

$$i_o = C_L \frac{dv_o}{dt} \tag{3.22}$$

The $R_o$–$C_L$ combination also acts as a low-pass filter, which introduces additional phase shift around the loop and can cause oscillation. The cure is to add a small resistor between $v_o$ and $C_L$, thus isolating $C_L$ from the feedback loop.

To achieve larger current outputs, the *current booster* is used. An ordinary op amp drives high-power transistors (on heat sinks if required). Then we can use the entire circuit as an op amp by connecting terminals $v_1$, $v_2$, and $v_o$ to external feedback networks. This places the booster section within the feedback loop and keeps distortion low.

## 3.15 PHASE-SENSITIVE DEMODULATORS

Figure 2.7 shows that a linear variable differential transformer requires a phase-sensitive demodulator to yield a useful output signal. A phase-sensitive demodulator does not measure phase but yields a full-wave-rectified output of the in-phase component of a sine wave. Its output is proportional to the amplitude of the input, but it changes sign when the phase shifts by 180°.

Figure 3.16 shows the functional operation of a phase-sensitive demodulator. Figure 3.16(a) shows a switching function that is derived from a *carrier oscillator* and causes the double-pole double-throw switch in Figure 3.16(b) to be in the upper position for +1 and in the lower position for −1. In effect, this multiplies the input signal $v_i$ by the switching function shown in Figure 3.16(a). The in-phase sine wave in Figure 3.16(c) is demodulated by this switch to yield the full-wave-rectified positive signal in Figure 3.16(d). The sine wave in Figure 3.16(e) is 180° out of phase, so it yields the negative signal in Figure 3.16(f).

Amplifier stray capacitance may cause an undesirable *quadrature voltage* that is shifted 90°, as shown in Figure 3.16(g). The demodulated signal in Figure 3.16(h) averages to zero when passed through a low-pass filter and is rejected. The dc signal shown in Figure 3.16(i) is demodulated to the wave shown in Figure 3.16(j) and is rejected. Any frequency component not locked to the

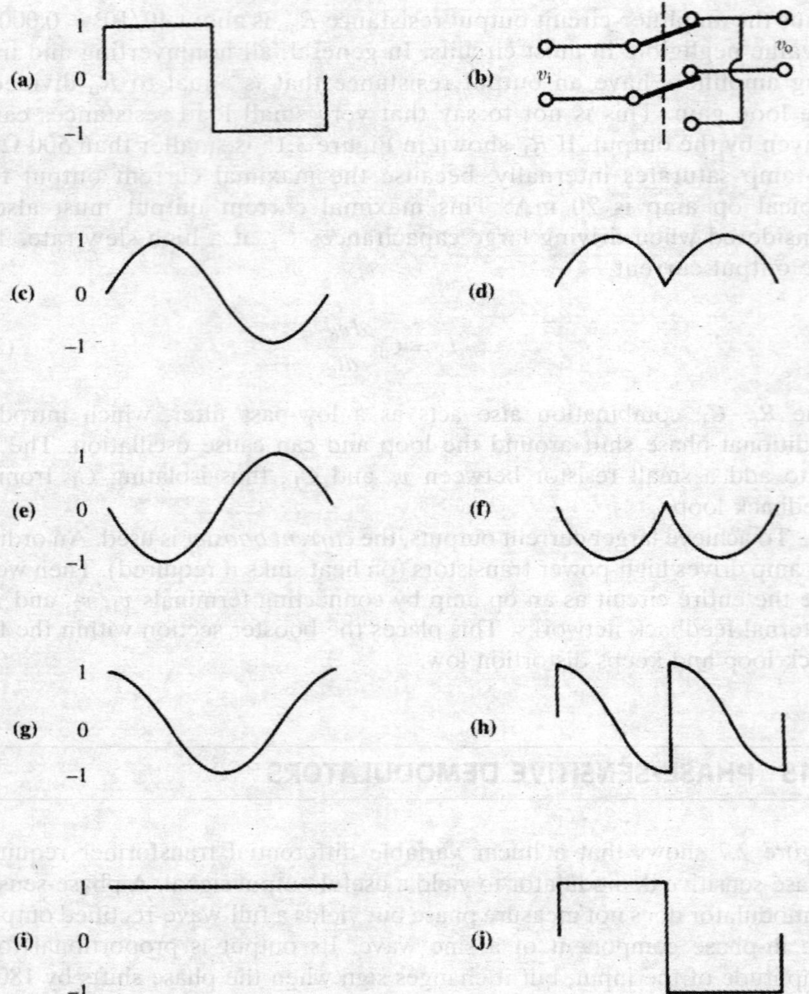


**Figure 3.16 Functional operation of a phase-sensitive demodulator** (a) Switching function. (b) Switchswitch. (c), (e), (g), (i) Several several input voltages. (d), (f), (h), (j) Corresponding corresponding output voltages.

carrier frequency is similarly rejected. Because the phase-sensitive demodulator has excellent noise-rejection capabilities, it is frequently used to demodulate the suppressed-carrier waveforms obtained from linear variable differential transformers (LVDTs) and the ac-excited strain-gage Wheatstone bridge (Section 2.3). A carrier system and phase-sensitive demodulator are also essential for operation of the electromagnetic blood flowmeter (Section 8.3). The noise-rejection capability may be improved by placing a tuned amplifier before the phase-sensitive demodulator, thus forming a lock-in amplifier (Aronson, 1977).

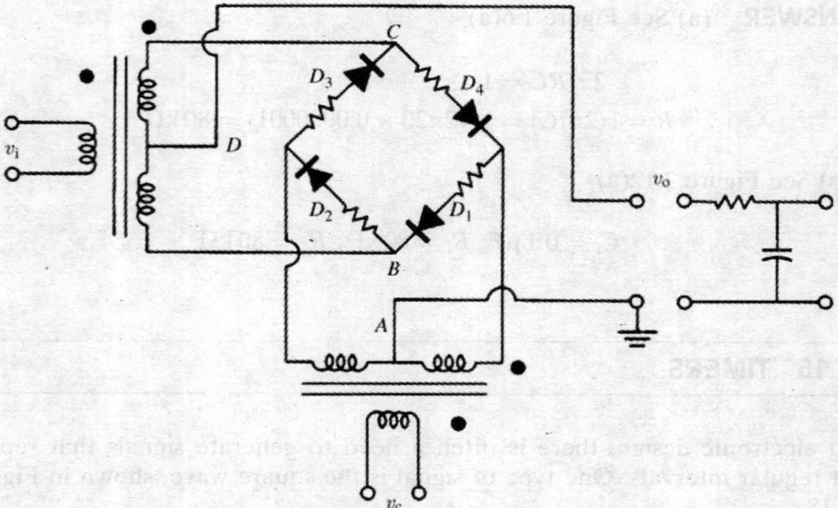


**Figure 3.17 A ring demodulator** This phase-sensitive detector produces a full-wave-rectified output $v_o$ that is positive when the input voltage $v_i$ is in phase with the carrier voltage $v_c$ and negative when $v_i$ is 180° out of phase with $v_c$.

A practical phase-sensitive demodulator is shown in Figure 3.17. This *ring demodulator* operates with the following action, provided that $v_c$ is more than twice $v_i$ If the carrier waveform $v_i$ is positive at the black dot, diodes $D_1$ and $D_2$ are forward-biased and $D_3$ and $D_4$ are reverse-biased. By symmetry, points A and B are at the same voltage. If the input waveform $v_i$, is positive at the black dot, this transforms to a voltage $v_{DB}$ that appears at $v_o$, as shown in the first half of Figure 3.16(d).

During the second half of the cycle, diodes $D_3$ and $D_4$ are forward-biased and $D_1$ and $D_2$ are reverse-biased. By symmetry, points A and C are at the same potential. The reversed polarity of $v_i$ yields a positive $v_{DC}$, which appears at $v_o$. Thus $v_o$ is a full-wave-rectified waveform. If $v_i$, changes phase by 180°, as shown in Figure 3.16(e), $v_o$ changes polarity. To eliminate ripple, the output is usually low-pass filtered by a filter the corner frequency of which is about one-tenth of the carrier frequency.

The ring demodulator has the advantage of having no moving parts. Also, because transformer coupling is used, $v_i$, $v_c$, and $v_c$ çan all be referenced to different dc levels. The availability of type 1495 solid-state double-balanced demodulators on a single chip (Jung, 1986) makes it possible to eliminate the bulky transformers but requires more care in biasing $v_i$, $v_c$, and $v_o$ at different dc levels.

**EXAMPLE 3.4** (a) For Figure 3.17, assume that the carrier frequency is 3 kHz. Design the *RC* output low-pass filter to have a corner frequency of 20 Hz and a reasonable value capacitor (100 nF). Use (b) a one-section active filter.

**ANSWER** (a) See Figure 1.6(a)

$$2\pi fRC = 1$$
$$R = 1(2\pi fC) = 1/(2\pi 20 \times 0.0000001) = 80\,\text{k}\Omega$$

(b) See Figure 3.12(a)

$$C_f = 0.1\,\mu\text{F},\ R_i = 80\,\text{k}\Omega,\ R_f = 80\,\text{k}\Omega$$

## 3.16 TIMERS

In electronic design, there is often a need to generate signals that repeat at regular intervals. One type of signal is the square wave, shown in Figure 3.18.

The voltage of a square wave is high for a fixed amount of time, $T_h$, then it drops to a lower voltage for a length of time $T_l$. This pattern of alternating high and low cycles continuously repeats. The total period of the square wave, the time it takes to repeat, is thus

$$T = T_h + T_l \tag{3.23}$$

The duty cycle of a square wave is defined as the percentage of the time that the square wave is at its higher output voltage. Thus

$$\text{Duty cycle} = \frac{T_h}{T} \times (100\%) \tag{3.24}$$

For example, a square wave in which $T_h = T_l$ is said to have a 50% duty cycle.

There are many ways to generate square waves. Digital systems use square waves with 50% duty cycles as clocks to synchronize digital logic; thus, there

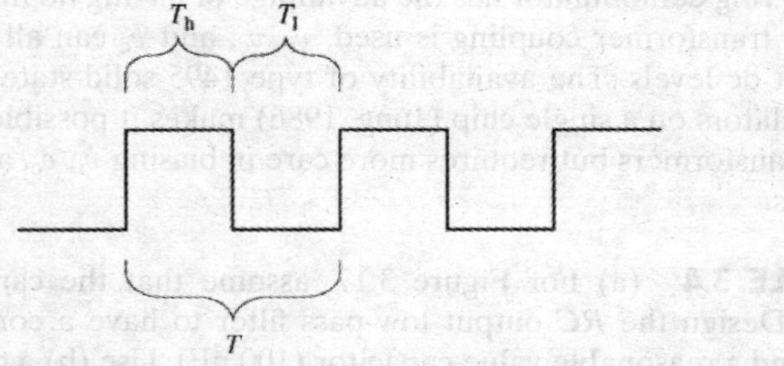


**Figure 3.18** A square wave of period $T$ oscillates between two values.

are many commercially available clock generator chips that yield square waves with 50% duty cycles.

Many times, however, we want to generate square waves with duty cycles other than 50%. A popular means of doing this is with a 555 timer. The 555 timer is an 8-pin integrated circuit, as shown in Figure 3.19(a). The 555 timers form the core of many different kinds of timing circuits. One popular configuration is shown in Figure 3.19(b). When powered, this circuit oscillates internally, alternately charging and discharging capacitor $C$. Figure 3.19(c) shows the output of the circuit. Note that the duty cycle of this circuit is always greater than 50% because $R_a$ must be nonzero. To get square waves with duty cycles less than 50%, the output of this circuit may be fed into an inverting amplifier or logic inverter.

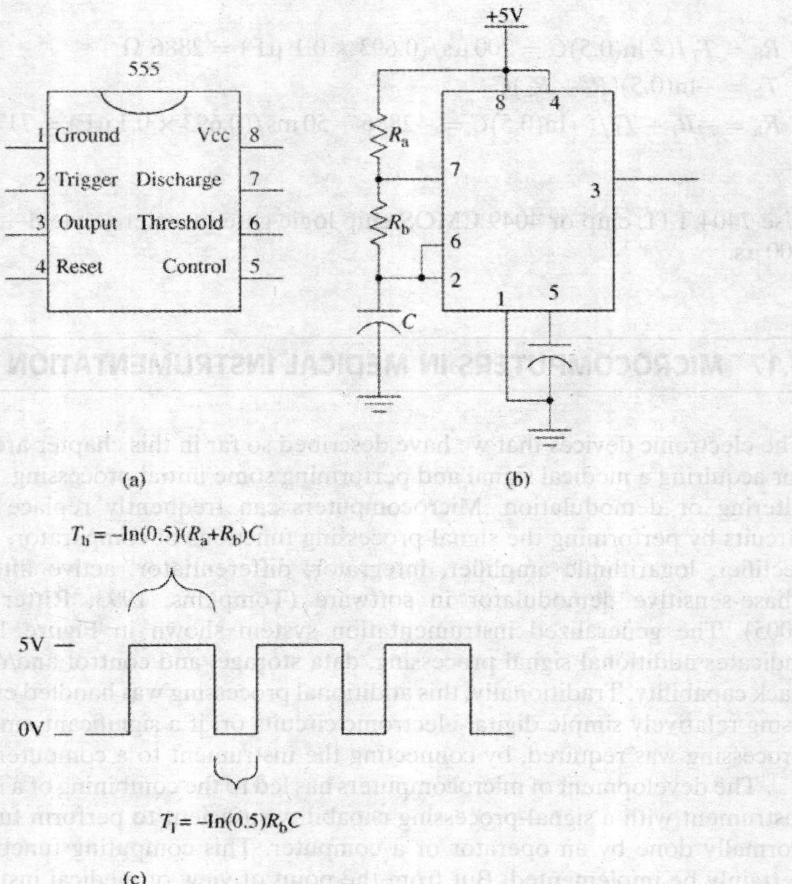


**Figure 3.19 The 555 timer** (a) Pinout for the 555 timer IC. (b) A popular circuit that utilizes a 555 timer and four external components creates a square wave with duty cycle > 50%. (c) The output from the 555 timer circuit shown in (b).

This method of generating square waves is simple and requires only a small integrated circuit (IC) and four external components. The circuit of Figure 3.19(b), however, is not very useful for precision timing applications, because of the difficulty of creating precision capacitors. Using typical off-the-shelf components, the period may vary by as much as 25% from the nominal values. Using variable resistances for $R_a$ and $R_b$, which allows fine-tuning of the time constants, can minimize this.

**EXAMPLE 3.5** Design a timer for a nerve stimulator that stimulates for 200 μs every 50 ms.

**ANSWER** Use the circuit shown in Figure 3.19(b). From Figure 3.19(c) $T_l = -\ln(0.5)R_bC$

$$R_b = T_l/(-\ln(0.5)C = 200\,\mu\text{s}/(0.693 \times 0.1\,\mu\text{F}) = 2886\ \Omega$$
$$T_h = -\ln(0.5)(R_l + R_h)C.$$
$$R_h = -R_l + T_h/(-\ln(0.5)C = -2886 + 50\,\text{ms}/(0.693 \times 0.1\,\mu\text{F}) = 717\ \text{k}\Omega.$$

Use 7404 TTL chip or 4049 CMOS chip logic gate inverter to yield +5 V for 200 μs.

## 3.17 MICROCOMPUTERS IN MEDICAL INSTRUMENTATION

The electronic devices that we have described so far in this chapter are useful for acquiring a medical signal and performing some initial processing, such as filtering or demodulation. Microcomputers can frequently replace analog circuits by performing the signal-processing functions of comparator, limiter, rectifier, logarithmic amplifier, integrator, differentiator, active filter, and phase-sensitive demodulator in software (Tompkins, 1993; Ritter *et al.*, 2005). The generalized instrumentation system shown in Figure 1.1 also indicates additional signal processing, data storage, and control and/or feedback capability. Traditionally, this additional processing was handled either by using relatively simple digital-electronic circuits or, if a significant amount of processing was required, by connecting the instrument to a computer.

The development of microcomputers has led to the combining of a medical instrument with a signal-processing capability sufficient to perform functions normally done by an operator or a computer. This computing function can certainly be implemented. But from the point of view of medical instrumentation, it is more instructive to view the microcomputer as a microcontroller. The use of a microcomputer generally results in fewer IC packages. This reduced complexity, together with the capability for self-calibration and detection of errors, enhances the reliability of the instrument. The most useful applications of microcomputers for medical instrumentation involve this controller function. Microcomputers can provide self-calibration for measurement systems, automatic sequencing of events, and an easy way to enter such patient data as height, weight, and sex for calculating expected or normal performance. All these functions are made possible by the basic structure of the microcomputer system. Further development has resulted in chip-based systems. For instance digital filters are now directly hard coded onto dedicated chips which result in significant computational savings The LabVIEW PC-based system provides modular software-based instruments for data acquisition. It permits graphical system design of embedded applications for microprocessor and microcontroller devices. Thus the LabVIEW developed software can be used in many new medical instruments after the purchase of one LabVIEW system that includes the Microprocessor SDK toolkit. (http://www.ni.com/labview/; Tompkins and Webster, 1981; Tompkins and Webster, 1988; Carr and Brown, 2001).

## PROBLEMS

**3.1** (a) Design an inverting amplifier with an input resistance of 20 kΩ and a gain of 10. (b) Include a resistor to compensate for bias current. (c) Design a summing amplifier such that $v_o = -(10v_1 + 2v_2 + 0.5v_3)$.

**3.2** The axon action potential (AAP) is shown in Figure 4.1. Design a dc-coupled one-op-amp circuit that will amplify the 100 mV to 50 mV input range to have the maximal gain possible without exceeding the typical guaranteed linear output range.

**3.3** Use the circuit shown in Figure E3.1 to design a dc-coupled one-op-amp circuit that will amplify the ±100 μV EOG to have the maximal gain possible without exceeding the typical guaranteed linear output range. Include a control that can balance (remove) series electrode offset potentials up to ±300 mV. Give all numerical values.

**3.4** Design a noninverting amplifier having a gain of 10 and $R_i$ of Figure 3.4(b) equal to 20 kΩ. Include a resistor to compensate for bias current.

**3.5** An op-amp differential amplifier is built using four identical resistors, each having a tolerance of ±5%. Calculate the worst possible CMRR.

**3.6** Design a three-op-amp differential amplifier having a differential gain of 5 in the first stage and 6 in the second stage.

**3.7** Design a comparator with hysteresis in which the hysteresis width extends from 0 to 2 V.

**3.8** For an inverting half-wave perfect rectifier, sketch the circuit. Plot the input–output characteristics for both the circuit output and the op-amp output, which are not the same point as in most op-amp circuits.

**3.9** Using the principle shown in Figure 3.8, design a signal compressor for which an input-voltage range of ±10 V yields an output-voltage range of ±4 V.

**3.10** Design an integrator with an input resistance of 1 MΩ. Select the capacitor such that when $v_i = +10$ V, $v_o$ travels from 0 to 10 V in 0.1 s.

**3.11** In Problem 3.10, if $v_i = 0$ and offset voltage equals 5 mV, what is the current through $R$? How long will it take for $v_o$ to drift from 0 V to saturation? Explain how to cure this drift problem.

**3.12** In Problem 3.10, if bias current is 200 pA, how long will it take for $v_o$ to drift from 0 V to saturation? Explain how to cure this drift problem.

**3.13** Design a differentiator for which $v_o = -10$ V when $dv_i/dt = 100$ V/s.

**3.14** Design a one-section high-pass filter with a gain of 20 and a corner frequency of 0.05 Hz. Calculate its response to a step input of 1 mV.

**3.15** Design a one-op-amp high-pass active filter with a high-frequency gain of 10 (not –10), a high-frequency input impedance of 10 MΩ, and a corner frequency of 10 Hz.

**3.16** Find $V_o(j\omega)/V_i(j\omega)$ for the bandpass filter shown in Figure 3.12(c).

**3.17** Figure 6.16 shows that the frequency range of the AAP is 110 to 10 kHz. Design a one-op-amp active bandpass filter that has a midband input impedance of approximately 10 kΩ, a midband gain of approximately 1, and a frequency response from 1 to 10 kHz (corner frequencies).

**3.18** Figure 6.16 shows the maximal single-peak signal and frequency range of the EMG. Design a one-op-amp bandpass filter circuit that will amplify the EMG to have the maximal gain possible without exceeding the typical guaranteed linear output range and will pass the range of frequencies shown.

**3.19** Using 411 op amps, explain how an amplifier with a gain of 100 and a bandwidth of 100 kHz can be designed.

**3.20** Refer to Figure 3.13. If the amplifier gain is 1000, what is the loop gain at 100 Hz?

**3.21** For the differentiator shown in Figure 3.11, ground the input, break the feedback loop at any point, and determine the phase shift in each section. Explain why the circuit tends to oscillate.

**3.22** For Problem 3.21, calculate the amplifier input and output resistances at 100 Hz, for inverting and noninverting amplifiers.

**3.23** For Figure 3.15, what is the maximal capacitive load $C_L$ that can be connected to a 411 without degrading the normal slew rate (15 V/μs) at the maximal current output (20 mA)?

**3.24** For Figure 3.17, if the forward drop of $D_1$ is 10% higher than that of the other diodes, what change occurs in $v_o$?

**3.25** Given an oscillator block, design (show the circuit diagram for) an LVDT, phase-sensitive demodulator and a first-order low-pass filter with a corner frequency of 100 Hz. Sketch waveforms at each significant location.

## REFERENCES

Aronson, M. H., "Lock-in and carrier amplifiers." *Med. Electron. Data*, 8(3), 1977, C1–C16.

Ary, J. P., "A head-mounted 24-channel evoked potential preamplifier employing low-noise operational amplifiers." *IEEE Trans. Biomed. Eng.*, BME-24, 1977, 293–297.

Carr, J. J., and J. M. Brown, *Introduction to Biomedical Equipment Technology*, 4th ed., Upper Saddle River, NJ: Prentice-Hall, 2001.

Franco, S., *Design with Operational Amplifiers and Analog Integrated Circuits*. 3rd ed., New York: McGraw-Hill, 2002.

Graeme, J. G., "Rectifying wide-range signals with precision, variable gain." *Electron.*, Dec. 12, 1974, 45(25), 107–109.

Horowitz, P., and W. Hill, *The Art of Electronics*, 2nd ed. Cambridge, England: Cambridge University Press, 1989.

Jung, W. G., *1C Op-Amp Cookbook*, 3rd ed. Indianapolis: Howard W. Sams, 1986.

Ritter, A. B., S. Reisman, and B. B. Michniak, *Biomedical Engineering Principles*. Boca Raton: CRC Press, 2005.

Shepard, R. R., "Active filters: Part 12, Short cuts to network design." *Electron.*, Aug. 18, 1969, 42(17), 82–92.

Tobey, G. E., J. G. Graeme, and L. P. Huelsman, *Operational Amplifiers: Design and Application*. New York: McGraw-Hill, 1971.

Tompkins, W. J. (ed.), *Biomedical Digital Signal Processing: C-Language Examples and Laboratory Experiments for the IBM PC*. Englewood Cliffs, NJ: Prentice Hall, 1993.

Tompkins, W. J., and J. G. Webster (eds.), *Design of Microcomputer-Based Medical Instrumentation*. Englewood Cliffs, NJ: Prentice-Hall, 1981.

Tompkins, W. J., and J. G. Webster (eds.), *Interfacing Sensors to the IBM PC*. Englewood Cliffs, NJ: Prentice-Hall, 1988.

Wait, J. V., L. P. Huelsman, and G. A. Korn, *Introduction to Operational Amplifier Theory and Applications*. New York: McGraw-Hill, 1975.

# 4

# THE ORIGIN OF BIOPOTENTIALS

John W. Clark Jr.

This chapter deals with the genesis of various bioelectric signals that are recorded routinely in modern clinical practice. Given adequate monitoring equipment, many forms of bioelectric phenomena can be recorded with relative ease. These phenomena include the electrocardiogram (ECG), electroencephalogram (EEG), electroneurogram (ENG), electromyogram (EMG), and electroretinogram (ERG).

Engineers generally have a good physical insight into the nature of electromagnetic fields produced by bioelectric sources, and, because of their comprehensive understanding of the physical problem, they may contribute to the solution of biological problems.

This chapter begins by introducing bioelectric phenomena at the cellular level. It proceeds to discuss volume-conductor potential distributions of simple bioelectric sources, and gradually more anatomically complex ones. The volume-conductor electric field problem provides the link (mapping) between microscopic electrical activity generated within the bioelectric source, the flow of action current through the conducting medium, and the macroscopic potential distribution produced at the surface of the body. We continue with a discussion of the functional organization of the peripheral nervous system (outside the brain and spinal cord), which leads to a discussion of the ENG and EMG. Finally, other bioelectric sources (and associated field potentials) are discussed including the active heart (ECG), retina (ERG), and brain (EEG).

## 4.1 ELECTRICAL ACTIVITY OF EXCITABLE CELLS

Bioelectric potentials are produced as a result of electrochemical activity of a certain class of cells, known as *excitable cells*, that are components of nervous, muscular, or glandular tissue. Electrically they exhibit a *resting potential* and, when appropriately stimulated, an *action potential,* as the following paragraphs explain.

### THE RESTING STATE

The individual excitable cell maintains a steady electrical potential difference between its internal and external environments. This resting potential of the internal medium lies in the range −40 to −90 mV, relative to the external medium.

Figure 4.1(a) shows how the resting potential is usually measured. A micromanipulator advances a microelectrode (see Section 5.8) close to the surface of an excitable cell and then, by small movements, pushes it through the cell membrane. For the membrane to seal properly around the penetrating tip, the diameter of the tip must be small relative to the size of the cell in which it is placed. Figure 4.1(b) shows a typical electrical recording from a single nerve fiber, including the dc offset potential (resting potential) that occurs upon penetration of the membrane. It also shows the transient disturbance of membrane potential (the action potential) when an adequate stimulus is given.

The cell membrane is a very thin (7 to 15 nm) lipoprotein complex that is essentially impermeable to intracellular protein and other organic anions ($A^-$). The membrane in the resting state is only slightly permeable to $Na^+$ and rather

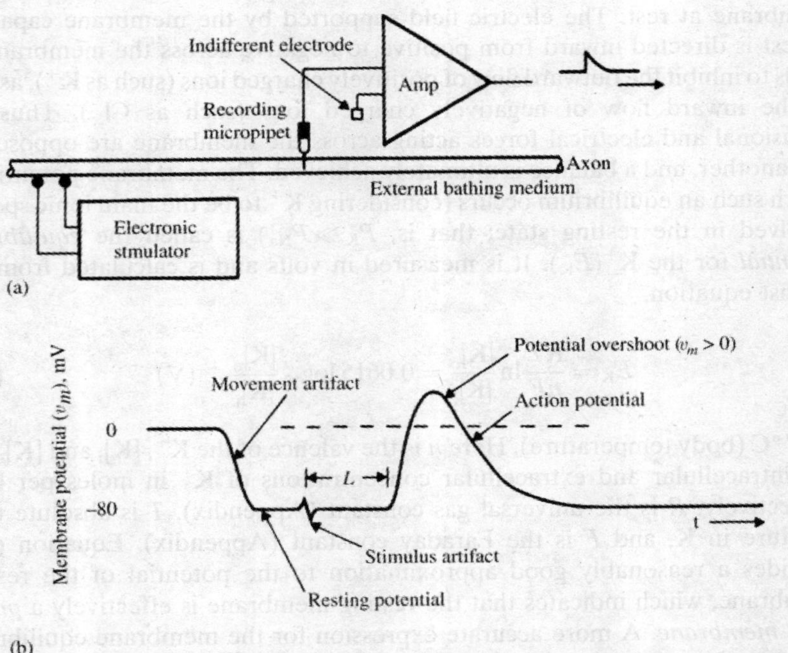


**Figure 4.1 Recording of action potential of an invertebrate nerve axon** (a) An electronic stimulator supplies a brief pulse of current to the axon, strong enough to excite the axon. A recording of this activity is made at a downstream site via a penetrating micropipette. (b) The movement artifact is recorded as the tip of the micropipette drives through the membrane to record resting potential. A short time later, an electrical stimulus is delivered to the axon; its field effect is recorded instantaneously at downstream measurement site as the stimulus artifact. The action potential however, proceeds along the axon with a constant conduction velocity. The time period $L$ is the *latent period* or transmission time from stimulus to recording site.

freely permeable to $K^+$ and $Cl^-$. The permeability of the resting membrane to potassium ion ($P_K$) is approximately 50 to 100 times larger than its permeability to sodium ion ($P_{Na}$).

Typically, the $K^+$ concentration of the internal medium (cytosol) is 140 mmol/liter, whereas that of the external (bathing) medium is 2.5 mmol/liter. The concentration difference creates a diffusion gradient that is directed outward across the membrane. The movement of the $K^+$ along this diffusion gradient (while the nondiffusible anion component stays within the cell) is in such a direction as to make the interior of the cell more negative relative to the external medium (that is, positive charge is removed from the interior). Consequently, a transmembrane potential difference is established. Electrically the membrane can be described as a leaky capacitor, since structurally it is comprised of a thin dielectric material (the lipoprotein complex) that acts as a charge separator, and yet it has transmembrane ion channels (pores) of different types, some of which allow a leakage flow of ions across the membrane at rest. The electric field supported by the membrane capacitor at rest is directed inward from positive to negative across the membrane. It tends to inhibit the outward flow of positively charged ions (such as $K^+$), as well as the inward flow of negatively charged ions (such as $Cl^-$). Thus the diffusional and electrical forces acting across the membrane are opposed to one another, and a balance is ultimately achieved. The membrane potential at which such an equilibrium occurs (considering $K^+$ to be the main ionic species involved in the resting state; that is, $P_K \gg P_{Na}$) is called the *equilibrium potential* for the $K^+ (E_K)$. It is measured in volts and is calculated from the Nernst equation,

$$E_K = \frac{RT}{nF} \ln \frac{[K]_o}{[K]_i} = 0.0615 \log_{10} \frac{[K]_o}{[K]_i} \quad (V) \qquad (4.1)$$

at 37 °C (body temperature). Here $n$ is the valence of the $K^+$, $[K]_i$ and $[K]_o$ are the intracellular and extracellular concentrations of $K^+$ in moles per liter, respectively, $R$ is the universal gas constant (Appendix), $T$ is absolute temperature in K, and $F$ is the Faraday constant (Appendix). Equation (4.1) provides a reasonably good approximation to the potential of the resting membrane, which indicates that the resting membrane is effectively a *potassium membrane*. A more accurate expression for the membrane equilibrium potential $E$, which accounts for the influence of other ionic species in the internal and external media was first developed by Goldman (1943) and later modified by Hodgkin and Katz (1949), who assumed a constant electric field across the membrane:

$$E = \frac{RT}{F} \ln \left\{ \frac{P_K[K]_o + P_{Na}[Na]_o + P_{Cl}[Cl]_i}{P_K[K]_i + P_{Na}[Na]_i + P_{Cl}[Cl]_o} \right\} \qquad (4.2)$$

Here $E$ is the equilibrium transmembrane (resting) potential when net current through the membrane is zero and $P_M$ is the *permeability coefficient* of the membrane for a particular ionic species M. It is called the *Goldman–Hodgkin–Katz* (GHK) *formulation.*

**EXAMPLE 4.1** For frog skeletal muscle, typical values for the intracellular and extracellular concentrations of the major ion species (in millimoles per liter) are as follows.

| Species | Intracellular | Extracellular |
|---|---|---|
| $Na^+$ | 12 | 145 |
| $K^+$ | 155 | 4 |
| $Cl^-$ | 4 | 120 |

Assuming room temperature (20 °C) and typical values of permeability coefficient for frog skeletal muscle ($P_{Na} = 2 \times 10^{-8}$ cm/s, $P_K = 2 \times 10^{-6}$ cm/s, and $P_{Cl} = 4 \times 10^{-6}$ cm/s), calculate the equilibrium resting potential for this membrane, using the Goldman equation.

**ANSWER** From (4.2),

$$E = 0.0581 \log_{10}\left[\frac{P_K(4) + P_{Na}(145) + P_{Cl}(4)}{P_K(155) + P_{Na}(12) + P_{Cl}(120)}\right]$$

$$= 0.0581 \log_{10}\left(\frac{26.9 \times 10^{-6}}{790.24 \times 10^{-6}}\right) = -85.3 \text{ mV}$$

which is close to typical measured values for the resting membrane potential in frog skeletal muscle.

Maintaining the steady-state ionic imbalance between the internal and external media of the cell requires continuous active transport of ionic species against their electrochemical gradients. The active transport mechanism is located within the membrane and is referred to as the *sodium–potassium pump*. It actively transports $Na^+$ out of the cell and $K^+$ into the cell in the ratio $3Na^+ : 2K^+$. The associated pump current $i_{NaK}$ is a net outward current that tends to increase the negativity of the intracellular potential. Energy for the pump is provided by a common source of cellular energy, adenosine triphosphate (ATP) produced by mitochondria in the cell.

Thus the factors influencing the flow of ions across the membrane are (1) diffusion gradients, (2) the inwardly directed electric field, (3) membrane structure (availability of pores), and (4) active transport of ions against an established electrochemical gradient. The charge separated by the cell membrane and the structure of this membrane ($P_K, P_{Na}, P_{Cl}$) account for the resting potential. $K^+$ diffuses outwardly according to its concentration gradient, whereas the nondiffusible organic anion component remains within the cell, creating a potential difference across the membrane. Electroneutrality is maintained within the bulk internal and external media, but due to the membrane capacitance, there is a monolayer of cations distributed on the outer membrane surface and a monolayer of anions along the inner surface. The number of ions responsible for the membrane potential, however, is very small relative to the total number present in the bulk media. The $Na^+$ influx does not compensate for the $K^+$ efflux because, in the resting state, $P_{Na} \ll P_K$. Chloride ion diffuses inward down its concentration gradient, but its movement is balanced by the electrical gradient.

**EXAMPLE 4.2** The giant axon of the squid is frequently used in electrophysiological investigations because of its size. Typically it has a diameter of 1000 μm, a membrane thickness of 7.5 nm, a specific membrane capacity of 1 μF/cm², and a resting transmembrane potential $v_m$ of 70 mV. Assume a uniform field within the membrane and calculate the magnitude and direction of the electric field intensity **E** within the membrane.

**ANSWER** The membrane is quite thin, serves as a charge separator, and can be represented by a parallel-plate capacitor with **E** directed inward.

$$\mathbf{E} = \frac{v_m}{d} = \frac{70 \times 10^{-3}}{7.5 \times 10^{-9}} = 9.33 \times 10^6 \text{ V/m}$$

## THE ACTIVE STATE

Another property of an excitable cell is its ability to conduct an action potential [Figure 4.1(b)] when adequately stimulated. An *adequate stimulus* is one that brings about the depolarization of a cell membrane that is sufficient to exceed its threshold potential and thereby elicit an all-or-none action potential (brief transient disturbance of the membrane potential), which travels in an unattenuated fashion and at a constant conduction velocity along the membrane. Because of the steady resting potential, the cell membrane is said to be *polarized*. A lessening of the magnitude of this polarization is called *depolarization*, whereas an increase in magnitude is referred to as *hyperpolarization*. The all-or-none property of the action potential means that the membrane potential goes through a very characteristic cycle: a change in potential from the resting level of a certain amount for a fixed duration of time. For a nerve fiber, $\Delta v \cong 120$ mV and the duration is approximately 1 ms. Further increases in intensity or duration of stimulus beyond that required for exceeding the threshold level produce only the same result.

The origin of the action potential lies in the voltage- and time-dependent nature of the membrane permeabilities (or equivalently, in electrical terms, membrane conductivities) to specific ions, notably $Na^+$ and $K^+$. As the *transmembrane potential* ($v_m$) is depolarized, the membrane permeability to sodium $P_{Na}$ (or, equivalently, the conductance of the membrane to sodium $g_{Na}$) is significantly increased. As a result, $Na^+$ rushes into the internal medium of the cell, bringing about further depolarization, which in turn brings about a further increase in $g_{Na}$ (i.e., $g_{Na}$ is dependent on transmembrane potential). If the membrane potential threshold is exceeded, this process is self-regenerative

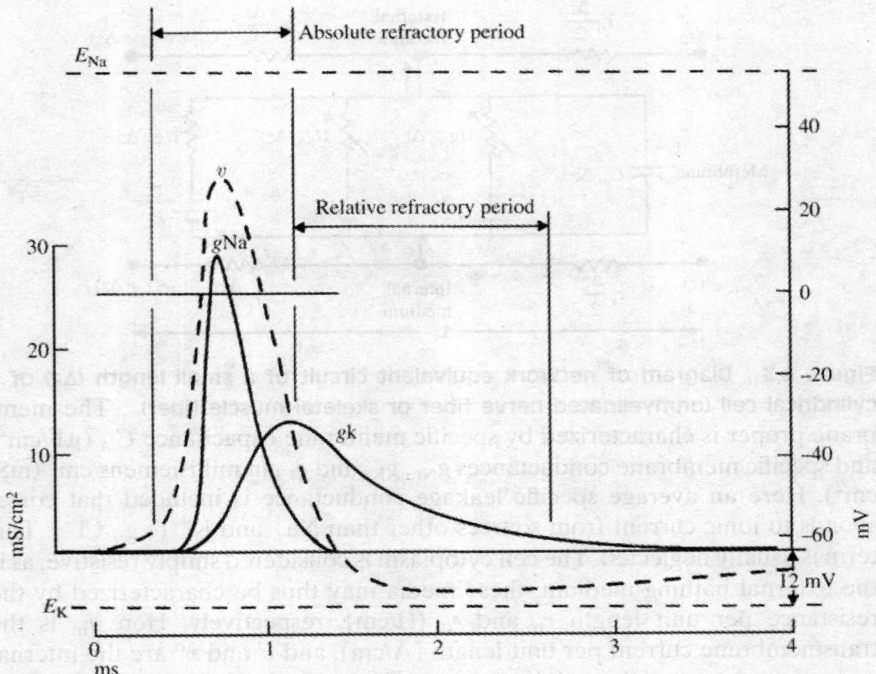


**Figure 4.2** Model-generated transmembrane potential ($v_m$) and membrane ionic conductance changes for sodium ($g_{Na}$) and potassium ($g_K$) during the action potential. These waveforms are obtained by solving the differential equations developed by Hodgkin and Huxley for the giant axon of the squid at a bathing medium temperature of 18.5 °C. $E_{Na}$ and $E_K$ are the Nernst *equilibrium potentials* for $Na^+$ and $K^+$ across the membrane. (Modified from A. L. Hodgkin and A. F. Huxley, "A quantitative description of membrane current and its application to conduction and excitation in nerve." *Journal of Physiology,* 1952, 117, 530.)

and leads to *runaway* depolarization. Under these conditions, $v_m$ tends to approach the equilibrium Nernst potential of sodium, $E_{Na}$, which has a value of about +60 mV.

However, $v_m$ never achieves this level because of two factors: (1) $g_{Na}$ is not only voltage dependent but also time dependent, and (as shown in Figure 4.2) it is relatively short-lived compared with the action potential. (2) There is a delayed increase in $g_K$ that acts as a hyperpolarizing influence, tending to restore $v_m$ to resting levels (Figure 4.2). As $v_m$ ultimately returns to the resting level, $g_K$ is still elevated with respect to its resting value and returns slowly along an exponential time course. Since $K^+$ continue to leave the cell during this time, the membrane hyperpolarizes and an undershoot is produced in the transmembrane potential waveform ($v_m$).

The calculated $g_{Na}$ and $g_K$ waveforms of Figure 4.2 are based on *voltage-clamp* data from squid axon. In voltage-clamp experiments, transmembrane potential $v_m$ is held at prescribed levels via a negative-feedback control circuit.

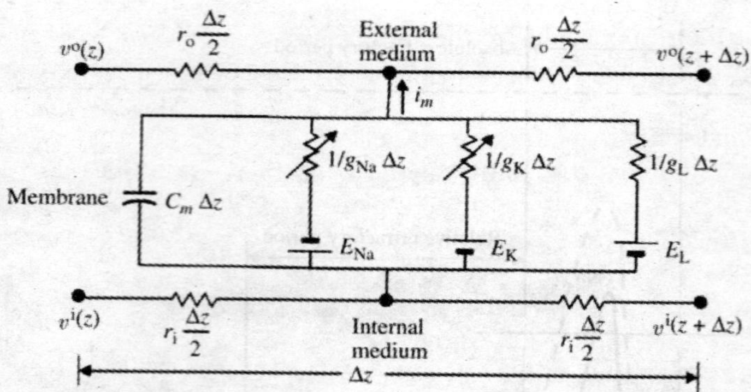


**Figure 4.3 Diagram of network equivalent circuit of a small length ($\Delta z$) of a cylindrical cell (unmyelinated nerve fiber or skeletal muscle fiber)** The membrane proper is characterized by specific membrane capacitance $C_m$ ($\mu F/cm^2$) and specific membrane conductances $g_{Na}$, $g_K$, and $g_{Cl}$ in millisiemens/cm$^2$ (mS/cm$^2$). Here an average specific leakage conductance is included that corresponds to ionic current from sources other than $Na^+$ and $K^+$ (e.g., $Cl^-$). This term is usually neglected. The cell cytoplasm is considered simply resistive, as is the external bathing medium; these media may thus be characterized by the resistance per unit length $r_i$, and $r_o$ ($\Omega$/cm), respectively. Here $i_m$ is the transmembrane current per unit length (A/cm), and $v^i$ and $v^o$ are the internal and external potentials at point $z$, respectively. Transmembrane potential at each point in $z$ is given by $v_m = v^i - v^o$. (Modified from A. L. Hodgkin and A. F. Huxley, "A quantitative description of membrane current and its application to conduction and excitation in nerve." *Journal of Physiology*, 1952, 117, 501.)

Membrane currents in response to step changes in $v_m$ are studied in order to determine the voltage- and time-dependent nature of $g_{Na}$ and $g_K$.

Figure 4.3 shows a network equivalent circuit describing the electrical behavior of a small unit area of membrane. The entire nerve axon membrane can be characterized in a distributed fashion by utilizing an iterative structure of this same basic form.

**EXAMPLE 4.3** Suppose that the electrical properties of an elongated excitable cell of cylindrical geometry (such as a nerve or skeletal muscle fiber) can be modeled fairly accurately with a distributed parameter "cable" model such as that of Figure 4.3. What should the temporal-membrane potential response to brief square pulses of stimulating current look like at some fixed distance from a particular stimulating electrode? As the separation distance between the particular stimulating electrode and the exploring micropipette is progressively increased, in what manner should the amplitude of the subthreshold response change?

**ANSWER** Figure 4.3 shows that each section of the distributed parameter model forms an *R–C* low-pass filter. Multiple sections form multiple low-pass filters. Thus the response due to the stimulating square-wave pulse is progressively smoothed and attenuated as the separation distance increases.

When an excitable membrane produces an action potential in response to an adequate stimulus, the ability of the membrane to respond to a second stimulus of any sort is markedly altered. During the initial portion of the action potential, the membrane cannot respond to any stimulus, no matter how intense. This interval is referred to as the *absolute refractory period*. It is followed by the *relative refractory period,* wherein an action potential can be elicited by an intense superthreshold stimulus (Figure 4.2). The existence of the refractory period produces an upper limit to the frequency at which an excitable cell may be repetitively discharged. For example, if a nerve axon has an absolute refractory period of 1 ms, it has an upper limit of repetitive discharge of less than 1000 impulses/s.

For an action potential propagating along a single unmyelinated nerve fiber, the region of the fiber undergoing a transition into the active state (the *active region*) at an instant of time is usually small relative to the length of the fiber. Figure 4.4(a) shows schematically the charge distribution along the fiber

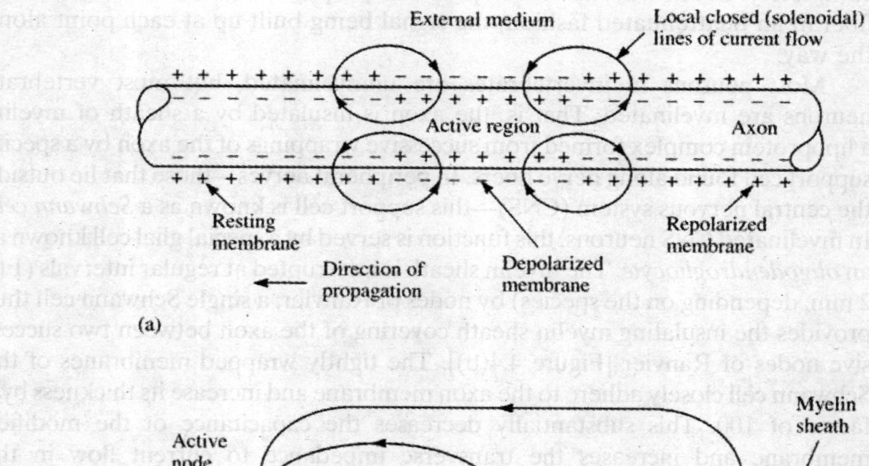


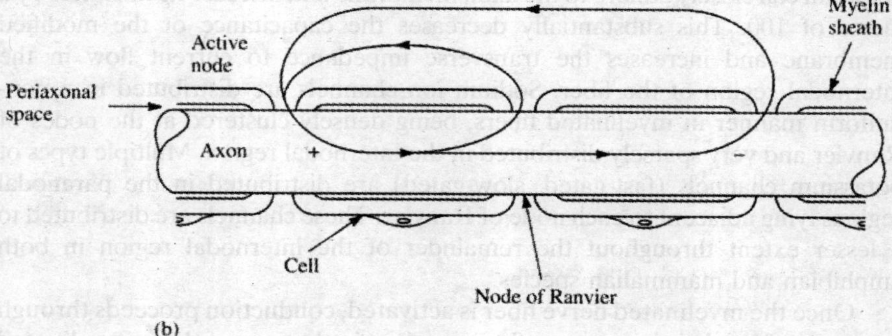


**Figure 4.4** (a) Charge distribution in the vicinity of the active region of an unmyelinated fiber conducting an impulse. (b) Local circuit current flow in the myelinated nerve fiber.

in the vicinity of the active region. Note that the direction of propagation of the action potential (considered frozen in time) is to the left, and the membrane lying ahead of the active region is polarized, as in the resting state. A reversal of polarity is shown within the active region because of depolarization of the membrane to positive values of potential. The membrane lying behind the active zone is repolarized membrane.

From the indicated charge distribution, *solenoidal* (closed-path) current flows in the pattern shown in Figure 4.4(a). In the region ahead of the active zone, the ohmic potential drop across the membrane caused by this solenoidal current flowing outward through the membrane is of such a polarity as to reduce the magnitude of $v_m$ i.e., depolarize the membrane. When $v_m$ is depolarized to the threshold level (about 20 mV more positive than the resting potential), this region becomes activated as well. The same current pattern flowing behind the active region is ineffective in re-exciting the membrane, which is in the refractory state. The nature of this process is therefore self-excitatory, each new increment of membrane being brought to the threshold level by lines of current from the active source region. The membrane stays in the active state for only a brief period of time and ultimately repolarizes completely. In this way, the action potential propagates down the length of the fiber in an unattenuated fashion, the signal being built up at each point along the way.

Most neurons in invertebrates are unmyelinated, but most vertebrate neurons are myelinated. That is, the axon is insulated by a sheath of myelin, a lipoprotein complex formed from successive wrappings of the axon by a special support cell found along nerve fibers. In peripheral nerves—those that lie outside the central nervous system (CNS)—this support cell is known as a *Schwann cell*. In myelinated CNS neurons, this function is served by a special glial cell known as an *oligodendrogliocyte*. The myelin sheath is interrupted at regular intervals (1 to 2 mm, depending on the species) by nodes of Ranvier; a single Schwann cell thus provides the insulating myelin sheath covering of the axon between two successive nodes of Ranvier [Figure 4.4(b)]. The tightly wrapped membranes of the Schwann cell closely adhere to the axon membrane and increase its thickness by a factor of 100. This substantially decreases the capacitance of the modified membrane and increases the transverse impedance to current flow in the internodal region of the fiber. Sodium ion channels are distributed in a non-uniform manner in myelinated fibers, being densely clustered at the nodes of Ranvier and very sparsely distributed in the internodal region. Multiple types of potassium channels (fast-gated, slow-gated) are distributed in the paranodal regions lying adjacent to each node of Ranvier. These channels are distributed to a lesser extent throughout the remainder of the internodal region in both amphibian and mammalian species.

Once the myelinated nerve fiber is activated, conduction proceeds through a process of local circuit current flow, much as in the case of the unmyelinated nerve fiber described earlier [Figure 4.4(a)]. There are differences, however, in that the sources for action current flow are localized at the nodes of Ranvier and are therefore not uniformly distributed along the axonal membrane, as in the case of the unmyelinated fiber. Myelination of the internode reduces leakage currents, decreases membrane capacitance, and improves the transmission properties of the cable-like myelinated fiber. Local circuit currents emanating from an active node have an exponentially diminishing magnitude over an axial distance spanning several internodal lengths. Accordingly, they contribute to a drop in nodal potential as current passes outward through a given inactive nodal membrane [Figure 4.4(b)].

Thus myelinated nerve fiber conduction proceeds via rapid, sequential activation of the nodes of Ranvier, and local circuit current provides the underlying mechanism for bringing the nodal membrane voltage to threshold. This process is frequently called *saltatory conduction* (from the Latin *saltare*, "to leap or dance"), because action potentials appear to leap from node to node. For an axon of a given diameter, myelination improves the conduction rate by a factor of approximately 20. By reason of its structure, the myelinated nerve fiber represents a more complicated bioelectric action current source than the unmyelinated nerve fiber. Mathematical modeling studies of conduction in both unmyelinated and myelinated nerve fibers have appeared in the literature (Moore *et al.*, 1978; Waxman and Brill, 1978; Halter and Clark, 1991; Moffit *et al.*, 2004).

## 4.2 VOLUME-CONDUCTOR FIELDS

A fundamental problem in electrophysiology is that of the single active cell immersed in a volume conductor (a salt solution simulating the composition of body fluids). A study of this simple problem lends considerable insight into other, more complex volume-conductor-field problems, including the ENG, EMG, and ECG.

The problem consists of two parts: (1) the bioelectric source and (2) its bathing medium or electrical load. The bioelectric source is the active cell, which behaves electrically as a constant-current source, delivering its solenoidal activation current to the resistive bathing medium over a large range of loading conditions. We consider the single active unmyelinated nerve fiber (bioelectric source) bathed by a volume conductor (specific resistivity $\rho$) whose dimensions are large relative to the spatial extent of the electric field surrounding the nerve fiber (infinite volume conductor). The lines of solenoidal current flow emanating from the active fiber into the bathing medium and returning to the fiber are indicated schematically in Figure 4.4(a). This pattern of current flow is consistent with the charge distribution shown in Figure 4.4(a).

We assume that the action potential travels down the fiber at a constant conduction velocity. Hence, the temporal waveform $v_m(t)$ can be converted easily to a spatial distribution $v_m(z)$, where $z$ is the axial distance along the fiber. For a simple monophasic action potential, the associated potential waveform at the outer surface of the membrane is (1) triphasic in nature,

(2) of greater spatial extent than the action potential, and (3) much smaller in peak-to-peak magnitude. The magnitude of the field potential in a large bathing medium falls off exponentially with increasing radial distance from the active fiber (potential zero within fifteen fiber radii). Field potential magnitude at the fiber surface depends on the amount of active cell membrane surface area (bioelectric source) contributing to the signal and is usually on the order of tens of microvolts (μV).

Changes in the properties of the volume conductor can also have an effect on the field potential magnitude. If its specific resistivity ($\rho$) is increased, the magnitude of the field potential measured at the outer membrane surface increases, as it would if the volume conductor is made smaller. In each case, the extracellular load resistance to current flow from the constant action current generator (membrane) is greater. From Ohm's law, potential is increased [by changing material properties of volume conductor ($\rho$) or its dimensions].

If instead, we consider the source to be an active nerve trunk with its thousands of component nerve fibers simultaneously activated, the extracellular field potential recorded in an infinite homogeneous bathing medium can appear quite similar to the triphasic response of the single fiber [Figure 4.5(b)].

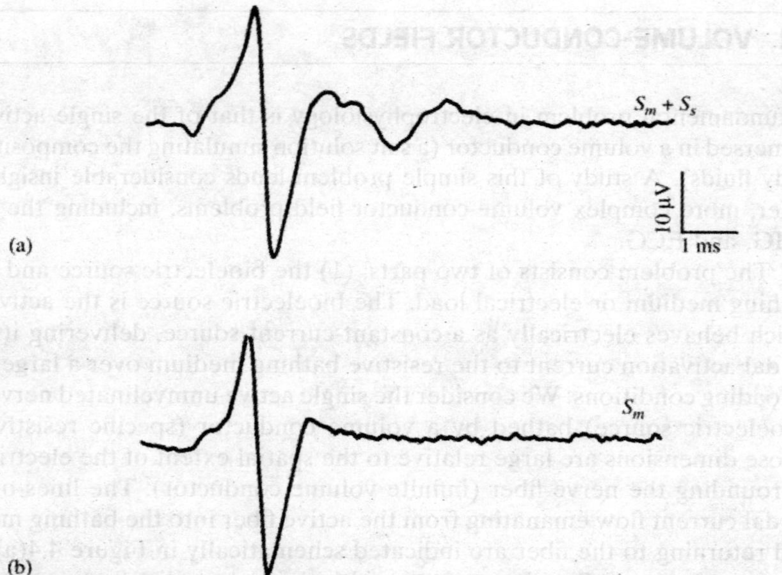


**Figure 4.5** Extracellular field potentials (average of 128 responses) were recorded at the surface of an active (1 mm-diameter) frog sciatic nerve in an extensive volume conductor. The potential was recorded with (a) both motor and sensory components excited ($S_m + S_s$), (b) only motor nerve components excited ($S_m$), and (c) only sensory nerve components excited ($S_s$).

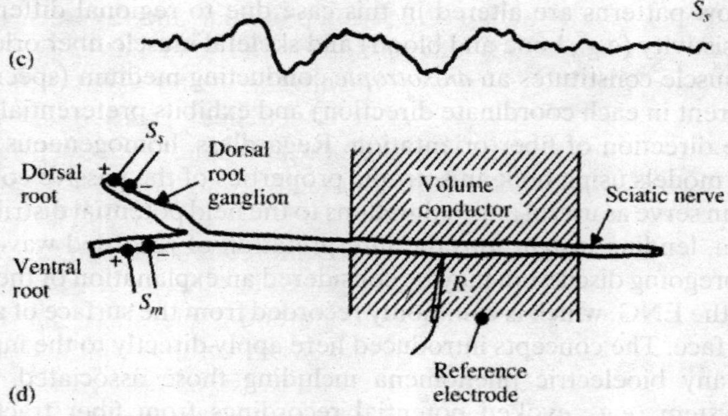


**Figure 4.5** (*Continued*)

Here, the extracellular field potential is formed from the superimposed electric fields of individual active fibers within the nerve trunk. The extracellular potential recorded at a field point in the volume conductor is triphasic, low-microvolt range in amplitude, and it diminishes in amplitude and high-frequency content as field point is moved to larger radial distances from the surface of the trunk. The frog sciatic nerve utilized in this experiment is a rather complex bioelectric source, consisting of large diameter motor fibers running from the spinal cord to the leg muscles, as well as large and small sensory fibers running from sensory receptors in the leg and skin to the spinal cord. In Figure 4.5(a), the entire nerve trunk (containing both motor and sensory fibers of different diameters) was simultaneously excited by a brief suprathreshold electric stimulus.

It is possible, however, to excite the motor and sensory components of the trunk separately by isolating the nerve trunk in the vicinity of the spinal cord. Here the nerve trunk divides into a sensory branch (the *dorsal root*) and a motor branch (the *ventral root*). The results of separate motor and sensory stimulation are shown in Figure 4.5(b) and (c). Stimulation of the many large-diameter motor fibers in the trunk provides the largest extracellular response (largest active membrane surface area), whereas stimulation of the sensory root excites at least two groups of sensory fibers—a group of larger, fast conducting fibers (group I) and a group of smaller, slower fibers (group II). Observing the extracellular waveform produced by combined stimulation [Figure 4.5(a)], we can see the approximate superposition of motor and sensory responses.

The volume-conductor load of the active nerve trunk can also be altered and made more complicated. A relatively simple variation is to increase the $\rho$ of the bathing medium or decrease the radial extent of the volume conductor, or both. These alterations produce larger extracellular potentials due to the constant nature of the bioelectric current source. Ultimately, the volume-conductor load can consist of a nonhomogeneous multilayered conducting medium containing skeletal muscle, blood vessels and bone (leg or arm).

Current flow patterns are altered in this case due to regional differences in specific resistivity (e.g., bone and blood) and skeletal muscle fiber orientation. Skeletal muscle constitutes an *anisotropic* conducting medium (specific resistivity different in each coordinate direction) and exhibits preferential conduction in the direction of fiber orientation. Regardless, homogeneous volume-conductor models using bulk anisotropic properties of the passive conducting medium can serve as useful approximations to the field potential distribution in such media, lending insight into the interpretation of recorded waveforms.

The foregoing discussion may be considered an explanation of the electrogenesis of the ENG, which is commonly recorded from the surface of an arm, a leg, or the face. The concepts introduced here apply directly to the interpretation of many bioelectric phenomena including those associated with the nervous system (e.g., evoked potential recordings from fiber tracts in the spinal cord and sensory centers in the brain), as well as active skeletal muscle (EMG), cardiac muscle (ECG), and smooth muscle (EGG).

## 4.3 FUNCTIONAL ORGANIZATION OF THE PERIPHERAL NERVOUS SYSTEM

### THE REFLEX ARC

The spinal nervous system is functionally organized on the basis of what is commonly called the *reflex arc* [Figure 4.6(a)]. The components of this arc are as follows:

1. A *sense organ,* consisting of many individual sense receptors that respond preferentially to an environmental stimulus of a particular kind, such as pressure, temperature, touch, or pain.
2. A *sensory nerve,* containing many individual nerve fibers that perform the task of transmitting information (encoded in the form of action potential frequency) from a peripheral sense receptor to other cells lying within the central system (brain and spinal cord).
3. The CNS, which in this case serves as a central integrating station. Here information is evaluated, and, if warranted, a "motor" decision is implemented. That is, action potentials are initiated in motor-nerve fibers associated with the motor-nerve trunk.
4. A *motor nerve,* serving as a communication link between the CNS and peripheral muscle.
5. The *effector organ,* which consists, in this case, of skeletal muscle fibers that contract (shorten) in response to the driving stimuli (action potentials) conducted by motor-nerve fibers.

The simplest example of the behavior of the reflex arc is the knee-jerk reflex, in which the patellar tendon below the knee is given a slight tap that stretches

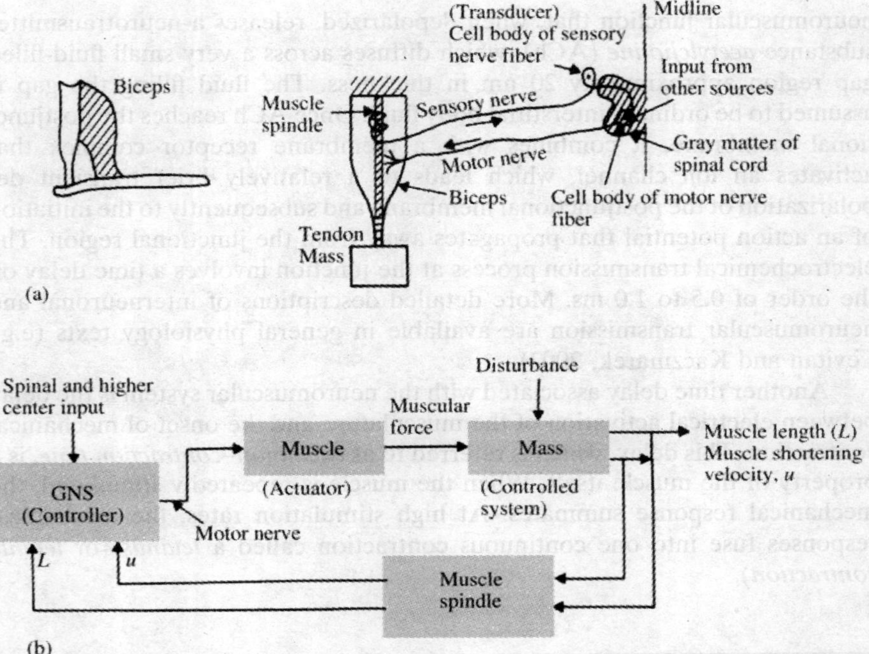


**Figure 4.6 Schematic diagram of a muscle-length control system for a peripheral muscle (biceps)** (a) anatomical diagram of limb system, showing interconnections and (b) block diagram of control system.

specialized length receptors, called *muscle spindles,* within the muscle and subsequently excites them. This excitation results in action potentials that propagate along the sensory nerve that enters the spinal cord and communicates with CNS cells, specifically motoneurons. The resultant motor activity reflexly brings about contraction of the muscle that was initially stimulated, and the shortening muscle jerks the limb, producing the well-known knee-jerk response. Note that the initial stimulus to the muscle was a stretch, whereas the response was a contraction of the muscle. This simple reflex arc has many of the features of a negative-feedback loop, in which the control variable is muscle length [Figure 4.6(b)]. The CNS acts as the controller, the muscle spindle as a feedback length sensor, and the muscle–limb system as the process to be controlled.

## JUNCTIONAL TRANSMISSION

Within the reflex arc there are intercommunicating links between neurons (neuro–neuro junctions) called *synapses*, as well as communicating links between neurons and muscle fibers called *neuromuscular junctions*. These occur at small, specialized regions of the muscle fiber referred to as an *end-plate regions.* The junctional transmission process in each of these cases is electrochemical in nature. There is a prejunctional fiber involved in the neuromuscular junction that, when depolarized, releases a neurotransmitter substance *acetylcholine* (ACh), which diffuses across a very small fluid-filled gap region approximately 20 nm in thickness. The fluid filling the gap is assumed to be ordinary interstitial body fluid. Once ACh reaches the postjunctional membrane, it combines with a membrane receptor complex that activates an ion channel, which leads to a relatively brief transient depolarization of the postjunctional membrane and subsequently to the initiation of an action potential that propagates away from the junctional region. The electrochemical transmission process at the junction involves a time delay on the order of 0.5 to 1.0 ms. More detailed descriptions of interneuronal and neuromuscular transmission are available in general physiology texts (e.g., Levitan and Kaczmarek, 2002).

Another time delay associated with the neuromuscular system is the delay between electrical activation of the musculature and the onset of mechanical contraction. This delay, which is referred to as *excitation–contraction time*, is a property of the muscle itself. When the muscle is repeatedly stimulated, the mechanical response summates. At high stimulation rates, the mechanical responses fuse into one continuous contraction called a *tetanus* (or *tetanic contraction*).

## 4.4 THE ELECTRONEUROGRAM

Conduction velocity in a peripheral nerve is measured by stimulating a motor nerve at two points a known distance apart along its course. Subtraction of the shorter latency from the longer latency (Figure 4.7) gives the conduction time

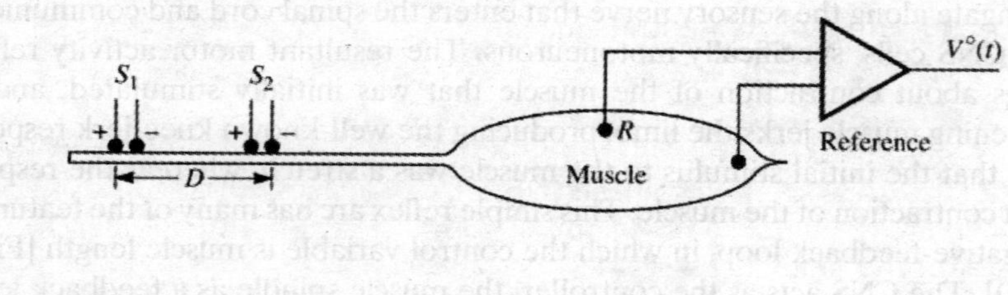


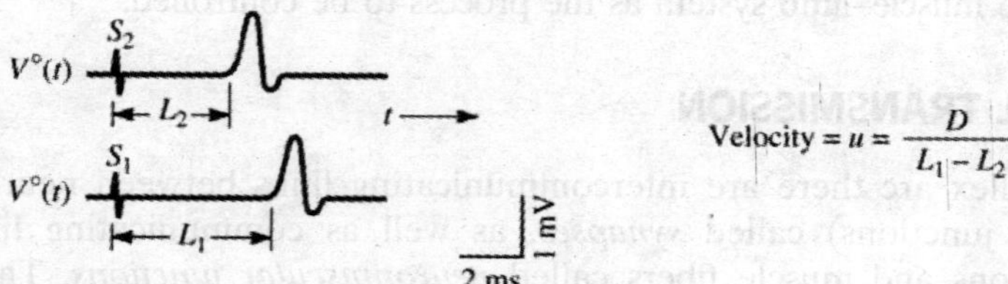


**Figure 4.7** Measurement of neural conduction velocity via measurement of latency of evoked electrical response in muscle. The nerve was stimulated at two different sites a known distance $D$ apart.

along the segment of nerve between the stimulating electrodes. Knowing the separation distance, we can determine the conduction velocity of the nerve, which has potential clinical value since, e.g., conduction velocity in a regenerating nerve fiber is slowed following nerve injury (Sinkjaer *et al.*, 2006).

Skeletal muscle fibers (70 μm diameter) are much larger than myelinated nerve fibers (2 to 20 μm); hence the amplitude of field potentials recorded from active nerve trunks are much smaller than field potentials recorded from groups of active muscle fibers (larger active membrane surface area). Such potentials can be recorded with either concentric needle electrodes or surface electrodes (Chap. 5). Nerve field potentials can also be evoked by applying stimuli to "mixed" nerves that contain both motor and sensory components (such as the ulnar nerve of the arm), in which case the resultant field potentials are derived from both types of active fibers. However, field potentials can also be elicited from purely sensory nerves (e.g., the sural nerve in the leg) or from sensory components of a mixed nerve, wherein stimulation is applied in a manner that does not excite the motor components of the nerve. In general, the study of evoked field potentials from sensory nerves has been shown to be of considerable value in diagnosing peripheral nerve disorders.

Although measurements of conduction velocity and latency are most useful in the assessment of peripheral nerve function, the characteristics of the field potentials evoked in muscle, as stimulated by its active motor nerve, are also important. When considering evoked muscle potentials, the duration of the response is frequently of interest, since slowed conduction in a few motor nerve fibers may lead to late activation of a portion of the muscle. The integrated field potential thus recorded may appear prolonged and polyphasic. If the component motor fibers of the muscle have a uniform conduction velocity, there will be a superposition of the recorded field potentials resulting in a larger amplitude, shorter duration triphasic response. Slowed conduction in some of the motor fibers may lead to partial fractionation of the integrated field potential waveform with a decrease in its magnitude and a broadening of its duration.

## FIELD POTENTIALS OF SENSORY NERVES

Extracellular field responses from sensory nerves can be easily measured from the median or ulnar nerves of the arm by using ring-stimulating electrodes applied to the fingers (Figure 4.8). Recording at two sites a known distance apart along the course of the nerve enables one to compute the conduction velocity of the sensory nerve. In the case of the ulnar nerve (roughly, it supplies the third and fourth fingers), evoked neural potentials can be recorded from different sites along the course of the nerve as high as the armpit. In the case of the median nerve (roughly, it supplies the index and the second fingers), field potentials can be recorded from the nerve at and above the elbow.

Long pulses cause muscle contractions, limb movement, and undesired signals (*artifacts*). These are avoided by positioning the limb in a comfortable, relaxed posture and applying a brief, intense stimulus (square pulse of approximately 100 V amplitude with a duration of 100 to 300 μs). Such a

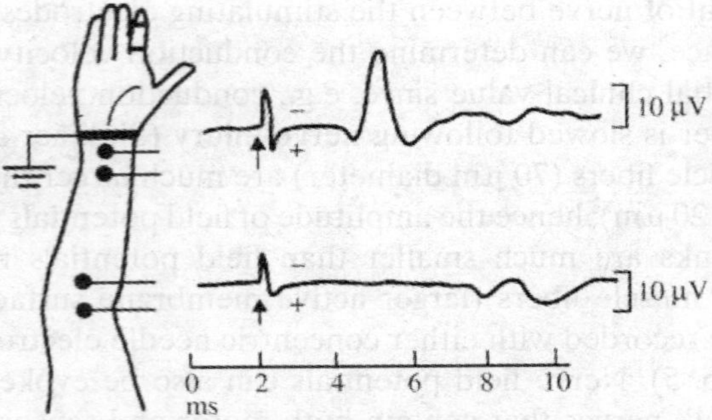


**Figure 4.8** Sensory nerve action potentials evoked from median nerve of a healthy subject at elbow and wrist after stimulation of index finger with ring electrodes. The potential at the wrist is triphasic and of much larger magnitude than the delayed potential recorded at the elbow. Considering the median nerve to be of the same size and shape at the elbow as at the wrist, we find that the difference in magnitude and waveshape of the potentials is due to the size of the volume conductor at each location and the radial distance of the measurement point from the neural source. (From J. A. R. Lenman and A. E. Ritchie, *Clinical Electromyography,* 2nd ed., Philadelphia: Lippincott, 1977. Reproduced by permission of the authors.)

stimulus excites the large, rapidly conducting sensory nerve fibers but not small pain fibers or surrounding muscle. To minimize artifacts caused by stimuli, we use a stimulus isolation unit (isolation transformer, diode-bridge circuit, optical coupler, and so on) to isolate the bipolar stimulating electrodes from ground. A patient ground is placed at the wrist between the stimulating and recording electrodes to provide a ground point for the passive electric field coupling from the stimulating electrodes. The skin should be abraded under both the stimulating and recording electrodes (Section 5.5) to reduce skin resistance and ensure good contact.

Clinically, field potentials are recorded using high-gain, high-input-impedance differential preamplifiers with good common-mode rejection capability and low inherent amplifier noise (Section 6.5). Figure 4.8 shows that the measured ENGs are on the order of 10 μV, and power-line interference is sometimes a problem even with good amplifier common-mode properties. The input leads should be properly twisted together and shielded. In addition, if warranted, the subject could be placed in an adequately shielded room or cage.

A further step we can use to enhance the signal-to-noise ratio in the presence of random noise (for the most part generated by the amplifier) is to use a *signal averager* (Section 6.8).

## MOTOR-NERVE CONDUCTION VELOCITY

*In vivo* measurement of the conduction velocity of a motor nerve may be obtained as shown in Figure 4.7. For example, the peroneal nerve of the left leg may be stimulated first behind the knee and second behind the ankle. A muscular response is obtained from the side of the foot, using surface or needle electrodes.

## REFLEXLY EVOKED FIELD POTENTIALS

When a peripheral nerve is stimulated and an evoked field potential is recorded in the muscle it supplies, it is sometimes possible to record a second potential that occurs later than the initial response. As the neural stimulus site is brought progressively closer to the muscle, the latency of the first response decreases, whereas the latency of the second response is increased. This behavior of the second response indicates that to activate the muscle, the stimulus must travel along the nerve toward the central nervous system (proximally) for some distance before ultimately traveling in the opposite direction (distally). The latency of the second response is such that the activity could have traveled proximally along sensory nerves as far as the spinal cord to elicit a spinal reflex.

If the posterior tibial nerve in the leg is stimulated, a late potential can be evoked from the triceps sural muscle (Figure 4.9). This long latency response has a low threshold and appears at stimulus intensities that are well below the levels required to elicit the conventional (short-latency) *M wave*. This long-latency potential—known as the *H* wave—was discovered by Hoffman (Figure 4.9). Its latency indicates that it is a spinal reflex. It is, in fact, the electrical homolog of the simple "ankle-jerk" reflex.

Thus, when a mixed peripheral nerve such as the posterior tibial nerve is stimulated by a stimulus of low intensity, only fibers of large diameter are stimulated because they have the lowest threshold. These large fibers are sensory

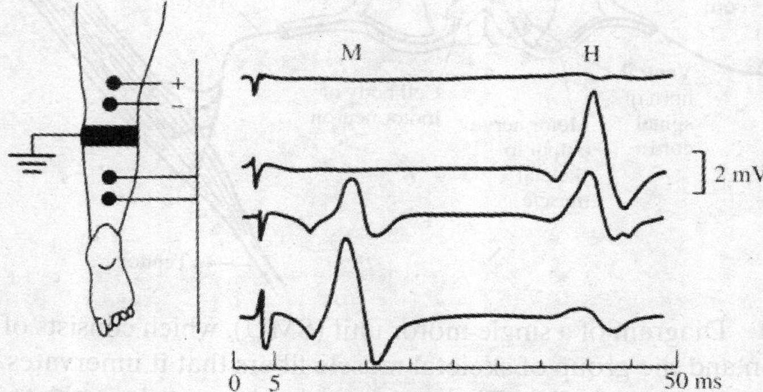


**Figure 4.9 The H reflex** The four traces show potentials evoked by stimulation of the medial popliteal nerve with pulses of increasing magnitude (the stimulus artifact increases with stimulus magnitude). The later potential or H wave is a low-threshold response, maximally evoked by a stimulus too weak to evoke the muscular response (M wave). As the M wave increases in magnitude, the H wave diminishes. (From J. A. R. Lenman and A. E. Ritchie, *Clinical Electromyography*, 2nd ed., Philadelphia: Lippincott, 1977; reproduced by permission of the authors.)

fibers from muscle spindles that conduct toward the CNS and ultimately connect with motor fibers in the spinal cord via a single synapse. The motoneurons discharge and produce a response in the gastrocnemius muscle of the leg (the H wave). With a stimulus of medium intensity, smaller motor fibers in the mixed nerve are stimulated in addition to the sensory fibers, producing a direct, short-latency muscle response, the M wave (Figure 4.9). With still stronger stimuli, impulses conducted centrally along the motor fibers may interfere with the production of the H wave (these excited motor fibers are in their refractory period) so that only an M wave is produced (Figure 4.9). The amplitude of the H response depends on the number of motoneurons discharged. Its amplitude is also somewhat variable as a result of fluctuating background neural conditions within the spinal cord. These neural disturbances are provided by the activity of other spinal and higher center neurons impinging on the motoneuron(s) involved in the reflex.

## 4.5 THE ELECTROMYOGRAM

Skeletal muscle is organized functionally on the basis of the *motor unit* (see Figure 4.10), which consists of a single motor nerve fiber and the bundle of

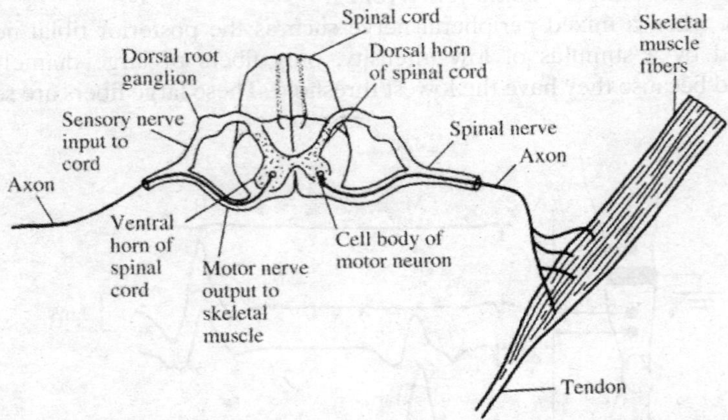


**Figure 4.10** Diagram of a single motor unit (SMU), which consists of a single motoneuron and the group of skeletal muscle fibers that it innervates. Length transducers [muscle spindles, Figure 4.6(a)] in the muscle activate sensory nerve fibers whose cell bodies are located in the dorsal root ganglion. These bipolar neurons send axonal projections to the spinal cord that divide into a descending and an ascending branch. The descending branch enters into a simple reflex arc with the motor neuron, whereas the ascending branch conveys information regarding current muscle length to higher centers in the CNS via ascending nerve fiber tracts in the spinal cord and brain stem. These ascending pathways are discussed in Section 4.8.

muscle fibers to which it is attached. The motor unit is the smallest unit that can be activated by a volitional effort, in which case all constituent muscle fibers are activated synchronously. The component fibers of the motor unit extend lengthwise in loose bundles along the muscle. In cross section, however, the fibers of a given motor unit are interspersed with fibers of other motor units. Thus, the active muscle fibers of the *single motor unit* (SMU) constitute a distributed bioelectric source located in a volume conductor that consists of all other fibers within the muscle (active and inactive), blood vessels and connective tissue. The evoked field potential from the active fibers of an SMU has a triphasic form of brief duration (3 to 15 ms) and an amplitude of 20 to 2000 $\mu$V, depending on the size of the motor unit. The frequency of discharge usually varies from 6 to 30 per second (De Luca, 2006).

One of the disadvantages of recording the EMG by using the convenient surface electrodes is that they can be used only with superficial muscles and are sensitive to electrical activity over too wide an area. Various types of monopolar, bipolar, and multipolar insertion-type electrodes are commonly used in electromyography for recording from deep muscles and from SMUs. These types of electrodes generally record local activity from small regions within the muscle in which they are inserted. Often a simple fine-tipped monopolar needle electrode can be used to record SMU field potentials even during powerful voluntary contractions. Bipolar recordings are also employed. Various types of electrodes are discussed in Chapter 5.

Figure 4.11 shows motor unit potentials from the normal dorsal interosseus muscle under graded levels of contraction. At high levels of effort, many superimposed motor unit responses give rise to a complicated response (the *interference pattern*) in which individual units can no longer be distinguished. In interpreting Figure 4.11, note that when a muscle contracts progressively under volition, active motor units increase their rate of firing and new (previously inactive) motor units are also recruited.

The shape of SMU potentials is considerably modified by disease. In peripheral neuropathies, partial denervation of the muscle frequently occurs and is followed by regeneration. Regenerating nerve fibers conduct more slowly than healthy axons. In addition, in many forms of peripheral neuropathy, the excitability of the neurons is changed and there is widespread slowing of nerve conduction. One effect of this is that neural impulses are more difficult to initiate and take longer in transit to the muscle, generally causing scatter or desynchronization in the EMG pattern.

A number of mathematical modeling studies of single-fiber and multiple-fiber (single motor unit) action potentials have appeared in the literature (Nandedkar *et al.,* 1985; Ganapathy *et al.,* 1987), as well as detailed volume-conductor-based simulations of surface EMG signals (Duchêne and Hogrel, 2000; Farina *et al.*, 2004). Signal processing methods have been

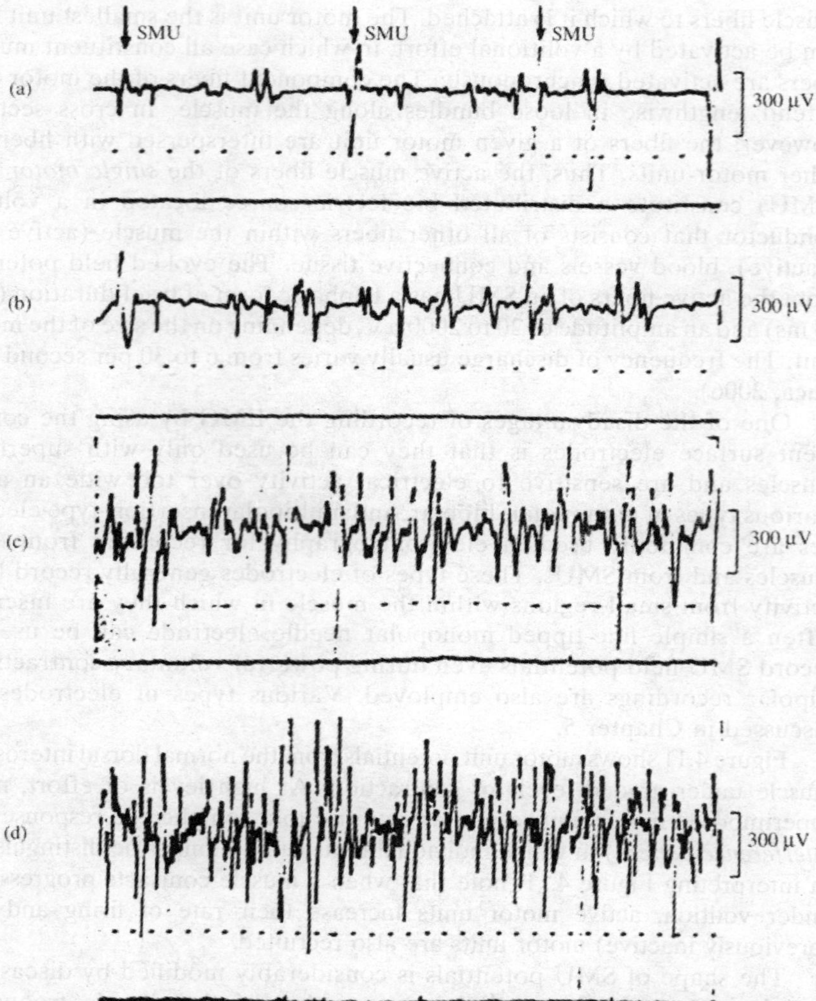


**Figure 4.11** Motor unit action potentials from normal dorsal interosseus muscle during progressively more powerful contractions. (c) In the interference pattern, individual units can no longer be clearly distinguished. (d) Interference pattern during very strong muscular contraction. Time scale is 10 ms per dot. (From J. A. R. Lenman and A. E. Ritchie, *Clinical Electromyography,* 2nd ed., Philadelphia: Lippincott, 1977; reproduced by permission of the authors.)

employed in the analysis of surface EMGs and SMU signals (Reucher *et al*., 1987; Farina *et al*., 2003), as have automatic techniques for the detection, decomposition, and analysis of EMG signals (Mambrito and De Luca, 1984; Stashuk 2001).

## 4.6 THE ELECTROCARDIOGRAM

### ANATOMY AND FUNCTION OF THE HEART

The heart serves as a four-chambered pump for the circulatory system (Figure 4.12). Its main pumping function is supplied by the ventricles. The atria are merely antechambers to store blood during the time the ventricles are pumping. The resting or filling phase of the heart cycle is referred to as *diastole,* whereas the contractile or pumping phase is called *systole.* The smooth, rhythmic contraction of the atria and ventricles has an underlying electrical precursor in the form of a well-coordinated series of electrical events that takes place within the heart. That this set of electrical events is intrinsic to the heart itself is well demonstrated when the heart (particularly that of cold-blooded vertebrates such as the frog or turtle) is removed from the body and placed in a nutrient medium (such as glucose-Ringer solution). The heart continues to beat rhythmically for many hours. Thus, the coordinated contraction of the atria and ventricles is set up by a specific pattern of electrical activation in the musculature of these structures. In humans, these electrical activation patterns in the walls of the atria and ventricles are initiated by a coordinated series of events within the *specialized conduction system* of the heart (Figure 4.12).

In relation to the heart as a whole, the specialized conduction system is very small and constitutes only a minute portion of the total mass of the heart. The wall of the left ventricle (Figure 4.12) is 2.5 to 3.0 times as thick as the right ventricular wall, and the intraventricular septum is nearly as thick as the left ventricular wall. Thus, the major portion of the muscle mass of the ventricles consists of the free walls of the right and left ventricles and the septum. Considering the heart as a bioelectric source, the source strength at each instant can be expected to be directly related to the active muscle mass at that moment (i.e., to the number of active myocardial cells). Hence, the active free walls of the atria and ventricles and the interventricular septum can be considered the major action current sources responsible for the production of external field potentials recorded from the heart (e.g., recorded within the thoracic volume-conductor medium or at the surface of the body).

### ELECTRICAL BEHAVIOR OF CARDIAC CELLS

The heart comprises several different types of tissues (SA and AV nodal tissue; atrial, Purkinje, and ventricular tissue). Representative cells of each type of tissue differ anatomically to a considerable degree. They are all electrically excitable, and each type of cell exhibits its own characteristic action potential (Figure 4.13).

### THE VENTRICULAR CELL

The ventricular myocardium is composed of millions of individual cardiac cells ($15 \times 15 \times 150\ \mu m$ long). Figure 4.14 is a drawing of a small section of cardiac muscle as seen under light microscopy. The individual cells are relatively long

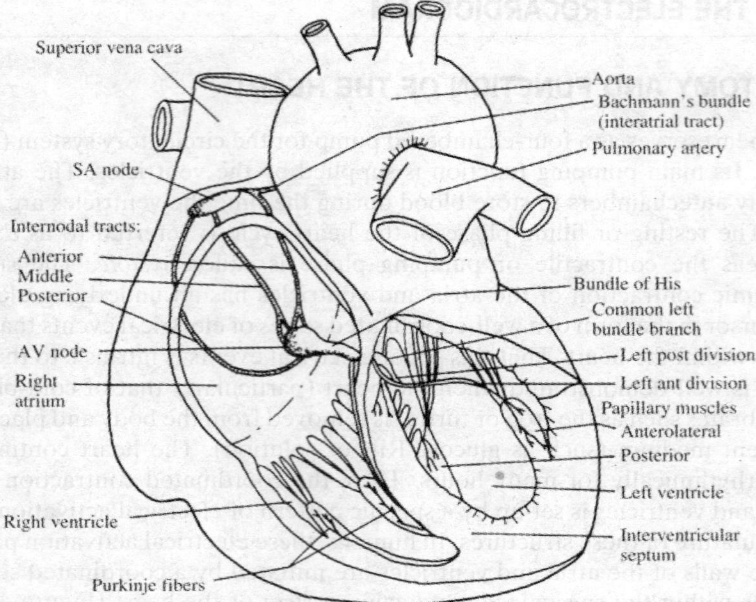


**Figure 4.12 Distribution of specialized conductive tissues in the atria and ventricles, showing the impulse-forming and conduction system of the heart** The rhythmic cardiac impulse originates in pacemaking cells in the sinoatrial (SA) node, located at the junction of the superior vena cava and the right atrium. Note the three specialized pathways (anterior, middle, and posterior internodal tracts) between the SA and atrioventricular (AV) nodes. Bachmann's bundle (interatrial tract) comes off the anterior internodal tract leading to the left atrium. The impulse passes from the SA node in an organized manner through specialized conducting tracts in the atria to activate first the right and then the left atrium. Passage of the impulse is delayed at the AV node before it continues into the bundle of His, the right bundle branch, the common left bundle branch, the anterior and posterior divisions of the left bundle branch, and the Purkinje network. The right bundle branch runs along the right side of the interventricular septum to the apex of the right ventricle before it gives off significant branches. The left common bundle crosses to the left side of the septum and splits into the anterior division (which is thin and long and goes under the aortic valve in the outflow tract to the anterolateral papillary muscle) and the posterior division (which is wide and short and goes to the posterior papillary muscle lying in the inflow tract). (From B. S. Lipman, E. Massie, and R. E. Kleiger, *Clinical Scalar Electrocardiography*. Copyright © 1972 by Yearbook Medical Publishers, Inc., Chicago. Used with permission.)

and thin, and although they run generally parallel to one another, there is considerable branching and interconnecting (*anastomosing*). The cells are surrounded by a plasma membrane that makes end-to-end contact with adjacent cells at a dense structure known as the *intercalated disk*

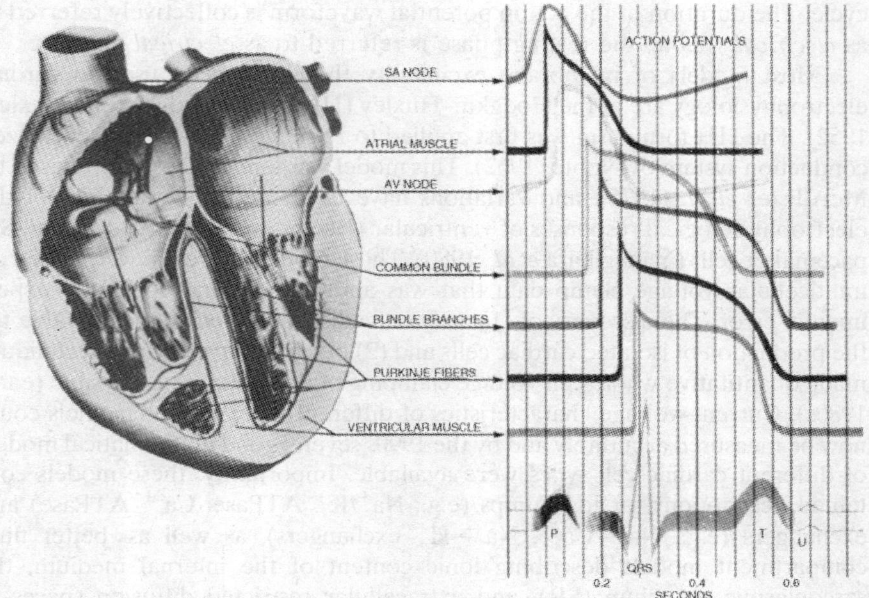


**Figure 4.13 Representative electric activity from various regions of the heart** The bottom trace is a scalar ECG, which has a typical QRS amplitude of 1 to 3 mV. (Copyright © 1969 CIBA Pharmaceutical Company, Division of CIBA-GEIGY Corp. Reproduced, with permission, from *The Ciba Collection of Medical Illustrations,* Frank H. Netter, M.D. All rights reserved.)

(Figure 4.14). Each fiber contains many contractile *myofibrils* that follow the axis of the cell from one end (intercalated disk) to the other. These myofibrils constitute the "contractile machinery" of the fiber. The component cells of cardiac tissue are in intimate contact at the intercalated disks, both electrically and mechanically, so the heart muscle functions as a unit (a *functional syncytium*).

Prior to excitation, the typical ventricular cell has a resting potential of approximately −85 mV. The initial rapid depolarization phase has a rate of rise that is usually greater than 150 V/s. This phase is followed by an initial rapid repolarization that leads to a maintained depolarizing plateau region lasting approximately 200 to 300 ms. A final repolarization phase restores membrane potential to the resting level and is maintained for the remainder of the cardiac

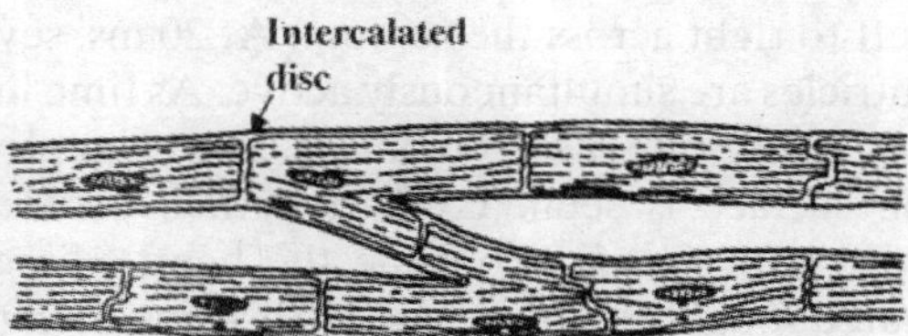


**Figure 4.14 The cellular architecture of myocardial fibers** Note the centroid nuclei and transverse intercalated disks between cells.

cycle. The duration of the action potential waveform is collectively referred to as *electrical systole;* the resting phase is referred to as *electrical diastole*.

Most models of membrane excitability that have been used in cardiac electrophysiology are of the Hodgkin–Huxley (HH) type (Hodgkin and Huxley, 1952). The HH formalism was first applied to Purkinje fibers of the specialized conduction system by Noble (1962). This model was later extensively revised by McAllister *et al.* (1975), and variations have been used in simulations of the electrophysiological responses of ventricular (Beeler and Reuter, 1977) and SA pacemaker cells (Yanagihara *et al.*, 1980). These models however, were based on multicellular voltage clamp data that was approximate and contained experimental error. The discovery of (1) enzymatic dispersion techniques suitable for the production of isolated cardiac cells and (2) patch clamp electrode techniques made quantitative whole-cell voltage clamping of individual cells possible (early 1980s). Current–voltage characteristics of different types of ion channels could now be measured accurately and by the 1990s several good mathematical models of different cardiac cell types were available. Importantly, these models contained descriptions for ion pumps (e.g., $Na^+/K^+$ ATPase, $Ca^{2+}$ ATPase) and exchangers (e.g., $Na^+-Ca^{2+}$, $Na^+-H^+$ exchangers), as well as, better fluid compartment models describing ionic content of the internal medium, the sarcoplasmic reticulum (SR), and extracellular restricted diffusion spaces in the intra- and extracellular media. The seminal model initiating these extensive changes in cardiac cell modeling was the Purkinje fiber model developed by DiFrancesco and Noble (1985). It still utilized some ion channel data derived from multicellular voltage clamp experiments, but nevertheless pointed the way to the development of modern day cardiac cell models for all cell types: SA node (Wilders *et al.*, 1991; Demir *et al.*, 1994); atrial cell (Nygren *et al.*, 1998); ventricular cell (Luo and Rudy, 1994; Puglisi and Bers, 2001).

## VENTRICULAR ACTIVATION

Investigators have conducted studies of ventricular activation on experimental animals using multiple "plunge-type" electrodes inserted into many sites in the heart (Spach *et al.*, 1972) (see Figure 4.15). The time of arrival of electrical activation is noted, and *isochronous* (synchronously excited) excitation surfaces can be mapped. Figure 4.15 shows a plot of isochronous lines of activation for the perfused heart of a human who died from a noncardiac condition. Note that activation first takes place on the septal surface of the left ventricle (5 ms into the QRS complex) and that the activity spreads with increasing time in a direction from left to right across the septum. At 20 ms, several regions of the right and left ventricles are simultaneously active. As time increases, excitation spreads and tends to become more confluent. For example, at 30 ms a nearly closed activation surface is seen. Excitation then proceeds in a relatively uniform fashion in an *epicardial* (outside the heart) direction. The apex of the heart is activated roughly in the period 30 to 40 ms, along with other sites on the right and left ventricular walls where "breakthrough" of activation has occurred. From both Figure 4.15 and data taken in other planes, we can see that the posterior-basal region of the heart is the last region activated.

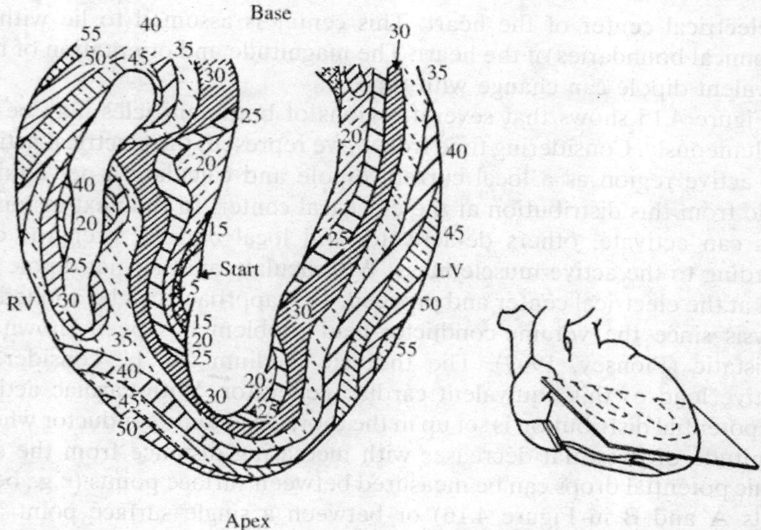


**Figure 4.15** **Isochronous lines of ventricular activation of the human heart** Note the nearly closed activation surface at 30 ms into the QRS complex. (Modified from "The Biophysical basis for electrocardiography," R. Plonsey. In *CRC Critical Reviews in Bioengineering,* 1(1), 1971, 5. © The Chemical Rubber Co., 1971. Used by permission of The Chemical Rubber Co. Based on data by D. Durrer, "Total excitation of the isolated human heart." *Circulation,* 41, 1970, 899–912, by permission of the American Heart Association, Inc.)

The isochronous electromotive surface propagates through the myocardium in an outward direction from the *endocardium* (the inside of the heart). The seat of this electromotive surface is, of course, the individual cardiac cell. In a localized region of the heart, however, many of these cells are active simultaneously because of the high degree of electrical interaction between cells. The anatomical substrate for this electrical interaction is the high degree of branching of individual cardiac cells and the low resistance of the intercalated disks at the junctions between cells (Barr *et al.*, 1965).

## BODY-SURFACE POTENTIALS

The preceding section dealt with the sequence of events involved in electrical activation of the ventricle. This activation sequence leads to the production of closed-line action currents that flow in the thoracic volume conductor (considered a purely passive medium containing no electric sources or sinks). Potentials measured at the outer surface of this medium—that is, on the body surface—are referred to as *electrocardiograms* (ECGs).

In the electrocardiographic problem, the heart is viewed as an electrical equivalent generator. A common assumption is that, at each instant of time in the sequence of ventricular activation, the electrical activity of the heart can be represented by a net equivalent current dipole located at a point that we call the electrical center of the heart. This center is assumed to lie within the anatomical boundaries of the heart. The magnitude and orientation of the net equivalent dipole can change with time.

Figure 4.15 shows that several regions of both ventricles may be active simultaneously. Considering time frozen, we represent the electrical activity of each active region as a local current dipole and calculate a net equivalent dipole from this distribution at the electrical center. In the next instant, new areas can activate, others de-activate, and local current strengths change according to the active muscle mass. We calculate another net dipole equivalent at the electrical center and proceed. This approach can be applied to the analysis since the volume-conductor-field problem has been shown to be quasistatic (Plonsey, 1969). The thoracic medium can be considered the resistive load of this equivalent cardiac generator. With cardiac activity, a field potential distribution is set up in the thoracic volume conductor where the magnitude of potential decreases with increasing distance from the source. Ohmic potential drops can be measured between surface points (e.g., between points A and B in Figure 4.16) or between a single surface point and an assigned reference point. The general volume-conductor problem is illustrated in a highly schematic fashion in Figure 4.16 in terms of current source and lumped resistive load.

A scalar "lead" gives the magnitude of a single body-surface potential difference plotted versus time. Figure 4.13 (bottom) shows a typical scalar electrocardiographic lead, where the significant features of the waveform are the (1) individual waves (P, Q, R, S, and T), (2) wave durations, and (3) specific time intervals (e.g., the P–R, S–T, and Q–T intervals). This figure also shows the temporal relationship between single transmembrane cellular activities in

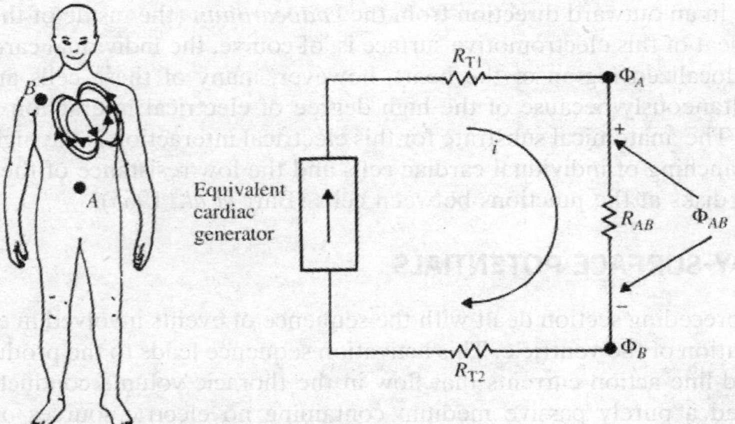


**Figure 4.16 The electrocardiographic problem** Points $A$ and $B$ are arbitrary observation points on the torso, $R_{AB}$ is the resistance between them, and $R_{T1}$, $R_{T2}$ are lumped thoracic medium resistances. The bipolar ECG scalar lead voltage $\Phi_{AB} = \Phi_A - \Phi_B$, where these voltages are both measured with respect to an indifferent reference potential.

various regions of the heart (atria, ventricles, and specialized conduction system) and this typical ECG waveform.

Clearly the P wave is produced by atrial depolarization, the QRS complex primarily by ventricular depolarization, and the T wave by ventricular repolarization. The manifestations of atrial repolarization are normally masked by the QRS complex. The P–R and S–T intervals are normally at zero potential, the P–R interval being caused mainly by conduction delay in the AV node. The S–T segment is related to the average duration of the plateau regions of individual ventricular cells. A small additional wave, called the U wave, is sometimes recorded temporally after the T wave. It is not always present and is believed to be the result of slow repolarization of ventricular papillary muscles.

Section 6.2 describes the 12 standard leads that constitute a diagnostic ECG, so they will not be considered further here.

## NORMAL AND ABNORMAL CARDIAC RHYTHMS

Each beat of the normal human heart originates in the SA node. The normal heart rate is approximately 70 beats per minute (bpm). The rate is slowed (*bradycardia*) during sleep and is accelerated (*tachycardia*) by emotion, exercise, fever, and many other stimuli. Detailed aspects of the control that the nervous system has over heart rate are beyond the scope of this book; the reader interested in further discussion is referred to Rowell (1993). Because many parts of the heart possess an inherent rhythmicity (e.g., nodal tissue, Purkinje fibers of the specialized conduction system, and atrial tissues), any part under abnormal conditions can become the dominant cardiac pacemaker. This can happen when the activity of the SA node is depressed, when the bundle of His is interrupted or damaged, or when an abnormal (ectopic) focus or site in the atria or in specialized conduction-system tissue in the ventricles discharges at a rate faster than the SA node.

When the bundle of His is interrupted completely, the ventricles beat at their own slow inherent rate (the *idioventricular rhythm*). The atria continue to beat independently at the normal sinus rate, and complete or third-degree block is said to occur [Figure 4.17(a)]. The idioventricular rate in human beings is approximately 30 to 45 bpm.

When the His bundle is not completely interrupted, incomplete heart block is present. In the case of *first-degree heart block*, all atrial impulses reach the ventricles, but the P–R interval is abnormally prolonged because of an increase in transmission time through the affected region [Figure 4.17(b)]. In the case of *second-degree heart block*, not all atrial impulses are conducted to the ventricles. There may be, for example, one ventricular beat every second or third atrial beat (2:1 block, 3:1 block, and so on).

In another form of incomplete heart block involving the AV node, the P–R interval progressively lengthens until the atrial impulse fails to conduct to the ventricle (*Wenckebach phenomenon*). The first conducted beat after the pause (or dropped beat) has a shorter P–R interval (sometimes of normal length) than any subsequent P–R interval. Then the process of the lengthening of the P–R interval begins anew, progressing over several cardiac cycles until another

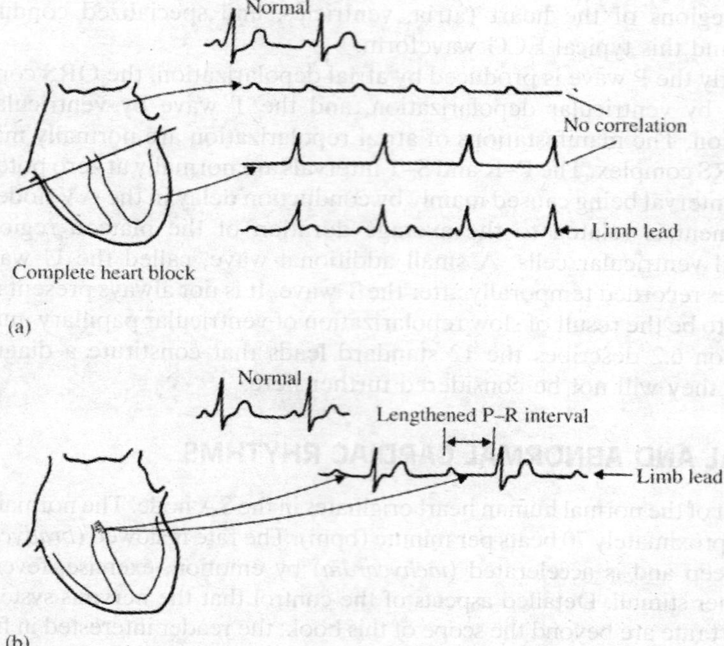


**Figure 4.17 Atrioventricular block** (a) Complete heart block. Cells in the AV node are dead and activity cannot pass from atria to ventricles. Atria and ventricles beat independently, ventricles being driven by an ectopic (other-than-normal) pacemaker. (b) AV block wherein the node is diseased (examples include rheumatic heart disease and viral infections of the heart). Although each wave from the atria reaches the ventricles, the AV nodal delay is greatly increased. This is first-degree heart block. (Adapted from Brendan Phibbs, The Human Heart, 3rd ed., St. Louis: The C.V. Mosby Company, 1975.)

beat is dropped. The electrocardiographic sequence starting with the ventricular pause and ending with the next blocked atrial beat constitutes a *Wenckebach period*. The ratio of the number of P waves to QRS complexes determines the block (for example, 6:5 or 5:4 Wenckebach periods).

When one branch of the bundle of His is interrupted, causing right- or left-bundle-branch block, excitation proceeds normally down the intact bundle and then sweeps back through the musculature to activate the ventricle on the blocked side. The ventricular rate is normal, but the QRS complexes are prolonged and deformed.

## ARRHYTHMIAS

A portion of the myocardium (or the AV node or specialized conduction system) sometimes becomes "irritable" and discharges independently. This site is then referred to as an *ectopic focus*. If the focus discharges only once, the result is a beat that occurs before the next expected normal beat, and the

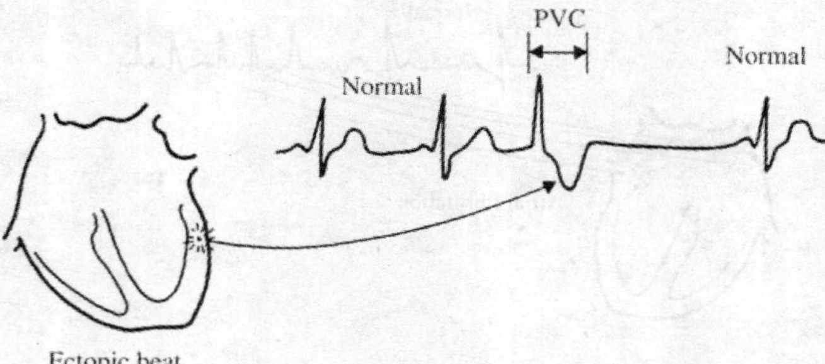


**Figure 4.18 Normal ECG followed by an ectopic beat** An irritable focus, or ectopic pacemaker, within the ventricle or specialized conduction system may discharge, producing an extra beat, or extrasystole, that interrupts the normal rhythm. This extrasystole is also referred to as a *premature ventricular contraction* (PVC). (Adapted from Brendan Phibbs, The Human Heart, 3rd ed., St. Louis: The C.V. Mosby Company, 1975.)

cardiac rhythm is therefore transiently interrupted. (With respect to atrial, nodal, or ventricular *ectopic beat*, see Figure 4.18.) If the focus discharges repetitively at a rate that exceeds that of the SA node, it produces rapid regular tachycardia. [With respect to atrial, nodal, or ventricular paroxysmal tachycardia or atrial flutter, see Figure 4.19(a) and (b).] A rapidly and irregularly discharging focus or, more likely, a group of foci in the atria or ventricles may

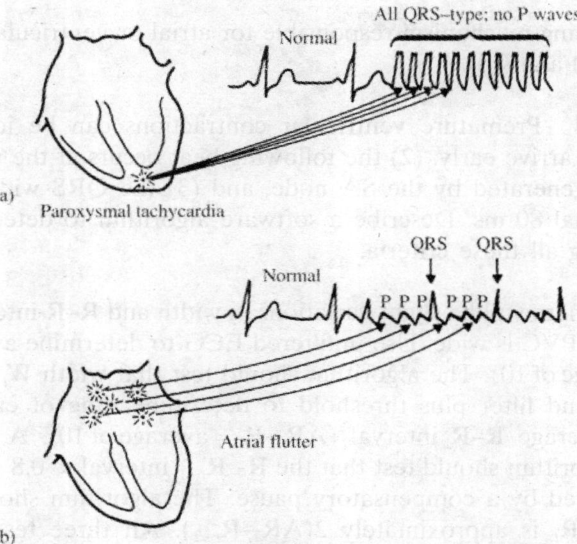


**Figure 4.19** (a) Paroxysmal tachycardia. An ectopic focus may repetitively discharge at a rapid regular rate for minutes, hours, or even days. (b) Atrial flutter. The atria begin a very rapid, perfectly regular "flapping" movement, beating at rates of 200 to 300 bpm. (Adapted from Brendan Phibbs, *The Human Heart*, 3rd ed., St. Louis: The C.V. Mosby Company, 1975.)

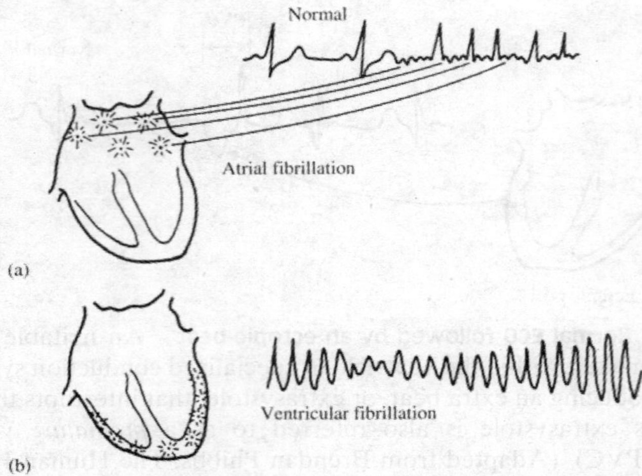


**Figure 4.20** (a) Atrial fibrillation. The atria stop their regular beat and begin a feeble, uncoordinated twitching. Concomitantly, low-amplitude, irregular waves appear in the ECG, as shown. This type of recording can be clearly distinguished from the very regular ECG waveform containing atrial flutter. (b) Ventricular fibrillation. Mechanically the ventricles twitch in a feeble, uncoordinated fashion with no blood being pumped from the heart. The ECG is likewise very uncoordinated, as shown. (Adapted from Brendan Phibbs, *The Human Heart*, 3rd ed., St. Louis: The C.V. Mosby Company, 1975.)

be the underlying mechanism responsible for atrial or ventricular fibrillation [Figure 4.20(a) and (b)].

**EXAMPLE 4.4** Premature ventricular contractions can be identified because (1) they arrive early, (2) the following beat occurs at the normal time, because it is generated by the SA node, and (3) the QRS width is greater than the normal 80 ms. Describe a software algorithm to detect and count PVCs by using all these criteria.

**ANSWER** There will be slight variations in width and R–R interval of QRS complexes. A PVC is wide. Use unfiltered ECG to determine average width (AW = average of 10). The algorithm should test that width $W_t > 1.3\text{AW}_{t-1}$. Use narrowband filter plus threshold to determine time of each R wave. Determine average R–R interval (AR–R = average of 10). A PVC occurs early. The algorithm should test that the $\text{R–R}_{t-1}$ interval $< 0.8\ \text{AR–R}_{t-2}$. A PVC is followed by a compensatory pause. The algorithm should test that $\text{R–R}_{t-1} + \text{R–R}_t$ is approximately $2(\text{AR–R}_{t-2})$. All three tests should be positive to yield a PVC.

Rhythm disturbances can arise from sources other than ectopic foci or competing pacemakers. A feasible alternative is a *circus re-excitation or*

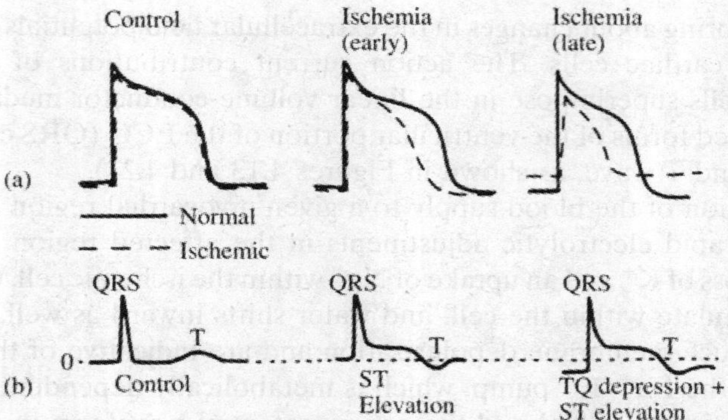


**Figure 4.21** (a) Action potentials recorded from normal (solid lines) and ischemic (dashed lines) myocardium in a dog. Control is before coronary occlusion. (b) During the control period prior to coronary occlusion, there is no ECG S–T segment shift; after ischemia, there is such a shift. (From Andrew G. Wallace, "Electrophysiology of the myocardium." In *Clinical Cardiopulmonary Physiology*, 3rd ed. New York: Grune & Stratton, 1969; used with permission of Grune & Stratton. Based on data by W. E. Sampson and H. M. Scher, "Mechanism of S–T segment alteration during acute myocardial injury," 1960, Circulation Research, 8, by permission of The American Heart Association.)

*re-entrant* mechanism (Allessie *et al.*, 1973). This concept assumes a region of depressed conductivity within the atrium, Purkinje system, or ventricle. It is therefore *ischemic* (deficient in its blood supply) relative to surrounding normal tissue. This brings about pronounced electrophysiological changes in the ischemic zone and a decreased velocity of conduction (see Figure 4.21).

Propagation in this area is slow enough to permit other areas to recover from initial excitation and be re-entered by the slowly emerging impulse. The re-entrant impulse may in turn re-excite the area of slow conduction to complete a circus-movement loop. Intermittent establishment of a re-entrant circuit would result in occasional ectopic beats (*extrasystoles*), and continuous propagation of impulses in the established circuit would underlie an episode of tachyarrhythmia.

## ALTERATION OF POTENTIAL WAVEFORMS IN ISCHEMIA

Of particular interest in Figure 4.21 is the change in the intracellular and extracellular potential waveforms in ischemia. Note particularly that in late ischemia (ischemia that occurs several minutes after induced coronary occlusion), there are decreases in the magnitudes of the resting potential, the velocity of the upstroke, and the height and duration of the action potential. (A decrease in upstroke velocity is indicative of a lowered velocity of conduction of the action-potential wave front through this ischemic region.) The slope of the potential during the plateau phase of the action potential is also altered in ischemia (increased). These changes in the action-potential waveform bring about changes in the extracellular field potentials produced by individual cardiac cells. The action current contributions of normal and ischemic cells superimpose in the linear volume-conductor medium to bring about altered forms of the ventricular portion of the ECG (QRS complex, S–T segment, and T wave, as shown in Figures 4.13 and 4.21).

Occlusion of the blood supply to a given myocardial region brings about relatively rapid electrolytic adjustments in the affected region. Specifically, there is a loss of $K^+$ and an uptake of $Na^+$ within the ischemic cell. $Ca^{2+}$ and $H^+$ also accumulate within the cell, and water shifts inward as well. These ionic shifts produce membrane depolarization and are indicative of the depressed activity of the $Na^+$–$K^+$ pump, which is metabolically dependent. Changes in the cell resting potential and the action potential waveform in ischemia are simply external manifestations of the underlying electrochemical changes brought about by an inadequate oxygen (blood) supply.

## 4.7 THE ELECTRORETINOGRAM

### ANATOMY OF VISION

The normal eye is an approximately spherical organ about 24 mm in diameter (Figure 4.22). The retina, located at the back of the eye, is the sensory portion of the eye.

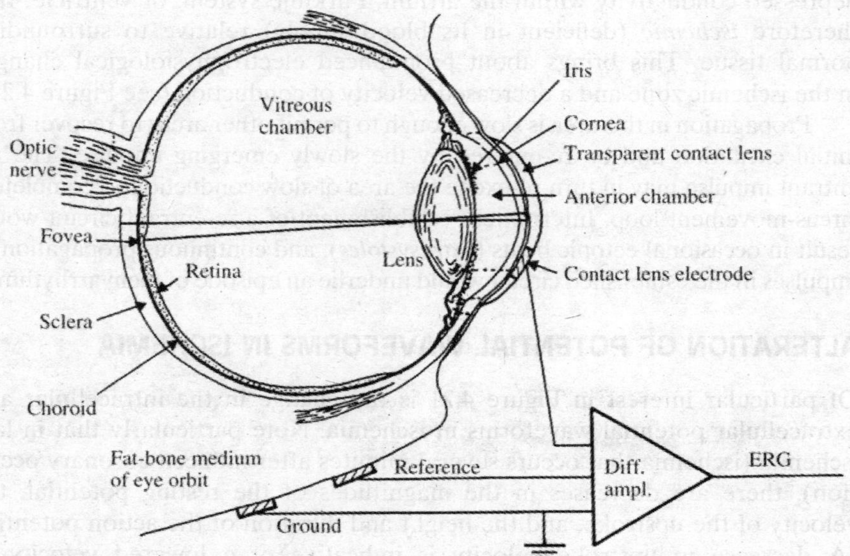


**Figure 4.22** The transparent contact lens contains one electrode, shown here on horizontal section of the right eye. Reference electrode is placed on the right temple.

The light-transmitting parts of the eye are the cornea, anterior chamber, lens, and vitreous chamber, named in the order in which these structures are traversed by light. A transparent fluid, the *aqueous humor*, is found in the anterior chamber. The vitreous chamber is filled by a transparent gel, the *vitreous body*. The aqueous humor provides a nutrient transport medium, but it is also of further optical significance. It is normally maintained at a pressure (20 to 25 mm Hg) that is adequate to inflate the eye against its resistive outer coats (the sclera and choroid). This makes possible the precise geometrical configuration of the retina and the optical pathway that is necessary to ensure formation of a clear visual image. In addition, the aqueous humor is the essential link between the circulatory system and the lens and cornea, which themselves lack blood vessels. To satisfy the respiratory and nutritive requirements of these two structures, there is a continual movement of fluid and solute material between the aqueous humor and contiguous blood vessels. Interference with this flow, in pathological conditions, not only leads to damage of the lens and cornea but may also result in the development of pressures within the eye that are high enough to injure the retina. *Glaucoma* is the term applied to this high-pressure condition.

In considering the neural organization of the retina, we need examine only five types of nerve cells: *photoreceptors* and *bipolar, horizontal, amacrine,* and *ganglion* cells. The ganglion cells, the axons of which produce the nerve fibers sweeping across the inner retinal surface to be collected at the optic disk (and which form the greater bulk of the nerve fibers of the optic nerve), are substantially fewer in number than the photoreceptors. There is a convergence in the neural pathways of the retina as a whole. [That is, many photoreceptors terminate on each bipolar cell ($n:1$), and many bipolar cells, in turn, terminate on a single ganglion cell. The degree of convergence varies considerably, being greater in the peripheral parts of the retina and minimal at the fovea (Figure 4.22). That is, the neural chain from photoreceptor to ganglion cell is 1 : 1 in the foveal region.] The synaptic interconnections between photoreceptors and bipolar cells and between bipolar cells and ganglion cells occur in two well-defined regions. The *external plexiform layer* is the region of contact between photoreceptor and bipolar cells, and the *internal plexiform layer* is the region of contact between bipolar and ganglion cells.

Lateral connections are also found in both layers. For example, horizontal cells interconnect rods and cones (defined below) at the level of the external plexiform layer, and amacrine cells provide a second horizontal network at the level of the inner plexiform layer. The retina may thus be considered functionally organized into two parts: an outer sensory layer containing the photoelectric sensors (photoreceptors) and an inner layer responsible for organizing and relaying electrical impulses generated in the photoreceptor layer to the brain.

Two types of photoreceptors occur in the human retina: *rods* (the agents of vision in dim light) and *cones* (the mediators of color vision in brighter light). Both rods and cones are differentiated into outer and inner segments. The inner segments are the major sites of metabolism and contain all the synaptic terminals. Outer segments—typically cylindrical and thin in rods and stout and conical in cones—are sites of visual excitation. The first stage in the transduction of light to neural messages is the absorption of photons by photopigments localized in the outer segments of the retina's photoreceptors. The photopigment localized in the compact membrane infolding of the rod's external segment is *rhodopsin*. It is easily isolated and has been extensively studied. Cones in human beings contain one of three photopigments and have photospectral absorption characteristics that differ from one another, and from the rod pigment rhodopsin. Cone pigments have proved very difficult to isolate in humans and other vertebrates, and hence their spectral characteristics have usually had to be measured by indirect means (e.g., reflection densitometry). Each cone pigment responds to a range of light wavelengths, but with maximal light absorption in the red, green, or blue regions of wavelength, respectively. Photopigments are embedded in the specialized membranes of the outer segments of the photoreceptors, and they are *photolabile*; that is, events initiated by light absorption result eventually in breakdown or "bleaching" of the photopigment.

For example, the photopigment in rods is rhodopsin (Rh), and it is comprised of two parts: a protein called *opsin* and *retinal*, a light-sensitive chromophore derived from vitamin A. In the absence of light, retinal is in its 11-cis form and is bound to opsin. With absorption of a photon, retinal straightens out to assume its all-trans form and dissociates. This process initiates a cascade of intramolecular reactions that brings about a conformational change in rhodopsin (now called *activated rhodopsin Rh**). $Rh^*$ in turn activates a G-protein coupled signal transduction cascade which targets closing of $Na^+$ channels on the external segment membrane. An important second messenger mediating this channel closing is cyclic guanosine 3,5-cyclic monophosphate (GMP). Turning off the $Na^+$ current that flows during the dark hyperpolarizes the cell membrane and reduces the release of neurotransmitter to downstream neurons in the visual pathway. Rhodopsin kinase and arrestin inactivate $Rh^*$ resetting the signal transduction pathway.

Details of the phototransduction process are beyond the scope of this book, but most physiology texts cover this subject intensively. Both intracellular and extracellular potential recordings have been made from isolated photoreceptors, as well as whole-cell voltage clamp recordings that provide quantitative descriptions of some of the membranes currents involved, e.g., Yagi and Macleish (1994).

## ELECTROPHYSIOLOGY OF THE EYE

When the retina is stimulated with a brief flash of light, a characteristic temporal sequence of changes in potential can be recorded between an exploring electrode—placed either on the inner surface of the retina or on the cornea—and an indifferent electrode placed elsewhere on the body (usually the temple, forehead, or earlobe). These potential changes are collectively known as the *electroretinogram* (ERG), and they are clinically

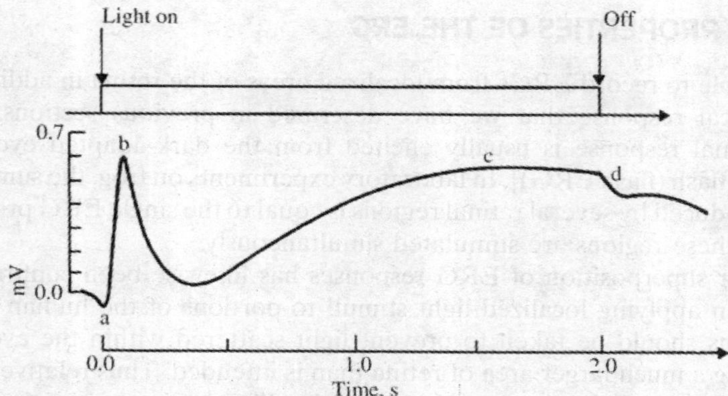


**Figure 4.23 Vertebrate ERG**

recorded with the aid of an Ag/AgCl electrode embedded in a special contact lens used as the exploring electrode. The saline-filled contact lens is in good contact with the cornea, which is very thin and in intimate contact with the aqueous humor and passive fluid medium of the inner eye. The contact lens is usually well tolerated by the subject and permits long examinations without discomfort. By considering the eye as a fluid-filled sphere and the retina as a thin sheetlike bioelectric source attached to the posterior pole of the sphere (Figure 4.22), we can easily visualize the volume-conductor problem in electroretinography.

Figure 4.23 shows a typical vertebrate ERG waveform in response to a 2 s light flash. The four most commonly identified components of the ERG waveform (the a, b, c, and d waves) are common to most vertebrates, including humans. The first part of the response to a brief light flash is the *early-receptor potential* (ERP) generated by the initial light-induced changes in the photopigment molecules. It appears almost instantaneously with the onset of the light stimulus. The second component, with a latency of 1 to 5 ms, is the *late-receptor potential* (LRP), which has been found to be maximal near the synaptic endings of the photoreceptors and therefore reflects the outputs of the receptors. Normally the ERP and LRP sum to form the leading edge of the a wave. The b wave is generated by activity of the bipolar and ganglion cells of the inner layers of the retina. This is best seen in laboratory experiments under conditions where the retinal artery supplying the inner layers of the retina is occluded, and the b wave is abolished. This experimental technique is useful since in the absence of the b wave, the entire time course of the early photoreceptor response (ERP + LRP) can be studied. The ERP is linear with light intensity; the LRP is already markedly nonlinear, varying approximately logarithmically with intensity. The c wave is not generated by the retina itself, but rather by the pigment epithelial layer in which the tips of the external segments are embedded. This is shown experimentally by chemically ablating the pigment epithelium or using an isolated retina preparation. The d wave is the off-response of the retina to the light stimulus.

## SPATIAL PROPERTIES OF THE ERG

It is possible to record ERGs from localized areas of the retina in addition to the classical response that we have described in previous sections. [This conventional response is usually elicited from the dark-adapted eye via a brief light flash (flash ERG)]. In laboratory experiments on frog, the sum of the ERGs produced by several retinal regions is equal to the single ERG produced when all these regions are stimulated simultaneously.

Linear superposition of ERG responses has likewise been confirmed in humans. In applying localized light stimuli to portions of the human retina, precautions should be taken to prevent light scattered within the eye from stimulating a much larger area of retina than is intended. Thus relatively high steady background illumination is supplied that illuminates most of the retina, and a localized stimulus is superimposed. The background illumination light causes the retina to adapt and renders it much less sensitive to light scattered from the stimulus region. In general, relatively high-background and low-stimulus intensities are preferred, making these locally generated ERG potentials low in amplitude and detectable with only average response calculations involving large numbers of responses. Without these special precautions, the resultant ERG represents the overall retinal response to light stimulation. Little is known about the actual nature of the light input to a particular retinal locus in the photoreceptive layer.

Despite the anatomical complexities of the retina, the problems of obtaining good records from untrained subjects, and the need for employing averaging techniques in obtaining spatially localized ERGs, the ERG has potential importance in assessing functional retinal behavior. It serves as an objective record of retinal function, is not dependent on the function of the optic nerve or the optic pathways, and is minimally affected by clouding of the optic pathway.

## THE ELECTRO-OCULOGRAM (EOG)

In addition to the transient potential recorded as the ERG, there is a steady corneal–retinal potential. This steady dipole may be used to measure eye position by placing surface electrodes to the left and right of the eye (e.g., on the nose and the temple). When the gaze is straight ahead, the steady dipole is symmetrically placed between the two electrodes, and the EOG output is zero. When the gaze is shifted to the left, the positive cornea becomes closer to the left electrode, which becomes more positive. There is an almost linear relationship between horizontal angle of gaze and EOG output up to approximately $\pm 30^\circ$ of arc. Electrodes may also be placed above and below the eye to record vertical eye movements.

The EOG, unlike other bipotentials, requires a dc amplifier. The signal is in the microvolt range, so recessed Ag/AgCl electrodes are required to prevent drift. It is necessary to abrade the skin to short out changes in the potential that exists between the inside and the outside of the skin. A noise is present that is compounded of effects from EEG, EMG, and the recording equipment; it is equivalent to approximately 1° of eye movement. Thus EOG data suffer from a lack of accuracy at the extremes. Specifically eye movements of less than 1° or 2° are difficult to record, whereas large eye movements (for example, greater than 30° of arc) do not produce bioelectric amplitudes that are strictly proportional to eye position. For an analysis of the accuracy and precision of electro-oculographic recordings, consult North (1965).

The EOG is frequently the method of choice for recording eye movements in sleep and dream research, in recording eye movements from infants and children, and in evaluating reading ability and visual fatigue. For a practical clinical EOG setup, see Niedermeyer and Lopes Da Silva (1999).

## 4.8 THE ELECTROENCEPHALOGRAM

The background electrical activity of the brain in unanesthetized animals was described qualitatively in the nineteenth century, but it was first analyzed in a systematic manner by the German psychiatrist Hans Berger, who introduced the term *electroencephalogram* (EEG) to denote the potential fluctuations recorded from the brain. Conventionally, the electrical activity of the brain is recorded with three types of electrodes—scalp, cortical, and depth electrodes. When electrodes are placed on the exposed surface (cortex) of the brain, the recording is called an *electrocorticogram* (ECoG). Thin insulated needle electrodes of various designs may also be advanced into the neural tissue of the brain, in which case the recording is referred to as a *depth recording.* (There is surprisingly little damage to the brain tissue when electrodes of appropriate size are employed.) Whether obtained from the scalp, cortex, or depths of the brain, the recorded fluctuating potentials represent a superposition of the field potentials produced by a variety of active neuronal current generators within the volume-conductor medium. Unlike the relatively simple bioelectric source considered in Section 4.2 (the nerve trunk with its enclosed bundles of circular cylindrical nerve axons), the sources generating these field potentials are aggregates of neuronal elements with complex interconnections. The neuronal elements mentioned previously are the dendrites, cell bodies (somata), and axons of nerve cells. Moreover, the architecture of the neuronal brain tissue is not uniform from one location to another in the brain. Therefore, prior to undertaking any detailed study of electroencephalography, we first discuss necessary background information regarding (1) the gross anatomy and function of the brain, (2) the ultrastructure of the cerebral cortex, (3) the field potentials of single neurons leading to an interpretation of extracellular potentials recorded in the cerebral cortex, and (4) typical clinical EEG waveforms recorded via scalp electrodes. We shall then focus on the general volume-conductor problem in electroencephalography and briefly discuss abnormal EEG waveforms (Sherman and Walterspacher, 2006).

## INTRODUCTION TO THE ANATOMY AND FUNCTION OF THE BRAIN

The central nervous system (CNS) consists of the spinal cord lying within the bony vertebral column and its continuation, the brain, lying within the skull [Figure 4.24]. The brain is the greatly modified and enlarged portion of the CNS, surrounded by three protective membranes (the *meninges*) and enclosed within the cranial cavity of the skull. The spinal cord is likewise surrounded by downward continuations of the meninges, and it is encased within the protective bony vertebral column. Both brain and spinal cord are bathed in a special extracellular fluid called *cerebral spinal fluid* (CSF).

Division of the brain into three main parts—*cerebrum, brainstem*, and *cerebellum*—provides a useful basis for the study of brain localization and function (Figure 4.24). The brainstem (*medulla, pons, midbrain, diencephalon*) is the oldest part of the brain. It is actually a short extension of the spinal cord and

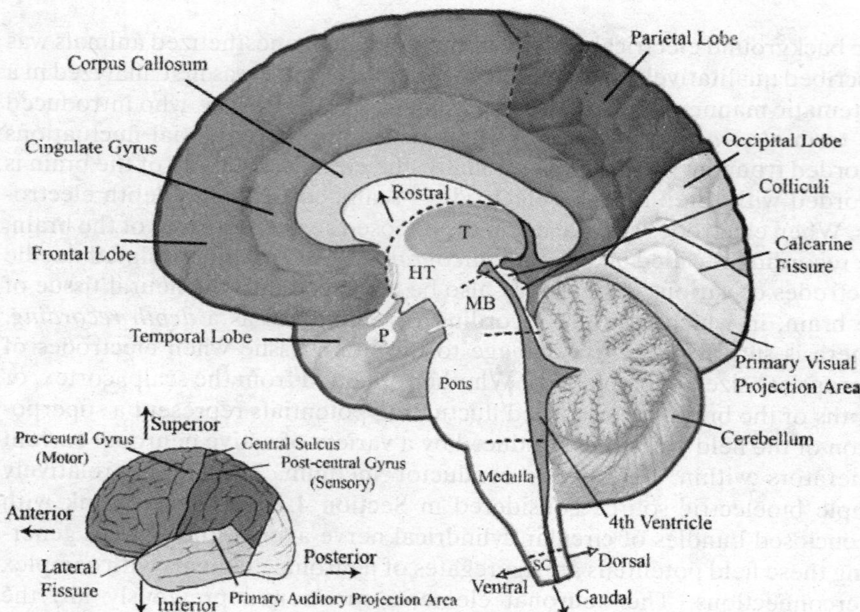


**Figure 4.24** Anatomical relationship of brainstem structures [medulla oblongata, pons, midbrain, and diencephalon (thalamus and hypothalamus)] to the cerebrum and cerebellum. General anatomic directions of orientation in the nervous system are superimposed on the diagrams. Here the terms *rostral* (toward head), *caudal* (toward tail), *dorsal* (back), and *ventral* (front) are associated with the brainstem; remaining terms are associated with the cerebrum. The terms *medial* and *lateral* imply nearness and remoteness, respectively, to or from the central midline axis of the brain. Symbols: T (thalamus), HT (hypothalamus), MB (midbrain), SC (spinal cord), P pituitary gland). (Adapted from John H. Martin, *Neuroanatomy: Text and Atlas*, 2nd ed., 1996, pp 14–15, with permission of Appleton and Lange, a Simon and Schuster Company.)

serves three major functions: (1) a connecting link between the cerebral cortex, spinal cord, and cerebellum; (2) an integrative center for several visceral functions (e.g., control of blood pressure and ventilation); and (3) an integration center for various motor reflexes. The *diencephalon* is the most superior portion of the brainstem; its chief component and largest structure is the *thalamus*. The thalamus serves as a major relay station and integration center for all of the general and special sensory systems, sending information to their respective cortical reception areas. It serves as the gateway to the cerebrum. Another major component of the diencephalon is the *hypothalamus*, which integrates functions of the autonomic nervous system and along with the pituitary gland, regulates functions of the thyroid, adrenal, and reproductive glands. The *cerebellum* is a coordinator in the voluntary (somatic) muscle system and acts in conjunction with the brainstem and cerebral cortex to maintain balance and provide harmonious muscle movements. The larger *cerebrum* occupies a special dominant position in the central nervous system, and conscious functions of the nervous system are localized within this structure.

Within the CNS there are *ascending* (*sensory*) nerve tracts that run from the spinal cord or brain stem to various areas of the brain, conveying information regarding changes in the external environment of the body that are reported by various peripheral biological sensors. There are a variety of such sensors, including the general sensors of temperature, pain, fine touch, pressure, as well as the special senses of vision, audition, equilibrium, taste, and olfaction. Figure 4.25 shows the basic plan associated with the general sense pathways from the periphery (e.g., skin, muscles) to the cortex. A three-neuron chain is involved in conveying information to the cortex where the *primary neuron* has its cell body in a ganglion outside the CNS and makes synaptic contact with a secondary neuron whose cell body is located in a nucleus within

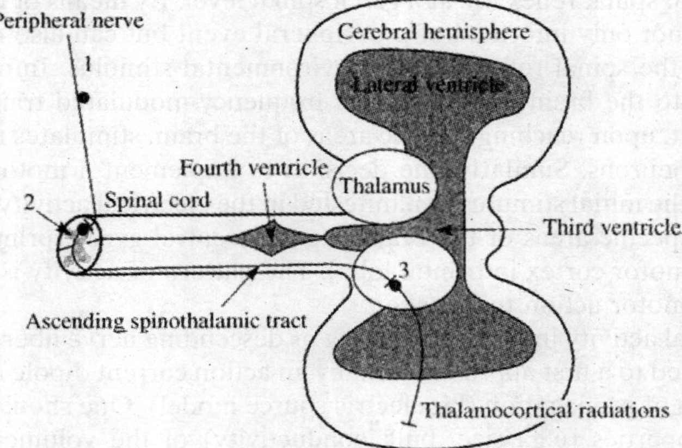


**Figure 4.25** A simplified diagram of the CNS showing a typical general sense pathway from the periphery (neuron 1) to the brain (neuron 3). Note that the axon of the secondary neuron (neuron 2) in the pathway decussates (crosses) to the opposite side of the cord. Descending (motor) pathways are also crossed (see text).

either the spinal cord [e.g., the dorsal horn or the brain stem (Figure 4.25)]. Note from Figure 4.25 that the axon of the *secondary neuron* crosses (decussates) to the other side of the cord and joins a nerve fiber tract bound for the thalamus. The *tertiary neuron* in the pathway is located in a thalamic nucleus, and its axon travels in the *thalamocortical radiations* to the *postcentral gyrus,* which is located just posterior to the *central sulcus* [Figure 4.24 (inset)]. Thus, the postcentral gyrus is the cortical projection area for the general senses.

Neural pathways for the special senses, particularly audition and vision, follow the same general ground plan; however, there are notable deviations from the scheme depicted in Figure 4.25. Usually, more than three neurons are involved in the pathway and not all of the "secondary neurons" decussate. Most of the neurons cross to the opposite (contralateral) side of the body, however a significant number ascend to the thalamus on the same (ipsilateral) side of the body. The auditory and visual pathways have their own special thalamic relay centers—the medial and lateral geniculate bodies, respectively, as well as their own cortical projection areas (Figure 4.24).

Likewise, within the CNS there are *descending* (*motor*) nerve tracts that originate in various brain structures such as the cerebrum and cerebellum (Figure 4.24) and terminate ultimately on motor neurons in the ventral horn of the spinal cord (Figure 4.10). These motoneurons, in turn, control the contractile activity of the skeletal musculature. For example, the corticospinal tract is a bundle of axons from the primary motor cortex [precentral gyrus, Figure 4.24 (inset)], which projects directly to motor neurons in the spinal cord. Since the ascending general sensory pathways are crossed, the descending corticospinal tracts each cross to the opposite side of the body prior to making synaptic contact with the spinal motor neurons.

Thus, two-way communication links exist between the brain and spinal cord that allow higher centers in the brain to control or modify the behavior of the elemental spinal reflex arc at a given spinal level. By means of these links, the brain is not only informed of a peripheral event but can also modify the response of the spinal reflex to that environmental stimulus. Information is transmitted to the brain by means of a frequency-modulated train of nerve impulses that, upon reaching specific areas of the brain, stimulates the activity of resident neurons. Similarly, the decision to implement a motor action in response to the initial stimulus is manifested in the electrical activity of cortical neurons in specific areas of the brain [e.g., precentral gyrus (primary motor cortex); premotor cortex in frontal lobe]. The pattern of activity is specific to the type of motor action to be taken.

Electrical activity in either ascending or descending nerve fiber tracts may be represented to a first approximation by an action current dipole oriented in the direction of propagation (bioelectric source model). One should be aware that the properties (e.g., size, bulk conductivity) of the volume-conductor medium can change along the length of a particular fiber tract between the spinal cord and the cortex, and the volume-conductor model adopted should be based on the particular measurement considered. The volume-conductor-field potential solutions can be used to both fit and interpret body surface potential measurements obtained clinically. Recording field potentials noninvasively from the relatively small volume of active nerve trunks, invariably requires the use of cumulative signal averaging techniques. In Figure 4.8, the median nerve was stimulated and compound action potentials were recorded from the subject's forearm. Although not shown in this figure, sensory fibers in the median nerve thus activated, initiate activity in the general sense pathways to the brain. Averaged field potential recordings can be taken at a variety of points along the ascending pathways [e.g., from spinal cord and brain stem tracts taking note of the crossed nature of the pathway, and finally at the cortex itself (postcentral gyrus)]. The field potentials associated with long nerve tracts depends to a large extent on (a) whether the tract is straight or bent and (b) the resistance (geometry and specific conductivity) of the surrounding volume-conductor media.

This important subject is discussed later; however, for the present, these different types of averaged field potentials are called collectively *somatosensory evoked potentials*. The subject of nerve tracts has been discussed previously; however, the activity of both nuclei in the ascending pathway and clusters of cells in the cortex, depends not only on the ensemble of neurons there, but also on the geometry of the ensemble and the different types of synaptic connections involved.

Averaged sensory evoked potentials in response to brief auditory "clicks" or flashes of light are also routinely recorded as the auditory evoked response (AER) and the visual evoked response (VER), respectively (Jacobson, 1994; Heckenlively and Arden, 1991). Using an electromagnetic stimulating device held over the primary motor cortex (just anterior to the central sulcus), it is also possible to induce currents that activate the corticospinal tract, making possible the recording of averaged field potentials from the descending motor pathways (York, 1987; Geddes, 1987; Esselle and Stuchly, 1992). The same volume-conductor principles are applicable to the analysis of these different types of evoked potential recordings. The cerebrum is a paired structure, with right and left cerebral hemispheres, each relating to the opposite side of the body. That is, voluntary movements of the right hand are "willed" by the left cerebral hemisphere. The surface layer of the hemisphere is called the *cortex*; it receives sensory information from skin, eyes, ears, and other receptors located generally on the opposite side of the body. This information is compared with previous experience and produces movements in response to these stimuli.

Each hemisphere consists of several layers. The outer layer is a dense collection of nerve cells that appear gray in color when examined in a fresh state. It is consequently called *gray matter*. This outer layer, roughly 1 cm thick, is called the *cerebral cortex*. It has a highly convoluted surface consisting of *gyri* (ridges) and *sulci* (valleys), the deeper sulci being termed *fissures*. The deeper layers of the hemisphere (beneath the cortex) consist of myelinated *axons* (or white matter) and collections of cell bodies termed *nuclei*. Some of the integrative functions of the cerebrum can be localized within certain regions of the cortex; others are more diffusely distributed.

A major dividing landmark of the cerebral cortex is the lateral fissure (Figure 4.24), which runs on the lateral (side) surface of the brain from the open end in front, posteriorly and dorsally (backward and upward). The lateral fissure defines a side lobe of cortex inferior to (below) it that is called the *temporal lobe* [Figure 4.24 (inset)]. The superior (upper) part of this lobe contains the *primary auditory cortex*, which is the part of the cortex that receives auditory impulses via neural pathways leading from the auditory receptors in the inner ear.

The visual system is another example of the projection of the senses onto the cerebral cortex. The *occipital lobe* at the back of the head is the primary visual cortex. Light flashed into the eye evokes large electrical potentials from electrodes placed over this area of the cortex.

Another major landmark of the cerebral cortex is the central sulcus [Figure 4.24 (inset)]. However, it is not so prominent and unvarying an anatomical landmark as the lateral fissure. The central sulcus runs from the medial surface (surface along the midline of the brain) over the convexity of the hemisphere to the lateral fissure. It also represents the posterior border of the frontal lobe. The gyrus lying just anterior (forward) to the central sulcus is the *precentral gyrus*, which functions as the *primary motor cortex*. From this gyrus, nerve signals run down through the brainstem to the spinal cord for control of skeletal muscles via neural control of motoneurons in the ventral horn of the spinal cord (Figure 4.10). Lesions (destruction) of part of the precentral gyrus cause partial paralysis on the opposite side of the body.

Immediately posterior to the central sulcus [Fig. 24 (inset)] is the primary *somatosensory cortex*, the *postcentral gyrus*. This region receives impulses from all the general sense receptors from the skin (such as pressure, touch, and pain receptors). Each little area along this gyrus is related to a particular part of the body (for example, the legs on the medial end, the hand in the center, and the face on the end next to the lateral fissure). If a recording electrode is placed appropriately during a neurosurgical procedure, a cortical response can be evoked by tactile stimuli delivered to the *contralateral* (opposite) hand. Likewise, if a stimulus is applied through the same electrode, the subject reports a tingling sensation in the contralateral hand. Higher-order sensory discrimination, such as the ability to recognize a number drawn on the palm of the hand, is organized solely in the parietal lobe of which the postcentral gyrus is a part. Destruction of the parietal lobe results in a loss of this discriminative ability. For example, a subject may still know that he or she is being touched but cannot tell where or what is being drawn on the palm of the hand. The parietal lobe is also responsible for a person's awareness of the general position of the body and its limbs in space.

## ULTRASTRUCTURE OF THE CEREBRAL CORTEX

The functional part of the cerebrum is the cerebral cortex (bark, outer covering), a relatively thin layer of gray matter (1.5 to 4.0 mm in thickness) covering the outer surface of the cerebrum, including its intricate convolutions.

Because it is the most recent phylogenetic acquisition of the brain, the cerebral cortex has undergone a relatively greater development than other parts of the brain. The greatest advance in relative growth has been the neocortex, which is present on the superior and lateral aspects of the cerebral hemispheres. The distinctly different type of cortex located on the medial surface and base of the brain is known as the *paleocortex*. We shall use the term *cortex* in this chapter to refer specifically to the neocortex.

Cortical architectures in vertebrates share several common features: (1) stratified layers containing cell bodies and fiber bundles; (2) an outermost layer that lacks neurons (layer I); (3) at least one inner layer containing neurons that give rise to large dendrites, which rise vertically to layer I and travel in that layer forming multiple branches (arborization). The human cortex is generally arranged in six such cortical layers. The neurons are of two main types: *pyramidal* and *nonpyramidal* (many subtypes have been identified). There are also a large number of horizontally oriented layers of nerve fibers that extend between adjacent regions of the cortex, as well as vertically oriented bundles that extend from the cortex to more distant regions of the cortex or downward to the brainstem and spinal cord.

Figure 4.26 shows a schematic drawing of a typical cortical pyramidal cell. The bodies of this type of cell are commonly triangular in shape, with the base down and the apex directed toward the cortical surface. (Pyramidal

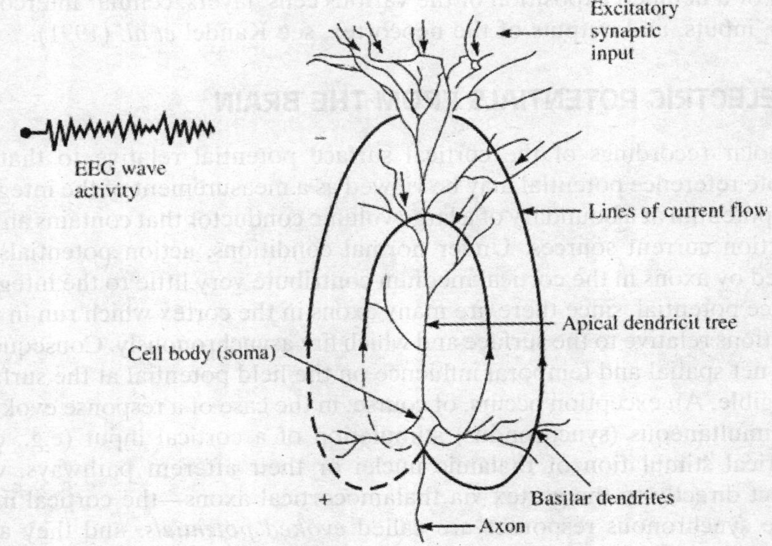


**Figure 4.26** Electrogenesis of cortical field potentials for a net excitatory input to the apical dendritic tree of a typical pyramidal cell. For the case of a net inhibitory input, polarity is reversed and the apical region becomes a source (+). Current flow to and from active fluctuating synaptic knobs on the dendrites produces wavelike activity. (See text.)

cell bodies vary greatly in size, from axial dimensions of $15 \times 10\,\mu m$ up to $120 \times 90\,\mu m$ or more for the giant pyramids of the motor cortex, which are called *Betz cells* after their discoverer.) These cells usually consist of the following parts: (1) a long apical dendrite (up to 2 mm in length) that ascends from the apex of the cell body through the overlaying cellular layers, and which frequently reaches and branches terminally within the outermost layer of the cortex; (2) dense dendritic arborization occurring at the base of the pyramid-shaped cell (largely horizontally—basilar dendrites); and (3) a single pyramidal cell axon which can emerge from the inner surface of the cortex as projection fibers to other areas of the cortex, or to other structures (e.g., the thalamus, cerebellum, or spinal cord). Frequently these axons send recurrent collateral (feedback) branches back on the cellular regions from which they sprang. Axons of some pyramidal cells turn back toward the cortical surface (never leaving the gray matter) to end via their many branches on the dendrites of other cells.

Nonpyramidal cells of the neocortex differ remarkably from pyramidal cells. Their cell bodies are small, and dendrites spring from them in all directions to ramify in the immediate vicinity of the cell. The axon may arise from a large dendrite; it commonly divides repeatedly to terminate on the cell bodies and dendrites of immediately adjacent cells. The axons of other nonpyramidal cells may turn upward toward the cortical surface, or they may leave the motor cortex (though this is not common).

For a detailed exposition of the various cells, layers, cellular interconnections, inputs, and outputs of the neocortex, see Kandel *et al.* (1991).

## BIOELECTRIC POTENTIALS FROM THE BRAIN

Unipolar recordings of the cortical surface potential relative to that of a remote reference potential may be viewed as a measurement of the integrated field potential at a boundary of a large volume conductor that contains an array of action current sources. Under normal conditions, action potentials conducted by axons in the cortical medium contribute very little to the integrated surface potential, since there are many axons in the cortex which run in many directions relative to the surface and which fire asynchronously. Consequently, their net spatial and temporal influence on the field potential at the surface is negligible. An exception occurs, of course, in the case of a response evoked by the simultaneous (synchronous) stimulation of a cortical input (e.g., direct electrical stimulation of thalamic nuclei or their afferent pathways, which project directly to the cortex via thalamocortical axons—the cortical input). These synchronous responses are called *evoked potentials,* and they are of relatively large amplitude. Synchronicity of the underlying fiber and cortical neuron activity is a major factor influencing surface potential magnitude. Unipolar field potentials recorded within the cortical layers have shown that the cortical surface potential is largely due to the net effect of local postsynaptic potentials of cortical cells (Figure 4.26). These may be of either sign (excitatory or inhibitory) and may occur directly underneath the electrode or at some distance from it. A potential change recorded at the surface is a measure of the net potential (current resistance $iR$) drop between the surface site and the distant reference electrode. It is obvious, however, that if all the cell bodies and dendrites of cortical cells were randomly arranged in the cortical medium, the net influence of synaptic currents would be zero. This would result in a "closed field" situation that produces relatively small far-field potentials (Lorente de No, 1947). Thus, any electrical change recorded at the surface must be due to the orderly and symmetric arrangement of some class of cells within the cortex.

Pyramidal cells of the cerebral cortex are oriented vertically, with their long apical dendrites running parallel to one another. Potential changes in one part of the cell relative to another part create "open" potential fields in which current may flow and potential differences can be measured at the cortical surface. Figure 4.26 illustrates this concept in diagrammatic fashion. Synaptic inputs to the apical dendritic tree cause depolarization of the dendritic membrane. As a result, subthreshold current flows in a closed path through the cytoplasmic core of the dendrites and cell body of the pyramidal cell, returning ultimately to the surface synaptic sites via the extracellular bathing medium. From the indicated direction of the lines of current flow, the extracellular medium about the soma behaves as a *source* (+), while the upper part of the apical dendritic tree behaves as a *sink* (−).

The influence of a particular dendritic *postsynaptic potential* (PSP) on the cortical surface recording depends on its sign [excitatory (−) or inhibitory (+)] and on its location relative to the measurement site. The effect of each PSP may be regarded as creating a radially oriented current dipole. Therefore, continuing synaptic input creates a series of potential dipoles and resulting current flows that are staggered but overlapped in space and time. Surface potentials of any form can be generated by one population of presynaptic fibers and the cells on which they terminate, depending on the proportion that are inhibitory or excitatory, the level of the postsynaptic cells in the cortex, and so forth.

Nonpyramidal cells in the neocortex, on the other hand, are unlikely to contribute substantially to surface records. Their spatially restricted dendritic trees are radially arranged around their cell bodies such that charge differences between the dendrites and the cell body produce fields of current flow that sum to zero when viewed from a relatively great distance on the cortical surface (closed-field situation).

Thus, to summarize, the apical dendrites of pyramidal cells constitute a meshwork of similarly oriented, densely packed units in the outer layers of the cortex. As multiple synaptic endings on the dendritic tree of each cell become active, current can flow in either direction between the dendritic process depending on whether the synapses are excitatory or inhibitory. The source–sink relationship between dendrite and cell is that of a constantly shifting current dipole, where variations in dipole orientation and strength produce wavelike fluctuations in the surface field potential (Figure 4.26). When the sum of dendritic activity is negative relative to the cell, the cell is depolarized and quite excitable. When it is positive, the cell is hyperpolarized and less excitable.

## RESTING RHYTHMS OF THE BRAIN

Electric recordings from the exposed surface of the brain or from the outer surface of the head demonstrate continuous oscillating electric activity within the brain. Both the intensity and the patterns of this electric activity are determined to a great extent by the overall excitation of the brain resulting from functions in the brainstem reticular activating system (RAS). The undulations in the recorded electric potentials (Figure 4.27) are called *brain waves*, and the entire record is called an *electroencephalogram* (EEG).

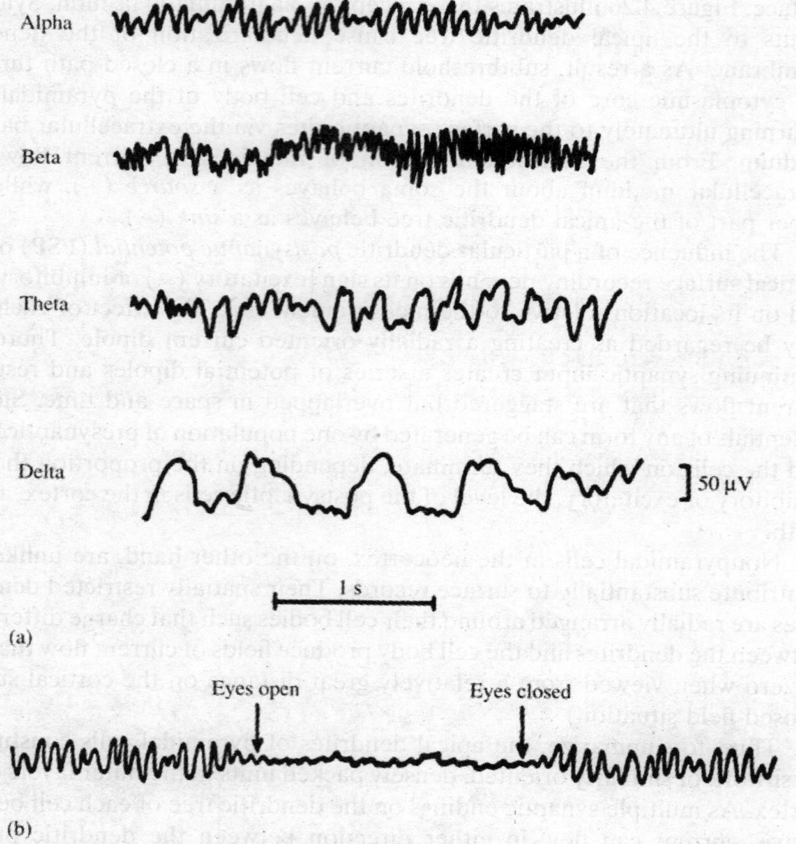


**Figure 4.27** (a) Different types of normal EEG waves. (b) Replacement of alpha rhythm by an asynchronous discharge when patient opens eyes. (c) Representative abnormal EEG waveforms in different types of epilepsy. (From A. C. Guyton, *Structure and Function of the Nervous System*, 2nd ed., Philadelphia: W.B. Saunders, 1972; used with permission.)

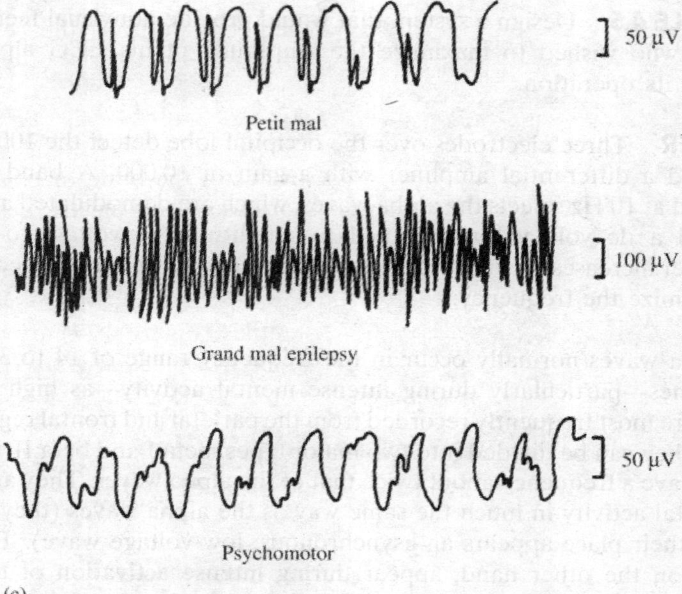


**Figure 4.27** (*Continued*)

The intensities of the brain waves on the surface of the brain (recorded relative to an indifferent electrode such as the earlobe) may be as large as 10 mV, whereas those recorded from the scalp have a smaller amplitude of approximately 100 μV. The frequencies of these brain waves range from 0.5 to 100 Hz, and their character is highly dependent on the degree of activity of the cerebral cortex. For example, the waves change markedly between states of wakefulness and sleep. Much of the time, the brain waves are irregular, and no general pattern can be observed. Yet at other times, distinct patterns do occur. Some of these are characteristic of specific abnormalities of the brain, such as epilepsy (discussed later). Others occur in normal persons and may be classified as belonging to one of four wave groups (*alpha, beta, theta,* and *delta*), which are shown in Figure 4.27(a).

Alpha waves are rhythmic waves occurring at a frequency between 8 and 13 Hz. They are found in EEGs of almost all normal persons when they are awake in a quiet, resting state of cerebration. These waves occur most intensely in the occipital region but can also be recorded, at times, from the parietal and frontal regions of the scalp. Their voltage is approximately 20 to 200 μV. When the subject is asleep, the alpha waves disappear completely. When the awake subject's attention is directed to some specific type of mental activity, the alpha waves are replaced by asynchronous waves of higher frequency but lower amplitude. Figure 4.27(b) demonstrates the effect on the alpha waves of simply opening the eyes in bright light and then closing them again. Note that the visual sensations cause immediate cessation of the alpha waves; these are replaced by low-voltage, asynchronous waves.

**EXAMPLE 4.5** Design a system that would provide nonvisual feedback to a subject who wished to maximize the amplitude of his EEG alpha waves. Explain its operation.

**ANSWER** Three electrodes over the occipital lobe detect the 100 μV EEG and feed a differential amplifier with a gain of 10,000. A band-pass filter centered at 10 Hz selects the alpha waves, which are demodulated and filtered to yield a dc voltage proportional to amplitude. A voltage-to-frequency converter increases the frequency of an acoustic tone, and the subject attempts to maximize the frequency.

Beta waves normally occur in the frequency range of 14 to 30 Hz, and sometimes—particularly during intense mental activity—as high as 50 Hz. These are most frequently recorded from the parietal and frontal regions of the scalp. They can be divided into two major types: beta I and beta II. The beta I waves have a frequency about twice that of the alpha waves. They are affected by mental activity in much the same way as the alpha waves (they disappear and in their place appears an asynchronous, low-voltage wave). The beta II waves, on the other hand, appear during intense activation of the central nervous system and during tension. Thus one type of beta activity is elicited by mental activity, whereas the other is inhibited by it.

Theta waves have frequencies between 4 and 7 Hz. These occur mainly in the parietal and temporal regions in children, but they also occur during emotional stress in some adults, particularly during periods of disappointment and frustration. For example, they can often be brought about in the EEG of a frustrated person by allowing the person to enjoy some pleasant experience and then suddenly removing the element of pleasure. This causes approximately 20 s of theta waves.

Delta waves include all the waves in the EEG below 3.5 Hz. Sometimes these waves occur only once every 2 or 3 s. They occur in deep sleep, in infancy, and in serious organic brain disease. They can also be recorded from the brains of experimental animals that have had subcortical transections producing a functional separation of the cerebral cortex from the reticular activating system. Delta waves can thus occur solely within the cortex, independent of activities in lower regions of the brain.

A single cortical cell can give rise only to small extracellular current, so large numbers of neurons must be synchronously active to give rise to the potentials recorded from the cerebral surface. The individual waves of the EEG are of long duration (for example, 30 to 500 ms), and one might well ask how they are produced. They can be long-lasting depolarizations of the cell membranes (for example, of the apical dendrites of pyramidal cells) or a summation of a number of shorter responses. In any event, a sufficiently large number of neurons must discharge together to give rise to these cortical potentials. The term *synchronization* is used to describe the underlying process that acts to bring a group of neurons into unified action. Synaptic interconnections are generally thought to bring about synchronization, although extracellular field interaction between cells has been proposed as a possible mechanism. Rhythmically firing neurons are very sensitive to voltage gradients in their surrounding medium.

Besides the synchronization required for each wave of resting EEG, the series of repeated waves suggests a rhythmic and a trigger or pacemaker process that initiates such rhythmic action. By means of knife cuts below the intact connective-tissue covering (*meningeal layer or pia matter*) of the brain, one may prepare *chronic islands* of cortex—with all neuronal connections cut, but with the blood supply via surface vessels intact. Only a low level of EEG activity remains in such islands. Though the isolated islands of cortex may not show spontaneous EEG activity, they still have the ability to respond rhythmically, which may be readily demonstrated by the rhythmic responses that are elicited by applying a single electrical stimulus. The inference is that various regions of the cortex, though capable of exhibiting rhythmic activity, require trigger inputs to excite rhythmicity. The RAS, mentioned earlier, appears to provide this pacemaker function.

## THE CLINICAL EEG

The system most often used to place electrodes for monitoring the clinical EEG is the International Federation 10–20 system shown in Figure 4.28. This system uses certain anatomical landmarks to standardize placement of EEG electrodes. The representation of the EEG channels is referred to as a *montage*. In the bipolar montage, each channel measures the difference between two adjacent electrodes. In the referential montage, each channel

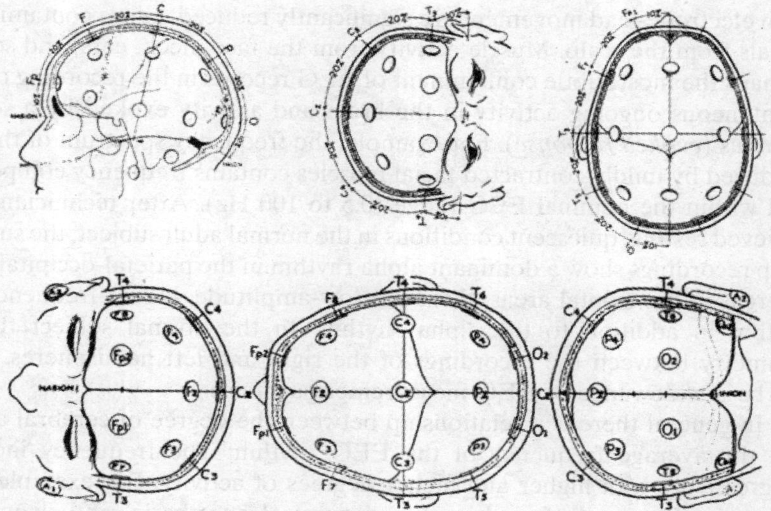


**Figure 4.28 The 10–20 electrode system** This system is recommended by the International Federation of EEG Societies. [From H. H. Jasper, "The ten–twenty electrode system of the International Federation in Electroencephalography and Clinical Neurophysiology." *EEG Journal*, 1958, 10 (Appendix), 371–375.]

measures the diffference between one electrode and a reference electrode, such as on the ear. In the average reference montage, each channel measures the difference between one electrode and the average of all other electrodes. In the Laplacian montage, each channel measures the difference between one electrode and a weighted average of the surrounding electrodes. The differential amplifier requires a separate ground electrode plus differential inputs to the electrode connections. The advantage of using a differential recording between closely spaced electrodes (between successive pairs in the standard system, for example) is cancellation of far-field activity common to both electrodes; one thereby obtains sharp localization of the response. Although the same electric events are recorded in each of the ways, they appear in a different format in each case. The potential changes that occur are amplified by high-gain, differential, capacitively coupled amplifiers. The output signals are recorded and displayed.

In the routine recording of clinical EEGs, the input electrodes are a problem. They must be small, they must be easily affixed to the scalp with minimal disturbance of the hair, they must cause no discomfort, and they must remain in place for extended periods of time. Technicians prepare the surface of the scalp, degrease the recording area by cleaning it with alcohol, apply a conducting paste, and glue nonpolarizable Ag/AgCl electrodes to the scalp with a glue (collodion) and hold them in place with rubber straps, or use a rubber cap that contains all electrodes.

The EEG is usually recorded with the subject awake but resting recumbent on a bed with eyes closed. With the patient relaxed in such a manner, artifacts from electrode-lead movement are significantly reduced, as are contaminating signals from the scalp. Muscle activity from the face, neck, ears, and so on is perhaps the most subtle contaminant of EEG records in the recording of both spontaneous ongoing activity in the brain and activity evoked by a sensory stimulus (*evoked response*). For example, the frequency spectrum of the field produced by mildly contracted facial muscles contains frequency components well within the nominal EEG range (0.5 to 100 Hz). After technicians have achieved resting, quiescent conditions in the normal adult subject, the subject's scalp recordings show a dominant alpha rhythm in the parietal-occipital areas, whereas in the frontal areas, there is a low-amplitude, higher-frequency beta rhythm in addition to the alpha rhythm. In the normal subject there is symmetry between the recordings of the right and left hemispheres. There can be a wide range of EEG measurement artifacts.

In general there is a relationship between the degree of cerebral activity and the average frequency of the EEG rhythm: The frequency increases progressively with higher and higher degrees of activity. For example, delta waves are frequently found in stupor, surgical anesthesia, and sleep; theta waves in infants; alpha waves during relaxed states; and beta waves during intense mental activity. However, during periods of mental activity, the waves usually become asynchronous rather than synchronous, so that the magnitude of the summed surface potential recording decreases despite increased cortical activity.

## SLEEP PATTERNS

When an individual in a relaxed, inattentive state becomes drowsy and falls asleep, the alpha rhythm is replaced by slower, larger waves (Figure 4.29). In deep sleep, very large, somewhat irregular delta waves are observed. Interspersed with these waves—during moderately deep sleep—are bursts of alpha-like activity called *sleep spindles*. The alpha rhythm and the patterns of the drowsy and sleeping subject are *synchronized*, in contrast with the low-voltage *desynchronized*, irregular activity seen in the subject who is in an alert state.

The high-amplitude, slow waves seen in the EEG of a subject who is asleep are sometimes replaced by rapid, low-voltage irregular activity resembling that obtained in alert subjects. However, the sleep of a subject with this irregular pattern is not interrupted; in fact, the threshold for arousal by sensory stimuli is elevated. This condition has therefore come to be called *paradoxical sleep*. During paradoxical sleep, the subject exhibits rapid, roving eye movements. For this reason, it is also called *rapid-eye-movement* sleep, or REM sleep. Conversely, *spindle* or synchronized sleep is frequently called *nonrapid-eye-movement* (NREM), or slow-wave sleep. Human subjects aroused at a time when their EEG exhibits a paradoxical (REM) sleep pattern generally report

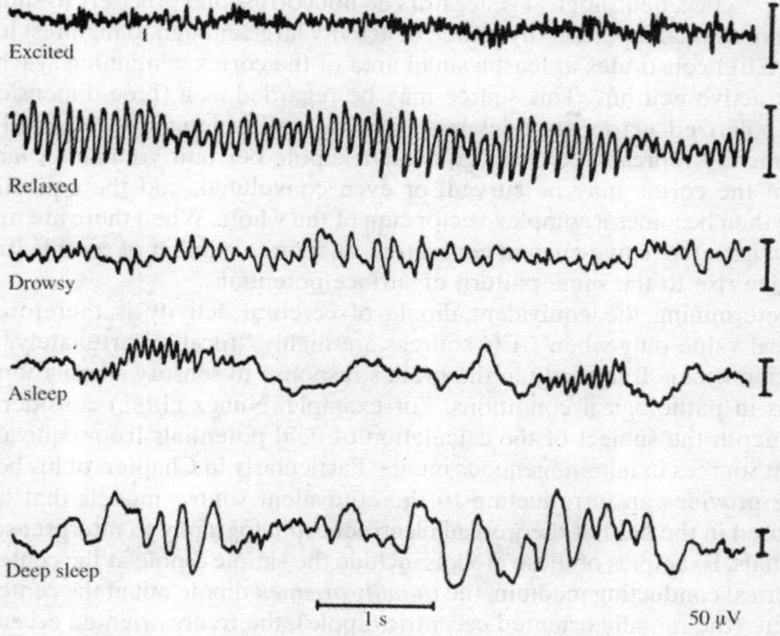


**Figure 4.29 The electroencephalographic changes that occur as a human subject goes to sleep** The calibration marks on the right represent 50 μV. (From H. H. Jasper, "Electrocephalography." In *Epilepsy and Cerebral Localization*, W. G. Penfield and T. C. Erickson (eds.). Springfield, IL: Charles C. Thomas, 1941.)

that they were dreaming, whereas individuals wakened from spindle sleep do not. This observation and other evidence indicate that REM sleep and dreaming are closely associated. It is interesting that during REM sleep, there is a marked reduction in muscle tone, despite the rapid eye movements.

## THE VOLUME-CONDUCTOR PROBLEM IN ELECTROENCEPHALOGRAPHY

Geometrically speaking, the brain approximates a sphere surrounded by concentric shells that differ in impedance and comprise the *meninges* (connective tissue coverings of the brain), cerebral spinal fluid, skull, and scalp. This model is inaccurate to the extent that the brain is not really a true sphere, and its coverings are irregular in shape and thickness. Such irregularities are insignificant for the upper half of the brain, but complications are introduced by the marked departure of the lower parts of the brain from a spherical shape, as well as by variations in impedance produced by the openings (to the spinal column) through the base of the shell. Various cerebral structures differ somewhat in specific resistivity. Resistivity also varies in relation to the predominant direction of the fibers within the white matter. Thus the brain is neither a homogeneous nor an isotropic conducting medium.

In practice, neurological generators do not correspond precisely to simple, one-dimensional dipoles. Any source of activity large enough to manifest itself in the EEG constitutes at least a small area of the cortex containing synchronously active neurons. This source may be regarded as a three-dimensional sheet polarized across its thickness. If it is small enough, it may still be conveniently represented as an equivalent dipole per unit volume. A larger area of the cortex may be curved, or even convoluted, and the equivalent dipole then becomes a complex vector sum of the whole. When there are many widely scattered active-current generators, an infinite number of combinations may give rise to the same pattern of surface potentials.

Determining the equivalent dipole of cerebral activity is therefore of practical value only when EEG sources are highly "focal." Fortunately, this condition occurs frequently in the brain's response to sensory stimulation, as well as in pathological conditions. For example, Nunez (1981) considers in some depth the subject of the calculation of field potentials from equivalent current sources in inhomogeneous media. Particularly in Chapter of his book, Nunez provides an introduction to the equivalent source models that have been used in the field of theoretical electroencephalography to interpret scalp potentials. Examples of these models include the simple dipole at the center of a spherical conducting medium, the *radially oriented* dipole not at the center of a sphere (the radially oriented eccentric dipole), the freely oriented eccentric dipole in a sphere, the dipole in a three-concentric spherical shell model, and a dipole current source below a multilayered planar conducting medium.

Considerable interest has arisen in determining the location of intracerebral sources of the potentials that are measured on the scalp. In general, nonuniqueness of this *inverse* problem is well known in that different configurations of sources can lead to the same surface distribution. The usual approach taken to obtaining an approximate solution to the inverse problem is as follows:

1. Assume a model (such as the eccentrically located dipole in a uniform, homogeneous spherical conducting medium. Assume that the electric field is quasistatic).
2. After obtaining a solution to the associated boundary-value problem (the forward problem), produce model-generated potential values at measurement points on the cortical surface.
3. Compare these theoretical potential values with particular discrete-time values of EEG waveforms measured at the same surface sites, and form a general least-squares reconstruction error function wherein the error is defined as the difference between predicted and measured potential at several selected cortical measurement sites.
4. Iteratively adjust the EEG dipolar source parameters at each discrete-time instant to obtain the best fit to sampled EEG waveforms in a least-squares sense. The optimal dipole location is assumed to be the dipole location obtained when the reconstruction error function is so minimized.

The influence of anisotropy on various EEG phenomena has been studied using models [Henderson *et al.* (1975); Cuffin (1991); Haueisen *et al.* (2002)]. These investigations, together with various *in vivo* studies, substantially agree that the presence of tissue anisotropy tends to attenuate and smear the pattern of scalp-recorded EEGs. However, this type of amplitude-related degradation apparently does not affect the model's ability to predict the locus of the EEG equivalent-dipole generator (although the dipole moment might be underestimated). This is important in the sense that one of the major objectives of electroencephalography is determination of source location—for localized or focal activity—because in case of evoked cortical potentials and deep-brain pathologies, this concept of an equivalent-dipole generator is of clinical value.

## THE ABNORMAL EEG

One of the more important clinical uses of the EEG is in the diagnosis of different types of epilepsy and in the location of the focus in the brain causing the epilepsy. Epilepsy is characterized by uncontrolled excessive activity by either a part or all of the CNS. A person predisposed to epilepsy has attacks when the basal level of excitability of all or part of the nervous system rises above a certain critical threshold. However, as long as the degree of excitability is held below this threshold, no attack occurs.

There are two basic types of epilepsy, *generalized epilepsy* and *partial epilepsy*. Generalized epilepsy involves the entire brain at once, whereas partial epilepsy involves a portion of the brain—sometimes only a minute focal spot and at other times a fair amount of the brain. Generalized epilepsy is further divided into *grand mal* and *petit mal* epilepsy.

Grand mal epilepsy is characterized by extreme discharges of neurons originating in the brainstem portion of the RAS. These discharges then spread throughout the cortex, to the deeper parts of the brain, and even to the spinal cord to cause generalized tonic convulsions of the entire body. They are followed near the end of the attack by alternating muscular contractions, called *clonic convulsions*. The grand mal seizure lasts from a few seconds to as long as 3 to 4 min and is characterized by postseizure depression of the entire nervous system. The subject may remain in a stupor for 1 min to as long as a day or more after the attack is over.

The middle recording in Figure 4.27(c) shows a typical EEG during a grand mal attack. This response can be recorded from almost any region of the cortex. The recorded potential is of a high magnitude, and the response is synchronous, with the same periodicity as normal alpha waves. The same type of discharge occurs on both sides of the brain at the same time, indicating that the origin of the abnormality is in the lower centers of the brain that control the activity of the cerebral cortex, not in the cortex itself. Electrical recordings from the thalamus and reticular formation of experimental animals during an induced grand mal attack indicate typical high-voltage synchronous activity in these areas, similar to that recorded from the cerebral cortex. Experiments on animals have further shown that a grand mal attack is caused by intrinsic hyperexcitability of the neurons that make up the RAS structures or by some abnormality of the local neural pathways of this system.

Petit mal epilepsy is closely allied to grand mal epilepsy. It occurs in two forms, the *myoclonic* form and the *absence* form. In the myoclonic form, a burst of neuronal discharges, lasting a fraction of a second, occurs throughout the nervous system. These discharges are similar to those that occur at the beginning of a grand mal attack. The person exhibits a single violent muscular jerk involving arms or head. The entire process stops immediately, however, and the attack is over before the subject loses consciousness or stops what he or she is doing. This type of attack often becomes progressively more severe until the subject experiences a grand mal attack. Thus the myoclonic form of petit mal is similar to a grand mal attack, except that some form of inhibitory influence promptly stops it.

The absence type of petit mal epilepsy is characterized by 5 to 20 s of unconsciousness, during which the subject has several twitchlike contractions of the muscles, usually in the head region. There is a pronounced blinking of the eyes, followed by a return to consciousness and continuation of previous activities. This type of epilepsy is also closely allied to grand mal epilepsy. In rare instances, it can initiate a grand mal attack.

Figure 4.27(c) shows a typical *spike-and-dome* pattern that is recorded during the absence type of petit mal epilepsy. The spike portion of the record is almost identical to the spikes occurring in grand mal epilepsy, but the dome portion is distinctly different. The spike-and-dome pattern can be recorded over the entire cortex, illustrating again that the seizure originates in the RAS.

Partial epilepsy can involve almost any part of the brain, either localized regions of the cerebral cortex or deeper structures of both the cerebrum and brainstem. Partial epilepsy almost always results from some organic lesion of the brain, such as a scar that pulls on the neuronal tissue, a tumor that compresses an area of the brain, or a destroyed region of the brain tissue. Lesions such as these can cause local neurons to fire very rapid discharges. When the rate exceeds approximately 1000/s, synchronous waves begin spreading over adjacent cortical regions. These waves presumably result from the activity of localized reverberating neuronal circuits that gradually recruit adjacent areas of the cortex into the "discharge," or firing, zone. The process spreads to adjacent areas at rates as slow as a few millimeters per minute to as fast as several centimeters per minute. When such a wave of excitation spreads over the motor cortex, it causes a progressive "march" of muscular contractions throughout the opposite side of the body, beginning perhaps in the leg region and marching progressively upward to the head region, or at other times marching in the opposite direction. This is called *Jacksonian epilepsy* or *Jacksonian march*.

Another type of partial epilepsy is the so-called *psychomotor seizure*, which may cause (1) a short period of amnesia, (2) an attack of abnormal rage, (3) sudden anxiety or fear, (4) a moment of incoherent speech or mumbling, or (5) a motor act of rubbing the face with the hand, attacking someone, and so forth. Sometimes the person does not remember his or her activities during the attack; at other times the person is completely aware of, but unable to control, his or her behavior. The bottom tracing of Figure 4.27(c) represents a typical EEG during a psychomotor seizure showing a low-frequency rectangular-wave response with a frequency between 2 and 4 Hz with superimposed 14 Hz waves.

The EEG frequently can be used to locate tumors and also abnormal spiking waves originating in diseased brain tissue that might predispose to epileptic attacks. Once such a focal point is found, surgical excision of the focus often prevents future epileptic seizures.

The EEG is also used to monitor the depth of anesthesia.

The EEG is also used as a brain–computer interface to enable disabled persons to communicate with a computer.

## 4.9 THE MAGNETOENCEPHALOGRAM

Active bioelectric sources in the brain generate magnetic as well as electric fields. However, the magnitude of the magnetic field associated with active cortex is extremely low. For example, it is estimated that the magnetic field of the alpha wave is approximately 0.1 pT at a distance of 5 cm from the surface of the scalp. By way of comparison, this biomagnetic field associated with the magnetoencephalogram (MEG) is roughly one hundred million times weaker than the magnetic field of the earth ($\sim$ 50 $\mu$T). Recent technological advances in the study of superconductivity have made measurement of these extremely low-strength magnetic fields possible. Specifically, the superconducting quantum interference device (SQUID) magnetometer, which is based on a superconducting effect at liquid helium temperature, has sensitivity on the order of 0.01 pT. Background fields such as the earth's magnetic field and urban magnetic noise fields (~10 to 100 nT) can be removed for all practical purposes by using a gradiometer technique.

Using the MEG offers a number of advantages: (1) The brain and overlying tissues can be characterized as a single medium having a constant magnetic permeability $\mu$. Therefore, the magnetic field (unlike the electric field) is not influenced by the shell-like anisotropic inhomogeneities (meninges, fluid layers, skull, muscle layer, and scalp) surrounding the brain. (2) The measurement is indirect in that electrodes are not necessary to record the MEG. That is, the SQUID detector does not need to touch the scalp, because the magnetic field does not disappear in air.

The magnetic vector potential **A** has the same orientation as the equivalent current dipole representing an active region of the brain. For a derivation of the vector potential in terms of the volume current density **J**, see Plonsey (1969). Because the magnetic field lies perpendicular to the vector potential, radially oriented current dipoles produce magnetic fields that are oriented tangentially to the sphere representing the head. Similarly, tangentially oriented brain dipoles produce radially oriented magnetic fields.

The local time dependence of biomagnetic fields can be recorded faithfully with SQUID detection systems, but in order to measure the field distribution over the surface of the scalp, measurements must be made at many locations. This is a time-consuming process. Superconducting quantum interference device (SQUID) magnetometer vendors have systems with well over 100 channels (Wiksow, 1995). Advances in material fabrication techniques in the field of superconductivity should yield smaller detector coils for better spatial resolution and, subsequently, more precise localization of intracerebral sources of activity.

## PROBLEMS

**4.1** What are the four main factors involved in the movement of ions across the cell membrane in the steady-state condition?

**4.2** Assume that life on Mars requires an interior cell potential of +100 mV and that the extracellular concentrations of the three major species are as given in Example 4.1. Choose *one* species that has the permeability coefficient given, and assume the other two permeabilities are zero. Design the cell by calculating the intracellular concentration of the chosen species.

**4.3** An excitable cell is impaled by a micropipette, and a second extracellular electrode is placed close by at the outer-membrane surface. Brief pulses of current are then passed between these electrodes, which may cause it to conduct an action potential. Explain how the polarity of the stimulating pair influences the membrane potential, and subsequently the activity, of the excitable cell.

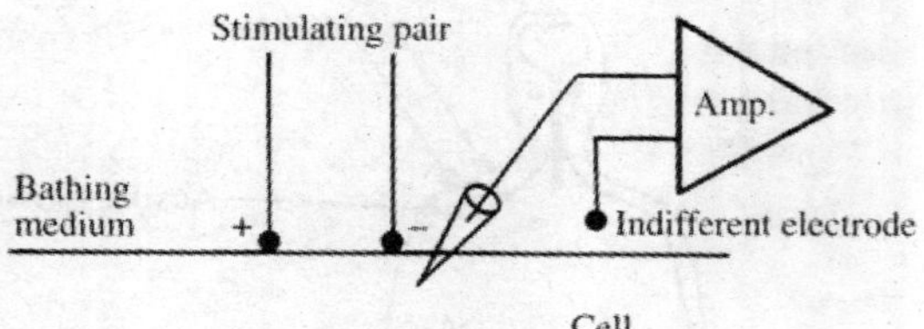


**Figure P4.1**

**4.4** Explain the subthreshold-membrane potential changes that would occur in the immediate vicinity of each of two extracellular stimulating electrodes placed at the outer-membrane surface of an excitable cell. (See Figure P4.1.) Assume that membrane potential is determined by impaling the cell with a micropipette at various points in the vicinity of the stimulating electrodes and recording the potential with respect to an indifferent extracellular electrode.

**4.5** If a stimulus of adequate strength is supplied to the stimulating pair of Problem 4.4, an action potential is generated. Explain by means of the concept of "local-circuit" current flow how the action potential is able to propagate in an unattenuated fashion down the fiber and away from the site of stimulation.

**4.6** If an elongated fiber is stimulated in the middle (as opposed to at either end), is an action potential propagated in both directions along the fiber? If so, would you expect any differences in the action-potential response measured at equal distances on either side of the stimulation site?

**4.7** Define the following terms: (a) absolute refractory period, (b) relative refractory period, (c) compound nerve-action potential, (d) synapse, (e) neuromyo junction, (f) motor unit, (g) reflex arc.

**4.8** An excised, active nerve trunk serves as a bioelectric source located on the axis of a circular cylindrical volume conductor. Field potentials are recorded at various radial distances from the nerve trunk from an appropriate electrode assembly connected to an amplifier. (a) Describe the behavior of the field potential with increasing radial distance from the nerve (angle and axial distance are fixed). (b) Describe the effect of increasing the specific resistivity $\rho$ of the bathing medium on the magnitude of the field potential, and explain how this change in $\rho$ might be accomplished experimentally. (c) In what manner would changing the radius of the surrounding volume-conductor affect the magnitude and waveshape of the extracellular field potential? (d) When can a volume conductor of finite dimensions be considered an essentially "infinite" volume conductor?

**4.9** The experimental situation posed in Problem 4.8 is roughly analogous to the problem of recording either surface or intramuscular potentials from the arm of a human subject whose ulnar or median nerve has been stimulated (see Figure 4.8, for instance). Explain in terms of changes in specific resistivity and geometry why potential waveforms recorded at the wrist may differ considerably from those recorded at the level of the forearm (see Figure 4.8).

**4.10** Define the M wave and the H reflex.

**4.11** In many forms of peripheral neuropathies, the excitability of some neurons is changed, and their conduction velocities are consequently altered.

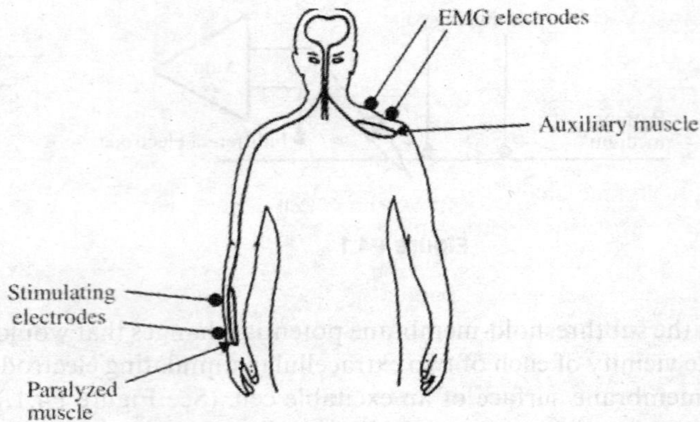


Figure P4.2

Describe the effect that this might have on an EMG recording and on muscular contraction.

**4.12** A muscle is paralyzed if its neural connection to, or within, the CNS is interrupted. A disconnection at the level of the motor neuron is called a *lower motoneuron lesion*. A disconnection higher in the spinal cord or brain is called an *upper motoneuron lesion*. In both cases, the contractility of the peripheral skeletal muscle is initially preserved, but after a period of disuse, the muscle atrophies. (Atrophy, however, is much delayed in the case of an upper motoneuron lesion.) Consider Figure P4.2 to represent schematically a quadriplegic patient with paralyzed extremities as shown. Suggest a scheme for using the EMG from an auxiliary intact muscle (for example, the left trapezius muscle) to aid in the control of stimulation of the paralyzed limb. (The motor nerve supply to the trapezius muscle is assumed to lie above the site of spinal-cord lesion and is therefore under volitional control. Draw a block diagram of the suggested control system. Label the anatomical structures serving as the plant (or controlled system), the controller, the feedback pathway, the actuator, and so forth. [*Hint*: The EMG signal is usually amplified, rectified, and low-pass filtered before it is used to modulate a stimulator. For further interesting discussions of the work in this area, see Vodovnik *et al.* (1981).]

**4.13** Conduct a search of the literature on the subject of the use of electromyography in the study of (a) the function of ocular muscles (the EMG yields valuable information regarding the synergistic action of the different ocular muscles, and it is of value in the interpretation of paralytic squint) and (b) myasthenia gravis and other disorders of neuromuscular transmission.

**4.14** Define the following cardiac anatomical terms: (a) internodal tracts, (b) subendocardial layer, (c) intercalated disk, (d) bundle branches, (e) ventricular activation.

**4.15** Draw a typical lead II electrocardiogram and label all waves (P, QRS, T) and intervals. Explain what is happening electrically within the heart during each wave or interval.

**4.16** The electrical activity of the His bundle normally is not present in the typical ECG recorded at the body surface because of its relatively small tissue mass. However, clinical recordings of His bundle activity could be of considerable importance in the analysis of various disorders of the conduction system. The His bundle signal can be enhanced for such analyses by successively averaging the surface electrocardiogram, or—better yet—by using an invasive technique wherein a small bipolar electrode is introduced into the right atrial chamber via conventional techniques of cardiac catheterization. Conduct a search of the literature on the topics of noninvasive and invasive methods of recording His bundle activity as well as on the use of this signal in diagnosing various disorders of the conduction system.

**4.17** Why is it necessary for the ventricular action potential to have a relatively long absolute refractory period?

**4.18** Draw and label a block diagram of the retina considered as a photoelectric sensor. What is the output at the ganglion cell layer and at the photoreceptive layer?

**4.19** Explain the components of the ERG in terms of retinal cell activity.

**4.20** Discuss, in terms of volume-conductor theory, the production of an ERG signal at a point on the corneal surface of the eye when the retinal bioelectric source is considered an array of current dipole sources per unit volume. Consider the possibility of (experimentally) exciting each of the elements of retinal dipole array individually, one at a time, by applying a localized spot of light superimposed on a background illumination that partially adapts the retina. What special technical considerations are involved?

**4.21** Discuss the use of the steady corneal–retinal potential of the eye to measure eye movements. How accurate is this technique? Discuss at least two applications of this method.

**4.22** Explain the functional role played by the following CNS structures.

**a.** The ascending pathways of the general sensory-nerve fibers and the descending pathways of the motor-nerve fibers
**b.** The ascending reticular formation (RAS)
**c.** The pre- and postcentral gyri
**d.** The primary auditory and visual cortices
**e.** The specific and nonspecific thalamic neural fibers to the cortex

**4.23** Relate EEG-wave activity recorded at the surface of the cortex to the underlying activity of cortical neurons.

**4.24** Discuss in general terms the design of a spectrum analyzer for automatic analysis of EEG waves.

**4.25** How might volume-conductor theory aid in the analysis of evoked cortical potentials produced by specific repetitive stimuli (auditory, visual, etc.)?

**4.26** Design the switches and resistor networks required, and show all connections between any four electrodes on the scalp (Fig. 4.28) and one differential amplifier, to record the EEG for each of the *three* types of electrode connections (monopolar, bipolar, and "average" potential recordings). See text associated with Figure 4.28.

## REFERENCES

Allessie, M. A., F. I. Bonke, and F. J. Shopman, "Circus movement in rabbit atrial muscle as a mechanism of tachycardia." *Circ. Res.*, 1973, 33, 54–62.

Barr, L., M. M. Dewey, and W. Berger, "Propagation of action potentials and the structure of the nexus in cardiac muscle." *J. Gen. Physiol.*, 1965, 48, 797–823.

Beeler, G. W., and H. Reuter, "Reconstruction of the action potential of ventricular myocardial fibres." *J. Physiol.*, 1977, 268, 177–210.

Clark, J. W., and R. Plonsey, "The extracellular potential field of the single active nerve fiber in a volume conductor." *Biophys. J.*, 1968, 8, 842–864.

Cuffin, N. "Eccentric spheres model of the head." *IEEE Trans. Biomed. Eng.*, 1991, 38, 871–878.

DeLuca, C., "Electromyography." In J. G. Webster (ed.), *Encyclopedia of Medical Devices and Instrumentation*. 2nd ed. New York: Wiley, 2006, Vol. 3, pp. 98–109.

Demir, S., J. W. Clark, C. Murphey, and W. Giles, "A mathematical model of a rabbit sinoatrial node cell." *Amer. J. Physiol.*, 1994, 266, C832–C852.

DiFrancesco, D., and D. Noble, "Model of cardiac electrical activity incorporating ionic pumps and concentration changes." *Phil. Trans. R. Soc.*, 1985, B307, 353–398.

Duchêne, J. and J. Y. Hogrel, "A model of EMG generation." *IEEE Trans. Biomed. Eng.*, 2000, 47, 192–201.

Esselle, K. P., and M. A. Stuchly, "Neural stimulation with magnetic fields." *IEEE Trans. Biomed. Eng.*, 1992, 39, 693–700.

Farina, D, L. Mesin, S. Martina, and R. Merletti, "A surface EMG generation model with multilayer cylindrical description of the volume conductor." *IEEE Trans. Biomed. Eng.*, 2004, 51, 415–426.

Farina, D., E. Schulte, R. Merletti, G. Rau, C. Disselhorst-Klug, "Single motor unit analysis from spatially filtered surface electromyogram signals: Parts I and II." *Med. Biol. Eng. Comput.*, 2003, 41, 330–345.

Ganapathy, N., J. W. Clark Jr., and O. B. Wilson, "Extracellular potentials from skeletal muscle." *Math. Biosciences*, 1987, 83, 61–96.

Geddes, L. A., "Optimal stimulus duration for extracranial cortical stimulation." *Neurosurgery*, 1987, 20, 94–99.

Goldman, D. E., "Potential, impedance and rectification in membranes." *J. Gen. Physiol*, 1943, 27, 37–60.

Halter, J. A., and J. W. Clark Jr., "A distributed-parameter model of the myelinated nerve fiber," *J. Theo. Biol.*, 1991, 148, 345–382.

Haueisen, J., D. S. Tuch, C. Ramon, P. H. Schimpf, V. J. Wedeen, J. S. George, and J. W. Belliveau, "The influence of brain tissue anisotropy on human EEG and MEG." *Neuroimage*, 2002, 15, 159–166.

Heckenlively, J. R., and G. B. Arden (eds.), *Principles and Practice of Clinical Electrophysiology of Vision*. St. Louis, MO: Mosby Year Book, 1991.

Henderson, C. J., S. R. Butler, and A. Glass, "The localization of equivalent dipoles of EEG sources by the application of electric field theory." *Electroencephalog. Clin. Neurophysiol.*, 1975, 39, 117–130.

Hodgkin, A. L., and A. F. Huxley, "A quantitative description of membrane current and its application to conduction and excitation in nerve." *J. Physiol.*, 1952, 117, 530.

Hodgkin, A. L., and B. Katz, "The effect of sodium ions on the electrical activity of the giant axon of the squid." *J. Physiol.*, 1949, 108, 37–77.

Jacobson, J. T., *Principles and Applications in Auditory Evoked Potentials*. Boston, MA: Allyn and Bacon, 1994.

Kandel, E. R., J. H. Schwartz, and T. M. Jessell, *Principles of Neural Science*, 3rd ed. New York: Elsevier Science, 1991.

Levitan I. B., and Kaczmarek, L. K., *The Neuron: Cell and Molecular Biology*, 3rd ed., New York: Oxford University Press, 2002.

Lorente de No, R., "Action potential of the motoneurons of the hypoglossus nucleus," *J. Cell. Comp. Physiol.*, 1947, 29, 207–287.

Luo, C. H., and Y. Rudy, "A dynamic model of the cardiac ventricular action potential I: Simulations of ionic currents and concentration changes," *Circ. Res.*, 1994, 74, 1097–1113.

Mambrito, B., and C. J. DeLuca, "A technique for the detection, decomposition and analysis of the EMG signal." *Electroencephalog. Clin. Neurophysiol.*, 1984, 58, 175–188.

McAllister, R. E., D. Noble, and R. W. Tsien, "Reconstruction of the electrical activity of cardiac Purkinje fibers." *J. Physiol.*, 1975, 251, 1–59.

Moffit, M. A., C. C. McIntyre, and W. M. Grill, "Prediction of myelinated nerve fiber stimulation thresholds: Limitations of linear models." *IEEE Trans. Biomed. Eng.*, 2004, 51, 229–236.

Moore, J. W., R. W. Joyner, M. H. Brill, S. G. Waxman, and M. Najar-Joa, "Simulations of conduction in uniform myelinated fibers." *Biophys. J.*, 1978, 21, 147–160.

Nandedkar, S. D., E. Stalberg, and D. B. Sanders, "Simulation techniques in electromyography." *IEEE Trans. Biomed. Eng.*, 1985, 32, 775–785.

Nazeran, H., "Electrocardiography, computers in." In J. G. Webster (ed.), *Encyclopedia of Medical Devices and Instrumentation*, 2nd ed. New York: Wiley, 2006, pp. 34–53.

Niedermeyer, E. and Lopes Da Silva, F. *Electroencephalography: Basic Principles, Clinical Applications and Related Fields*, 4th ed. Philadelphia: Lippincott, Williams and Wilkins, 1999.

Noble, D., "A modification of the Hodgkin–Huxley equations applicable to Purkinje fiber action and pacemaker potentials." *J. Physiol.*, 1962, 160, 317–352.

North, A. W., "Accuracy and precision of electro-oculographic recording." *Invest. Ophthalmol.*, 1965, 4, 343–348.

Nunez, P. L., *Electric Fields of the Brain: The Neurophysics of the EEG*. New York: Oxford University Press, 1981.

Nygren, A., C. Fiset, L. Firek, J. W. ClarkJr., D. S. Lindblad, R. B. Clark, and W. R. Giles, "Mathematical model of an adult human atrial cell: The role of $K^+$ currents in repolarization." *Circ. Res.*, 1998, 82, 63–81.

Plonsey, R., and R. C. Barr, *Bioelectricity: A Quantitative Approach*, 3rd ed. New York: Springer, 2007.

Plonsey, R., *Bioelectric Phenomena*. New York: McGraw-Hill, 1969.

Puglisi, J. L., and D. M. Bers, "LabHEART: an interactive computer model of rabbit ventricular myocyte ion channels and Ca transport." *Amer. J. Physiol.*, 2001, 281, C2049–2060.

Reucher, H., G. Rau, and J. Silny, "Spatial filtering of noninvasive multielectrode EMG: Parts I and II." *IEEE Trans. Biomed. Eng.*, 1987, 34, 98–113.

Rowell, L. B., *Human Cardiovascular Control*. New York: Oxford University Press, 1993.

Sherman, D., and D. Walterspacher, "Electroencephalography." In J. G. Webster (ed.), *Encyclopedia of Medical Devices and Instrumentation*. 2nd ed., New York: Wiley, 2006, Vol. 3, pp. 62–83.

Sinkjaer, T., K. Yoshida, W. Jensen, and V. Schnabel, "Electroneurography." In J. G. Webster (ed.), *Encyclopedia of Medical Devices and Instrumentation*. 2nd ed. New York: Wiley, 2006, Vol. 3, pp. 109–132.

Spach, M. S., R. C. Barr, G. A. Serwer, J. M. Kootsey, E. A. Johnson, "Extracellular potentials related to intracellular action potentials in the dog Purkinje system." *Circ. Res.*, 1972, 30, 505–519.

Stashuk, D., "EMG signal decomposition: how can it be accomplished and used?" *J. Electromyogr. Kinesiol.*, 2001, 11, 151–173.

Vodovnik, L., T. Bajd, A. Kralj, F. Gracanin, and P. Strojnik, "Functional electrical stimulation for control of locomotor systems." *CRC Crit. Rev. Bioeng.*, 1981, 6, 63–151.

Waxman, S. G., and M. H. Brill, "Conduction through demyelinated plaques in multiple sclerosis: Computer simulations of facilitation by short internodes." *J. Neural., Neurosurg. and Psychiat.*, 1978, 41, 408–416.

Wikswo, J. P., Jr., "SQUID magnetometers for biomagnetism and nondestructive testing: important questions and initial answers." *IEEE Trans. Appl. Superconductivity*, 1995, 5, 74–120.

Wilders, R., H. J. Jongsma, and A. C van Ginneken, "Pacemaker activity of the rabbit sincatrial node. A comparison of mathematical models." *Biophys. J.*, 1991, 60, 1202–1216.

Yagi T. and P. R. Macleish, "Ionic conductances of monkey solitary cone inner segments." *J. Neurophysiol.*, 1994, 71, 656–665.

Yanagihara, K., A. Noma, and H. Irisawa, "Reconstruction of sino-atrial node pacemaker potential based on the voltage clamp experiments." *Japan J. Physiol.*, 1980, 30, 841–857.

York, D. H., "Review of descending motor pathways involved with transcranial stimulation." *Neurosurgery*, 1987, 20, 70–73.

# 5

# BIOPOTENTIAL ELECTRODES

Michael R. Neuman

In order to measure and record potentials and, hence, currents in the body, it is necessary to provide some interface between the body and the electronic measuring apparatus. Biopotential electrodes carry out this interface function. In any practical measurement of potentials, current flows in the measuring circuit for at least a fraction of the period of time over which the measurement is made. Ideally this current should be very small. However, in practical situations, it is never zero. Biopotential electrodes must therefore have the capability of conducting a current across the interface between the body and the electronic measuring circuit.

Our first impression is that this is a rather simple function to achieve and that biopotential electrodes should be relatively straightforward. But when we consider the problem in more detail, we see that the electrode actually carries out a transducing function, because in the body current is carried by ions, whereas in the electrode and its lead wire it is carried by electrons. Thus the electrode must serve as a transducer to change an ionic current into an electronic current. This greatly complicates electrodes and places constraints on their operation. We shall briefly examine the basic mechanisms involved in the transduction process and shall look at how they affect electrode characteristics. We shall next examine the principal electrical characteristics of biopotential electrodes and discuss electrical equivalent circuits for electrodes based on these characteristics. We shall then cover some of the different forms that biopotential electrodes take in various types of medical instrumentation systems. Finally, we shall look at electrodes used for measuring the ECG, EEG, EMG, and intracellular potentials.

## 5.1 THE ELECTRODE–ELECTROLYTE INTERFACE

The passage of electric current from the body to an electrode can be understood by examining the electrode–electrolyte interface that is schematically illustrated in Figure 5.1. The electrolyte represents the body fluid containing ions. A net current that crosses the interface, passing from the electrode to the electrolyte, consists of (1) electrons moving in a direction opposite to that of

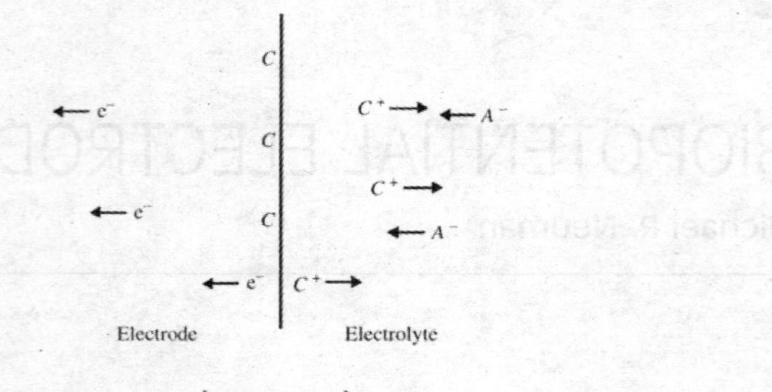


**Figure 5.1 Electrode–electrolyte interface** The current crosses it from left to right. The electrode consists of metallic atoms $C$. The electrolyte is an aqueous solution containing cations of the electrode metal $C^+$ and anions $A^-$.

the current in the electrode, (2) cations (denoted by $C^+$) moving in the same direction as the current, and (3) anions (denoted by $A^-$) moving in a direction opposite to that of the current in the electrolyte.

For charge to cross the interface—there are no free electrons in the electrolyte and no free cations or anions in the electrode—something must occur at the interface that transfers the charge between these carriers. What actually occur are chemical reactions at the interface, which can be represented in general by the following reactions:

$$C \rightleftarrows C^{n+} + ne^- \tag{5.1}$$

$$A^{m-} \rightleftarrows A + me^- \tag{5.2}$$

where $n$ is the valence of $C$ and $m$ is the valence of $A$. Note that in (5.1) we are assuming that the electrode is made up of some atoms of the same material as the cations and that this material in the electrode at the interface can become oxidized to form a cation and one or more free electrons. The cation is discharged into the electrolyte; the electron remains as a charge carrier in the electrode.

The reaction involving the anions is given in (5.2). In this case an anion coming to the electrode–electrolyte interface can be oxidized to a neutral atom, giving off one or more free electrons to the electrode.

Note that both reactions are often reversible and that reduction reactions (going from right to left in the equations) can occur as well. As a matter of fact, when no current is crossing the electrode–electrolyte interface, these reactions often still occur. But the rate of oxidation reactions equals the rate of reduction reactions, so the net transfer of charge across the interface is zero. When the current flow is from electrode to electrolyte, as indicated in Figure 5.1, the oxidation reactions dominate. When the current is in the opposite direction, the reduction reactions dominate.

To further explore the characteristics of the electrode–electrolyte interface, let us consider what happens when we place a piece of metal into a solution containing ions of that metal. These ions are cations, and the solution, if it is to maintain neutrality of charge, must have an equal number of anions. When the metal comes in contact with the solution, the reaction represented by (5.1) begins immediately. Initially, the reaction goes predominantly either to the left or to the right, depending on the concentration of cations in solution and the equilibrium conditions for that particular reaction. The local concentration of cations in the solution at the interface changes, which affects the anion concentration at this point as well. The net result is that neutrality of charge is not maintained in this region. Thus the electrolyte surrounding the metal is at a different electric potential from the rest of the solution. A potential difference known as the *half-cell potential* is determined by the metal involved, the concentration of its ions in solution, and the temperature, as well as other second-order factors. Knowledge of the half-cell potential is important for understanding the behavior of biopotential electrodes.

The distribution of ions in the electrolyte in the immediate vicinity of the metal–electrolyte interface has been of great interest to electrochemists, and several theories have been developed to describe it. Geddes (1972) compares the charges and potential distributions for four of these theories, whereas Cobbold (1974), in a discussion of the half-cell potential, considers the Stern model. Rather than analyze these theories here, we shall accept their general conclusion. Some separation of charges at the metal–electrolyte interface results in an electric double layer, wherein one type of charge is dominant on the surface of the metal, and the opposite charge is distributed in excess in the immediately adjacent electrolyte. This charge distribution at the electrode–electrolyte interface can affect electrode performance, as we will see in Section 5.3.

It is not possible to measure the half-cell potential of an electrode because—unless we use a second electrode—we cannot provide a connection between the electrolyte and one terminal of the potential-measuring apparatus. Because this second electrode also has a half-cell potential, we merely end up measuring the difference between the half-cell potential of the metal and that of the second electrode. There would of course be a very large number of combinations of pairs of electrodes, so tabulations of such differential half-cell potentials would be very extensive. To avoid this problem, electrochemists have adopted the standard convention that a particular electrode—the hydrogen electrode—is defined as having a half-cell potential of zero under conditions that are achievable in the laboratory. We can then measure the half-cell potentials of all other electrode materials with respect to this electrode.

Table 5.1 lists several common materials that are used for electrodes and gives their half-cell potentials. Table 5.1 also gives the oxidation–reduction reactions that occur at the surfaces of these electrodes and enable us to arrive at the potentials. The hydrogen electrode is based on the reaction

$$H_2 \rightleftarrows 2H \rightleftarrows 2H^+ + 2e^- \tag{5.3}$$

**Table 5.1 Half-cell Potentials for Common Electrode Materials at 25 °C**
The metal undergoing the reaction shown has the sign and potential $E^0$ when referenced to the hydrogen electrode

| Metal and Reaction | Potential $E^0$ (V) |
|---|---|
| $Al \rightarrow Al^{3+} + 3e^-$ | −1.706 |
| $Zn \rightarrow Zn^{2+} + 2e^-$ | −0.763 |
| $Cr \rightarrow Cr^{3+} + 3e^-$ | −0.744 |
| $Fe \rightarrow Fe^{2+} + 2e^-$ | −0.409 |
| $Cd \rightarrow Cd^{2+} + 2e^-$ | −0.401 |
| $Ni \rightarrow Ni^{2+} + 2e^-$ | −0.230 |
| $Pb \rightarrow Pb^{2+} + 2e^-$ | −0.126 |
| $H_2 \rightarrow 2H^+ + 2e^-$ | 0.000 by definition |
| $Ag + Cl^- \rightarrow AgCl + e^-$ | +0.223 |
| $2Hg + 2Cl^- \rightarrow Hg_2Cl_2 + 2e^-$ | +0.268 |
| $Cu \rightarrow Cu^{2+} + 2e^-$ | +0.340 |
| $Cu \rightarrow Cu^+ + e^-$ | +0.522 |
| $Ag \rightarrow Ag^+ + e^-$ | +0.799 |
| $Au \rightarrow Au^{3+} + 3e^-$ | +1.420 |
| $Au \rightarrow Au^+ + e^-$ | +1.680 |

SOURCE: Data from *Handbook of Chemistry and Physics,* 55th ed., Cleveland, OH: CRC Press, 1974–1975, with permission.

where $H_2$ gas bubbled over a platinum electrode is the source of hydrogen molecules. The platinum also serves as a catalyst for the reaction on the left-hand side of the equation and as an acceptor of the generated electrons.

## 5.2 POLARIZATION

The half-cell potential of an electrode is described in Section 5.1 for conditions in which no electric current exists between the electrode and the electrolyte. If, on the other hand, there is a current, the observed half-cell potential is often altered. The difference is due to polarization of the electrode. The difference between the observed half-cell potential and the equilibrium zero-current half-cell potential is known as the *overpotential.* Three basic mechanisms contribute to this phenomenon, and the overpotential can be separated into three components: the ohmic, the concentration, and the activation overpotentials.

The *ohmic overpotential* is a direct result of the resistance of the electrolyte. When a current passes between two electrodes immersed in an electrolyte, there is a voltage drop along the path of the current in the electrolyte as a result of its resistance. This drop in voltage is proportional to the current and the resistivity of the electrolyte. The resistance between the electrodes can itself vary as a function of the current. Thus the ohmic overpotential does not necessarily have to be linearly related to the current. This is especially true in electrolytes having low concentrations of ions. This situation, then, does not necessarily follow Ohm's law.

The *concentration overpotential* results from changes in the distribution of ions in the electrolyte in the vicinity of the electrode–electrolyte interface. Recall that the equilibrium half-cell potential results from the distribution of ionic concentration in the vicinity of the electrode–electrolyte interface when no current flows between the electrode and the electrolyte. Under these conditions, reactions (5.1) and (5.2) reach equilibrium, so the rates of oxidation and reduction at the interface are equal. When a current is established, this equality no longer exists. Thus it is reasonable to expect the concentration of ions to change. This change results in a different half-cell potential at the electrode. The difference between this and the equilibrium half-cell potential is the concentration overpotential.

The third mechanism of polarization results in the *activation overpotential.* The charge-transfer processes involved in the oxidation–reduction reaction (5.1) are not entirely reversible. In order for metal atoms to be oxidized to metal ions that are capable of going into solution, the atoms must overcome an energy barrier. This barrier, or *activation energy,* governs the kinetics of the reaction. The reverse reaction—in which a cation is reduced, thereby plating out an atom of the metal on the electrode—also involves an activation energy, but it does not necessarily have to be the same as that required for the oxidation reaction. When there is a current between the electrode and the electrolyte, either oxidation or reduction predominates, and hence the height of the energy barrier depends on the direction of the current. This difference in energy appears as a difference in voltage between the electrode and the electrolyte, which is known as the *activation overpotential.*

These three mechanisms of polarization are additive. Thus the net overpotential of an electrode is given by

$$V_{\mathrm{p}} = E^0 + V_{\mathrm{r}} + V_{\mathrm{c}} + V_{\mathrm{a}} \tag{5.4}$$

where

$V_{\mathrm{p}}$ = total potential, or polarization potential, of the electrode
$E^0$ = half-cell potential
$V_{\mathrm{r}}$ = ohmic overpotential
$V_{\mathrm{c}}$ = concentration overpotential
$V_{\mathrm{a}}$ = activation overpotential

When an ion-selective semipermeable membrane separates two aqueous ionic solutions of different concentration, an electric potential exists across this membrane. It can be shown (Plonsey and Barr, 2007) that this potential is given by the Nernst equation

$$E = -\frac{RT}{nF}\ln\frac{a_1}{a_2} \tag{5.5}$$

where $a_1$ and $a_2$ are the activities of the ions on each side of the membrane. [Other terms are defined in (4.1) and the Appendix.] In dilute solutions, ionic activity is approximately equal to ionic concentration. When intermolecular effects become significant, which happens at higher concentrations, the activity of the ions is less than their concentration.

The half-cell potentials listed in Table 5.1 are known as the standard half-cell potentials because they apply to standard conditions. When the electrode–electrolyte system no longer maintains this standard condition, half-cell potentials different from the standard half-cell potential are observed. The differences in potential are determined primarily by temperature and ionic activity in the electrolyte. *Ionic activity* can be defined as the availability of an ionic species in solution to enter into a reaction.

The standard half-cell potential is determined at a standard temperature; the electrode is placed in an electrolyte containing cations of the electrode material having unity activity. As the activity changes from unity (as a result of changing concentration), the half-cell potential varies according to the Nernst equation:

$$E = E^0 + \frac{RT}{nF}\ln(a_{c^{n+}}) \tag{5.6}$$

where

$E$ = half-cell potential

$E^0$ = standard half-cell potential

$n$ = valence of electrode material

$a_{c^{n+}}$ = activity of cation $C^{n+}$

Equation (5.6) represents a specific application of the Nernst equation to the reaction of (5.1). The more general form of this equation can be written for a general oxidation–reduction reaction as

$$\alpha A + \beta B \rightleftarrows \gamma C + \delta D + ne^- \tag{5.7}$$

where $n$ electrons are transferred. The general Nernst equation for this situation is

$$E = E^0 = \frac{RT}{nF}\ln\frac{a_C^{\gamma}a_D^{\delta}}{a_A^{\alpha}a_B^{\beta}} \tag{5.8}$$

where the $a$'s represent the activities of the various constituents of the reaction.

An electrode–electrolyte interface is not required for a potential difference to exist. If two electrolytic solutions are in contact and have different concentrations of ions with different ionic mobilities, a potential difference, known as a *liquid-junction potential,* exists between them. For solutions of the same composition but different activities, its magnitude is given by

$$E_j = \frac{\mu_+ - \mu_-}{\mu_+ + \mu_-} \frac{RT}{nF} \ln \frac{a'}{a''} \tag{5.9}$$

where $\mu_+$ and $\mu_-$ are the mobilities of the positive and negative ions, and $a'$ and $a''$ are the activities of the two solutions. Though liquid-junction potentials are generally not so high as electrode–electrolyte potentials, they can easily be of the order of tens of millivolts. For example, two solutions of sodium chloride, at 25 °C, with activities that vary by a factor of 10, have a potential difference of approximately 12 mV. Note that you can generate potentials of the order of some biological potentials by merely creating differences in concentration in an electrolyte. This is a factor to consider when you are examining actual electrode systems used for biopotential measurements.

**EXAMPLE 5.1** An electrode consisting of a piece of Zn with an attached wire and another electrode consisting of a piece of Ag coated with a layer of AgCl and an attached wire are placed in a 1 M $ZnCl_2$ solution (activities of $Zn^{2+}$ and $Cl^-$ are approximately unity) to form an electrochemical cell that is maintained at a temperature of 25 °C.

**a.** What chemical reactions might you expect to see at these electrodes?
**b.** If a very high input impedance voltmeter were connected between these electrodes, what would it read?
**c.** If the lead wires from the electrodes were shorted together, would a current flow? How would this affect the reactions at the electrodes?
**d.** How would you expect the voltage between the electrodes to differ from the equilibrium open-circuit voltage of the cell immediately following removal of the short circuit?

**ANSWER**

**a.** Zinc is much more chemically active than Ag, so the atoms on its surface oxidize to $Zn^{2+}$ ions according to the reaction: $Zn \rightleftarrows Zn^{2+} + 2e^-$, which according to Table 5.1 has an $E^0$ of –0.763 V.

At the Ag electrode, Ag can be oxidized to form $Ag^+$ ions according to the reaction: $Ag \rightleftarrows Ag^+ + 1e^-$. These ions immediately react with the $Cl^-$ ions in solution to form AgCl, $Ag^+ + Cl^- \rightleftarrows AgCl\downarrow$. Most of this precipitates out of solution due to this salt's low solubility. This reaction has an $E^0$ of 0.223 V at 25 °C.

**b.** When no current is drawn from or supplied to either electrode, and the concentration of ions is uniform throughout the solution, the difference in voltage between the electrodes is the difference between the half-cell potentials:

$$V = E^0_{Zn} - E^0_{Ag} = -0.763\ V - 0.233\ V = -0.986\ V$$

Because Zn oxidizes at a higher potential, the electrons remaining in it are at a higher energy than those in the Ag. Thus the Zn electrode has a negative voltage with respect to the Ag electrode.

**c.** There is a potential difference between the two electrodes, so there will be a current when they are shorted together. The flow of electrons is from the Zn to the Ag, because the Zn electrons are at a higher energy. Thus Zn is consumed and yields electrons, and AgCl absorbs electrons and plates out metallic Ag.

**d.** When the electrodes are connected, they must be at the same potential at the point of connection. Thus the 0.986 V half-cell potential difference must be opposed by polarization overpotentials and ohmic losses in the electrodes and connecting wires. When the connection is broken and the current stops, the ohmic overpotential and electrode losses become zero, but the concentration overpotential remains until the gradient of the ionic concentration at the electrode surfaces returns to its equilibrium value for zero current. Thus the difference in voltage between the two electrodes is less than 0.986 V when the circuit is opened but rises to that value asymptotically with time.

## 5.3 POLARIZABLE AND NONPOLARIZABLE ELECTRODES

Theoretically, two types of electrodes are possible: those that are perfectly polarizable and those that are perfectly nonpolarizable. This classification refers to what happens to an electrode when a current passes between it and the electrolyte. *Perfectly polarizable electrodes* are those in which no actual charge crosses the electrode–electrolyte interface when a current is applied. Of course, there has to be current across the interface, but this current is a displacement current, and the electrode behaves as though it were a capacitor. *Perfectly nonpolarizable electrodes* are those in which current passes freely across the electrode–electrolyte interface, requiring no energy to make the transition. Thus, for perfectly nonpolarizable electrodes there are no overpotentials.

Neither of these two types of electrodes can be fabricated; however, some practical electrodes can come close to acquiring their characteristics. Electrodes made of noble metals such as platinum come closest to behaving as perfectly polarizable electrodes. Because the materials of these electrodes are relatively inert, it is difficult for them to oxidize and dissolve. Thus current passing between the electrode and the electrolyte changes the concentration primarily of ions at the interface, so a majority of the overpotential seen from this type of electrode is a result of $V_c$, the concentration overpotential. The electrical characteristics of such an electrode show a strong capacitive effect.

### THE SILVER/SILVER CHLORIDE ELECTRODE

The silver/silver chloride (Ag/AgCl) electrode is a practical electrode that approaches the characteristics of a perfectly nonpolarizable electrode and can

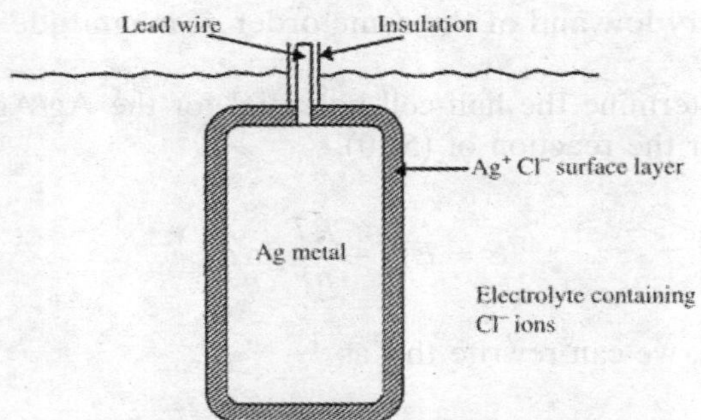


**Figure 5.2** A silver/silver chloride electrode, shown in cross section.

be easily fabricated in the laboratory. It is a member of a class of electrodes each of which consists of a metal coated with a layer of a slightly soluble ionic compound of that metal with a suitable anion. The whole structure is immersed in an electrolyte containing the anion in relatively high concentrations.

The structure is shown in Figure 5.2. A silver metal base with attached insulated lead wire is coated with a layer of the ionic compound AgCl. (This material—AgCl—is only very slightly soluble in water, so it remains stable.) The electrode is then immersed in an electrolyte bath in which the principal anion of the electrolyte is $Cl^-$. For best results, the electrolyte solution should also be saturated with AgCl so that there is little chance for any of the surface film on the electrode to dissolve.

The behavior of the Ag/AgCl electrode is governed by two chemical reactions. The first involves the oxidation of silver atoms on the electrode surface to silver ions in solution at the interface.

$$Ag \rightleftarrows Ag^+ + e^- \tag{5.10}$$

$$Ag^+ + Cl^- \rightleftarrows AgCl \downarrow \tag{5.11}$$

The second reaction occurs immediately after the formation of $Ag^+$ ions. These ions combine with $Cl^-$ ions already in solution to form the ionic compound AgCl. As mentioned before, AgCl is only very slightly soluble in water, so most of it precipitates out of solution onto the silver electrode and contributes to the silver chloride deposit. Silver chloride's rate of precipitation and of returning to solution is a constant $K_s$ known as the *solubility product.*

Under equilibrium conditions the ionic activities of the $Ag^+$ and $Cl^-$ ions must be such that their product is the solubility product.

$$a_{Ag^+} \times a_{Cl^-} = K_s \tag{5.12}$$

In biological fluids the concentration of $Cl^-$ ions is relatively high, which gives it an activity just a little less than unity. The solubility product for AgCl, on the other hand, is of the order of $10^{-10}$. This means that, when an Ag/AgCl electrode is in contact with biological fluids, the activity of the $Ag^+$

ion must be very low and of the same order of magnitude as the solubility product.

We can determine the half-cell potential for the Ag/AgCl electrode by writing (5.6) for the reaction of (5.10).

$$E = E^0_{\mathrm{Ag}} + \frac{RT}{nF} \ln a_{\mathrm{Ag}^+} \tag{5.13}$$

By using (5.12), we can rewrite this as

$$E = E^0_{\mathrm{Ag}} + \frac{RT}{nF} \ln \frac{K_s}{a_{\mathrm{Cl}^-}} \tag{5.14}$$

or

$$E = E^0_{\mathrm{Ag}} + \frac{RT}{nF} \ln K_s - \frac{RT}{nF} \ln a_{\mathrm{Cl}^-} \tag{5.15}$$

The first and second terms on the right-hand side of (5.15) are constants; only the third is determined by ionic activity. In this case, it is the activity of the $Cl^-$ ion, which is relatively large and not related to the oxidation of Ag, which is caused by the current through the electrode. The half-cell potential of this electrode is consequently quite stable when it is placed in an electrolyte containing $Cl^-$ as the principal anion, provided the activity of the $Cl^-$ remains stable. Because this is the case in the body, we shall see in later sections of this chapter that the Ag/AgCl electrode is relatively stable in biological applications.

There are several procedures that can be used to fabricate Ag/AgCl electrodes (Janz and Ives, 1968). Two of them are of particular importance in biomedical electrodes. One is the electrolytic process for forming Ag/AgCl electrodes. An electrochemical cell is made up in which the Ag electrode on which the AgCl layer is to be deposited serves as anode and another piece of Ag—having a surface area much greater than that of the anode—serves as cathode. A 1.5 V battery serves as the energy source, and a series resistance limits the peak current, thereby controlling the maximal rate of reaction. A milliammeter can be placed in the circuit to observe the current, which is proportional to the rate of reaction.

The reactions of (5.10) and (5.11) begin to occur as soon as the battery is connected, and the current jumps to its maximal value. As the thickness of the deposited AgCl layer increases, the rate of reaction decreases and the current drops. This situation continues, and the current approaches zero asymptotically. Theoretically, the reaction is not complete until the current drops to zero. In practice this never occurs because of other processes going on that conduct a current. Therefore the reaction can be stopped after a few minutes, once the current has reached a relatively stable low value—of the order of 10 μA for most biological electrodes.

**EXAMPLE 5.2** An AgCl surface is grown on an Ag electrode by the electrolytic process described in the previous paragraph. The current passing through the cell is measured and recorded during the growth of the AgCl layer and is found to be represented by the equation

$$I = 100\,\text{mA}\,e^{-t/10\,\text{s}} \tag{E5.1}$$

**a.** If the reaction is allowed to run for a long period of time, so that the current at the end of this period is essentially zero; how much charge is removed from the battery during this reaction?

**b.** How many grams of AgCl are deposited on the Ag electrode's surface by this reaction?

**c.** The chloride electrode is now placed into a beaker containing 1 liter of 0.9 molar NaCl solution. How much AgCl will be dissolved?

**ANSWER**

**a.** The total charge crossing the electrode–electrolyte interface during the reaction is

$$q = \int_0^\infty i\,dt = 100\,\text{mA} \int_0^\infty e^{-t/10}\,dt = 1\,\text{C} \tag{E5.2}$$

**b.** One molecule of AgCl is deposited for each electron. The number of atoms deposited is

$$N = \frac{1\,\text{C}}{1.6 \times 10^{-19}\,\text{C/atom}} = 6.25 \times 10^{8}\ \text{atoms} \tag{E5.3}$$

The number of moles can be found by dividing by Avogadro's number.

$$N = \frac{6.25 \times 10^{18}}{6.03 \times 10^{23}} = 1.036 \times 10^{-5}\ \text{mol} \tag{E5.4}$$

The molecular weight of AgCl is 143.2, therefore the mass of AgCl formed is

$$142.3 \times 1.036 \times 10^{-5} = 1.47 \times 10^{-3}\ \text{g} \tag{E5.5}$$

**c.** For AgCl the solubility product is $K_s = 1.56 \times 10^{-10}$ at 25 °C. The activity and concentration are about the same at these low concentrations. Thus

$$[\text{Ag}^+][\text{Cl}^-] = 1.56 \times 10^{-10} \tag{E5.6}$$

Since $[\text{Cl}^-]$ in the NaCl solution is 0.9 mole/liter, the dissolved Ag will be

$$[\text{Ag}^+] = 1.73 \times 10^{-10}\ \text{mol/liter}$$

In terms of mass this will be $1.73 \times 10^{-10} \times 142.3 = 2.46 \times 10^{-8}$ g.

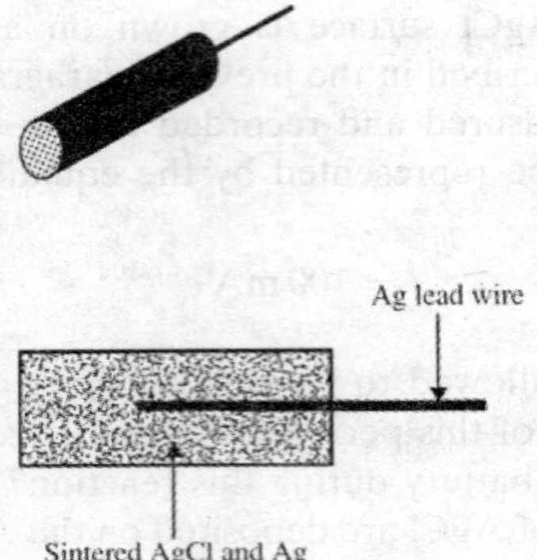


**Figure 5.3** Sintered Ag/AgCl electrode

The second process for producing Ag/AgCl electrodes useful in medical instrumentation is a sintering process that forms pellet electrodes, as shown in Figure 5.3. The electrode consists of an Ag lead wire surrounded by a sintered Ag/AgCl cylinder. It is formed by placing the cleaned lead wire in a die that is then filled with a mixture of powdered Ag and AgCl. The die is compressed in an arbor press to form the powdered components into a pellet, which is then removed from the die and baked at 400 °C for several hours. These electrodes tend to have a greater endurance than the electrolytically deposited AgCl electrodes, and they are best applied when repeated usage is necessary. The electrolytically deposited AgCl has a tendency to flake off under mechanical stress, leaving portions of metallic Ag in contact with the electrolyte, which can cause the electrode's half-cell, potential to be unstable and noisy.

Silver chloride is not a very good conductor of an electric current. If the powder that was compressed to make the sintered electrode consisted only of finely ground silver chloride, this would result in a high-resistance electric connection between the electrolytic solution and the silver wire in the center of the sintered electrode. Electrochemists found that they could increase the conductivity of the silver chloride pellet by including metallic silver powder along with the silver chloride powder. The amount of metallic silver is small enough to make highly unlikely any direct connection from the silver wire to the electrode through silver particles. Instead, there is always some silver chloride between the silver particles, but the presence of the silver particles makes it easier for current to pass through the silver chloride.

A similar situation occurs in the electrolytically prepared silver/silver chloride electrode. Although the silver chloride layer is much thinner in this case than it is for the sintered electrode, it remains a pure silver chloride layer for only a short time after it is deposited. Silver chloride is a silver-halide salt, and these materials are photosensitive. Light striking these salts can cause the silver ions to be reduced to metallic silver atoms. Thus, for all practical purposes, the electrolytically deposited silver chloride layer contains fine silver particles as well. Evidence of their presence appears when the layer is grown and immediately becomes dark gray because of the fine silver particles (pure silver chloride is amber colored).

In addition to its nonpolarizable behavior, the Ag/AgCl electrode exhibits less electric noise than the equivalent metallic Ag electrodes. Geddes and Baker (1989) showed that electrodes with the AgCl layer exhibited far less noise than was observed when the AgCl layer was removed. Also, a majority of the noise for the purely metallic electrodes was at low frequencies. This would provide the most serious interference for low-frequency, low-voltage recordings, such as the EEG.

A second kind of electrode that has characteristics approaching those of the perfectly nonpolarizable electrode is the *calomel electrode.* It is used primarily as a reference electrode for electrochemical determinations and is frequently applied as the reference electrode when pH is measured (see Section 10.2). The calomel electrode is often constructed as a glass tube with a porous glass plug at its base filled with a paste of mercurous chloride or calomel ($Hg_2Cl_2$) mixed with a saturated potassium chloride (KCl) solution. Like AgCl, the $Hg_2Cl_2$ is only slightly soluble in water, so most of it retains its solid form. A layer of elemental mercury is placed on top of the paste layer with an electric lead wire within it. This entire assembly is then positioned in the center of a larger glass tube with a porous glass plug at its base. The tube is filled with a saturated KCl solution so that the $Hg_2Cl_2$ layer of the inner tube is in contact with this electrolyte through the porous plug of the inner tube. We have a half-cell made up of Hg in intimate contact with an $Hg_2Cl_2$ layer that is in contact with the saturated KCl electrolyte. The porous plug at the bottom of the electrode assembly is used to make contact between the internal KCl solution and the solution in which the electrode is immersed. This is actually a liquid–liquid junction that can result in a liquid–liquid junction potential, which will add to the electrode half-cell potential.

Silver/silver chloride electrodes can be fabricated in the same form as the calomel electrode and used for electroanalytical chemical measurements. In this case, the mercury is replaced by silver and AgCl replaces the $Hg_2Cl_2$ in the electrode structure.

Using the same argument as that used for the Ag/AgCl electrode, we can show that the half-cell potential of this electrode is dependent on the $Cl^-$ activity in the saturated KCl solution. This is stable at a given temperature, because the solution is saturated and therefore has a stable chloride ion activity. In application, the tip of this electrode assembly that contains the porous plug is dipped into the electrolytic solution that it is to contact. In pH measurements, a pH electrode is also dipped into the solution, and the potential difference between the two electrodes is measured.

**EXAMPLE 5.3** To measure the potential across the rectal mucosa (inner surface of the rectum), a technique has been developed whereby an Ag/AgCl reference electrode is placed at some convenient point on the skin surface of the body away from the anal orifice. Another Ag/AgCl electrode is placed against the inner wall of the rectum about 8 cm up from the anus. The potential difference between these two electrodes is measured with a high-input impedance voltmeter, and the result recorded. The rectal electrode is then removed and immediately touched to the skin surrounding the anus, as close to it as possible. Another potential difference is measured and recorded. The difference between the two measurements is then determined. This is considered the true potential across the rectal mucosa.

At first glance, this appears to be a rather difficult way to make a simple measurement. We may wonder why we couldn't simply place one of the Ag/AgCl electrodes on the skin surrounding the anus and the other in the rectum and merely measure the potential difference between them. Explain why the biomedical engineer who developed this procedure considered the simpler approach inadequate and chose the more complicated, two-measurement technique.

**ANSWER** Although theoretically every Ag/AgCl electrode should have the same half-cell potential, there are usually differences from one to another. These differences should be quite small, of the order of millivolts. However, occasions can arise in which the differences can be as high as tens—or in extreme cases, even hundreds—of millivolts. When we are measuring the potential difference between two Ag/AgCl electrodes, the difference between the half-cell potentials of each electrode enters into the measured value. When both half-cell potentials are equal, the differences cancel out. However if the half-cell potentials are different, errors are introduced into the measurements. The engineer who designed this measurement knew that this was a possibility and therefore used a single electrode, instead of two different Ag/AgCl electrodes, to measure the potential across the rectal mucosa. With this technique, the half-cell potential when the electrode is in the rectum and the half-cell potential when it is on the perianal skin are identical; they cancel out completely.

## 5.4 ELECTRODE BEHAVIOR AND CIRCUIT MODELS

The electrical characteristics of electrodes have been the subject of much study. Often the current–voltage characteristics of the electrode–electrolyte interface are found to be nonlinear, and, in turn, nonlinear elements are required for modeling electrode behavior. Specifically, the characteristics of an electrode are sensitive to the current passing through the electrode, and the electrode characteristics at relatively high current densities can be considerably different from those at low current densities. The characteristics of electrodes are also waveform dependent. When sinusoidal currents are used to measure the electrode's circuit behavior, the characteristics are also frequency dependent.

The characterization of electrode–electrolyte interfacial impedances has been well reviewed by Geddes (1972), Cobbold (1974), Ferris (1974), and

Schwan (1963). It is only summarized here. For sinusoidal inputs, the terminal characteristics of an electrode have both a resistive and a reactive component. Over all but the lowest frequencies, this situation can be modeled as a series resistance and capacitance. We should not be surprised to see a capacitance entering into this model, because the half-cell potential described earlier was the result of the distribution of ionic charge at the electrode–electrolyte interface that had been considered a double layer of charge. This, of course, should behave as a capacitor—hence the capacitive reactance seen for real electrodes.

The series resistance–capacitance equivalent circuit breaks down at the lower frequencies, where this model would suggest an impedance going to infinity as the frequency approaches dc. To avoid this problem, we can convert this series $RC$ circuit to a parallel $RC$ circuit that has a purely resistive impedance at very low frequencies. If we combine this circuit with a voltage source representing the half-cell potential and a series resistance representing the interface effects and resistance of the electrolyte, we can arrive at the biopotential electrode equivalent circuit model shown in Figure 5.4.

In this circuit, $R_d$ and $C_d$ represent the resistive and reactive components just discussed. These components are still frequency and current-density dependent. In this configuration it is also possible to assign physical meaning to the components. $C_d$ represents the capacitance across the double layer of charge at the electrode–electrolyte interface. The parallel resistance $R_d$ represents the leakage resistance across this double layer. All the components of this equivalent circuit have values determined by the electrode material and its geometry, and—to a lesser extent—by the material of the electrolyte and its concentration.

The equivalent circuit of Figure 5.4 demonstrates that the electrode impedance is frequency dependent. At high frequencies, where $1/\omega C \ll R_d$, the impedance is constant at $R_s$. At low frequencies, where $1/\omega C \gg R_d$, the impedance is again constant but its value is larger, being $R_s + R_d$. At frequencies between these extremes, the electrode impedance is frequency dependent.

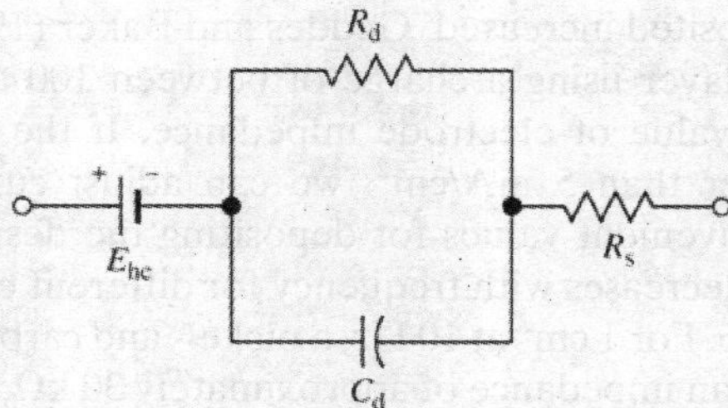


**Figure 5.4** Equivalent circuit for a biopotential electrode in contact with an electrolyte $E_{hc}$ is the half-cell potential, $R_d$ and $C_d$ make up the impedance associated with the electrode–electrolyte interface and polarization effects, and $R_s$ is the series resistance associated with interface effects and is due to resistance in the electrolyte.

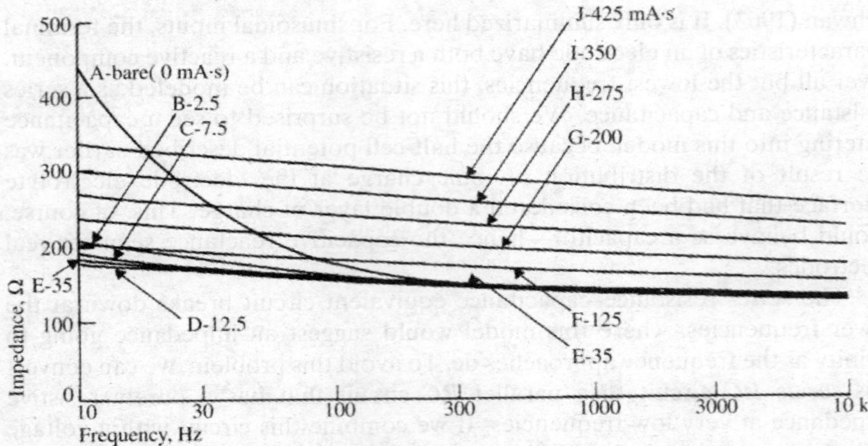


**Figure 5.5** Impedance as a function of frequency for Ag electrodes coated with an electrolytically deposited AgCl layer. The electrode area is 0.25 cm². Numbers attached to curves indicate number of mA·s for each deposit. (From L. A. Geddes, L. E. Baker, and A. G. Moore, "Optimum electrolytic chloriding of silver electrodes." *Medical and Biological Engineering,* 1969, 7, 49–56.)

The impedance of Ag/AgCl electrodes varies significantly from that of a pure silver electrode at frequencies under 100 Hz. Geddes *et al.* (1969) demonstrated this; their data are reproduced in Figure 5.5.

A metallic silver electrode having a surface area of 0.25 cm² had the impedance characteristic shown by curve A. At a frequency of 10 Hz, the magnitude of its impedance was almost three times the value at 300 Hz. This indicates a strong capacitive component to the equivalent circuit. Electrolytically depositing 2.5 mA·s of AgCl greatly reduced the low-frequency impedance, as reflected in curve B. Depositing thicker AgCl layers had minimal effects until the charge deposited exceeded approximately 100 mA·s. The curves were then seen to shift to higher impedances in a parallel fashion as the amount of AgCl deposited increased. Geddes and Baker (1989) point out that depositing an AgCl layer using a charge of between 100 and 500 mA·s/cm² provides the lowest value of electrode impedance. If the current density is maintained at greater than 5 mA/cm², we can adjust current and time to provide the most convenient values for depositing the desired layer.

The impedance decreases with frequency for different electrode materials as shown in Figure 5.6. For 1 cm² at 10 Hz, a nickel- and carbon-loaded silicone rubber electrode has an impedance of approximately 30 kΩ, whereas Ag/AgCl has an impedance of less than 10 Ω (Das and Webster, 1980).

**EXAMPLE 5.4** We want to develop an electrical model for a specific biopotential electrode studies in the laboratory. The electrode is

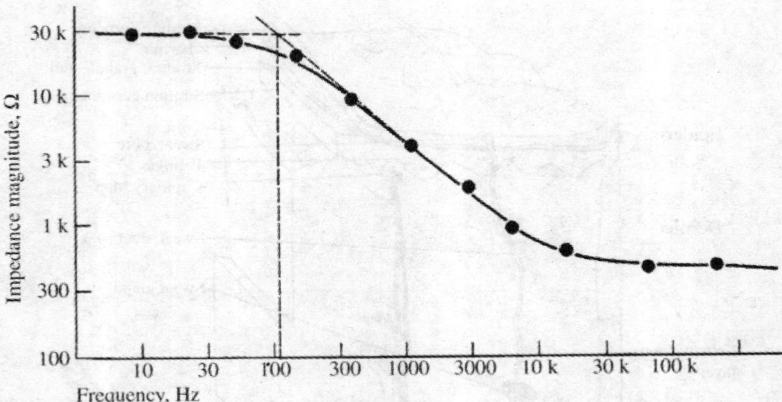


**Figure 5.6** Experimentally determined magnitude of impedance as a function of frequency for electrodes.

characterized by placing it in a physiological saline bath in the laboratory, along with an Ag/AgCl electrode having a much greater surface area and a known half-cell potential of 0.233 V. The dc voltage between the two electrodes is measured with a very-high-impedance voltmeter and found to be 0.572 V with the test electrode negative. The magnitude of the impedance between the two electrodes is measured as a function of frequency at very low currents; it is found to be that given in Figure 5.6. From these data, determine a circuit model for the electrode.

**ANSWER** The very large surface area of the Ag/AgCl reference electrode makes its impedance very small compared to that of the test electrode, so we can neglect it. We cannot, however, neglect its half-cell potential, which is unaffected by surface area. The half-cell potential of the test electrode is $E_x^0 = 0.223\text{ V} - 0.572\text{ V} = -0.349\text{ V}$.

At frequencies above about 20 kHz, the electrode impedance is constant because $C_d$ in Figure 5.4 is short-circuited. Thus $R_s = 500\ \Omega$. At frequencies less than 50 Hz, the electrode impedance is constant because $C_d$ is open-circuited. Thus $R_s + R_d = 30\text{ k}\Omega$. Thus $R_d = 29.5\text{ k}\Omega$. The corner frequency is 100 Hz. Thus $C_d = 1/(2\pi f R_d) = 1/(2\pi 100 \times 29500) = 5.3 \times 10^{-8}\text{ F}$.

## 5.5 THE ELECTRODE–SKIN INTERFACE AND MOTION ARTIFACT

In Section 5.1 we examined the electrode–electrolyte interface and saw how it influenced the electrical properties that are seen in practical electrodes. When biopotentials are recorded from the surface of the skin, we must consider an additional interface—the interface between the electrode–electrolyte and the skin—in order to understand the behavior of the electrodes. In coupling an electrode to the skin, we generally use transparent electrolyte gel containing

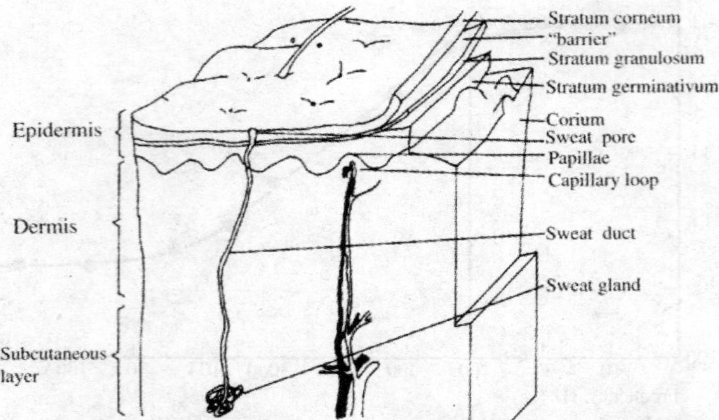


**Figure 5.7** **Magnified section of skin, showing the various layers** (Copyright © 1977 by The Institute of Electrical and Electronics Engineers. Reprinted, with permission, from *IEEE Trans. Biomed. Eng.*, March 1977, vol. BME-24, no. 2, pp. 134–139.)

$Cl^-$ as the principal anion to maintain good contact. Alternatively, we may use an electrode cream, which contains $Cl^-$ and has the consistency of hand lotion. The interface between this gel and the electrode is an electrode–electrolyte interface, as described above. However, the interface between the electrolyte and the skin is different and requires some explanation. Before we give this explanation, let us briefly review the structure of the skin.

Figure 5.7 shows a cross-sectional diagram of the skin. The skin consists of three principal layers that surround the body to protect it from its environment and that also serve as appropriate interfaces. The outermost layer, or *epidermis,* plays the most important role in the electrode–skin interface. This layer, which consists of three sublayers, is constantly renewing itself. Cells divide and grow in the deepest layer, the *stratum germinativum,* and are displaced outward as they grow by the newly forming cells underneath them. As they pass through the *stratum granulosum,* they begin to die and lose their nuclear material. As they continue their outward journey, they degenerate further into layers of flat keratinous material that forms the *stratum corneum,* or horny layer of dead material on the skin's surface. These layers are constantly being worn off and replaced at the stratum granulosum by new cells. The epidermis is thus a constantly changing layer of the skin, the outer surface of which consists of dead material that has different electrical characteristics from live tissue.

The deeper layers of the skin contain the vascular and nervous components of the skin as well as the sweat glands, sweat ducts, and hair follicles. These layers are similar to other tissues in the body and, with the exception of the sweat glands, do not bestow any unique electrical characteristics on the skin.

To represent the electric connection between an electrode and the skin through the agency of electrolyte gel, our equivalent circuit of Figure 5.4 must be expanded, as shown in Figure 5.8. The electrode–electrolyte interface

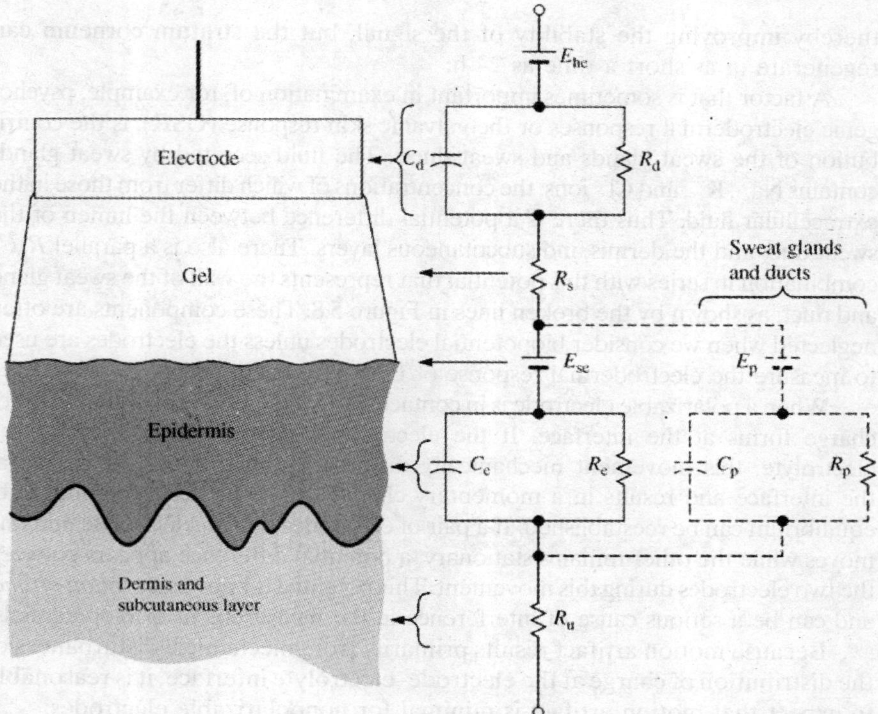


**Figure 5.8** A body-surface electrode is placed against skin, showing the total electrical equivalent circuit obtained in this situation. Each circuit element on the right is at approximately the same level at which the physical process that it represents would be in the left-hand diagram.

equivalent circuit is shown adjacent to the electrode–gel interface. The series resistance $R_s$ is now the effective resistance associated with interface effects of the gel between the electrode and the skin. We can consider the epidermis, or at least the stratum corneum, as a membrane that is semipermeable to ions, so if there is a difference in ionic concentration across this membrane, there is a potential difference $E_{se}$, which is given by the Nernst equation. The epidermal layer is also found to have an electric impedance that behaves as a parallel $RC$ circuit, as shown. For 1 $cm^2$, skin impedance reduces from approximately 200 kΩ at 1 Hz to 200 Ω at 1 MHz (Rosell *et al.*, 1988). The dermis and the subcutaneous layer under it behave in general as pure resistances. They generate negligible dc potentials.

Thus we see that—if the effect of the stratum corneum can be reduced—a more stable electrode will result. We can minimize the effect of the stratum corneum by removing it, or at least a part of it, from under the electrode. There are many ways to do this, ranging from vigorous rubbing with a pad soaked in acetone to abrading the stratum corneum with sandpaper to puncture it. In all cases, this process tends to short out $E_{se}$, $C_e$, and $R_e$, as shown in Figure 5.8, thereby improving the stability of the signal, but the stratum corneum can regenerate in as short a time as 24 h.

A factor that is sometimes important in examination of, for example, psychogenic electrodermal responses or the galvanic skin response (GSR), is the contribution of the sweat glands and sweat ducts. The fluid secreted by sweat glands contains $Na^+$, $K^+$, and $Cl^-$ ions, the concentrations of which differ from those in the extracellular fluid. Thus there is a potential difference between the lumen of the sweat duct and the dermis and subcutaneous layers. There also is a parallel $R_pC_p$ combination in series with this potential that represents the wall of the sweat gland and duct, as shown by the broken lines in Figure 5.8. These components are often neglected when we consider biopotential electrodes unless the electrodes are used to measure the electrodermal response or GSR (Boucsein, 1992).

When a polarizable electrode is in contact with an electrolyte, a double layer of charge forms at the interface. If the electrode is moved with respect to the electrolyte, this movement mechanically disturbs the distribution of charge at the interface and results in a momentary change of the half-cell potential until equilibrium can be reestablished. If a pair of electrodes is in an electrolyte and one moves while the other remains stationary, a potential difference appears between the two electrodes during this movement. This potential is known as *motion artifact* and can be a serious cause of interference in the measurement of biopotentials.

Because motion artifact results primarily from mechanical disturbances of the distribution of charge at the electrode–electrolyte interface, it is reasonable to expect that motion artifact is minimal for nonpolarizable electrodes.

Observation of the motion-artifact signals reveals that a major component of this noise is at low frequencies. Section 6.6 and Figure 6.16 will show that different biopotential signals occupy different portions of the frequency spectrum. Figure 6.16 shows that low-frequency artifact does not affect signals such as the EMG or axon action potential (AAP) nearly so much as it does the ECG, EEG, and EOG. In the former case, filtering can be effectively used to minimize the contribution of motion artifact on the overall signal. But in the latter case, such filtering also distorts the signal. Consequently, it is important in these applications to use a nonpolarizable electrode to minimize motion artifact stemming from the electrode–electrolyte interface.

This interface, however, is not the only source of motion artifact encountered when biopotential electrodes are applied to the skin. The equivalent circuit in Figure 5.8 shows that, in addition to the half-cell potential $E_{hc}$, the electrolyte gel–skin potential $E_{se}$ can also cause motion artifact if it varies with movement of the electrode. Variations of this potential indeed do represent a major source of motion artifact in Ag/AgCl skin electrodes (Tam and Webster, 1977). They have shown that this artifact can be significantly reduced when the stratum corneum is removed by mechanical abrasion with a fine abrasive paper. This method also helps to reduce the epidermal component of the skin impedance. Tam and Webster (1977) also point out, however, that removal of the body's outer protective barrier makes that region of skin more susceptible to irritation from the electrolyte gel. Therefore, the choice of a gel material is important. Remembering the dynamic nature of the epidermis, note also that the stratum corneum can regenerate itself in as short a time as 24 h, thereby renewing the source of motion artifact. This is a factor to be taken into account if the electrodes are to be used for chronic recording. A potential between the inside and outside of the skin can be measured (Burbank and Webster, 1978). Stretching the skin changes this skin potential by 5 to 10 mV, and this change appears as motion artifact. Ten 0.5 mm skin punctures through the barrier layer short-circuits the skin potential and reduces the stretch artifact to less than 0.2 mV. De Talhouet and Webster (1996) provide a model for the origin of this skin potential and show how it can be reduced by stripping layers of the skin using Scotch tape.

## 5.6 BODY-SURFACE RECORDING ELECTRODES

Over the years many different types of electrodes for recording various potentials on the body surface have been developed. This section describes the various types of these electrodes and gives an example of each. The reader interested in more extensive examples should consult Geddes (1972).

### METAL-PLATE ELECTRODES

Historically, one of the most frequently used forms of biopotential sensing electrodes is the metal-plate electrode. In its simplest form, it consists of a metallic conductor in contact with the skin. An electrolyte soaked pad or gel is used to establish and maintain the contact.

Figure 5.9 shows several forms of this electrode. A limb electrode for use with an electrocardiograph is shown in Figure 5.9(a). It consists of a flat metal plate that has been bent into a cylindrical segment. A terminal is placed on its

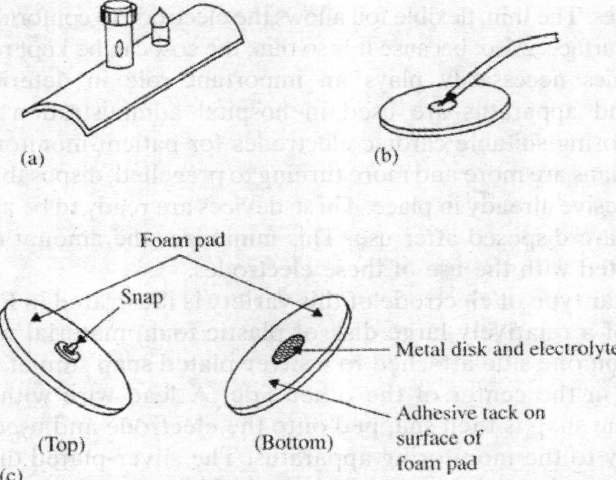


**Figure 5.9 Body-surface biopotential electrodes** (a) Metal-plate electrode used for application to limbs. (b) Metal-disk electrode applied with surgical tape. (c) Disposable foam-pad electrodes often used with electrocardiographic monitoring apparatus.

outside surface near one end; this terminal is used to attach the lead wire to the electrocardiograph. The electrode is traditionally made of German silver (a nickel–silver alloy). Before it is attached to the body with a rubber strap or tape, its concave surface is covered with electrolyte gel. Similarly arranged flat metal disks are also used as electrodes. Although based upon preceding sections of this chapter, one would expect that better electrode designs could be used with electrocardiographs today, these traditional electrodes are still occasionally used.

A more common variety of metal-plate electrode is the metal disk illustrated in Figure 5.9(b). This electrode, which has a lead wire soldered or welded to the back surface, can be made of several different materials. Sometimes a layer of insulating material, such as epoxy or polyvinylchloride, protects the connection between lead wire and electrode. This structure can be used as a chest electrode for recording the ECG or in cardiac monitoring for long-term recordings. In these applications the electrode is often fabricated from a disk of Ag that may have an electrolytically deposited layer of AgCl on its contacting surface. It is coated with electrolyte gel and then pressed against the patient's chest wall. It is maintained in place by a strip of surgical tape or a plastic foam disk with a layer of adhesive tack on one surface.

This style of electrode is also popular for surface recordings of EMG or EEG. In recording EMGs, investigators use stainless steel, platinum, or gold-plated disks to minimize the chance that the electrode will enter into chemical reactions with perspiration or the gel. These materials produce polarizable electrodes, and motion artifact can be a problem with active patients. Electrodes used in monitoring EMGs or EEGs are generally smaller in diameter than those used in recording ECGs. Disk-shaped electrodes such as these have also been fabricated from metal foils (primarily silver foil) and are applied as single-use disposable electrodes. The thin, flexible foil allows the electrode to conform to the shape of the body surface. Also, because it is so thin, the cost can be kept relatively low.

Economics necessarily plays an important role in determining what materials and apparatus are used in hospital administration and patient care. In choosing suitable cardiac electrodes for patient-monitoring applications, physicians are more and more turning to pregelled, disposable electrodes with the adhesive already in place. These devices are ready to be applied to the patient and are disposed after use. This minimizes the amount of personnel time associated with the use of these electrodes.

A popular type of electrode of this variety is illustrated in Figure 5.9(c). It consists of a relatively large disk of plastic foam material with a silver-plated disk on one side attached to a silver-plated snap similar to that used on clothing in the center of the other side. A lead wire with the female portion of the snap is then snapped onto the electrode and used to connect the assembly to the monitoring apparatus. The silver-plated disk serves as the electrode and may be coated with an AgCl layer. A layer of electrolyte gel covers the disk. The electrode side of the foam is covered with an adhesive material that is compatible with the skin. A protective cover or strip of release paper is placed over this side of the electrode and foam, and the complete electrode is packaged in a foil envelope so that the water component of the gel will not evaporate away. To apply the electrode to the patient, the clinician has only to clean the area of skin on which the electrode is to be placed, open the electrode packet, snap the lead wire on to the electrode, remove the release paper from the tack, and press the electrode against the patient's skin. This procedure is quickly accomplished and no special technique need be learned.

## SUCTION ELECTRODES

A modification of the metal-plate electrode that requires no straps or adhesives for holding it in place is the suction electrode illustrated in Figure 5.10. Such electrodes are frequently used in electrocardiography as the precordial (chest) leads, because they can be placed at particular locations and used to take a recording. They consist of a hollow metallic cylindrical electrode that makes contact with the skin at its base. An appropriate terminal for the lead wire is attached to the metal cylinder, and a rubber suction bulb fits over its other base. Electrolyte gel is placed over the contacting surface of the electrode, the bulb is squeezed, and the electrode is then placed on the chest wall. The bulb is released and applies suction against the skin, holding the electrode assembly in place. This electrode can be used only for short periods of time; the suction and the pressure of the contact surface against the skin can cause irritation. Although the electrode itself is quite large, Figure 5.10 shows that the actual contacting area is relatively small. This electrode thus tends to have a higher source impedance than the relatively large-surface-area metal-plate electrodes used for ECG limb electrodes, as shown in Figure 5.9(a).

## FLOATING ELECTRODES

In the previous section, we noted that one source of motion artifact in biopotential electrodes is the disturbance of the double layer of charge at

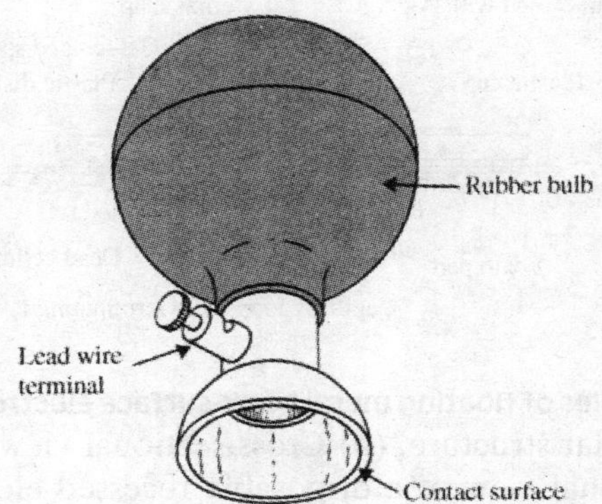


**Figure 5.10** A metallic suction electrode is often used as a precordial electrode on clinical electrocardiographs.

the electrode–electrolyte interface. The use of nonpolarizable electrodes, such as the Ag/AgCl electrode, can greatly diminish this artifact. But it still can be present, and efforts to stabilize the interface mechanically can reduce it further. *Floating electrodes* offer a suitable technique to do so.

Figure 5.11 shows examples of these devices. Figure 5.11(a) depicts a floating electrode known as a *top-hat* electrode; its internal structure is illustrated in cross section in Figure 5.11(b). The principal feature of the electrode is that the actual electrode element or metal disk is recessed in a cavity so that it does not come in contact with the skin itself. Instead, the element is surrounded by electrolyte gel in the cavity. The cavity and hence the gel does not move with respect to the metal disk, so it does not produce any mechanical disturbance of the double layer of charge. In practice, the electrode is filled with electrolyte gel and then attached to the skin surface by means of a double-sided adhesive-tape ring, as shown in Figure 5.11. The electrode element can be a disk made of a metal such as silver coated with AgCl. Another frequently encountered form of the floating electrode uses a sintered Ag/AgCl pellet instead of a metal disk. These electrodes are found to be quite stable and are reusable after appropriate cleaning between uses.

A single-use, disposable modification of the floating electrode is shown in cross section in Figure 5.11(c). Its structure is basically the same as that of the

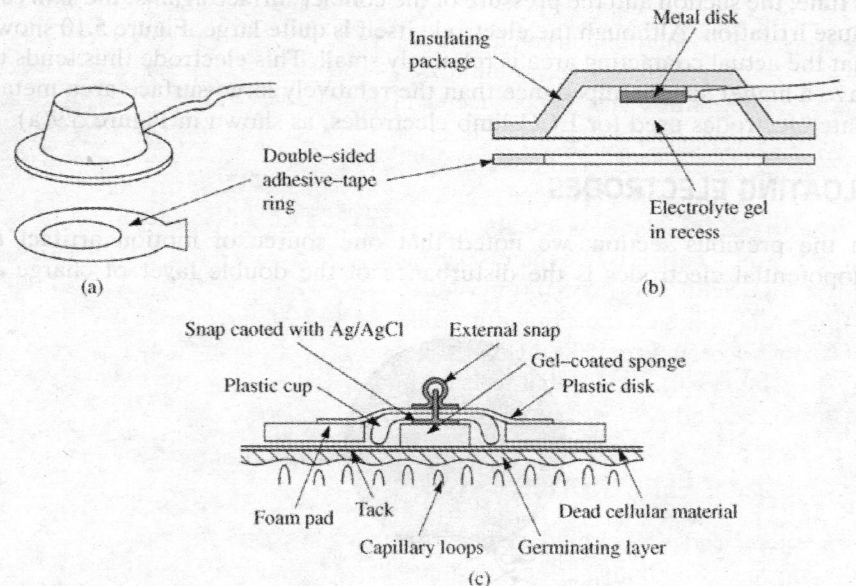


**Figure 5.11 Examples of floating metal body-surface electrodes** (a) Recessed electrode with top-hat structure. (b) Cross-sectional view of the electrode in (a). (c) Cross-sectional view of a disposable recessed electrode of the same general structure shown in Figure 5.9(c). The recess in this electrode is formed from an open foam disk, saturated with electrolyte gel, and placed over the metal electrode.

disposable metal-plate electrode shown in Figure 5.9(c), but it has one added component—a disk of thin, open-cell foam saturated with electrolyte gel. The foam is firmly affixed to the metal-disk electrode, thereby providing an intermediate electrolyte-gel layer between the electrode and the skin. Because the foam is fixed to the metal disk, the gel contained within it at the disk interface is mechanically stable. The other surface of the foam that is placed against the skin is able to move with the skin, thereby diminishing the motion artifact that sometimes results from differential movement between the skin and the electrolyte gel.

Coosemans et al. (2006) have made electrodes and antenna out of textile materials integrated into the baby's pajamas to measure the ECG of children with an increased risk of sudden infant death syndrome (SIDS). The three knitted and woven stainless steel electrodes (called Textrodes) yielded larger motion artifacts than disposable Ag/AgCl electrodes, but they could measure heart rate.

Kang et al. (2008) used both hand- and screen-printing thick-film techniques to develop fabric active electrodes that provide the comfort required for clothing. They used nonstretchable nonwoven (Evolon 100) as the flexible fabric substrate and a silver filled polymer ink (Creative Materials CMI 112-15) to form an electrode layer and conductive lines on the fabrics.

## ELECTRODE STANDARDS

During defibrillation, large currents may flow through the electrodes, greatly change the electrode overpotential, and make it difficult to determine whether the defibrillation has been successful. In general Ag/AgCl electrodes are satisfactory, whereas polarizable electrodes are not. Standards for pregelled disposable electrodes (Anonymous, 2005) require face-to-face bench testing to ensure that the offset voltage is less than 100 mV, the noise is less than 150 μV, the 10 Hz impedance is less than 2 kΩ, the defibrillation overload recovery to four 2 mC charges is less than 100 mV, and the bias current tolerance to 200 nA for 8 h yields less than 100 mV offset (McAdams, 2006). The defibrillation recovery voltage versus time for 12 electrode materials shows that the optimal recovery occurs for 500 mC/cm$^2$ of AgCl electrodeposited on Ag (Das and Webster, 1980). Additional tests on humans can assess motion artifact, adhesive tack, and skin irritation (Webster, 1984a; ibid., 1984b).

## FLEXIBLE ELECTRODES

The electrodes described so far are solid and either are flat or have a fixed curvature. The body surface, on the other hand, is irregularly shaped and can change its local curvature with movement. Solid electrodes cannot conform to this change in body-surface topography, which can result in additional motion artifact. To avoid such problems, flexible electrodes have been developed, examples of which are shown in Figure 5.12.

One type of flexible electrode is a woven, stretchable, nylon fabric impregnated with silver particles. Lead wire bonding is achieved by the use of epoxy. Gel pads are used for short-term monitoring.

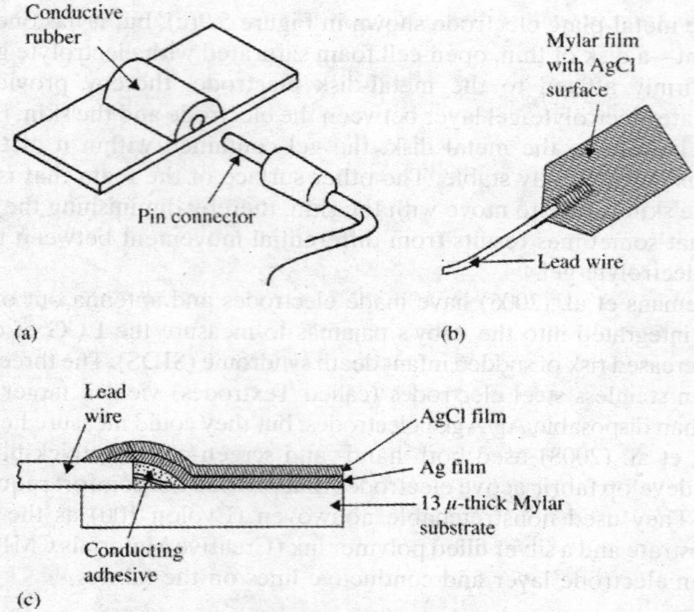


**Figure 5.12 Flexible body-surface electrodes** (a) Carbon-filled silicone rubber electrode. (b) Flexible thin-film neonatal electrode [after Neuman (1973)]. (c) Cross-sectional view of the thin-film electrode in (b). [Parts (b) and (c) are from International Federation for Medical and Biological Engineering. *Digest of the 10th ICMBE,* 1973.]

Figure 5.12(a) shows another technique employed to provide flexible electrodes. A carbon-filled silicone rubber compound in the form of a thin strip or disk is used as the active element of an electrode. The carbon particles in the silicone make it an electric conductor. A pin connector is pushed into the lead connector hole, and the electrode is used in the same way as a similar type of metal-plate electrode.

Flexible electrodes are especially important for monitoring premature infants. Electrodes for detecting the ECG and respiration by the impedance technique are attached to the chest of premature infants, who usually weigh less than 2500 g. Conventional electrodes are not appropriate; they cannot conform to the shape of the infant's chest and can cause severe skin ulceration at pressure points. They must also be removed when chest x rays are taken of the infant, because they are opaque and can obstruct the view of significant portions of the thoracic cavity. Neuman (1973) developed flexible, thin-film electrodes for use on newborn infants that minimize these problems. The basic electrode consists of a 13 μm-thick Mylar film on which an Ag and AgCl film have been deposited, as shown in Figure 5.12(b). The actual structure of the electrode is illustrated in cross section in Figure 5.12(c). The flexible lead wire is attached to the Mylar substrate by means of a conducting adhesive, and a silver film approximately 1 μm thick is deposited over this and the Mylar. An

AgCl layer is then grown on the surface of the silver film via the electrolytic process.

In addition to the advantage of being flexible and conforming to the shape of the newborn's chest, these electrodes have a layer of silver thin enough to be essentially x-ray transparent, so they need not be removed when chest x rays of the infant are taken. All that shows up on the x rays is the lead wire. Consequently, the infant's skin is also protected from the irritation caused by removing and reapplying the adhesive tape that holds the electrode in place. This has been demonstrated to reduce the occurrence of skin irritation significantly in nurseries in which flexible, thin-film electrodes have been used.

The flexible electrodes we have described require some type of adhesive tape to hold them in place against the skin. New electrolytic hydrogel materials have been developed that are in the form of a thin, flexible slab of gelatinous material. This substance has a sticky surface that is similar to the adhesive tack on the tape used to hold electrodes in place. By virtue of the mobile ions that it contains, it is also electrically conductive. A piece of this material the same size as the flexible electrode can be secured on the electrode's surface and used to hold it in place against the skin. Because the electrode and this interface material are both flexible, a good, mechanically secure electric contact can be made between the electrode and the skin. One drawback of this material is its relatively high electric resistance, compared to that of the electrolyte gel routinely used with electrodes. Hydrogels are less effective at hydrating the dry epidermal layer (Jossinet and McAdams, 1990). This is not a severe problem anymore, however, because the amplifiers used with these electrodes now have input impedances of the order of 10 MΩ or higher, which is much greater than the resistance of the electrolytic material. Often there is less motion artifact when these electrodes are used.

## 5.7 INTERNAL ELECTRODES

Electrodes can also be used within the body to detect biopotentials. They can take the form of *percutaneous electrodes,* in which the electrode itself or the lead wire crosses the skin, or they may be entirely *internal electrodes,* in which the connection is to an implanted electronic circuit such as a radiotelemetry transmitter. These electrodes differ from body-surface electrodes in that they do not have to contend with the electrolyte–skin interface and its associated limitations, as described in Section 5.5. Instead, the electrode behaves in the way dictated entirely by the electrode–electrolyte interface. No electrolyte gel is required to maintain this interface, because extracellular fluid is present.

There are many different designs for internal electrodes. An investigator studying a particular bioelectric phenomenon by using internal electrodes frequently designs his or her electrodes for that specific purpose. The following paragraphs describe some of the more common forms of these electrodes and give examples of their application.

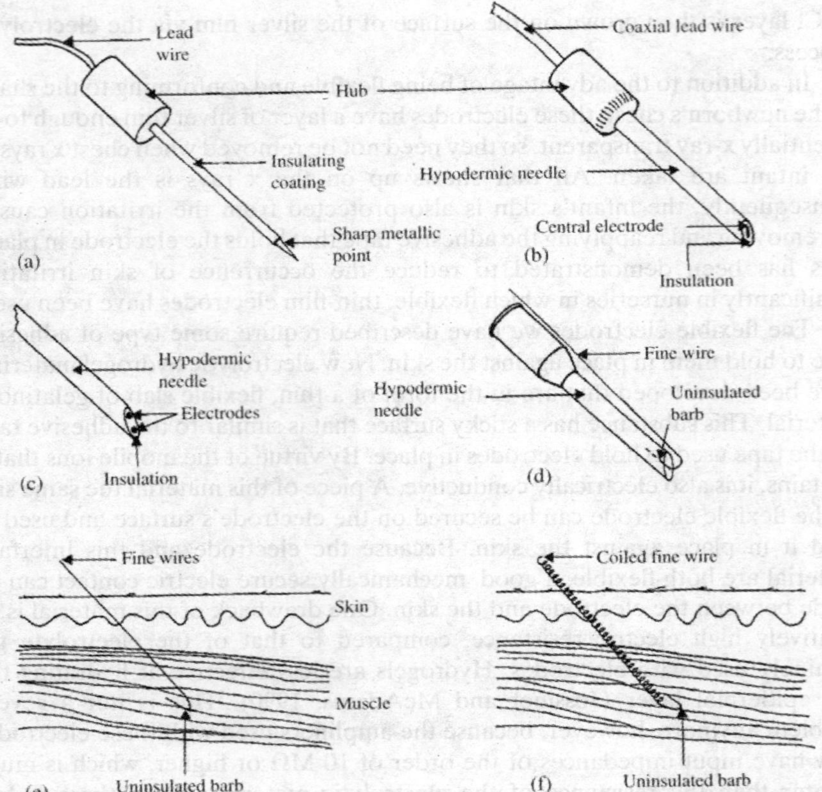


**Figure 5.13 Needle and wire electrodes for percutaneous measurement of biopotentials** (a) Insulated needle electrode. (b) Coaxial needle electrode, (c) Bipolar coaxial electrode. (d) Fine-wire electrode connected to hypodermic needle, before being inserted. (e) Cross-sectional view of skin and muscle, showing fine-wire electrode in place. (f) Cross-sectional view of skin and muscle, showing coiled fine-wire electrode in place.

Figure 5.13 shows different types of percutaneous needle and wire electrodes. The basic needle electrode consists of a solid needle, usually made of stainless steel, with a sharp point. The shank of the needle is insulated with a coating such as an insulating varnish; only the tip is left exposed. A lead wire is attached to the other end of the needle, and the joint is encapsulated in a plastic hub to protect it. This electrode, frequently used in electromyography, is shown in Figure 5.13(a). When it is placed in a particular muscle, it obtains an EMG from that muscle acutely and can then be removed.

A shielded percutaneous electrode can be fabricated in the form shown in Figure 5.13(b). It consists of a small-gage hypodermic needle that has been modified by running an insulated fine wire down the center of its lumen and filling the remainder of the lumen with an insulating material such as an epoxy resin. When the resin has set, the tip of the needle is filed to its original bevel, exposing an oblique cross section of the central wire, which serves as the active electrode. The needle itself is connected to ground through the shield of a coaxial cable, thereby extending the coaxial structure to its very tip.

Multiple electrodes in a single needle can be formed as shown in Figure 5.13(c). Here two wires are placed within the lumen of the needle and can be connected differentially so as to be sensitive to electrical activity only in the immediate vicinity of the electrode tip.

The needle electrodes just described are principally for acute measurements, because their stiffness and size make them uncomfortable for long-term implantation. When chronic recordings are required, percutaneous wire electrodes are more suitable. There are many different types of wire electrodes and schemes for introducing them through the skin. [The interested reader should refer to Geddes (1972) for a more detailed review.] The principle can be illustrated, however, with the help of Figure 5.13(d). A fine wire—often made of stainless steel ranging in diameter from 25 to 125 μm—is insulated with an insulating varnish to within a few millimeters of the tip. This non-insulated tip is bent back on itself to form a J-shaped structure. The tip is introduced into the lumen of the needle, as shown in Figure 5.13(d). The needle is inserted through the skin into the muscle at the desired location, to the desired depth. It is then slowly withdrawn, leaving the electrode in place, as shown in Figure 5.13(e). Note that the bent-over portion of wire serves as a barb holding the wire in place in the muscle. To remove the wire, the technician applies a mild uniform force to straighten out the barb and pulls it out through the wire's track.

Caldwell and Reswick (1975) have described a variation on this basic approach. Realizing that wire electrodes chronically implanted in active muscles undergo a great amount of flexing as the muscle moves (which can cause the wire to slip as it passes through the skin and increase the irritation and risk of infection at this point, or even cause the wire to break), they developed the helical electrode and lead wire shown in Figure 5.13(f). It, too, is made from a very fine insulated wire coiled into a tight helix of approximately 150 μm diameter that is placed in the lumen of the inserting needle. The uninsulated barb protrudes from the tip of the needle and is bent back along the needle before insertion. It holds the wire in place in the tissue when the needle is removed from the muscle. Of course, the external end of the electrode now passes through the needle and the needle must be removed—or at least protected—before the electrode is connected to the recording apparatus.

Another group of percutaneous electrodes are those used for monitoring fetal heartbeats. In this case it is desirable to get the electrocardiogram from the fetus during labor by direct connection to the presenting part (usually the head) through the uterine cervix (the mouth of the uterus). The fetus lies in a bath of amniotic fluid that contains ions and is conductive, so surface electrodes generally do not provide an adequate ECG as a result of the shorting effect of the amniotic fluid. Thus electrodes used to obtain the fetal ECG must penetrate the skin of the fetus.

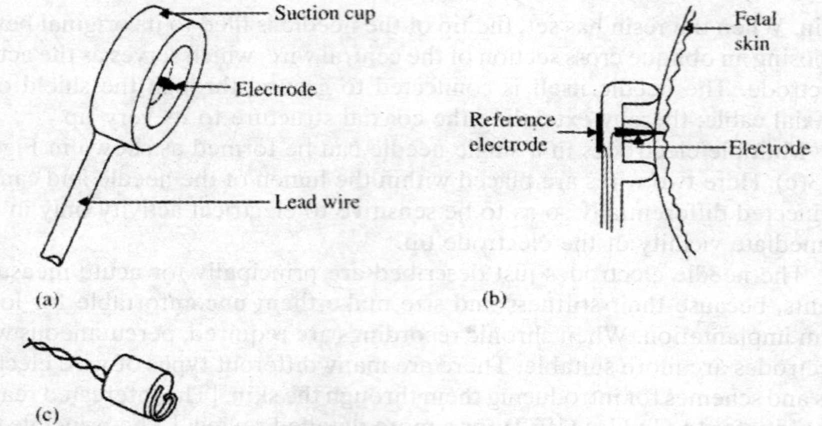


**Figure 5.14 Electrodes for detecting fetal electrocardiogram during labor, by means of intracutaneous needles** (a) Suction electrode. (b) Cross-sectional view of suction electrode in place, showing penetration of probe through epidermis. (c) Helical electrode that is attached to fetal skin by corkscrew-type action.

An example of a suction electrode that does this is shown in Figure 5.14(a). A sharp-pointed probe in the center of a suction cup can be applied to the fetal presenting part, as shown in Figure 5.14(b). When suction is applied to the cup after it has been placed against the fetal skin, the surface of the skin is drawn into the cup and the central electrode pierces the stratum corneum, contacting the deeper layers of the epidermis. On the back of the suction electrode is a reference electrode that contacts the fluid, and the signal seen between these two electrodes is the voltage drop across the resistance of the stratum corneum. Thus, although the amniotic fluid essentially places all the body surface of the fetus at a common potential, the potentials beneath the stratum corneum can be different, and fetal ECGs that have peak amplitudes of the order of 50 to 700 $\mu$V can be reliably recorded.

Another intradermal electrode that is widely applied for detecting fetal ECG during labor is the helical electrode developed by Hon (1972). It consists of a stainless steel needle, shaped approximately like one turn of a helix, mounted on a plastic hub. [See Figure 5.14(c).] The back surface of the hub contains an additional stainless steel reference electrode. When labor has proceeded far enough, this electrode can be attached to the fetal presenting part by rotating it so that the needle twists just beneath the surface of the skin as would a corkscrew shallowly penetrating a cork. This electrode remains firmly attached, and because of the shortness of the helical needle, it does not penetrate deep enough into the skin to cause significant risk to the fetus. It operates on the same basic principle as the suction electrode.

Often when implantable wireless transmission is used, we want to implant electrodes within the body and not penetrate the skin with any wires. In this case the radio transmitter is implanted in the body. A wide variety of electrodes can be used in this application. Only a few examples are given here.

The simplest electrode for this application is shown in Figure 5.15(a). Insulated multistranded stainless steel or platinum wire suitable for

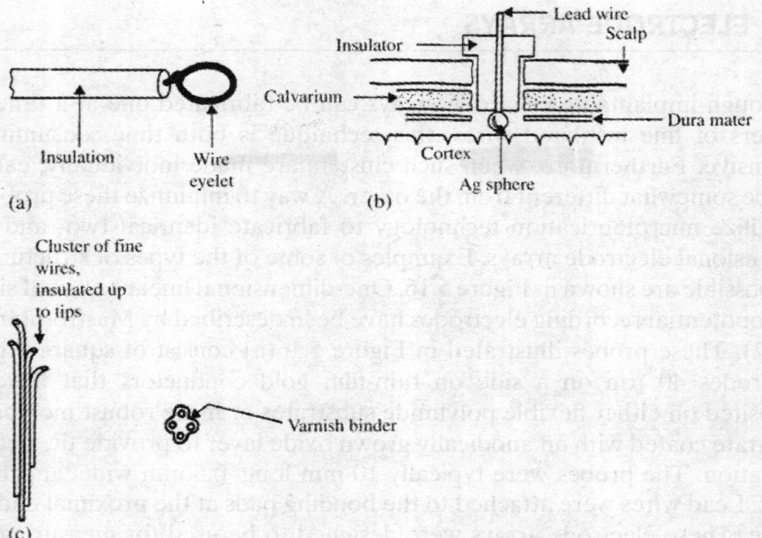


**Figure 5.15 Implantable electrodes for detecting biopotentials** (a) Wire-loop electrode. (b) platinum-sphere cortical-surface potential electrode. (c) Multi-element depth electrode.

implantation has one end stripped so that an eyelet can be formed from the strands of wire. This is best done by individually taking each strand and forming the eyelet either by twisting the wires together one by one at the point at which the insulation stops or by spot-welding each strand to the wire mass at this point. The eyelet can then be sutured to the point in the body at which electric contact is to be established. Silver should not be used for this type of electrode due to the toxicity of this metal and its effects on surrounding tissue.

Figure 5.15(b) shows another example of an implantable electrode for obtaining cortical-surface potentials from the brain. Critchfield *et al.* (1971) applied this electrode for the radiotelemetry of subdural EEGs. The electrode consists of a 2 mm-diameter metallic sphere located at the tip of the cylindrical Teflon insulator through which the electrode lead wire passes. The calvarium is exposed through an incision in the scalp, and a burr hole is drilled. A small slit is made in the exposed dura, and the silver sphere is introduced through this opening so that it rests on the surface of the cerebral cortex. The assembly is then cemented in place onto the calvarium by means of a dental acrylic material.

Deep cortical potentials can be recorded from multiple points using the technique described by Delgado (1964), as shown in Figure 5.15(c). This kind of electrode consists of a cluster of fine insulated wires held together by a varnish binder. Each wire has been cut transversely to expose an uninsulated cross section that serves as the active electrode surface. By staggering the ends of the wires as shown, we can produce electrodes located at known differences in depth in an array. The other ends of the electrodes can be attached to appropriate implantable electronic devices or to a connector cemented on the skull to allow connection to an external recording apparatus.

## 5.8 ELECTRODE ARRAYS

Although implantable electrode arrays can be fabricated one at a time using clusters of fine insulated wires, this technique is both time-consuming and expensive. Furthermore, when such clusters are made individually, each one will be somewhat different from the other. A way to minimize these problems is to utilize microfabrication technology to fabricate identical two- and three-dimensional electrode arrays. Examples of some of the types of structures that are possible are shown in Figure 5.16. One-dimensional linear arrays of six pairs of biopotential recording electrodes have been described by Mastrototaro *et al.* (1992). These probes illustrated in Figure 5.16(a) consist of square Ag/AgCl electrodes 40 μm on a side on thin-film gold conductors that have been deposited on either flexible polyimide substrates or more robust molybdenum substrate coated with an anodically grown oxide layer to provide the necessary insulation. The probes were typically 10 mm long, 0.5 mm wide, and 125 μm thick. Lead wires were attached to the bonding pads at the proximal end of the probe. These electrode arrays were designed to be used for measuring transmural potential distributions in the beating myocardium. Their flexibility was important to minimize tissue damage as the muscle contracts and relaxes.

Two-dimensional electrode arrays for mapping the electrical potentials across a region of the surface of an organ such as the heart are shown in Figure 5.16(b). These electrodes essentially represent an extension of the approach used for the one-dimensional arrays described above. A pattern of miniature electrodes is formed on a rigid or flexible surface and connected by conductors to the associated instrumentation. This interconnection can be quite a problem because large arrays require many connections. Sock electrodes consisting of individual silver spheres roughly 1 mm in diameter incorporated into a fabric sock that fits snugly over the heart have been used to map epicardial potentials. Each sphere is at the tip of an insulated wire that connects it to the recording apparatus. Needless to say, an array of a large number of electrodes of this type is difficult to build and awkward to use due to the large number of wires coming from the sock.

Ash *et al.* (1992) have shown that this process can be simplified by using a multilayer ceramic integrated circuit package as the electrode array. They have used this structure to map epicardial potentials. These investigators have also used thin-film microfabrication technology to form arrays of 144 miniature Ag/AgCl electrodes on polyimide substrates [Figure 5.16(b)]. The thin gold films serve as conductors as well as the bases for the Ag/AgCl electrodes. The interconnections were completed by using a miniature ribbon cable designed for surface mount microelectronic applications. Olsson *et al.* (2005) have taken this concept a step further by incorporating amplifiers in their electrode array probes. These have been used for extracellular recording of neural signals in animal studies.

Three-dimensional electrode arrays fabricated using silicon microfabrication technology have been described by Campbell *et al.* (1991), Branner *et al.* (2004), and others. Their devices have the appearance of a two-dimensional

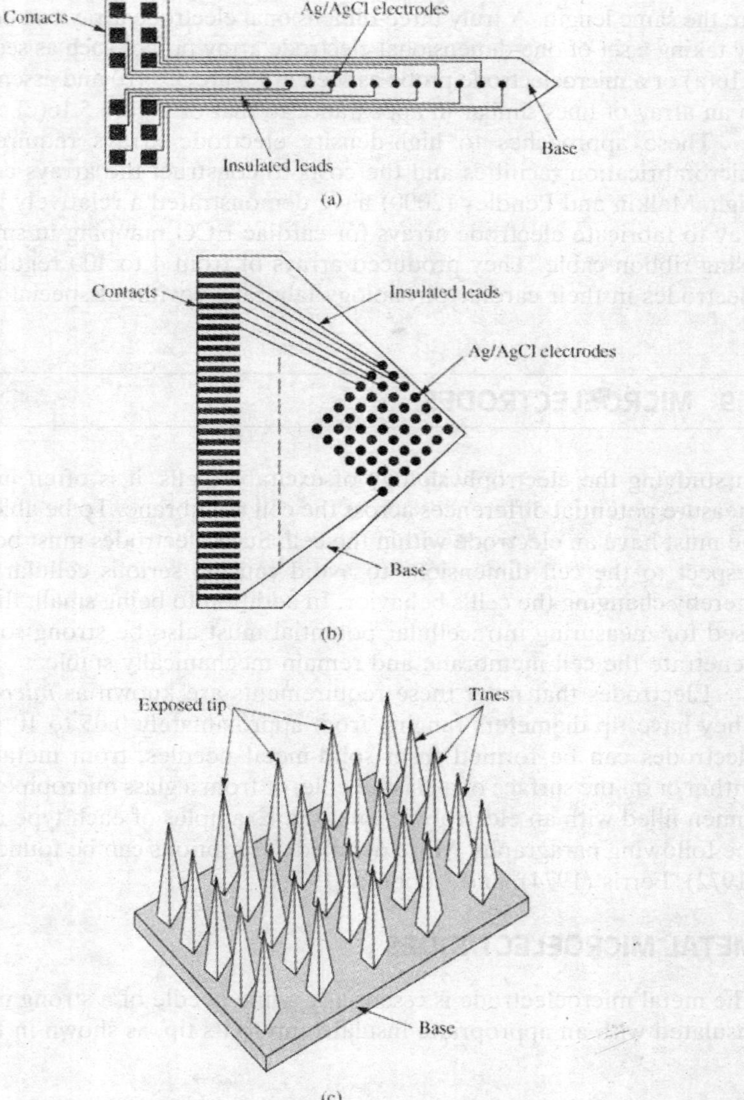


**Figure 5.16 Examples of microfabricated electrode arrays** (a) one-dimensional plunge electrode array [after Mastrototaro *et al.* (1992)], (b) two-dimensional array, and (c) three-dimensional array [after Campbell *et al.* (1991)].

comb [Figure 5.16(c)] with each tine being roughly 1.5 mm long and surrounded with insulating material up to the tip. The exposed tip serves as the electrode, and a wire connection on the base of the structure was needed to make contact with each tine electrode. Although this array is a three-dimensional structure, it really only measures from a two-dimensional array of electrodes because all of the tines are the same length. A truly three-dimensional electrode array can be fabricated by taking a set of one-dimensional electrode array probes such as seen in Figure 5.16(a) or a microelectrode probe as seen in Figure 5.20(b) and assembling them in an array of tines similar in appearance to that of Figure 5.16(c).

These approaches to high-density electrode arrays require extensive microfabrication facilities and the costs to construct the arrays can be quite high. Malkin and Pendley (2000) have demonstrated a relatively inexpensive way to fabricate electrode arrays for cardiac ECG mapping in small rodents using ribbon cable. They produced arrays of from 4 to 400 regularly spaced electrodes in their cardiac physiology laboratory without special equipment.

## 5.9 MICROELECTRODES

In studying the electrophysiology of excitable cells, it is often important to measure potential differences across the cell membrane. To be able to do this, we must have an electrode within the cell. Such electrodes must be small with respect to the cell dimensions to avoid causing serious cellular injury and thereby changing the cell's behavior. In addition to being small, the electrode used for measuring intracellular potential must also be strong so that it can penetrate the cell membrane and remain mechanically stable.

Electrodes that meet these requirements are known as *microelectrodes.* They have tip diameters ranging from approximately 0.05 to 10 μm. Microelectrodes can be formed from solid-metal needles, from metal contained within or on the surface of a glass needle, or from a glass micropipette having a lumen filled with an electrolytic solution. Examples of each type are given in the following paragraphs. More detailed descriptions can be found in Geddes (1972), Ferris (1974), and Cobbold (1974).

### METAL MICROELECTRODES

The metal microelectrode is essentially a fine needle of a strong metal that is insulated with an appropriate insulator up to its tip, as shown in Figure 5.17.

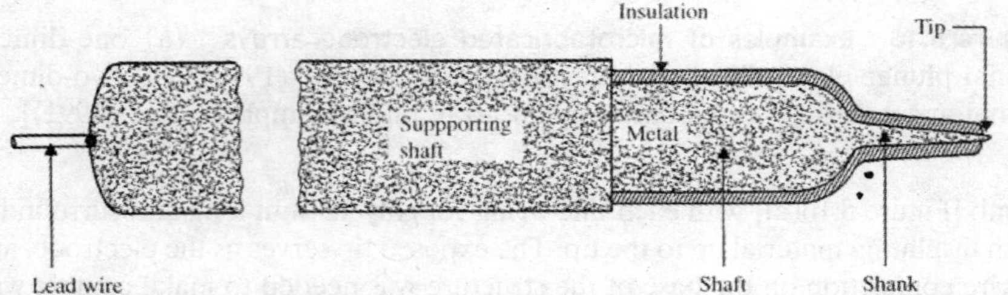


**Figure 5.17** The structure of a metal microelectrode for intracellular recordings.

The metal needle is prepared in such a way as to produce a very fine tip. This is usually done by electrolytic etching, using an electrochemical cell in which the metal needle is the anode. The electric current etches the needle as it is slowly withdrawn from the electrolyte solution. Very fine tips can be formed in this way, but a great deal of patience and practice are required to gain the skill to make them. Suitable strong metals for these microelectrodes are stainless steel, platinum–iridium alloy, and tungsten. The compound tungsten carbide is also used because of its great strength.

The etched metal needle is then supported in a larger metallic shaft that can be insulated. This shaft serves as a sturdy mechanical support for the microelectrode and as a means of connecting it to its lead wire. The microelectrode and supporting shaft are usually insulated by a film of some polymeric material or varnish. Only the extreme tip of the electrode remains uninsulated.

## SUPPORTED-METAL MICROELECTRODES

The properties of two different materials are used to advantage in supported-metal microelectrodes. A strong insulating material that can be drawn to a fine point makes up the basic support, and a metal with good electrical conductivity constitutes the contacting portion of the electrode.

Figure 5.18 shows examples of supported metal microelectrodes. The classic example of this form is a glass tube drawn to a micropipette structure with its lumen filled with an appropriate metal. Often this type of microelectrode, as shown in Figure 5.18(a), is prepared by first filling a glass tube with a metal that has a melting point near the softening point of the glass. The tube can then be heated to the softening point and pulled to form a narrow constriction. When it is broken at the constriction, two micropipettes filled with metal are formed. In this type of structure, the glass not only provides the mechanical support but also serves as the insulation. The active tip is the only metallic area exposed in cross section where the pipette was broken away.

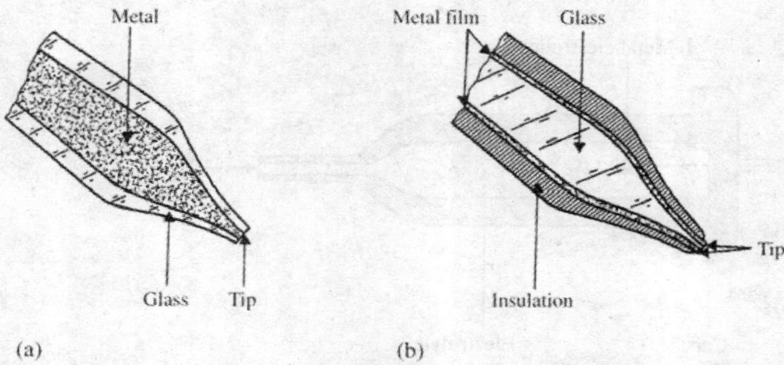


**Figure 5.18 Structures of two supported metal microelectrodes** (a) Metal-filled glass micropipette. (b) Glass micropipette or probe, coated with metal film.

Metals such as silver-solder alloy and platinum and silver alloys are used. In some cases metals with low melting points, such as indium or Wood's metal, are used.

New supported-metal electrode structures have been developed using techniques employed in the semiconductor microelectronics industry. Figure 5.18(b) shows the cross section of the tip of a deposited-metal-film microelectrode. A solid glass rod or glass tube is drawn to form the micropipette. A metal film is deposited uniformly on this surface to a thickness of the order of tenths of a micrometer. A polymeric insulation is then coated over this, leaving just the tip, with the metal film exposed.

## MICROPIPETTE ELECTRODES

Glass micropipette microelectrodes are fabricated from glass capillaries. The central region of a piece of capillary tubing, as shown in Figure 5.19(a), is heated with a burner to the softening point. It is then rapidly stretched to produce the constriction shown in Figure 5.19(b). Special devices, known as *microelectrode pullers*, that heat and stretch the glass capillary in a uniform reproducible way to fabricate micropipettes are commercially available. The two halves of the stretched capillary structure are broken apart at the constriction to produce a pipette structure that has a tip diameter of the order of 1 μm. This pipette is fabricated into the electrode form shown in Figure 5.19(c). It is filled with an electrolyte solution that is frequently 3$M$ KCl. A cap containing a metal electrode is then sealed to the pipette, as shown. The metal electrode contacts the electrolyte within the pipette. The

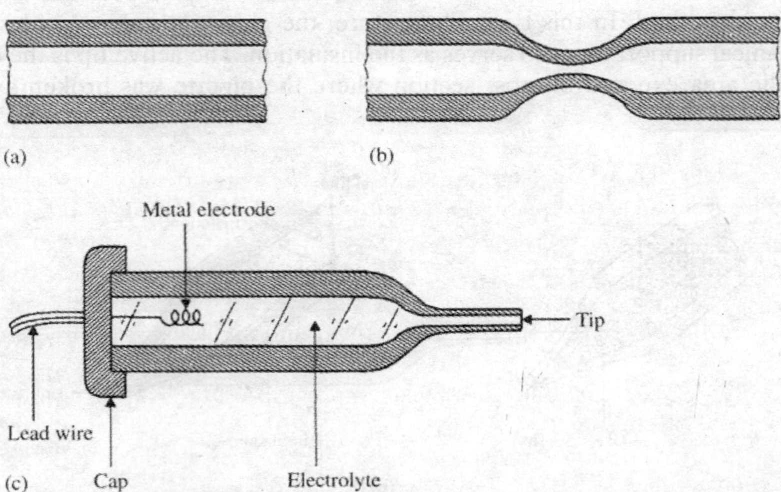


**Figure 5.19 A glass micropipette electrode filled with an electrolytic solution** (a) Section of fine-bore glass capillary. (b) Capillary narrowed through heating and stretching. (c) Final structure of glass-pipette microelectrode.

electrode is frequently a silver wire prepared with an electrolytic AgCl surface. Platinum or stainless steel wires are also occasionally used.

## MICROELECTRODES BASED ON MICROELECTRONIC TECHNOLOGY

The technology used to produce transistors and integrated circuits can also be used to micromachine small mechanical structures. This technique has been used by several investigators to produce metal microelectrodes. The structure shown in Figure 5.20(a) uses the technology for fabricating beam-lead transistors (Wise *et al.*, 1990). The basic structure consists of narrow gold strips deposited on a silicon substrate the surface of which has been first insulated by growing an $SiO_2$ film. The gold strips are then further insulated by depositing $SiO_2$ over their surface. The silicon substrate is next etched to a thin, narrow structure that is just wide enough to accommodate the gold strips in the region of the tip. The silicon substrate is etched a millimeter or two back from the tip so that only the gold strips and their $SiO_2$ insulation remain. The insulation is

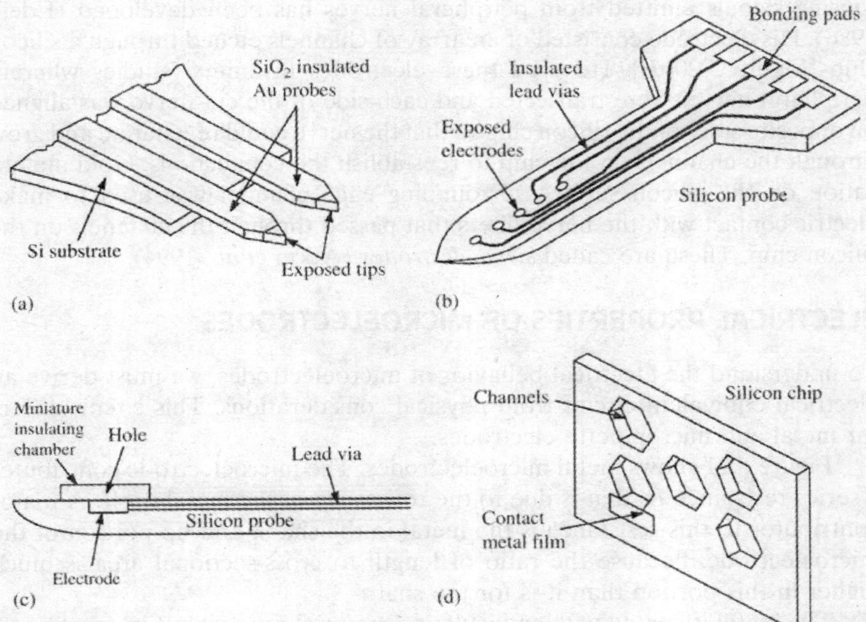


**Figure 5.20 Different types of microelectrodes fabricated using microelectronic technology** (a) Beam-lead multiple electrode. (Based on Figure 7 in K. D. Wise, J. B. Angell, and A. Starr, "An integrated circuit approach to extracellular microelectrodes." Reprinted with permission from *IEEE Trans. Biomed. Eng.*, 1970, BME-17, 238–246. Copyright 1970 by the Institute of Electrical and Electronics Engineers.) (b) Multielectrode silicon probe after Drake *et al.* (c) Multiple-chamber electrode after Prohaska *et al.* (d) Peripheral-nerve electrode based on the design of Edell.

etched away from the very tip of the gold strips to expose the contacting surface of the electrodes. Although this technology cannot produce tips as small as can be produced with the glass micropipette technique previously described, it is possible to make multielectrode arrays and to maintain very precisely the geometry between individual electrodes in the array. The high reproducibility of microelectronic processing allows many electrodes to be made that all have very similar geometric properties. Thus the characteristics vary little from one electrode array to the next.

Several other designs for sensing and stimulating electrodes have been developed through the use of microelectronic technology. An array of multisite microelectrodes can be grown on a thin silicon probe [Figure 5.20(b)] that can be placed in the cortex of the brain to detect local potentials (Drake *et al.*, 1988; Kovacs *et al.*, 1994). A similar design was utilized by Prohaska *et al.* (1986), but here the actual gold or silver/silver chloride electrode was located in a very small chamber filled with an electrolytic solution such as sodium chloride and was made from an insulating film with a small hole to allow communication with the nervous tissue in which it was placed [Figure 5.20(c)]. A novel electrode for sensing signals emitted from peripheral nerves has been developed (Edell, 1986). His electrode consisted of an array of channels etched through a silicon chip [Figure 5.20(d)]. He used these electrodes in animal studies wherein peripheral nerves were transected and each side of the cut nerve was aligned on opposite sides of the silicon chip so that the nerve could regenerate and grow through the channels on the chip to reestablish the connections. Gold metalization on the silicon surface surrounding each channel was used to make electric contact with the nerve fibers that passed through the channels on the silicon chip. These are called *sieve electrodes* (Atkin *et al.*, 1994).

## ELECTRICAL PROPERTIES OF MICROELECTRODES

To understand the electrical behavior of microelectrodes, we must derive an electrical equivalent circuit from physical considerations. This circuit differs for metal and micropipette electrodes.

Figure 5.21 shows metal microelectrodes. The microelectrode contributes a series resistance $R_s$ that is due to the resistance of the metal itself. A major contributor to this resistance is the metal in the shank and tip portion of the microelectrode, because the ratio of length to cross-sectional area is much higher in this portion than it is for the shaft.

The metal is coated with an insulating material over all but its most distal tip, so a capacitance is set up between the metal and the extracellular fluid. This is a distributed capacitance $C_d$ that we can represent in lumped form by separating the shank and tip from the shaft. In the shank region, we can consider the microelectrode to be a coaxial cylinder capacitor; the capacitance per unit length (F/m) is given by

$$\frac{C_{dl}}{L} = \frac{2\pi\varepsilon_r\varepsilon_0}{\ln D/d} \tag{5.16}$$

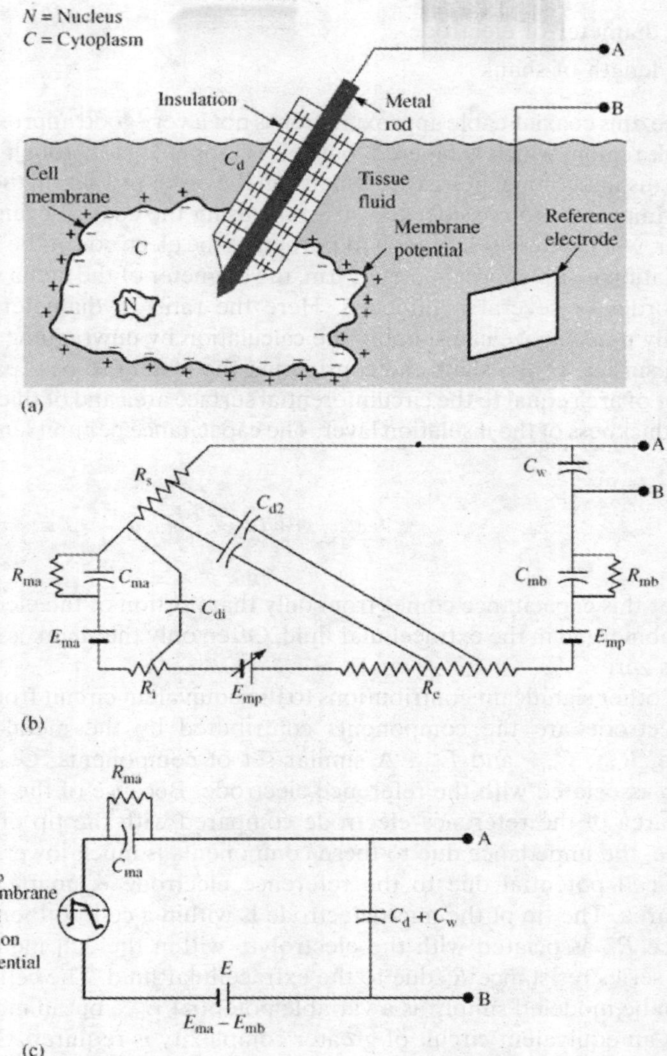


**Figure 5.21 Equivalent circuit of metal microelectrode** (a) Electrode with tip placed within a cell, showing origin of distributed capacitance. (b) Equivalent circuit for the situation in (a). (c) Simplified equivalent circuit. (From L. A. Geddes, *Electrodes and the Measurement of Bioelectric Events,* Wiley-Interscience, 1972. Used with permission of John Wiley and Sons, New York.)

where

$\varepsilon_0$ = dielectric constant of free space (Appendix A.1)

$\varepsilon_r$ = relative dielectric constant of insulation material

$D$ = diameter of cylinder consisting of electrode plus insulation

$d$ = diameter of electrode

$L$ = length of shank

Of course, this coaxial-cable approximation is not a very good approximation for the shank region, which is tapered, but it is reasonable for a rough calculation. Because insulation thicknesses are usually on the order of 1 μm in the shank and tip, it is important to consider the structure using the coaxial cylinder analog. However, when we consider the shaft portion of the electrode, if the thickness of the insulation is still approximately 1 μm, the diameter of the metal shaft can be on the order of several millimeters. Here the ratio of diameters would be practically unity, so we can simplify the calculation by unwrapping the circumferential surface of the shaft and considering the system to be a parallel-plate capacitor of area equal to the circumferential surface area and of thickness equal to $t$, the thickness of the insulation layer. The capacitance per unit length (F/m) is given by

$$\frac{C_{d2}}{L} = \frac{\varepsilon_r \varepsilon_0 \pi d}{t} \tag{5.17}$$

Note that this capacitance comes from only that portion of the electrode shaft that is submerged in the extracellular fluid. Often only the shank is submerged, so $C_{d2}$ is zero.

The other significant contributions to the equivalent circuit from the metal microelectrode are the components contributed by the metal–electrolyte interface, $R_{ma}$, $C_{ma}$, and $E_{ma}$. A similar set of components, $C_{mb}$, $R_{mb}$, and $E_{mb}$, are associated with the reference electrode. Because of the much larger surface area of the reference electrode compared with the tip of the microelectrode, the impedance due to these components is much lower. Of course, the half-cell potential due to the reference electrode is unaffected by the surface area. The tip of the microelectrode is within a cell, so there is a series resistance $R_i$, associated with the electrolyte within the cell membrane and another series resistance $R_e$ due to the extracellular fluid. The cell membrane itself can be modeled simply as a variable potential $E_{mp}$, but in more detailed analyses an equivalent circuit of greater complexity is required. Some of the distributed capacitance of the shank, $C_{d1}$, is between the microelectrode and the extracellular fluid, as shown in the equivalent circuit, whereas the remainder of it is between the microelectrode and the intracellular fluid.

There is also a capacitance associated with the lead wires, $C_w$. The physical basis for this equivalent circuit is shown in Figure 5.21(a); the actual equivalent circuit is shown in Figure 5.21(b). Often it is acceptable to simplify this equivalent circuit to that shown in Figure 5.21(c), which neglects the impedance of the reference electrode and the series-resistance contribution from the intracellular and extracellular fluid and lumps all the distributed capacitance together. Under circumstances in which the input impedance of the amplifier connected to this electrode is not sufficiently large, we see that this circuit can behave as a high-pass filter and significant waveform distortion can result.

The effective impedance of metal microelectrodes is frequency dependent and can be of the order of 10 to 100 MΩ. We can, however, lower this impedance by increasing the effective surface area of the tip of the microelectrode through the application of platinum black, as we did in the case of the hydrogen electrode. Impedance reduction of one or two orders of magnitude can be achieved in this way. At lower frequencies, the impedance can be reduced by applying an Ag/AgCl surface to the electrode tip. Care must be taken in doing this, however, because of the mechanically fragile nature of this film and its tendency to flake off, and the few silver ions that dissolve in the cell might affect its behavior.

The equivalent circuit for the micropipette electrode is somewhat more complicated than that of the metal microelectrode. The physical situation is illustrated in Figure 5.22(a), and the resulting equivalent circuit is shown in Figure 5.22(b). The internal electrode in the micropipette gives the metal–electrolyte interface components $R_{ma}$, $C_{ma}$, and $E_{ma}$. In series with this is a resistive element $R_t$ corresponding to the resistance of the electrolyte in the shank and tip region of the microelectrode. Connected to this is the distributed capacitance $C_d$ corresponding to the capacitance across the glass in this region. The distributed capacitance due to the shaft region has been neglected, because the glass wall of the electrode is much thicker in this region and the capacitive contribution is quite small.

There are two potentials associated with the tip of the micropipette microelectrode. The *liquid-junction potential* $E_j$ corresponds to the liquid junction set up between the electrolyte in the micropipette and the intracellular fluid. In addition, a potential known as the tip potential $E_t$ arises because the thin glass wall surrounding the tip region of the micropipette behaves like a glass membrane and has an associated membrane potential.

The equivalent circuit also includes resistances corresponding to the intracellular $R_i$ and extracellular $R_e$ fluids. These are coupled to the microelectrode through the distributive capacitance $C_d$, as is the case for the metal microelectrode. The equivalent circuit for the reference electrode remains unchanged from that shown in Figure 5.21(b).

Unlike the metal microelectrode, the micropipette's major impedance contribution is resistive. This can be illustrated by approximating the equivalent circuit to give that shown in Figure 5.22(c). Here the overall series resistance of the electrode is lumped together as $R_t$. This resistance generally ranges in value from 1 to 100 MΩ. The total distributed capacitance is lumped together to form $C_t$, which can be on the order of tens of picofarads. All the associated dc potentials are lumped together in the source $E_m$, which is given by

$$E_m = E_j + E_t + E_{ma} - E_{mb} \tag{5.18}$$

Note that the micropipette-type microelectrode behaves as a low-pass filter. The high series resistance and distributed capacitance cause the electrode output to respond slowly to rapid changes in cell-membrane potential. To

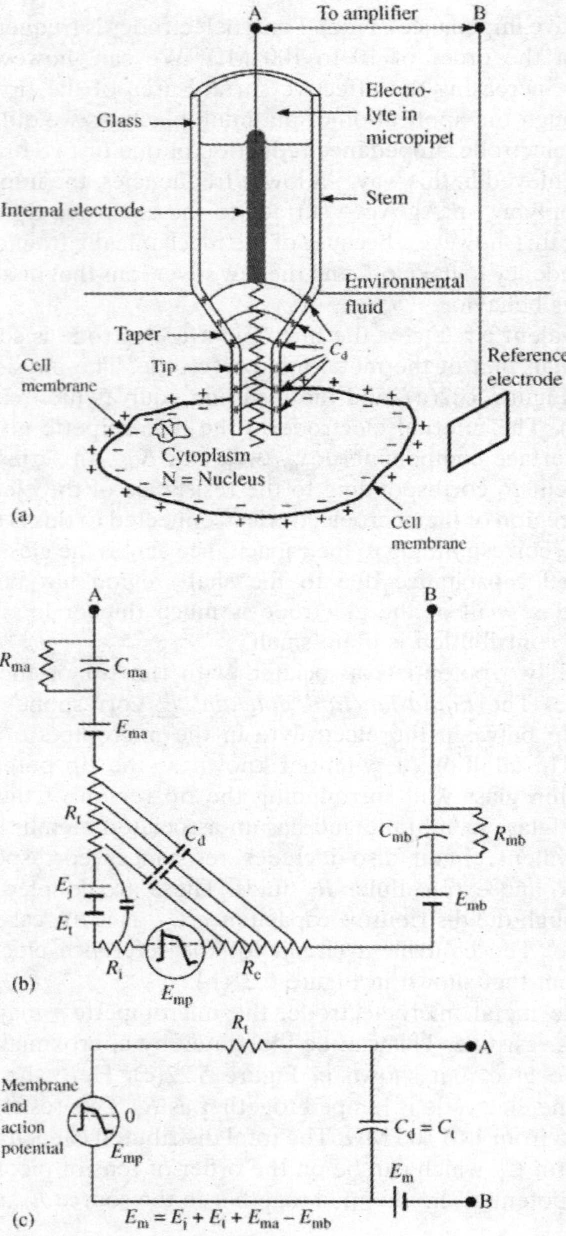


**Figure 5.22 Equivalent circuit of glass micropipette microelectrode** (a) Electrode with its tip placed within a cell, showing the origin of distributed capacitance. (b) Equivalent circuit for the situation in (a). (c) Simplified equivalent circuit. (From L. A. Geddes, *Electrodes and the Measurement of Bioelectric Events,* Wiley-Interscience, 1972. Used with permission of John Wiley and Sons, New York.)

reduce this problem, positive-feedback, negative-capacitance amplifiers (see Section 6.6) are used to reduce the effective value of $C_t$.

## 5.10 ELECTRODES FOR ELECTRIC STIMULATION OF TISSUE

Electrodes used for the electric stimulation of tissue follow the same general design as those used for the recording of bioelectric potentials. They differ in that currents as large as milliamperes cross the electrode–electrolyte interface in stimulating electrodes. Examples of specific electrodes used in cardiac pacemakers, other functional electric stimulators, and cardiac defibrillators (where currents are even larger) are given in Chapter 13. Other types of stimulating electrodes are of the same form as the potential recording electrodes described in this chapter.

In considering stimulating electrodes, we must bear in mind that the net current across the electrode–electrolyte interface is not always zero. When a biphasic stimulating pulse is used, the average current over long periods of time should be zero. However, over the stimulus cycle, there are periods of time during which the net current across the electrode is in one direction at one time and in the other direction at a different time. Also, the magnitudes of the currents in the two directions may be unequal. In studying the electrical characteristics of the electrode–electrolyte interface under such circumstances, we may well imagine that the equivalent circuit changes as the stimulus progresses. Thus the effective equivalent circuit for the electrode is determined by the stimulus parameters, principally the current and the duration of the stimulus.

Rectangular biphasic or monophasic pulses are frequently used for electric stimulation. However, other waveshapes, such as decaying exponentials, trapezoids, or sine waves, have also been used. Frequently a stimulus is used that is either constant current or constant voltage during the pulse. The response of a typical electrode to this type of stimulus is illustrated in Figure 5.23.

A constant-current stimulus pulse is applied to the stimulating electrodes in Figure 5.23(a), giving the voltage response shown. Note that the resulting voltage pulse is not constant. This is understandable when we consider that there is a strong reactive component to the electrode–electrolyte interface, or in other words, polarization occurs. The initial rise in voltage corresponding to the leading edge of the current pulse is due to the voltage drop across the resistive components of the electrode–electrolyte interface, but we see that the voltage continues to rise with the constant current. This is due to the establishment of a change in the distribution of charge concentration at the electrode–electrolyte interface—in other words, to a change in polarization resulting from the unidirectional current. As stated in the description of the simplified electrode–electrolyte equivalent circuit of Figure 5.4, this polarization effect can be represented by a capacitor. Again it is important to remember that the size of this capacitor is determined by several factors, one of which is the

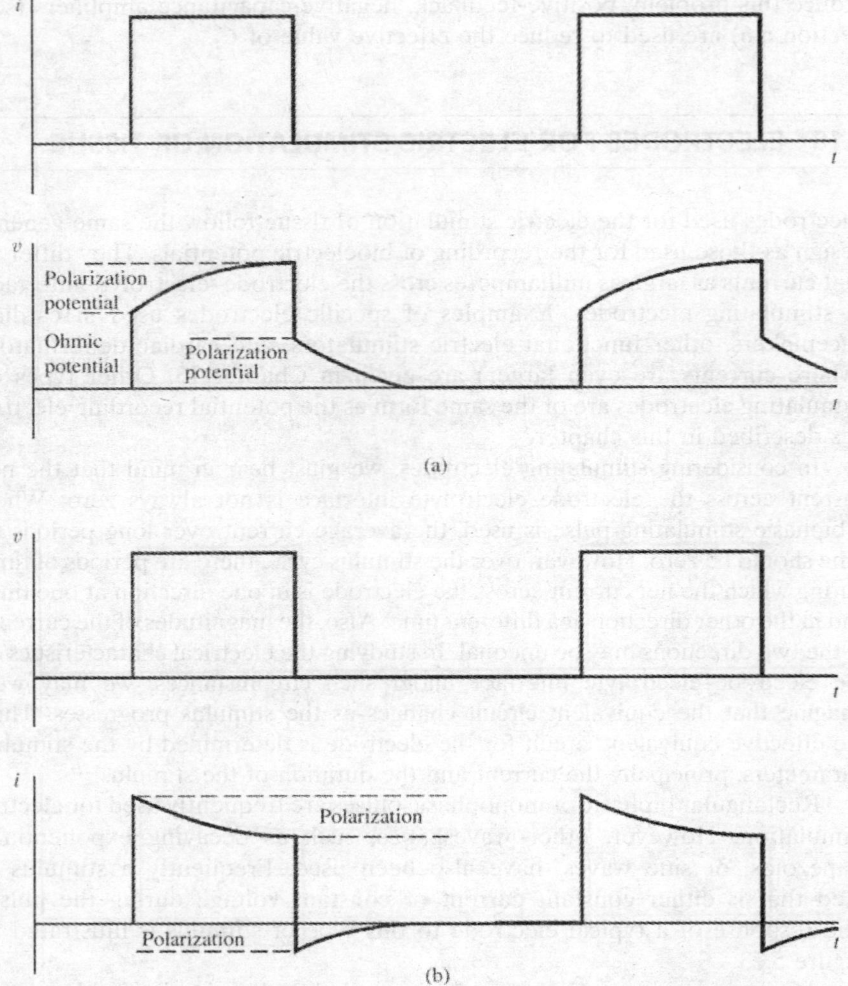


**Figure 5.23 Current and voltage waveforms seen with electrodes used for electric stimulation** (a) Constant-current stimulation. (b) Constant-voltage stimulation.

current density at the interface, so the equivalent circuit for stimulating electrodes changes with the stimulus.

When the current falls back to its low value, the voltage across the electrodes drops, but not back to its initial value. Instead, after the initial steep fall, there is a slower decay corresponding to the dissipation of the polarization charge at the interface.

Constant-voltage stimulation of the electrodes is shown in Figure 5.23(b). In this case the current corresponding to the rising edge of the voltage pulse is seen to jump in a large step and, as the distribution of the polarization charge becomes established, to fall back to a lower steady-state value. When the voltage pulse falls, the current is seen to change direction and then slowly return to its initial zero value. This is a result of the dissipation of the polarization charge built up at the electrode–electrolyte interface.

In choosing materials for stimulating electrodes, we must take into consideration chemical reactions occurring at the electrode–electrolyte interface. If a stimulating current causes the material of the electrode to be oxidized, the electrode is consumed, which limits its lifetime and also increases the concentration of the ions of electrode material in the vicinity of the electrode. This could be toxic to the tissue. When electrodes such as the Ag/AgCl electrode are used, the stimulating current can result in either the formation of additional $Cl^-$ or the reduction of what is already formed, thereby greatly changing the characteristics of the electrode. Thus the best stimulating electrodes are made from noble metals (or at least stainless steel), which undergo only minimal chemical reactions. It is also possible in this case that the chemical reaction involves water in the vicinity of the electrodes. Thus the local activity of hydrogen or hydroxyl ions in the vicinity of the electrode can greatly change. These changes in acidity or alkalinity can produce tissue damage that limits the overall effectiveness of the noble-metal electrodes. Of course, the polarization of these electrodes is large, and the waveforms, such as those shown in Figure 5.23, are less rectangular than they would be with nonpolarizable electrodes. In extreme cases, electrode voltage and current density can result in the electrolysis of water that leads to the evolution of small bubbles of hydrogen or oxygen gas. Clearly, this is a situation that should be avoided.

Carbon-filled silicone rubber electrodes are used for transcutaneous stimulation used in clinical pain management (McAdams, 2006). Arzbaecher (1982) describes a pill electrode that can either record a large P wave or pace the heart from the esophagus. A stimulating electrode based upon the iridium/iridium oxide system [Robblee *et al.* (1983)] has been shown to inject charge into biologic tissue. This type of electrode has been found to provide maximal current density for biphasic stimuli while minimizing chemical changes that could lead to tissue damage. The passage of charge from the electrode to tissue and in the reverse direction results in a chemical change in the iridium oxide chemical composition as opposed to injecting iridium ions into solution or reducing them. Cogan (2008) has reviewed recent techniques for electrically stimulating and recording neural tissue and the underlying electrochemistry that can lead to safer and more efficient interfaces with the nervous system.

## 5.11 PRACTICAL HINTS IN USING ELECTRODES

In using metal electrodes for measurement and stimulation, we should understand a few practical points not mentioned elsewhere in this chapter. The first point is the importance of constructing the electrode and any parts of the lead wire that may be exposed to the electrolyte *all of the same material.* Furthermore, a third material such as solder should not be used to connect the electrode to its lead wire unless it is certain that this material will not be in contact with the electrolyte. It is far better either to weld the lead wire to the electrode or at least to form a mechanical bond through crimping or peening. Dissimilar metals should not be used in contact because their half-cell potentials are different. Since they are electrically connected and in contact with the same electrolyte, it is more than likely that an electrochemical reaction will be set up between them that can result in additional polarization and often in corrosion of one of the metals. This factor also tends to make half-cell potentials less stable, thereby contributing to increased electric artifact from the electrode.

When pairs of electrodes are used for measuring differential voltages, such as in detecting surface potentials on the body or internal potentials within it, it is recommended to use the same material for each electrode, because the half-cell potentials are approximately equal. This means that the net dc potential seen at the input to the amplifier connected to the electrodes is relatively small, possibly even zero. This minimizes possible saturation effects in the case of high-gain direct-coupled amplifiers.

Electrodes placed on the skin's surface have a tendency to come off. Frequently, this is due to a loss of effectiveness of the adhesive tack holding the electrodes in place. However, this is not the only cause of this problem. Lead wires to surface electrodes should be extremely flexible yet strong. If they are, only tension on the lead wire can apply a force that is likely to separate the electrode from the skin. If the lead wire remains loose, it cannot apply any forces to the electrode because of its high flexibility. It is helpful to provide additional relief from strain by taping the lead wire to the skin a few cm from the electrode with some slack or even a loop in the wire so that tension in the wire is not transferred to the electrode.

The point at which the lead wire enters the electrode is a point of frequent failure. Even though the insulation appears intact, the wire within may be broken as a result of severe repeated flexing at this point. Well-designed electrodes minimize this problem by providing strain relief at this point, so that there is a gradual transition between the flexible wire and the solid material of the electrode. Using a tapered region of insulation that gradually increases from the diameter of the wire to a shape that is closer to that of the electrode often minimizes this problem and distributes the flexing forces over a greater portion of the wire.

Another point to consider is that the insulation of the lead wire and the electrode can also present problems. Electrodes are often in a high-humidity environment or are continually soaked in extracellular fluid or even in cleaning solution (if they are of the reusable type). The insulation of these electrodes is usually made of a polymeric material, so it can absorb water. Some of these materials can become more conductive when they absorb water, and in the case of implantable electrodes, this may result in a high-resistance connection between tissue and the lead wire as well as the contact at the electrode itself. If the lead wire is made of a material different from that of the electrode, the electrolytic problems described at the beginning of this section can result, thereby increasing the observed electric artifact and possibly leading to a weakening of the lead wires due to corrosion. Thus it is important to understand the insulation material used with the electrode and to make sure that there is a layer of it thick enough to prevent this problem from occurring.

When large intermittent currents in the frequency range around 500 kHz from an electrosurgical unit flow through ECG electrodes, the nonlinear current–voltage characteristics of the electrodes can cause them to act as rectifiers and yield large intermittent dc voltage shifts. These cause large low-frequency interference in the ECG that cannot be removed by filtering (Miller and Harrison, 1974, p. 152).

One final point regarding electrodes for measuring biopotentials: In deriving the equivalent circuit for electrodes such as those shown in Figure 5.4, we stressed that for high-fidelity recordings of the measured biopotential, the input impedance of the amplifier to which the electrodes are connected must be much higher than the source impedance represented by the electrodes' equivalent circuit. If this condition is not met, not only will the amplitude of the recorded signal be less than it should be, but significant distortion also will be introduced into the waveform of the signal. This is demonstrated by Geddes and Baker (1989) for electrodes used to record electrocardiograms. They show how lowering the input impedance of the amplifier causes the recorded signal to take on a more and more biphasic character as well as a reduced amplitude.

## PROBLEMS

**5.1** A set of biopotential electrodes made of silver is attached to the chest of a patient to detect the electrocardiogram. When current passes through the anode, it causes silver to be oxidized, producing silver ions in solution. There is a 10 μA leakage current between these electrodes. Determine the number of silver ions per second entering the solution at the electrode–electrolyte interface.

**5.2** Design a system for electrolytically forming Ag/AgCl electrodes. Give the chemical reactions that occur at *both* electrodes.

**5.3** Design an Ag/AgCl electrode that will pass 150 mC (millicoulombs) of charge without removing all the AgCl. Calculate the mass of AgCl required. Show the electrode in cross section and give the active area.

**5.4** When electrodes are used to record the electrocardiogram, an electrolyte gel is usually put between them and the surface of the skin. This makes it possible for the metal of the electrode to form metallic ions that move into the electrolyte gel. Often, after prolonged use, this electrolyte gel begins to dry out and change the characteristic of the electrodes. Draw an equivalent circuit for the electrode while the electrolyte gel is fresh. Then discuss and illustrate the way you expect this equivalent circuit to change as the electrolyte gel dries out. In the extreme case where there is no electrolyte gel left, what does the equivalent circuit of the electrode look like? How can this affect the quality of the recorded electrocardiogram?

**5.5** Design the electrode of the smallest area that has an impedance of 10 Ω at 100 Hz. State your source of information, describe construction of the electrode, and calculate its area.

**5.6** A pair of biopotential electrodes is used to detect the electrocardiogram of an adult male. It has become necessary to determine the equivalent-source impedance of this electrode pair so that a particular experiment can be performed. Describe an experimental procedure that can be used to determine this quantity, using a minimum of test equipment.

**5.7** Using test equipment found in most labs, design (show a block diagram and wiring connections) a test facility for measuring the impedance versus frequency of 1 $cm^2$ electrodes. It should use the largest current density that does not cause a change in the impedance.

**5.8** A pair of biopotential electrodes is placed in a saline solution and connected to a stimulator that passes a direct current through the electrodes. It is noted that the offset potentials from the two electrodes are different. Explain why this happens during the passage of current. Sketch the distribution of ions about each electrode while the current is on.

**5.9** Electrodes having a source resistance of 4 kΩ each are used in a bipolar configuration with a differential amplifier having an input impedance of 70 kΩ. What will be the percentage reduction in the amplitude of the biopotential signal? How can this distortion of the signal be reduced?

**5.10** A nurse noticed that one electrode of a pair of Ag/AgCl cardiac electrodes used on a chronic cardiac monitor was dirty and cleaned it by scraping it with steel wool (Brillo) until it was shiny and bright. The nurse then placed the electrode back on the patient. How did this procedure affect the signal observed from the electrode and electrode impedances?

**5.11** A metal microelectrode has a tip that can be modeled as being cylindrical. The metal itself is 1 μm in diameter, and the tip region is 3 mm long. The metal has a resistivity of $1.2 \times 10^{-5}$ Ω·cm and is coated over its circumference with an insulation material 0.2 μm thick. The insulation material has a relative dielectric constant of 1.67. Only the base of the cylinder is free of insulation.

**a.** What is the resistance associated with the tip of this microelectode?

**b.** What is the area of the surface of the electrode that contacts the electrolytic solution within the cell? The resistance associated with the electrode–electrolyte interface of this material is $10^3$ Ω for 1 $cm^2$. What is the resistance due to this microelectrode's contact with the electrolyte?

**c.** What is the capacitance associated with the tip of the microelectrode when the capacitances at the interface of the electrode–electrolytic solution are neglected?

**d.** Draw an approximate equivalent circuit for the tip portion of this microelectrode.

**e.** At what frequencies do you expect to see distortions when the electrode is connected to an amplifier having a purely resistive input impedance of 10 MΩ? You may assume that the reference electrode has an impedance low enough so that it will not enter into the answer to this question. If the amplifier's input impedance is raised to 100 MΩ, how does this affect the frequency response of the system? Is this difference significant for most intracellular biological applications?

**5.12** A micropipette electrode has a lumenal diameter of 3 μm at its tip. At this point, the glass wall is only 0.5 μm thick and 2 mm long. The resistance of the electrolyte in the tip is 40 MΩ. The glass has a relative dielectric constant of 1.63. Estimate the frequency response of this electrode when it is connected to an infinite-input-impedance amplifier. How can this frequency response be improved?

**5.13** A pair of biopotential electrodes are used to monitor a bioelectric signal from the body. The monitoring electronic circuit has a low-input impedance that is of the same order of magnitude as the source impedance in the electrodes.

**a.** Sketch an equivalent circuit for this situation.

**b.** Describe qualitatively what you expect the general characteristics of the frequency response of this system to be. It is not necessary to plot an analytic Bode plot.

**5.14** A pair of identical stainless steel electrodes is designed to be used to stimulate skeletal muscles. The stimulus consists of a rectangular constant-voltage pulse applied to the electrodes. The pulse has an amplitude of 5 V with a duration of 10 ms. Draw, on the basis of the equivalent circuits of each of the electrodes, an equivalent circuit for the load seen by the constant-voltage pulse generator. Simplify your circuit as much as possible. What is the waveshape of the current at the generator terminals? Remember that a constant-voltage generator has a source impedance of zero. Explain and sketch the resulting current waveform.

**5.15** An exotic new animal, recently discovered, has an unusual electrolyte makeup in that its major anion is $Br^-$ rather than $Cl^-$. Scientists want to measure the EEG of this animal, which is less than 25 μV. Electrodes made of Ag/AgCl seem to be noisy. Can you suggest a better electrode system and explain why it is better?

**5.16** Needle-type EMG electrodes are placed directly in a muscle. Figure P5.1 shows their simplified equivalent circuit and also the equivalent circuit of the

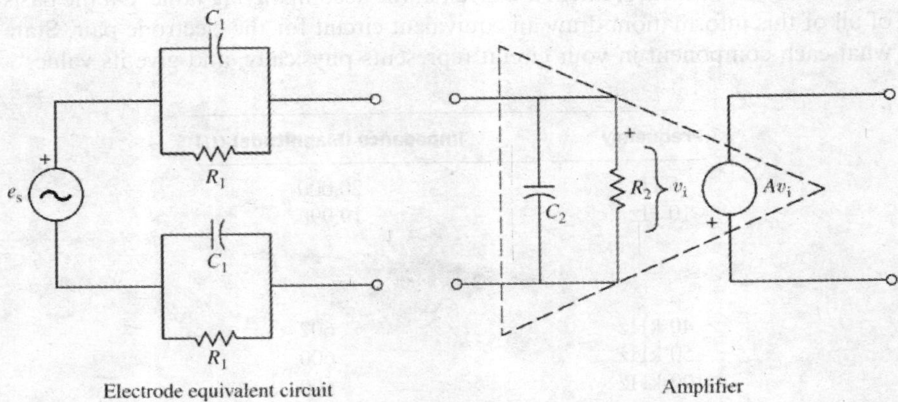


**Figure P5.1**

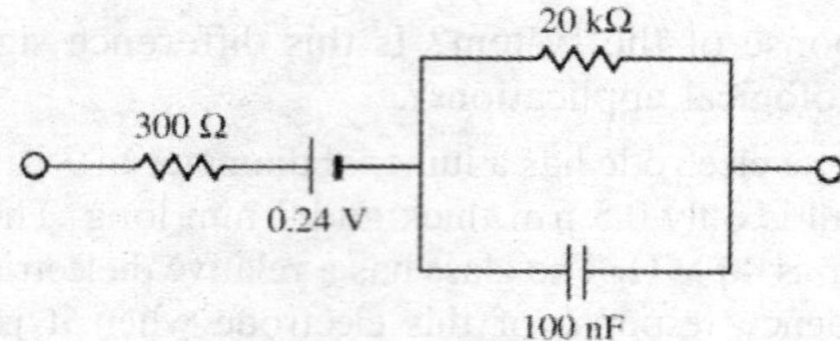


**Figure P5.2**

input stage of an amplifier. The value of the capacitor $C_2$ in the amplifier may be varied to any desired quantity.

**a.** Assuming $C_2 = 0$ and the amplifier gain is $A$, write an equation showing the output voltage of the amplifier as a function of $e_s$ (the signal) and frequency.

**b.** Determine a value for $C_2$ that gives electrode–amplifier characteristics that are independent of frequency.

**c.** What is the amplifier's output voltage in part (b) when the signal is $e_s$?

**5.17** Figure P5.2 shows the equivalent circuit of a biopotential electrode. A pair of these electrodes are tested in a beaker of physiological saline solution. The test consists of measuring the magnitude of the impedance between the electrodes as a function of frequency via low-level sinusoidal excitation so that the impedances are not affected by the current crossing the electrode–electrolyte interface. The impedance of the saline solution is small enough to be neglected. Sketch a Bode plot (log of impedance magnitude versus log of frequency) of the impedance between the electrodes over a frequency range of 1 to 100,000 Hz.

**5.18** A pair of biopotential electrodes are implanted in an animal to measure the electrocardiogram for a radiotelemetry system. One must know the equivalent circuit for these electrodes in order to design the optimal input circuit for the telemetry system. Measurements made on the pair of electrodes have shown that the polarization capacitance for the pair is 200 nF and that the half-cell potential for each electrode is 223 mV. The magnitude of the impedance between the two electrodes was measured via sinusoidal excitation at several different frequencies. The results of this measurement are given in the accompanying table. On the basis of all of this information, draw an equivalent circuit for the electrode pair. State what each component in your circuit represents physically, and give its value.

| Frequency | Impedance (Magnitude) (Ω) |
|---|---|
| 5 Hz | 20,000 |
| 10 Hz | 19,998 |
| . | . |
| . | . |
| . | . |
| 40 kHz | 602 |
| 50 kHz | 600 |
| 100 kHz | 600 |

## REFERENCES


Anonymous, Disposable ECG electrodes, American National Standard ANSI/AAMI EC12:2000/(R)2005, Arlington, VA: Association for the Advancement of Medical Instrumentation, 2005.

Arzbaecher, R., "New applications of the pill electrode for cardiac recording and pacing." *Proc. Annu. Int. Conf. IEEE Eng. Med. Biol. Soc.*, 1982, 4, 508–510.

Ash, R. B., T. A. Johnson, and H. T. Nagle, "Application of a multilevel ceramic integrated circuit package for epicardial mapping." *Proc. Annu. Int. Conf. IEEE Eng. Med. Biol. Soc.*, 1992, 2392.

Atkin, T., K. Najafi, R. H. Smoke, and R. M. Bradley, "A micromachined silicon sieve electrode for nerve regeneration applications." *IEEE Trans. Biomed. Eng.*, 1994, 41, 305–313.

Boucsein, W., *Electrodermal Activity*. New York: Plenum Press, 1992.

Branner A., R. B. Stein, E. Fernandez, Y. Aoyagi, and R. A. Normann, "Long-term stimulation and recording with a penetrating microelectrode array in cat sciatic nerve." *IEEE Trans. Biomed. Eng.*, 2004, 51(1), 146–157.

Burbank, D. P., and J. G. Webster, "Reducing skin potential motion artefact by skin abrasion." *Med. Biol. Eng. Comput.*, 1978, 16, 31–38.

Caldwell, C. W., and J. B. Reswick, "A percutaneous wire electrode for chronic research use." *IEEE Trans. Biomed. Eng.*, 1975, BME-22, 429–432.

Campbell, P. K., K. E. Jones, R. J. Huber, K. W. Horch, and R. A. Normann, "A silicon-based, three-dimensional neural interface: Manufacturing processes for an intracortical interface." *IEEE Trans. Biomed. Eng.*, 1991, 38, 758–768.

Cobbold, R. S. C, *Transducers for Biomedical Measurements: Principles and Applications*. New York: Wiley, 1974.

Cogan, S. F., "Neural stimulation and recording electrodes." *Annu. Rev. Biomed. Eng.*, 2008, 10, 275–309.

Coosemans, J., B. Hermans, and R. Puers, "Integrating wireless ECG monitoring in textiles." *Sens. Actuators A: Phys.*, 2006, 130–131, 48–53.

Critchfield, F. H., C. Xinteras, B. Johnson, and M. R. Neuman, "Surgical and engineering techniques for the supracephalic mounting of a multichannel EEG telemeter." *Dig. Int. Conf. Med. Biol. Eng.*, 1971, paper no. 22-4.

Das, D. P., and J. G. Webster, "Defibrillation recovery curves for different electrode materials." *IEEE Trans. Biomed. Eng.*, 1980, BME-27, 230–233.

De Talhouet, H., and J. G. Webster, "The origin of skin-stretch-caused motion artifacts under electrodes." *Physiol. Meas.*, 1996, 17, 81–93.

Delgado, J. M. R., "Electrodes for extracellular recording and stimulation." In W. L. Nastuk (ed.), *Physical Techniques in Biological Research*. New York: Academic, 1964, Vol. 5A.

Drake, K. L., K. D. Wise, J. Farraye, D. J. Anderson, and S. L. BeMent, "Performance of planar multisite microprobes in recording extracellular single-unit intracortical activity." *IEEE Trans. Biomed. Eng.*, 1988, 35, 719–732.

Edell, D. J., "A peripheral nerve information transducer for amputees: Long-term multichannel recordings from rabbit peripheral nerves." *IEEE Trans. Biomed. Eng.*, 1986, BME-33, 203–214.

Ferris, C. D., *Introduction to Bioelectrodes*. New York: Plenum, 1974.

Geddes, L. A., *Electrodes and the Measurement of Bioelectric Events*. New York: Wiley, 1972.

Geddes, L. A., and L. E. Baker, *Principles of Applied Biomedical Instrumentation*, 3rd ed., New York: John Wiley & Sons, 1989.

Geddes, L. A., L. E. Baker, and A. G. Moore, "Optimum electrolytic chloriding of silver electrodes." *Med. Biol. Eng.*, 1969, 7, 49–56.

Hon, E. H., R. H. Paul, and R. W. Hon, "Electronic evaluation of fetal heart rate. XI: Description of a spiral electrode." *Obstet. Gynecol.*, 1972, 40, 362–363.

Janz, G. J., and D. J. G. Ives, "Silver-silver chloride electrodes." *Ann. N.Y. Acad. Sci.*, 1968, 148, 210–221.

Jossinet, J., and E. McAdams, "Hydrogel electrodes in biosignal recording." *Proc. Annu. Int. Conf. IEEE Eng. Med. Biol. Soc.*, 1990, 12, 1490–1491.

Kang T. H., C. R. Merritt, E. Grant, B. Pourdeyhimi, and H. T. Nagle. "Nonwoven fabric active electrodes for biopotential measurement during normal daily activity." *IEEE Trans. Biomed. Eng.*, 2008, 55(1): 188–195.

Kovacs, G. T. A., C. W. Storment, M. Halks-Miller, C. R. Belczynski, Jr., C. C. D. Santina, E. R. Lewis, and N. I. Maluf, "Silicon-substrate microelectrode arrays for parallel recording of neural activity in peripheral and cranial nerves." *IEEE Trans. Biomed. Eng.*, 1994, 41, 567–577.

Malkin RA, and B. D. Pendley, "Construction of a very high-density extracellular electrode array." *Amer. J. Physiol.. Heart Circulatory Physiol.*, 2000, 279(1), H 437–442.

Mastrototaro, J. J., H. Z. Massoud, T. C. Pilkington, and R. E. Ideker, "Rigid and flexible thin-film multielectrode arrays for transmural cardiac recording." *IEEE Trans. Biomed. Eng.*, 1992, 39, 271–279.

McAdams, E., "Bioelectrodes." In J. G. Webster (ed.), *Encyclopedia of Medical Devices and Instrumentation*, 2nd ed., New York: Wiley, 2006, Vol. 1, pp. 120–166.

Miller, H. A., and D. C. Harrison (eds.), *Biomedical Electrode Technology*. New York: Academic, 1974.

Neuman, M. R., "Flexible thin film skin electrodes for use with neonates." *Dig. Int. Conf. Med. Biol. Eng.*, 1973, paper no. 35.11.

Olsson, R. H., III, D. L. Buhl, A. M. Sirota, G. Buzsaki, and K. D. Wise, "Band-tunable and multiplexed integrated circuits for simultaneous recording and stimulation with microelectrode arrays." *IEEE Trans. Biomed. Eng.*, 2005, 52(7), 1303–1311.

Plonsey, R., and R. C. Barr, *Bioelectricity a Quantitative Approach*, 3rd ed. New York: Springer, 2007.

Prohaska, O. J., F. Olcaytug, P. Pfundner, and H. Dragaun, "Thin-film multiple electrode probes: Possibilities and limitations." *IEEE Trans. Biomed. Eng.*, 1986, BME-33, 223–229.

Robblee, R. S., J. L. Lefko, and S. B. Brummer, "Activated iridium: an electrode suitable for reversible charge injection in saline solution." *J. Electrochem. Soc.*, 1983, 1130, 731–733.

Rosell, J., J. Colominas, P. Riu, R. Pallas-Areny, and J. G. Webster, "Skin impedance from 1 Hz to 1 MHz." *IEEE Trans. Biomed. Eng.*, 1988, 35, 649–651.

Schwan, H. P., "Determination of biological impedances." In W. L. Nastuk (ed), *Physical Techniques in Biological Research.* New York: Academic, 1963, pp. 323–407.

Tam, H. W., and J. G. Webster, "Minimizing electrode motion artifact by skin abrasion." *IEEE Trans. Biomed. Eng.*, 1977, BME-24, 134–139.

Webster, J. G., "Reducing motion artifacts and interference in biopotential recording." *IEEE Trans. Biomed. Eng.*, 1984a, BME-31, 823–826.

Webster, J. G., "What is important in biomedical electrodes? " *Proc. Annu. Conf. Eng. Med. Biol.*, 1984b, 26, 96.

Wise, K. D., K. Najafi, J. Ji, J. F. Hetke, S. J. Tanghe, A. Hoogerwerf, D. J. Anderson, S. L. BeMent, M. Ghazzi, W. Baer, T. Hull, and Y. Yang. "Micromachined silicon microprobes for CNS recording and stimulation." *Proc. Annu. Int. Conf. IEEE Eng. Med. Biol. Soc.*, 1990, 12, 2334–2335.

# 6

# BIOPOTENTIAL AMPLIFIERS

Michael R. Neuman

Amplifiers are an important part of modern instrumentation systems for measuring biopotentials. Such measurements involve voltages that often are at low levels, have high source impedances, or both. Amplifiers are required to increase signal strength while maintaining high fidelity. Amplifiers that have been designed specifically for this type of processing of biopotentials are known as *biopotential amplifiers*. In this chapter we examine some of the basic features of biopotential amplifiers and also look at specialized systems.

## 6.1 BASIC REQUIREMENTS

The essential function of a biopotential amplifier is to take a weak electric signal of biological origin and increase its amplitude so that it can be further processed, recorded, or displayed. Usually such amplifiers are in the form of voltage amplifiers, because they are capable of increasing the voltage level of a signal. Nonetheless, voltage amplifiers also serve to increase power levels, so they can be considered power amplifiers as well. In some cases, biopotential amplifiers are used to isolate the load from the source. In this situation, the amplifiers provide only current gain, leaving the voltage levels essentially unchanged.

To be useful biologically, all biopotential amplifiers must meet certain basic requirements. They must have high input impedance, so that they provide minimal loading of the signal being measured. The characteristics of biopotential electrodes can be affected by the electric load they see, which, combined with excessive loading, can result in distortion of the signal. Loading effects are minimized by making the amplifier input impedance as high as possible, thereby reducing this distortion. Modern biopotential amplifiers have input impedances of at least 10 MΩ.

The input circuit of a biopotential amplifier must also provide protection to the organism being studied. Any current or potential appearing across the amplifier input terminals that is produced by the amplifier is capable of affecting the biological potential being measured. In clinical systems, electric currents from the input terminals of a biopotential amplifier can result in microshocks or macroshocks in the patient being studied—a situation that can have grave consequences. To avoid these problems, the amplifier should have isolation and protection circuitry, so that the current through the electrode circuit can be kept at safe levels and any artifact generated by such current can be minimized.

The output circuit of a biopotential amplifier does not present so many critical problems as the input circuit. Its principal function is to drive the amplifier load, usually an indicating or recording device, in such a way as to maintain maximal fidelity and range in this readout. Therefore, the output impedance of the amplifier must be low with respect to the load impedance, and the amplifier must be capable of supplying the power required by the load.

Biopotential amplifiers must operate in that portion of the frequency spectrum in which the biopotentials that they amplify exist. Because of the low level of such signals, it is important to limit the bandwidth of the amplifier so that it is just great enough to process the signal adequately. In this way, we can obtain optimal signal-to-noise ratios (SNRs). Biopotential signals usually have amplitudes of the order of a few millivolts or less. Such signals must be amplified to levels compatible with recording and display devices. This means that most biopotential amplifiers must have high gains—of the order of 1000 or greater.

Very frequently biopotential signals are obtained from bipolar electrodes. These electrodes are often symmetrically located, electrically, with respect to ground. Under such circumstances, the most appropriate biopotential amplifier is a differential one. Because such bipolar electrodes frequently have a common-mode voltage with respect to ground that is much larger than the signal amplitude, and because the symmetry with respect to ground can be distorted, such biopotential differential amplifiers must have high common-mode-rejection ratios to minimize interference due to the common-mode signal.

A final requirement for biopotential amplifiers that are used both in medical applications and in the laboratory is that they make quick calibration possible. In recording biopotentials, the scientist and clinician need to know not only the waveforms of these signals but also their amplitudes. To provide this information, the gain of the amplifier must be well calibrated. Frequently biopotential amplifiers have a standard signal source that can be momentarily connected to the input, automatically at the start of a measurement or manually at the push of a button, to check the calibration. Biopotential amplifiers that need to have adjustable gains usually have a switch by which different, carefully calibrated fixed gains can be selected, rather than having a continuous control (such as the volume control of an audio amplifier) for adjusting the gain. Thus the gain is always known, and there is no chance of its being accidentally varied by someone bumping the gain control.

Biopotential amplifiers have additional requirements that are application-specific and that can be ascertained from an examination of each application. To illustrate some of these, let us first consider the electrocardiogram (ECG), the most frequently used application of biopotential amplifiers.

## 6.2 THE ELECTROCARDIOGRAPH

To learn more about biopotential amplifiers, we shall examine a typical clinical electrocardiograph. First, let us review the ECG itself.

### THE ECG

As we learned in Section 4.6, the beating heart generates an electric signal that can be used as a diagnostic tool for examining some of the functions of the heart. This electric activity of the heart can be approximately represented as a vector quantity. Thus we need to know the location at which signals are detected, as well as the time dependence of the amplitude of the signals. Electrocardiographers have developed a simple model to represent the electric activity of the heart. In this model, the heart consists of an electric dipole located in the partially conducting medium of the thorax. Figure 6.1 shows a typical example. Of course in reality the heart is a much more complicated electrophysiological entity, and far more complex models are needed to represent it.

This particular field and the dipole that produces it represent the electric activity of the heart at a specific instant. At the next instant the dipole can change its magnitude and its orientation, thereby causing a change in the electric field. Once we accept this simplified model, we need not draw a field plot every time we want to discuss the dipole field of the heart. Instead, we can represent it by its dipole moment, a vector directed from the negative charge to the positive charge and having a magnitude proportional to the amount of charge (either positive or negative) multiplied by the separation of the two charges. In electrocardiography this dipole moment, known as the *cardiac vector*, is represented by **M**, as shown in Figure 6.1. As we progress through a cardiac cycle, the magnitude and direction of **M** vary because the dipole field varies.

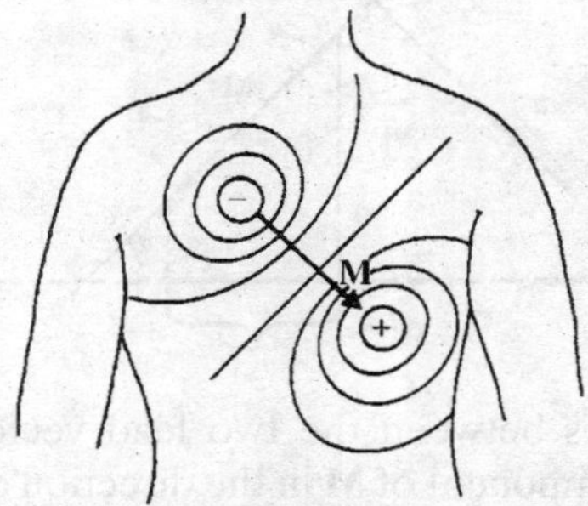


**Figure 6.1 Rough sketch of the dipole field of the heart when the R wave is maximal** The dipole consists of the points of equal positive and negative charge separated from one another and denoted by the dipole moment vector **M**.

The electric potentials generated by the heart appear throughout the body and on its surface. We determine potential differences by placing electrodes on the surface of the body and measuring the voltage between them, being careful to draw little current (ideally there should be no current at all, because current distorts the electric field that produces the potential differences). If the two electrodes are located on different equal-potential lines of the electric field of the heart, a nonzero potential difference or voltage is measured. Different pairs of electrodes at different locations generally yield different voltages because of the spatial dependence of the electric field of the heart. Thus it is important to have certain standard positions for clinical evaluation of the ECG. The limbs make fine guideposts for locating the ECG electrodes. We shall look at this in more detail later.

In the simplified dipole model of the heart, it would be convenient if we could predict the voltage, or at least its waveform, in a particular set of electrodes at a particular instant of time when the cardiac vector is known. We can do this if we define a *lead vector* for the pair of electrodes. This vector is a unit vector that defines the direction a constant-magnitude cardiac vector must have to generate maximal voltage in the particular pair of electrodes. A pair of electrodes, or combination of several electrodes through a resistive network that gives an equivalent pair, is referred to as a *lead*.

For a cardiac vector **M**, as shown in Figure 6.2, the voltage induced in a lead represented by the lead vector $\mathbf{a}_1$ is given by the component of **M** in the direction of $\mathbf{a}_1$. In vector algebra, this can be denoted by the dot product

$$v_{a1} = \mathbf{M} \cdot \mathbf{a}_1 \quad \text{or} \quad v_{a1} = |\mathbf{M}| \cos\theta \tag{6.1}$$

Where $v_{a1}$ is the scalar voltage seen in the lead that has the vector $\mathbf{a}_1$. Let us consider another lead, represented by the lead vector $\mathbf{a}_2$, as seen in Figure 6.2. In this case, the vector is oriented in space so as to be perpendicular to the

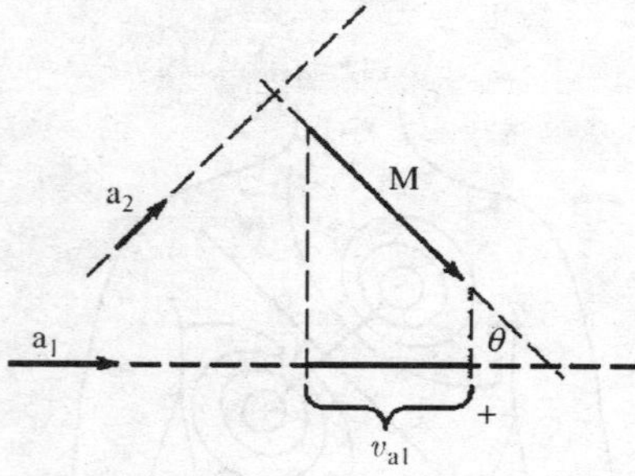


**Figure 6.2** Relationships between the two lead vectors $\mathbf{a}_1$ and $\mathbf{a}_2$ and the cardiac vector **M**. The component of **M** in the direction of $\mathbf{a}_1$ is given by the dot product of these two vectors and denoted on the figure by $v_{a1}$. Lead vector $\mathbf{a}_2$ is perpendicular to the cardiac vector, so no voltage component is seen in this lead.

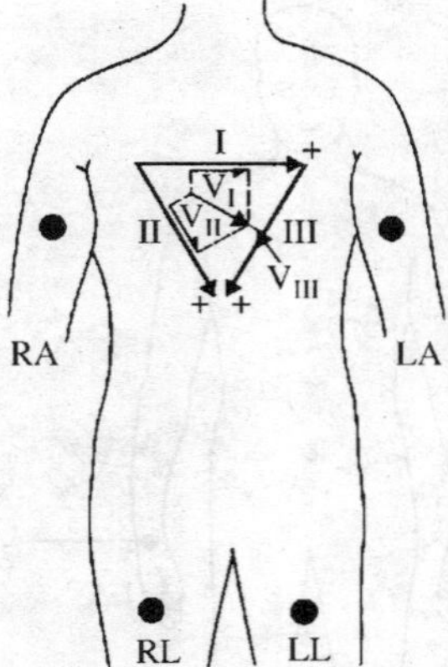


**Figure 6.3** Cardiologists use a standard notation such that the direction of the lead vector for lead I is 0°, that of lead II is 60°, and that of lead III is 120°. An example of a cardiac vector at 30° with its scalar components seen for each lead is shown.

cardiac vector **M**. The component of **M** along the direction of $\mathbf{a}_2$ is zero, so no voltage is seen in this lead as a result of the cardiac vector. If we measured the ECG generated by **M** using one of the two leads shown in Figure 6.2 alone, we could not describe the cardiac vector uniquely. However, by using two leads with different lead vectors, both of which lie in the same plane as the cardiac vector such as $\mathbf{a}_1$ and $\mathbf{a}_2$, we can describe **M**.

In clinical electrocardiography, more than one lead must be recorded to describe the heart's electric activity fully. In practice, several leads are taken in the *frontal plane* (the plane of your body that is parallel to the ground when you are lying on your back) and the *transverse plane* (the plane of your body that is parallel to the ground when you are standing erect).

Three basic leads make up *the frontal-plane* ECG. These are derived from the various permutations of pairs of electrodes when one electrode is located on the right arm (RA in Figure 6.3), the left arm (LA), and the left leg (LL). Very often an electrode is also placed on the right leg (RL) and grounded or connected to special circuits, as shown in Figure 6.15. The resulting three leads are lead I, LA to RA; lead II, LL to RA; and lead III, LL to LA. The lead vectors that are formed can be approximated as an equilateral triangle, known as *Einthoven's triangle*, in the frontal plane of the body, as shown in Figure 6.3. Because the scalar signal on each lead of Einthoven's triangle can be represented as a voltage source, we can write Kirchhoff's voltage law for the three leads.

$$\mathrm{I} - \mathrm{II} + \mathrm{III} = 0 \tag{6.2}$$

The components of a particular cardiac vector can be determined easily by placing the vector within the triangle and determining its projection along each

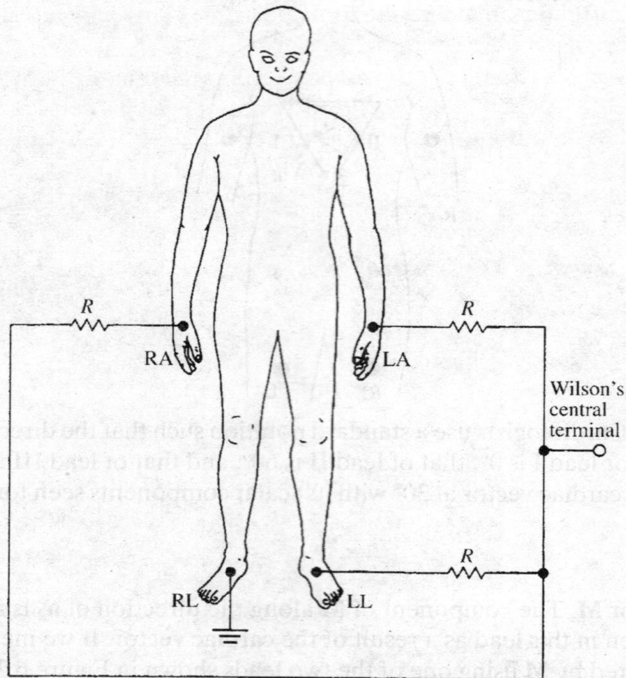


**Figure 6.4 Connection of electrodes to the body to obtain Wilson's central terminal**

side. The process can also be reversed, which enables us to determine the cardiac vector when we know the components along the three lead vectors, or at least two of them. It is this latter problem that usually concerns the electrocardiographer.

Three additional leads in the frontal plane—as well as a group of leads in the transverse plane—are routinely used in taking clinical ECGs. These leads are based on signals obtained from more than one pair of electrodes. They are often referred to as *unipolar leads*, because they consist of the potential appearing on one electrode taken with respect to an equivalent reference electrode, which is the average of the signals seen at two or more electrodes.

One such equivalent reference electrode is the *Wilson central terminal*, shown in Figure 6.4. Here the three limb electrodes just described are connected through equal-valued resistors to a common node. The voltage at this node, which is the Wilson central terminal, is the average of the voltages at each electrode. In practice, the values of the resistors should be at least 5 MΩ so that the loading of any particular lead will be minimal. Thus, a more practical approach is to use buffers (voltage followers, see Section 3.3) between each electrode and the equal-valued resistors. The signal between LA and the central point is known as VL, that at RA as VR, and that at the left foot as VF. Note that for each of these leads, one of the resistances *R* shunts the circuit between the central terminal and the limb electrode. This tends to reduce the amplitude of the signal observed, and we can modify these leads to *augmented leads* by removing the connection between the limb being measured and the central terminal. This does not affect the direction of the lead vector but results in a 50% increase in amplitude of the signal.

The augmented leads—known as aVL, aVR, and aVF—are illustrated in Figure 6.5, which also illustrates their lead vectors, along with those of leads I, II, and III. Note that when the negative direction for aVR is considered with

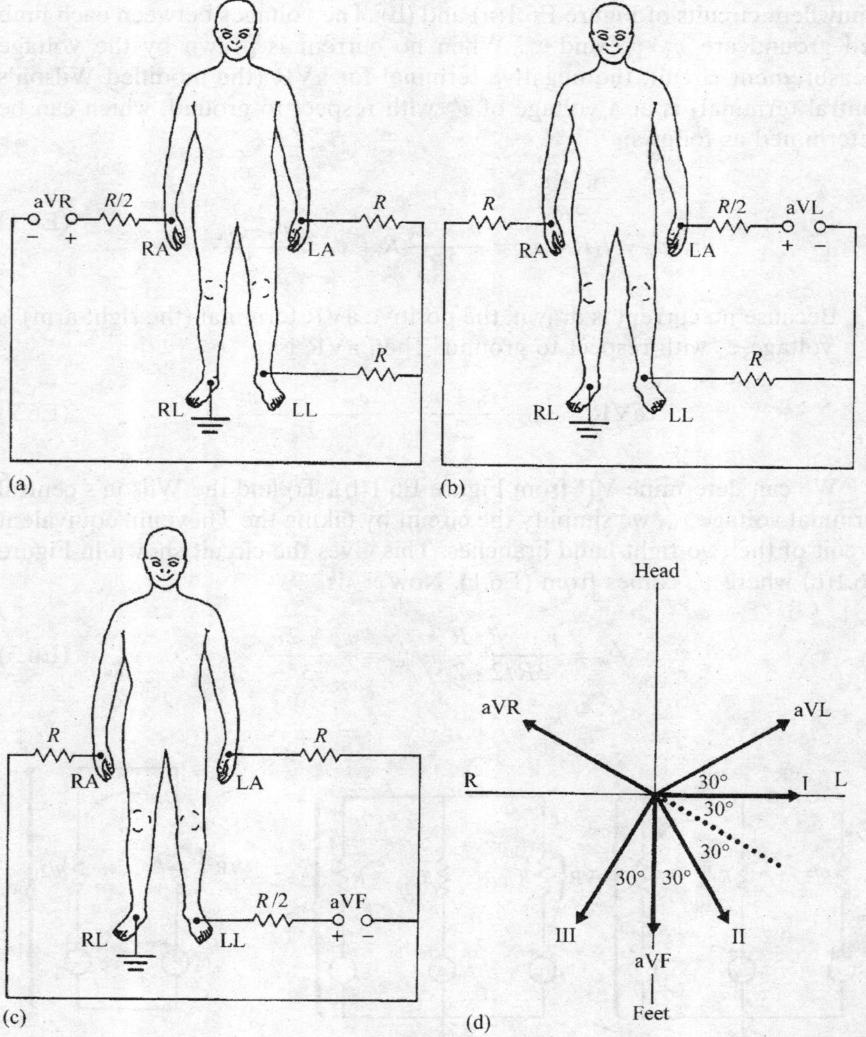


**Figure 6.5** (a), (b), (c) Connections of electrodes for the three augmented limb leads. (d) Vector diagram showing standard and augmented lead-vector directions in the frontal plane.

the other five, all six vectors are equally spaced, by 30°. It is thus possible for the cardiologist looking at an ECG consisting of these six leads to estimate the position of the cardiac vector by seeing which of the six leads has the greatest signal amplitude at that point in the cardiac cycle.

**EXAMPLE 6.1** Show that the voltage in lead aVR is 50% greater than that in lead VR at the same instant.

**ANSWER** Considering the connections for aVR and VR, we can draw the equivalent circuits of Figure E6.1(a) and (b). The voltages between each limb and ground are $v_a$, $v_b$, and $v_c$. When no current is drawn by the voltage measurement circuit, the negative terminal for aVR (the modified Wilson's central terminal) is at a voltage of $v'_w$ with respect to ground, which can be determined as follows:

$$\begin{aligned} i_1 &= \frac{v_b - v_c}{2R} \\ v'_w &= i_1 R + v_c = \frac{v_b - v_c}{2R} R + v_c = \frac{v_b - v_c}{2} \end{aligned} \quad \text{(E6.1)}$$

Because no current is drawn, the positive aVR terminal (the right arm) is at a voltage $v_a$ with respect to ground. Then aVR is

$$\text{aVR} = v_a - \frac{v_b + v_c}{2} = \frac{2v_a - v_b - v_c}{2} \quad \text{(E6.2)}$$

We can determine VR from Figure E6.1(b). To find the Wilson's central terminal voltage $v_w$, we simplify the circuit by taking the Thévenin equivalent circuit of the two right-hand branches. This gives the circuit shown in Figure E6.1(c) where $v'_w$ comes from (E6.1). Now $v_w$ is

$$v_w = \frac{v_a - v'_w}{3R/2} \frac{R}{2} + v'_w = \frac{v_a + 2v'_w}{3} \quad \text{(E6.3)}$$

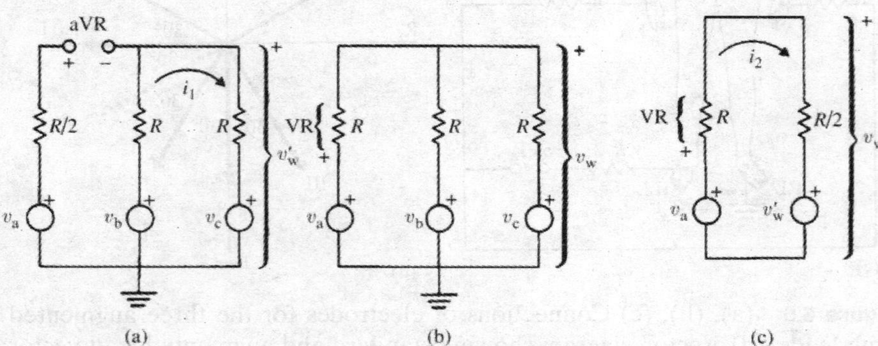


**Figure E6.1** (a) aVR, (b) VR, and (c) simplified circuit of (a).

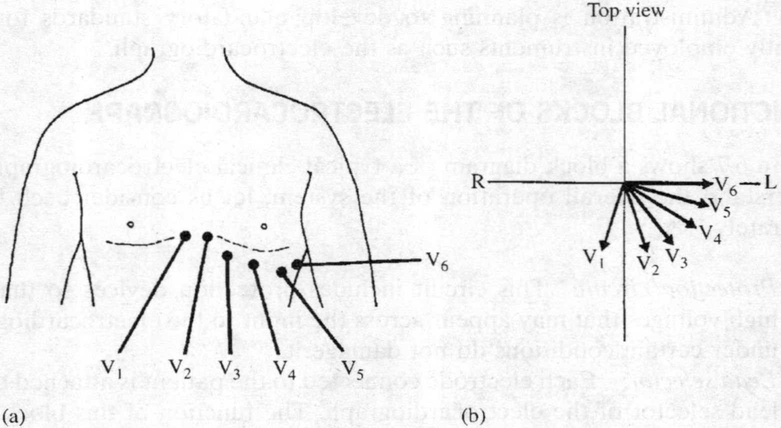


**Figure 6.6** (a) Positions of precordial leads on the chest wall. (b) Directions of precordial lead vectors in the transverse plane.

$$v_w = \frac{v_a + 2(v_b + v_c)/2}{3} = \frac{v_a + v_b + v_c}{3} \quad \text{(E6.4)}$$

Thus

$$VR = v_a - v_w = \frac{2v_a - v_b - v_c}{3} \quad \text{(E6.5)}$$

which shows that

$$aVR = \frac{3}{2} VR$$

When physicians look at the ECG in the transverse plane, they use *precordial* (chest) leads. They place an electrode at various anatomically defined positions on the chest wall, as shown in Figure 6.6. The potential between this electrode and Wilson's central terminal is the electrocardiogram for that particular lead. Figure 6.6 also shows the lead-vector positions. Physicians can obtain ECGs from the posterior side of the heart by means of an electrode placed in the esophagus. This structure passes directly behind the heart, and the potential between the esophageal electrode and Wilson's central terminal gives a posterior lead.

## SPECIFIC REQUIREMENTS OF THE ELECTROCARDIOGRAPH

Because the electrocardiograph is widely used as a diagnostic tool and there are several manufacturers of this instrument, standardization is necessary. Standard requirements for electrocardiographs have been developed over the years (Bailey *et al.* 1990; Anonymous, 1991). Table 6.1 gives a summary of performance requirements from the most recent of these (Anonymous, 1991). These recommendations are a part of a voluntary standard. The Food and

Drug Administration is planning to develop mandatory standards for frequently employed instruments such as the electrocardiograph.

## FUNCTIONAL BLOCKS OF THE ELECTROCARDIOGRAPH

Figure 6.7 shows a block diagram of a typical clinical electrocardiograph. To understand the overall operation of the system, let us consider each block separately.

1. *Protection circuit:* This circuit includes protection devices so that the high voltages that may appear across the input to the electrocardiograph under certain conditions do not damage it.
2. *Lead selector:* Each electrode connected to the patient is attached to the lead selector of the electrocardiograph. The function of this block is to determine which electrodes are necessary for a particular lead and to connect them to the remainder of the circuit. It is this part of the electrocardiograph in which the connections for the central terminal are made. This block can be controlled by the operator or by the

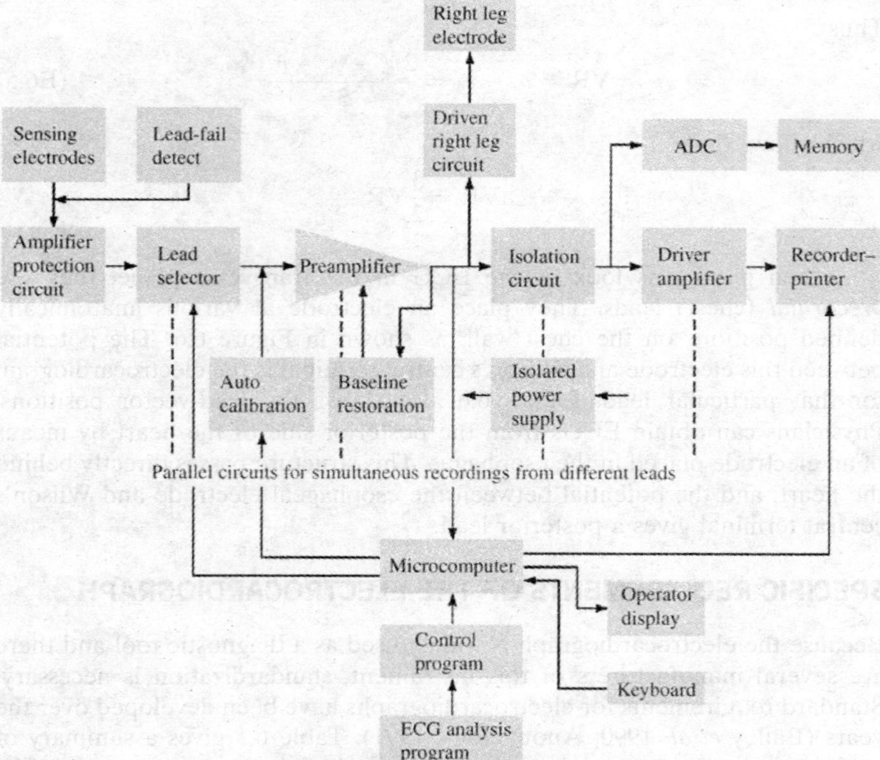


**Figure 6.7** Block diagram of an electrocardiograph

microcomputer of the electrocardiograph when it is operated in automatic mode. It selects one or more leads to be recorded. In automatic mode, each of the 12 standard leads is recorded for a short duration such as 10 s.

3. *Calibration signal:* A 1 mV calibration signal is momentarily introduced into the electrocardiograph for each channel that is recorded.
4. *Preamplifier:* The input preamplifier stage carries out the initial amplification of the ECG. This stage should have very high input impedance and a high common-mode-rejection ratio (CMRR). A typical preamplifier stage is the differential amplifier that consists of three operational amplifiers (op amps), shown in Figure 3.5. A gain-control switch is often included as a part of this stage.
5. *Isolation circuit:* The circuitry of this block contains a barrier to the passage of current from the power line (50 or 60 Hz). For example, if the patient came in contact with a 120 V line, this barrier would prevent dangerous currents from flowing from the patient through the amplifier to the ground of the recorder or microcomputer.
6. *Driven-right-leg circuit:* This circuit provides a reference point on the patient that normally is at ground potential. This connection is made to an electrode on the patient's right leg. Details on this circuit are given in Section 6.5.
7. *Driver amplifier:* Circuitry in this block amplifies the ECG to a level at which it can appropriately record the signal on the recorder. Its input should be ac coupled so that offset voltages amplified by the preamplifier are not seen at its input. These dc voltages, when amplified by this stage, might cause it to saturate. This stage also carries out the bandpass filtering of the electrocardiograph to give the frequency characteristics described in Table 6.1. Also it often has a zero-offset control that is used to position the signal on the recorder. This control adjusts the dc level of the output signal.
8. *Memory system:* Many modern electrocardiographs store electrocardiograms in memory as well as printing them out on a recorder. The signal is first digitized by an analog-to-digital converter (ADC), and then samples from each lead are stored in memory. Patient information entered via the keyboard is also stored. The microcomputer controls this storage activity.
9. *Microcomputer:* The microcomputer controls the overall operation of the electrocardiograph. The operator can select several modes of operation by invoking a particular program. For example, she or he can ask the microcomputer to generate the standard 12-lead electrocardiogram by selecting three simultaneous 10 s segments of the six frontal plane leads followed by three 10 s segments of the six transverse plane leads. The microcomputer in some machines can also perform a preliminary analysis of the electrocardiogram to determine the heart rate, recognize some types of arrhythmia, calculate the axes of various features of the electrocardiogram, and determine intervals between these features. A keyboard and an alphanumeric display enable the operator to communicate with the microcomputer.

**Table 6.1 Summary of Performance Requirements for Electrocardiographs (Anonymous, 1991)**

| Section | Requirement Description | Min/max | Units | Min/Max Value |
|---|---|---|---|---|
| 3.2.1 | Operating conditions: | | | |
| | Line voltage | Range | V rms | 104 to 1127 |
| | Frequency | Range | Hz | 60 ± 1 |
| | Temperature | Range | °C | 25 ± 10 |
| | Relative humidity | Range | % | 50 ± 20 |
| | Atmospheric pressure | Range | Pa | $7 \times 10^4$ to $10.6 \times 10^4$ |
| 3.2.2 | Lead definition (number of leads): | NA | NA | Table 3 |
| | Single-channel | Min | NA | 7 |
| | Three-channel | Min | NA | 12 |
| 3.2.3 | Input Dynamic Range: | | | |
| | Range of linear operations of input signal | Min | mV | ±5 |
| | Slew rate change | Max | mV/s | 320 |
| | DC offset voltage range | Min | mV | ±300 |
| | Allowed variation of amplitude with dc offset | Max | % | ±5 |
| 3.2.4 | Gain control, accuracy, and stability: | | | |
| | Gain selections | Min | mm/mV | 20, 10, 5 |
| | Gain error | Max | % | 5 |
| | Manual override of automatic gain control | NA | NA | NA |
| | Gain change rate/min | Max | %/min | ±0.33 |
| | Total gain change/h | Max | % | ±3 |
| 3.2.5 | Time base selection and accuracy: | | | |
| | Time base selections | Min | mm/s | 25, 50 |
| | Time base error | Max | % | ±5 |
| 3.2.6 | Output display: | | | |
| | General | NA | NA | per 3.2.3 |
| | Width of display | Min | mm | 40 |
| | Trace visibility (writing rates) | Max | mm/s | 1600 |
| | Trace width (permanent record only) | Max | mm | 1 |
| | Departure from time axis alignment | Max | mm | 0.5 |
| | | Max | ms | 10 |
| | Preruled paper division | Min | div/cm | 10 |
| | Error of rulings | Max | % | ±2 |
| | Time marker error | Max | % | ±2 |
| 3.2.7 | Accuracy of input signal reproduction: | | | |
| | Overall error for signals | Max | % | ±5 |
| | Up to ±5 mV and 125 mV/s | Max | μV | ±40 |

**Table 6.1** *(Continued)*

| Section | Requirement Description | Min/max | Units | Min/Max Value |
|---|---|---|---|---|
| | Upper cut-off frequency (3 dB) | Min | Hz | 150 |
| | Response to 20 ms, 1.5 mV triangular input | Min | mm | 13.5 |
| | Response after 3 mV, 100 ms impulse | Max | mV | 0.1 |
| | | Max | mV/s | 0.30 |
| | Error in lead weighting factors | Max | % | 5 |
| | Hysteresis after 15 mm deflection from baseline | Max | mm | 0.5 |
| 3.2.8 | Standardizing voltage: | | | |
| | Nominal value | NA | mV | 1.0 |
| | Rise time | Max | ms | 1 |
| | Decay time | Min | s | 100 |
| | Amplitude error | Max | % | ±5 |
| 3.2.9 | Input impedance at 10 Hz (each lead) | Min | megohms | 2.5 |
| 3.2.10 | DC current (any input lead) | Max | μA | 0.1 |
| | DC current (any patient electrode) | Max | μA | 1.0 |
| 3.2.11 | Common-Mode Rejection: | | | |
| | Allowable noise with 20 V, 60 Hz and ±300 mV dc and 51 kΩ | Max | mm | 10 |
| | Imbalance | Max | mV | 1 |
| 3.2.12 | System noise: | | | |
| | RTI, *p-p* | Max | μV | 30 |
| | Multichannel crosstalk | Max | % | 2 |
| 3.2.13 | Baseline control and stability: | | | |
| | Return time after reset | Max | s | 3 |
| | Return time after lead switch | Max | s | 1 |
| | Baseline stability: | | | |
| | Baseline drift rate RTI | Max | μV/s | 10 |
| | Total baseline drift RTI (2 min period) | Max | μV | 500 |
| 3.2.14 | Overload protection: | | | |
| | No damage from differential voltage, 60 Hz, 1 Vp-p, 10 s application | Min | V | 1 |
| | No damage from simulated defibrillator discharges: | | | |
| | *Overvoltage* | N/A | V | 5000 |
| | *Energy* | N/A | J | 360 |
| | Recovery time | Max | s | 8 |
| | Energy reduction by defibrillator shunting | Max | % | 10 |
| | Transfer of charge through defibrillator chassis | Max | μC | 100 |

*(Continued)*

**Table 6.1** *(Continued)*

| Section | Requirement Description | Min/max | Units | Min/Max Value |
|---|---|---|---|---|
| | ECG display in presence of pacemaker pulses: | | | |
| | *Amplitude* | Range | mV | 2 to 250 |
| | *Pulse duration* | Range | ms | 0.1 to 2.0 |
| | *Rise time* | Max | μs | 100 |
| | *Frequency* | Max | pulses/min | 100 |
| 3.2.15 | Risk current (isolated patient connection) | Max | μA | 10 |
| | | As per applicable document 2.11 | | |
| 3.2.16 | Auxiliary output (if provided): | | | |
| | No damage from short circuit risk | Max | μA | 10 |
| | Current (isolated patient connection) | As per applicable document 2.1.1 | | |

**10.** *Recorder–printer:* This block provides a hard copy of the recorded ECG signal. It also prints out patient identification, clinical information entered by the operator, and the results of the automatic analysis of the electrocardiogram. Although analog oscillograph-type recorders were employed for this function in the past, modern electrocardiographs make use of thermal or electrostatic recording techniques in which the only moving part is the paper being transported under the print head (Vermariën, 2006). Digitized electrocardiograms can also be stored in permanent memory such as flash memory or optically based disk media such as CDs or DVDs.

## 6.3 PROBLEMS FREQUENTLY ENCOUNTERED

There are many factors that must be taken into consideration in the design and application of the electrocardiograph as well as other biopotential amplifiers. These factors are important not only to the biomedical engineer, but also to the individual who operates the instrument and the physician who interprets the recorded information. In the following paragraphs, we shall describe a few of the more common problems encountered and shall indicate some of their causes.

### FREQUENCY DISTORTION

The electrocardiograph does not always meet the frequency-response standards we have described. When this happens, frequency distortion is seen in the ECG.

*High-frequency distortion* rounds off the sharp corners of the waveforms and diminishes the amplitude of the QRS complex.

An instrument that has a frequency response of 1 to 150 Hz shows *low-frequency distortion*. The baseline is no longer horizontal, especially immediately following any event in the tracing. Monophasic waves in the ECG appear to be more biphasic.

## SATURATION OR CUTOFF DISTORTION

High offset voltages at the electrodes or improperly adjusted amplifiers in the electrocardiograph can produce saturation or cutoff distortion that can greatly modify the appearance of the ECG. The combination of input-signal amplitude and offset voltage drives the amplifier into saturation during a portion of the QRS complex (Section 3.2). The peaks of the QRS complex are cut off because the output of the amplifier cannot exceed the saturation voltage.

In a similar occurrence, the lower portions of the ECG are cut off. This can result from negative saturation of the amplifier. In this case only a portion of the S wave may be cut off. In extreme cases of this type of distortion even the P and T waves may be below the cutoff level such that only the R wave appears.

## GROUND LOOPS

Patients who are having their ECGs taken on either a clinical electrocardiograph or continuously on a cardiac monitor are often connected to other pieces of electric apparatus. Each electric device has its own ground connection either through the power line or, in some cases, through a heavy ground wire attached to some ground point in the room.

A *ground loop* can exist when two machines are connected to the patient. Both the electrocardiograph and a second machine have a ground electrode attached to the patient. The electrocardiograph is grounded through the power line at a particular socket. The second machine is also grounded through the power line, but it is plugged into an entirely different outlet across the room, which has a different ground. If one ground is at a slightly higher potential than the other ground, a current from one ground flows through the patient to the ground electrode of the electrocardiograph and along its lead wire to the other ground. In addition to this current's presenting a safety problem, it can elevate the patient's body potential to some voltage above the lowest ground to which the instrumentation is attached. This produces common-mode voltages on the electrocardiograph that, if it has a poor CMRR, can increase the amount of interference seen.

## OPEN LEAD WIRES

Frequently one of the wires connecting a biopotential electrode to the electrocardiograph becomes disconnected from its electrode or breaks as a result of excessively rough handling, in which case the electrode is no longer connected to the electrocardiograph. Relatively high potentials can often be induced in the open wire as a result of electric fields emanating from the power lines or other sources in the vicinity of the machine. This causes a wide, peak-to-peak deflection of the trace on the recorder at the power-line frequency, as well as, of course, signal loss. Such a situation also arises when an electrode is not making good contact with the patient. A circuit for detecting poor electrode contact is described in Section 6.9.

## ARTIFACT FROM LARGE ELECTRIC TRANSIENTS

In some situations in which a patient is having an ECG taken, cardiac defibrillation may be required (Section 13.2). In such a case, a high-voltage high-current electric pulse is applied to the chest of the patient so that transient potentials can be observed across the electrodes. These potentials can be several orders of magnitude higher than the normal potentials encountered in the ECG. Other electric sources can cause similar transients. When this situation occurs, it can cause an abrupt deflection in the ECG, as shown in Figure 6.8. This is due to the saturation of the amplifiers in the electrocardiograph caused by the relatively high-amplitude pulse or step at its input. This pulse is sufficiently large to cause the buildup of charge on coupling capacitances in the amplifier, resulting in its remaining saturated for a finite period of time following the pulse and then slowly drifting back to the original baseline with a time constant determined by the low corner frequency of the amplifier. An example of the slowly recovering waveform is shown in Figure 6.8 at a reduced amplitude and time scale to demonstrate the transient.

Transients of the type just described can be generated by means other than defibrillation. Serious artifact caused by motion of the electrodes can produce variations in potential greater than ECG potentials. Another source of artifact is the patient's encountering a built-up static electric charge that can be partially discharged through the body. Older electrocardiographs exhibit a similar transient when they are switched manually from one lead

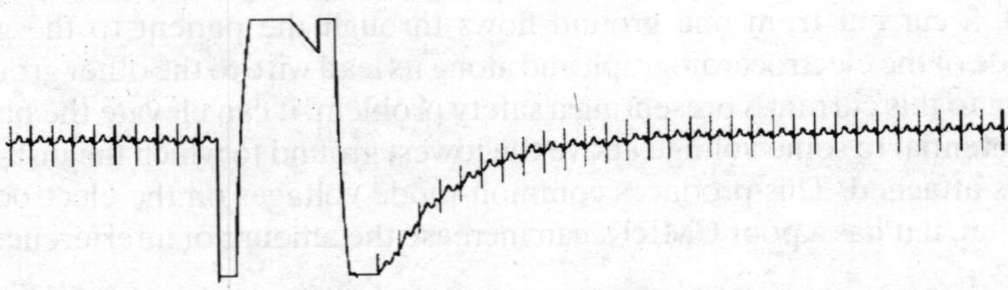

**Figure 6.8** Effect of a voltage transient on an ECG recorded on an electrocardiograph in which the transient causes the amplifier to saturate and a finite period of time is required for the charge to bleed off enough to bring the ECG back into the amplifier's active region of operation. This is followed by a first-order recovery of the system.

to another, because there are different offset potentials at each electrode. This is usually not seen on newer machines that switch leads automatically, because voltages due to excess charge are discharged during the switching process.

This problem is greatly alleviated by reducing the source of the artifact. Because we do not have time to disconnect an electrocardiograph when a patient is being defibrillated, we can include electronic protection circuitry, such as that described in Section 6.4, in the machine itself. In this way, we can limit the maximal input voltage across the ECG amplifier so as to minimize the saturation and charge buildup effects due to the high-voltage input signals. This results in a more rapid return to normal operation following the transient. Such circuitry is also important in protecting the electrocardiograph from any damage that might be caused by these pulses.

Artifact caused by static electric charge on personnel can be lessened noticeably by reducing the buildup of static charge through the use of conductive clothing, shoes, and flooring, as well as by having personnel touch the bed before touching the patient. Motion artifact from the electrodes can be decreased by using the techniques described in Chapter 5.

**EXAMPLE 6.2** An electrocardiograph has a broad frequency response so that its amplifier has a first-order time constant of 16 s. The electrocardiograph amplifier has a broad dynamic range of input voltages, but any input voltage greater than $\pm 2\,\text{mV}$ will be out the range of its display and cut off. While recording the ECG of a patient, a transient occurs that has an amplitude of 10 mV, and this causes the ECG to fall out of the range of the instrument's display. If the ECG R wave has an amplitude of 1 mV, how long will it take for the entire signal to be visible on the display?

**ANSWER** For the entire amplitude range of the ECG to be visible on the display, its baseline must be at a voltage of $2\,\text{mV} - 1\,\text{mV} = 1\,\text{mV}$. The recovery voltage at the amplifier will follow first-order exponential decay as given by

$$v = 10\,\text{mV}\, e^{-t/16\,\text{s}} \tag{E6.6}$$

This voltage must drop to 1 mV for the entire ECG waveform to be visible, so

$$\begin{aligned} 1\,\text{mV} &= 10\,\text{mV}\, e^{-t/16\,\text{s}} \\ 0.1 &= e^{-t/16\,\text{s}} \end{aligned} \tag{E6.7}$$

Solving for $t$, we find

$$\ln(0.1) = -\frac{t}{16\,\text{s}} = -2.303 \tag{E6.8}$$

and

$$t = 36.8\,\text{s}.$$

## INTERFERENCE FROM ELECTRIC DEVICES

A major source of interference when one is recording or monitoring the ECG is the electric-power system. Besides providing power to the electrocardiograph itself, power lines are connected to other pieces of equipment and appliances in the typical hospital room or physician's office. There are also power lines in the walls, floor, and ceiling running past the room to other points in the building. These power lines can affect the recording of the ECG and introduce interference at the line frequency in the recorded trace, as illustrated in Figure 6.9(a). Such interference appears on the recordings as a result of two mechanisms, each operating singly or, in some cases, both operating together.

*Electric-field* coupling between the power lines and the electrocardiograph and/or the patient is a result of the electric fields surrounding main power lines and the power cords connecting different pieces of apparatus to electric outlets. These fields can be present even when the apparatus is not turned on, because current is not necessary to establish the electric field. These fields couple into the patient, the lead wires, and the electrocardiograph itself. It is almost as though small capacitors joined these entities to the power lines, as shown by the crude model in Figure 6.10.

The current through the capacitance $C_3$ coupling the ungrounded side of the power line and the electrocardiograph itself flows to ground and does not cause interference. $C_1$ represents the capacitance between the power line and one of the leads. Current $i_{d1}$ does not flow into the electrocardiograph because of its high input impedance, but rather through the skin–electrode impedances $Z_1$ and $Z_G$ and the subject being measured to ground. Similarly, $i_{d2}$ flows through $Z_2$ and $Z_G$ and the subject to ground. Body impedance, which is about 500 Ω, can be neglected when compared with the other

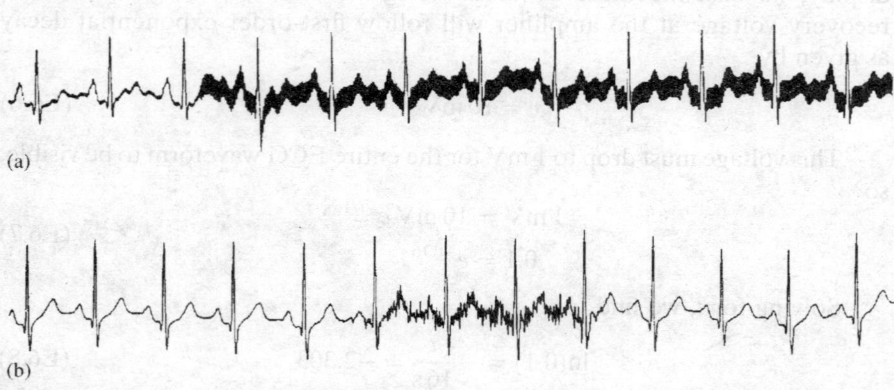


**Figure 6.9** (a) A 60 Hz power-line interference. (b) Electromyographic interference on the ECG. Severe 60 Hz interference is also shown on the bottom tracing in Figure 4.13.

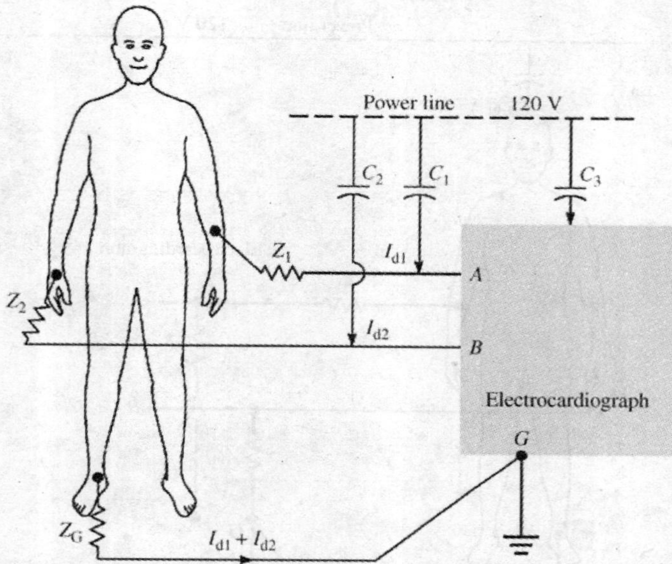


**Figure 6.10** A mechanism of electric-field pickup of an electrocardiograph resulting from the power line. Coupling capacitance between the hot side of the power line and lead wires causes current to flow through skin–electrode impedances on its way to ground.

impedances shown. The voltage amplified is that appearing between inputs A and B, $v_A - v_B$.

$$v_A - v_B = i_{d1}Z_1 - i_{d2}Z_2 \tag{6.3}$$

Huhta and Webster (1973) suggest that if the two leads run near each other, $i_{d1} \cong i_{d2}$. In this case,

$$v_A - v_B = i_{d1}(Z_1 - Z_2) \tag{6.4}$$

Values measured for 9 m cables show that $i_d \cong 6$ nA, although this value will be dependent on the room and the location of other equipment and power lines. Skin–electrode impedances may differ by as much as 20 kΩ. Hence

$$v_A - v_B = (6\,\text{nA})(20\,\text{k}\Omega) = 120\,\mu\text{V} \tag{6.5}$$

which would be an objectionable level of interference. This can be minimized by shielding the leads and grounding each shield at the electrocardiograph. This is done, in fact, in most modern electrocardiographs. Lowering skin–electrode impedances is also helpful.

Figure 6.11 shows that current also flows from the power line directly into the body. This displacement current $i_{db}$ flows through the ground impedance

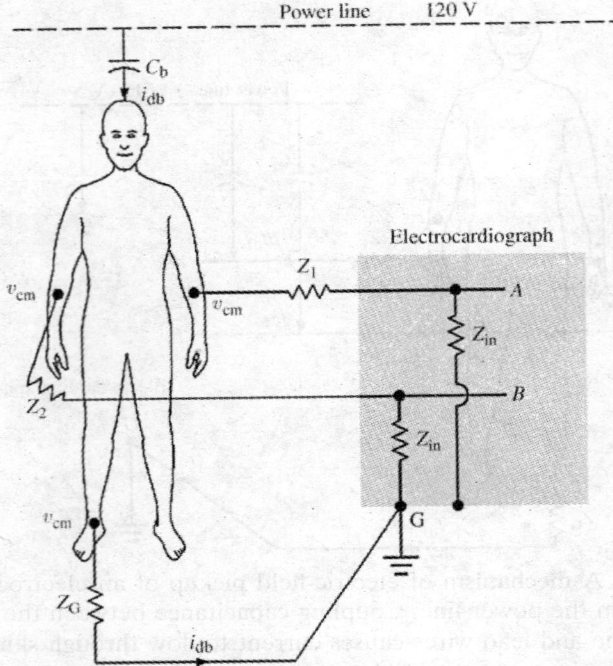


**Figure 6.11** Current flows from the power line through the body and ground impedance, thus creating a common-mode voltage everywhere on the body. $Z_{in}$ is not only resistive but, as a result of RF bypass capacitors at the amplifier input, has a reactive component as well.

$Z_G$ to ground. The resulting voltage drop causes a common-mode voltage $v_{cm}$ to appear throughout the body.

$$v_{cm} = i_{db} Z_G \tag{6.6}$$

Substituting typical values yields

$$v_{cm} = (0.2\,\mu\text{A})(50\,\text{k}\Omega) = 10\,\text{mV} \tag{6.7}$$

In poor electrical environments in which $i_{db} > 1\,\mu\text{A}$, $v_{cm}$ can be greater than 50 mV. For a perfect amplifier, this would cause no problem, because a differential amplifier rejects common-mode voltages (Section 3.4). However, real amplifiers have finite input impedances $Z_{in}$. Thus $v_{cm}$ is decreased because of the attenuator action of the skin–electrode impedances and $Z_{in}$. That is,

$$v_A - v_B = v_{cm}\left(\frac{Z_{in}}{Z_{in} + Z_1} - \frac{Z_{in}}{Z_{in} + Z_2}\right) \tag{6.8}$$

Because $Z_1$ and $Z_2$ are much less than $Z_{in}$,

$$v_A - v_B = v_{cm}\left(\frac{Z_2 - Z_1}{Z_{in}}\right) \tag{6.9}$$

Substituting typical values yields

$$v_A - v_B = (10\,\text{mV})(20\,\text{k}\Omega/5\,\text{M}\Omega) = 40\,\mu\text{V} \qquad \text{E6.10}$$

which would be noticeable on an ECG and would be very objectionable on an EEG. This interference can be minimized by lowering skin–electrode impedance and raising amplifier input impedance.

Thus we see that the difference between the skin–electrode impedances is an important consideration in the design of biopotential amplifiers. Some common-mode voltage is always present, so the input imbalance and $Z_{in}$ are critical factors determining the common-mode rejection, no matter how good the differential amplifier itself is.

**EXAMPLE 6.3** A clinical staff member has attached a patient to an electroencephalograph (EEG machine) for a sleep study that continuously displays that patient's EEG on a computer screen and stores it in memory. This staff member accidently used two different types of electrodes for the EEG lead, and each electrode had a different source impedance. One had a relatively low impedance of 1500 Ω at EEG frequencies, while the other had a higher impedance of 4700 Ω. A ground electrode having an impedance of 2500 Ω was also used. The input impedance of each differential input of the EEG machine to ground was 10 MΩ, and the instrument had a CMRR of 80 dB. The power-line displacement current to the patient was measured at 400 nA. The amplitude of the patient's EEG was 12 μV.

**a.** How much common-mode voltage will be seen on this patient and will it significantly interfere with the EEG signal?

**b.** How much power-line interference will be seen on the patient's EEG?

**ANSWER** The common-mode voltage will be determined by the displacement current through the ground electrode impedance $Z_G$ [see (6.6)].

**a.**

$$v_{cm} = 400 \times 10^{-9}\,\text{A}(2500\,\Omega) = 10^{-3}\,\text{V} \tag{E6.9}$$

The EEG machine's CMRR is 80 dB, which means that its differential gain is $10^4$ times greater than its common-mode gain. Thus even though the signal-to-common-mode-noise ratio is 12/1000 at the EEG machine's input, it will be 120/1 at its readout. This should be sufficiently high to allow clinical interpretation of the EEG signal.

**b.** Since the common-mode interference is low, any power-line interference seen will be the result of the unbalanced impedances of the EEG electrodes. This will result in a differential signal as determined by 6.17.

$$v_a - v_b = 10^{-3}\left(\frac{4{,}700\ \Omega - 1{,}500\ \Omega}{10^6\ \Omega}\right) = 3.2 \times 10^{-6}\ \text{V} = 3.2\ \mu\text{V} \qquad \text{(E6.10)}$$

This is small compared to the 100 μV amplitude of the EEG signal and would be noticeable but tolerable interference.

The other source of interference from power lines is magnetic induction. Current in power lines establishes a *magnetic field* in the vicinity of the line. Magnetic fields can also sometimes originate from transformers and ballasts in fluorescent lights or electric appliances and other apparatus. If such magnetic fields pass through the effective single-turn coil produced by the electrocardiograph, lead wires, and the patient, as shown in Figure 6.12, a voltage is induced in this loop. This voltage is proportional to the magnetic-field strength and the area of the effective single-turn coil. It can be reduced (1) by reducing the magnetic field through the use of magnetic shielding, (2) by keeping the electrocardiograph and leads away from potential magnetic-field regions (both of which are rather difficult to achieve in practice), or (3) by reducing the effective area of the single-turn coil.

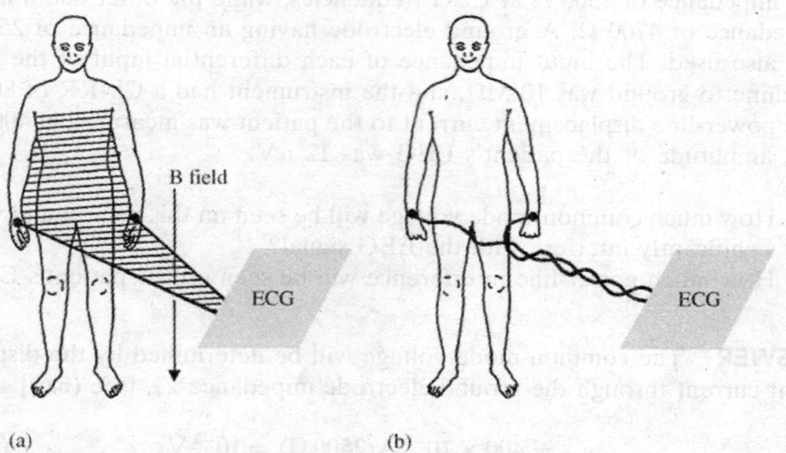


**Figure 6.12 Magnetic-field pickup by the electrocardiograph** (a) Lead wires for lead I make a closed loop (shaded area) when patient and electrocardiograph are considered in the circuit. The change in magnetic field passing through this area induces a current in the loop. (b) This effect can be minimized by twisting the lead wires together and keeping them close to the body in order to subtend a much smaller area.

This last approach can be achieved easily by twisting the lead wires together over as much as possible of the distance between the electrocardiograph and the patient.

## OTHER SOURCES OF ELECTRIC INTERFERENCE

Electric interference from sources other than the power lines can also affect the electrocardiograph. *Electromagnetic interference* from nearby high-power radio, television, or radar facilities can be picked up and rectified by the *p–n* junctions of the transistors in the electrocardiograph and sometimes even by the electrode–electrolyte interface on the patient. Lower power electromagnetic interference can arise from local sources such as wireless devices including mobile telephones and wireless computing networks. The lead wires and the patient serve as an antenna in either case. Once the signal is detected, the demodulated signal appears as interference on the electrocardiogram. It was thought that such interference from mobile telephones could interfere with patient monitoring equipment in hospitals, but a study at the Mayo Clinic has shown this not to be a problem at their institution (Tri *et al.,* 2007).

Electromagnetic interference can also be generated by high-frequency generators in the hospital itself. Electrosurgical and diathermy (Section 13.9) equipment is a frequent offender. Grobstein and Gatzke (1977) show both the proper use of electrosurgical equipment and the design of an ECG amplifier required to minimize interference. Electromagnetic radiation can be generated from x-ray machines or switches and relays on heavy-duty electric equipment in the hospital as well. Even arcing in a fluorescent light that is flickering and in need of replacement can produce serious interference.

Electromagnetic interference can usually be minimized by shunting the input terminals to the electrocardiograph amplifier with a small capacitor of approximately 200 pF. The reactance of this capacitor is quite high over the frequency range of the ECG, so it does not appreciably lower the input impedance of the electrocardiograph. However, with today's modern high-input-impedance machines, it is important to make sure that this is really the case. At radiofrequencies, its reactance is low enough to cause effective shorting of the electromagnetic interference picked up by the lead wires and to keep it from reaching the transistors in the amplifier.

There is also a source of electric interference located within the body itself that can have an effect on ECGs. There is always some skeletal muscle located between the electrodes making up a lead of the electrocardiograph. Any time this muscle is contracting, it generates its own electromyographic signal that can be picked up by the lead along with the ECG and can result in interference on the ECG, as shown in Figure 6.9(b). When we look only at the ECG and not at the patient, it is sometimes difficult to determine whether interference of this type is muscle interference or the result of electromagnetic radiation. However, while the ECG is being taken, we can easily separate the two sources, because the EMG interference is associated with the patient's muscle contractions that can be observed when we look at the patient.

## 6.4 TRANSIENT PROTECTION

The isolation circuits described in Section 14.9 are primarily for the protection of the patient in that they eliminate the hazard of electric shock resulting from interaction among the patient, the electrocardiograph, and other electric devices in the patient's environment. There are also times when other equipment attached to the patient can present a risk to the machine. For example, in the operating suite, patients undergoing surgery usually have their ECGs continuously monitored during the procedure. If the surgical procedure involves the use of an electrosurgical unit (Section 13.9), it can introduce onto the patient relatively high voltages that can enter the electrocardiograph or cardiac monitor through the patient's electrodes. If the ground connection to the electrosurgical unit is faulty or if higher-than-normal resistance is present, the patient's voltage with respect to ground can become quite high during coagulation or cutting. These high potentials enter the electrocardiograph or cardiac monitor and can be large enough to damage the electronic circuitry. They can also cause severe transients, of the type shown in Figure 6.8.

Ideally, cardiac monitors and electrocardiographs should be designed so that they are unaffected by such transients. Unfortunately, this cannot be achieved completely. However, it is possible to reduce the effects of these electric transients and to protect the equipment from serious damage. Figure 6.13 shows the basic arrangement of such protective circuits. Two-terminal voltage-limiting devices are connected between each patient electrode and electric ground.

Figure 6.14(a) shows the typical current–voltage characteristic of such a device. At voltages less than $V_b$, the breakdown voltage, the device allows very little current to flow and ideally appears as an open circuit. Once the voltage across the device attempts to exceed $V_b$, the characteristics of the device sharply change, and current passes through the device to such an extent that the voltage cannot exceed $V_b$ as a result of the voltage drop across the

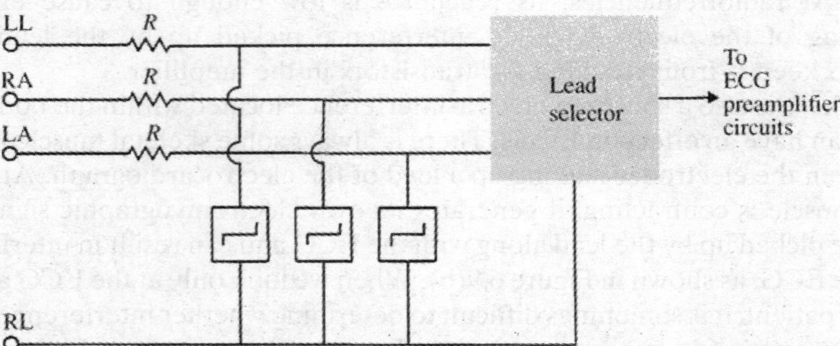


**Figure 6.13** A voltage-protection scheme at the input of an electrocardiograph to protect the machine from high-voltage transients. Circuit elements connected across limb leads on left-hand side are voltage-limiting devices.

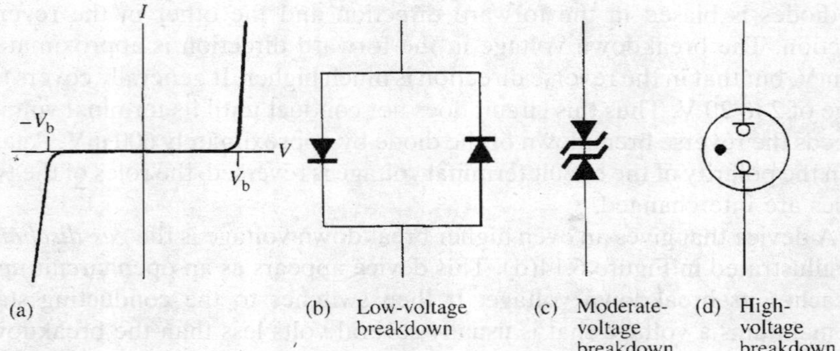


**Figure 6.14 Voltage-limiting devices** (a) Current–voltage characteristics of a voltage-limiting device. (b) Parallel silicon-diode voltage-limiting circuit. (c) Back-to-back silicon zener-diode voltage-limiting circuit. (d) Gas-discharge tube (neon light) voltage-limiting circuit element.

series resistors $R$ (in Figure 6.13). Under these conditions, the device appears to behave as a short circuit in series with a constant-voltage source of magnitude $V_b$.

In practice, there are several ways to achieve a characteristic approaching this idealized characteristic. Figure 6.14 indicates three of these. *Parallel silicon diodes*, as shown in Figure 6.14(b), give a characteristic with a breakdown voltage of approximately 600 mV. The diodes are connected such that the terminal voltage on one has a polarity opposite that on the other. Thus, when the voltage reaches approximately 600 mV, one of the diodes is forward-biased. And even though the other is reverse-biased, its bias voltage is limited to the forward voltage drop. When the voltage across the network is reversed, the roles of the two diodes are reversed, again limiting the voltage across the network to approximately 600 mV. The transition from nonconducting state to conducting state, however, is not so sharp as shown in the characteristic curve, and signal distortion can begin to appear from these diodes at voltages of approximately 300 mV. Although the ECG itself does not approach such a voltage, it is possible under extreme conditions for dc-offset potentials of that order of magnitude to result from faulty electrodes. The main advantage of this circuit is its low breakdown voltage; the maximal transients at the amplifier input are only approximately 600 mV peak amplitude.

Because the breakdown voltage of this circuit is too small, it is usually increased simply by connecting two or three diodes in series instead of using single diodes in each branch. This has the advantage of not only increasing the breakdown voltage by multiplying the initial 600 mV by the number of diodes in series but also increasing the resistance of the circuit, both in the conducting and the nonconducting state.

When we want higher breakdown voltages, we can use the circuit of Figure 6.14(c). This circuit consists of two silicon diodes, usually *zener diodes*, connected back to back. When a voltage is connected across this circuit, one of the diodes is biased in the forward direction and the other in the reverse direction. The breakdown voltage in the forward direction is approximately 600 mV, but that in the reverse direction is much higher. It generally covers the range of 2 to 20 V. Thus this circuit does not conduct until its terminal voltage exceeds the reverse breakdown of the diode by approximately 600 mV. Again, when the polarity of the circuit terminal voltage is reversed, the roles of the two diodes are interchanged.

A device that gives an even higher breakdown voltage is the *gas-discharge tube* illustrated in Figure 6.14(d). This device appears as an open circuit until it reaches its breakdown voltage. It then switches to the conducting state and maintains a voltage that is usually several volts less than the breakdown voltage. Breakdown voltages ranging from 50 to 90 V are typical for this device. This breakdown voltage is considered high for the input to most electrocardiographic amplifiers. Thus it is important to include a circuit element such as a resistor between the gas-discharge tube and the amplifier input to limit the amplifier's input current.

Designers of biopotential amplifiers often use miniature neon lamps as voltage limiters. They are essentially gas discharge tubes and are very inexpensive and have a symmetric characteristic, requiring only a single device per electrode pair. Their resistance in the nonconducting state is nearly infinite, so there is no loading effect on the electrodes—a feature that is most desirable when the biopotential amplifier has very high input impedance.

## 6.5 COMMON-MODE AND OTHER INTERFERENCE-REDUCTION CIRCUITS

As we noted earlier, common-mode voltages can be responsible for much of the interference in biopotential amplifiers. Although having an amplifier with a high CMRR minimizes the effects of common-mode voltages, a better approach to this problem is to discover the source of the voltage and try to eliminate it. In this section, we shall look at some of the sources of this and other types of interference to discover ways in which they can be minimized.

### ELECTRIC- AND MAGNETIC-FIELD INTERFERENCE

As we saw in Section 6.3, electric interference can be introduced in systems of biopotential measurement through capacitive coupling and magnetic induction. We can minimize these interfering signals by trying to eliminate the sources of the signals via shielding techniques. Electrostatic shielding is accomplished by placing a grounded conducting plane between the source of the electric field and the measurement system. The measurement of very-low-level biopotentials, such as the EEG, has traditionally been carried out in a shielded enclosure containing either continuous solid-metal panels or at least grounded copper screening to minimize interference. Today, high-quality differential instrumentation amplifiers with high CMRRs make such shielding unnecessary.

This type of shielding is ineffective for magnetic fields unless the metal panels have a high permeability (such as sheet steel or mumetal, a high permeability alloy). In other words, the panels must be good magnetic conductors as well as good electric conductors. Such rooms are available to provide magnetic shielding, but a much less expensive way of achieving a reduction of magnetically induced signals is to reduce the effective surface area between the differential inputs to the biopotential amplifier, in the case of differential signals, and between the inputs and ground, in the case of common-mode signals. Something as simple as a twisted pair of lead wires, as illustrated in Figure 6.12(b), may greatly improve the situation.

## DRIVEN-RIGHT-LEG SYSTEM

In most modern electrocardiographic systems, the patient is not grounded at all. Instead, the right-leg electrode is connected (as shown in Figure 6.15) to the output of an auxiliary op amp. The common-mode voltage on the body is sensed by the two averaging resistors $R_a$, inverted, amplified, and fed back to the right leg. This negative feedback drives the common-mode voltage to a

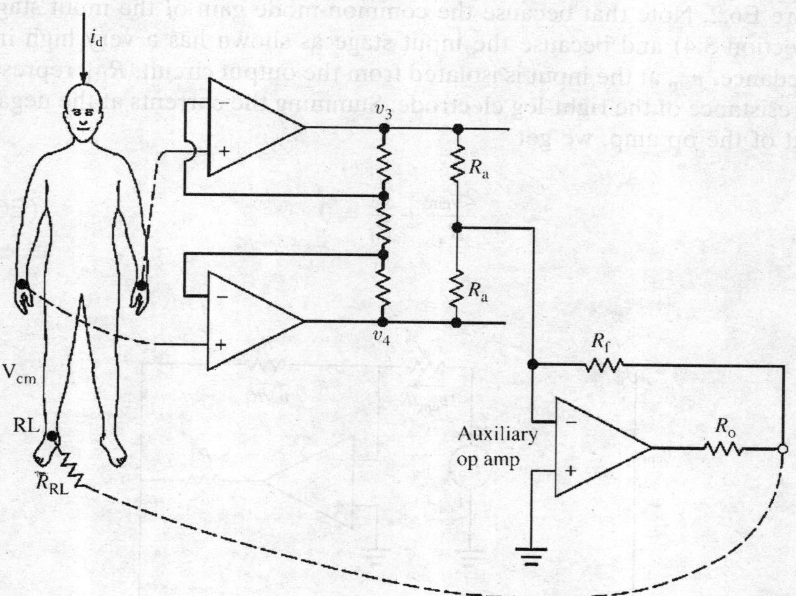


**Figure 6.15 Driven-right-leg circuit for minimizing common-mode interference** The circuit derives common-mode voltage from a pair of averaging resistors connected to $v_3$ and $v_4$ in Figure 3.5. The right leg is not grounded but is connected to output of the auxiliary op amp.

low value. The body's displacement current flows not to ground but rather to the op-amp output circuit. This reduces the interference as far as the ECG amplifier is concerned and effectively grounds the patient (Winter and Webster, 1983).

The circuit can also provide some electric safety. If an abnormally high voltage should appear between the patient and ground as a result of electric leakage or other cause, the auxiliary op amp in Figure 6.15 saturates. This effectively ungrounds the patient, because the amplifier can no longer drive the right leg. Now the parallel resistances $R_f$ and $R_o$ are between the patient and ground. They can be several megohms in value—large enough to limit the current. These resistances do not protect the patient, however, because 120 V on the patient would break down the op-amp transistors of the ECG amplifier, and large currents would flow to ground.

**EXAMPLE 6.4** Determine the common-mode voltage $v_{cm}$ on the patient in the driven-right-leg circuit of Figure 6.15 when a displacement current $i_d$ flows to the patient from the power lines. Choose appropriate values for the resistances in the circuit so that the common-mode voltage is minimal and there is only a high-resistance path to ground when the auxiliary op amp saturates. What is $v_{cm}$ for this circuit when $i_d = 0.2\ \mu A$?

**ANSWER** The equivalent circuit for the circuit of Figure 6.15 is shown in Figure E6.2. Note that because the common-mode gain of the input stage is 1 (Section 3.4) and because the input stage as shown has a very high input impedance, $v_{cm}$ at the input is isolated from the output circuit. $R_{RL}$ represents the resistance of the right-leg electrode. Summing the currents at the negative input of the op amp, we get

$$\frac{2v_{cm}}{R_a} + \frac{v_o}{R_f} = 0 \qquad \text{(E6.11)}$$

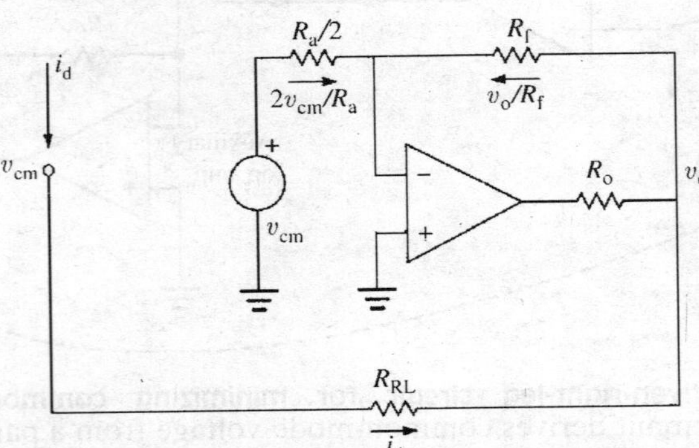


**Figure E6.2** Equivalent circuit of driven-right-leg system of Figure 6.15.

This gives

$$v_o = -\frac{2R_f}{R_a} v_{cm} \tag{E6.12}$$

but

$$v_{cm} = R_{RL} i_d + v_o \tag{E6.13}$$

Thus, substituting (E6.2) into (E6.3) yields

$$v_{cm} = \frac{R_{RL} i_d}{1 + 2R_f/R_a} \tag{E6.14}$$

The effective resistance between the right leg and ground is the resistance of the right-leg electrode divided by 1 plus the gain of the auxiliary op-amp circuit. When the amplifier saturates, as would occur during a large transient $v_{cm}$, its output appears as the saturation voltage $v_s$. The right leg is now connected to ground through this source and the parallel resistances $R_f$ and $R_o$. To limit the current, $R_f$ and $R_o$ should be large. Values as high as 5 MΩ are used.

When the amplifier is not saturated, we would like $v_{cm}$ to be as small as possible or, in other words, to be an effective low-resistance path to ground. This can be achieved by making $R_f$ large and $R_a$ relatively small. $R_f$ can be equal to $R_o$, but $R_a$ can be much smaller.

A typical value of $R_a$ would be 25 kΩ. A worst-case electrode resistance $R_{RL}$ would be 100 kΩ. The effective resistance between the right leg and ground would then be

$$\frac{100\,\text{k}\Omega}{1 + \dfrac{2 \times 5\,\text{M}\Omega}{25\,\text{k}\Omega}} = 249\,\Omega$$

For the 0.2 μA displacement current, the common-mode voltage is

$$v_{cm} = 249\,\Omega \times 0.2\,\mu\text{A} = 50\,\mu\text{V}$$

## 6.6 AMPLIFIERS FOR OTHER BIOPOTENTIAL SIGNALS

Up to this point we have stressed biopotential amplifiers for the ECG. Amplifiers for use with other biopotentials are essentially the same. However, other signals do put different constraints on some aspects of the amplifier. The frequency content of different biopotentials covers different portions of the spectrum. Some biopotentials have higher amplitudes than others. Both these facts place gain and

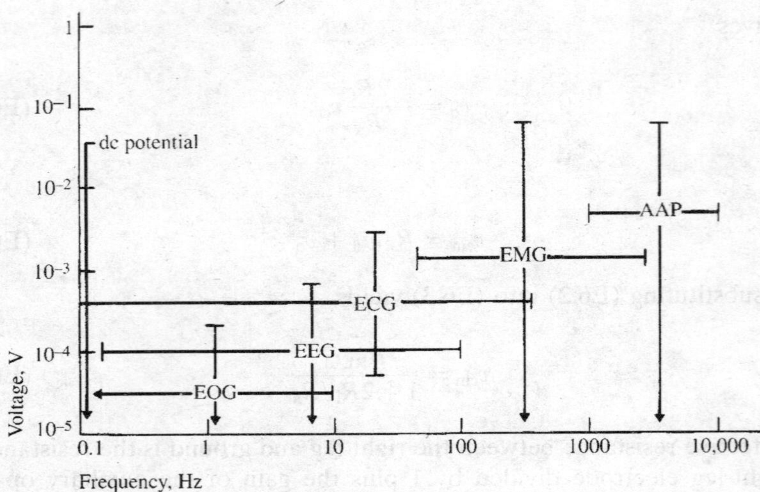


**Figure 6.16** Voltage and frequency ranges of some common biopotential signals; dc potentials include intracellular voltages as well as voltages measured from several points on the body. EOG is the electro-oculogram, EEG is the electroencephalogram, ECG is the electrocardiogram, EMG is the electromyogram, and AAP is the axon action potential. [From J. M. R. Delgado, "Electrodes for Extracellular Recording and Stimulation." In W. L. Nastuk (ed.), *Physical Techniques in Biological Research*. New York: Academic Press, 1964.]

frequency-response constraints on the amplifiers used. Figure 6.16 shows the ranges of amplitudes and frequencies covered by several of the common biopotential signals. Depending on the signal, frequencies range from dc to about 10 kHz. Amplitudes can range from tens of microvolts to approximately 100 mV. The amplifier for a particular biopotential must be designed to handle that potential and to provide an appropriate signal at its output.

The electrodes used to obtain the biopotential place certain constraints on the amplifier input stage. To achieve the most effective signal transfer, the amplifier must be matched to the electrodes. Also, the amplifier input circuit must not promote the generation of artifact by the electrode, as could occur with excessive bias current. Let us look at a few requirements placed on different types of biopotential amplifiers by the measurement being made.

## ELECTROMYOGRAPHY AMPLIFIER

Figure 6.16 shows that electromyographic signals range in frequency from 25 Hz to several kilohertz. Signal amplitudes range from 100 μV to 90 mV, depending on the type of signal and electrodes used. Thus electromyography (EMG) amplifiers must have a wider frequency response than ECG amplifiers, but they do not have to cover so low a frequency range as the ECGs. This is desirable because motion artifact contains mostly low frequencies that can be filtered more effectively in EMG amplifiers than in ECG amplifiers without affecting the signal.

If skin-surface electrodes are used to detect the EMG, the levels of signals are generally low, having peak amplitudes of the order of 0.1 to 1 mV. Electrode impedance is relatively low, ranging from about 200 to 5000 Ω, depending on the type of electrode, the electrode–electrolyte interface, and the frequency at which the impedance is determined. Thus the amplifier must have somewhat higher gain than the ECG amplifier for the same output-signal range, and its input characteristics should be almost the same as those of the ECG amplifier. When intramuscular needle electrodes are used, the EMG signals can be an order of magnitude stronger, thus requiring an order of magnitude less gain. Furthermore, the surface area of the EMG needle electrode is much less than that of the surface electrode, so its source impedance is higher. Therefore, a higher amplifier input impedance is desirable for quality signal reproduction.

## AMPLIFIERS FOR USE WITH GLASS MICROPIPETTE INTRACELLULAR ELECTRODES

Intracellular electrodes or microelectrodes that can measure the potential across the cell membrane generally detect potentials on the order of 50 to 100 mV. Their small size and small effective surface-contact area give them a very high source impedance, and their geometry results in a relatively large shunting capacitance. These features place on the amplifier the constraint of requiring an extremely high input impedance. Furthermore, the high shunting capacitance of the electrode itself affects the frequency-response characteristics of the system. Often positive-feedback schemes are used in the biopotential amplifier to provide an effective negative capacitance that can compensate for the high shunt capacitance of the source.

The frequency response of microelectrode amplifiers must be quite wide. Intracellular electrodes are often used to measure the dc potential difference across a cell membrane, so the amplifier must be capable of responding to dc signals. When excitable cell-membrane potentials are to be measured, such as in muscle cells and nerve cells, rise times can contain frequencies of the order of 10 kHz, and the amplifiers must be capable of passing these, too. The fact that the potentials are relatively high means that the voltage gain of the amplifier does not have to be as high as in previous examples.

A preamplifier circuit that is especially useful with microelectrodes is the negative-input-capacitance amplifier shown in Figure 6.17. The basic circuit consists of a low-gain, very-high-input-impedance, noninverting amplifier with a capacitor $C_f$ providing positive feedback to the input. If we look at the equivalent circuit for this amplifier [Figure 6.17(b)], we can relate the input voltage and current:

$$v_i = \frac{1}{C_f}\int i_i\,dt + A_v v_i \qquad (6.11)$$

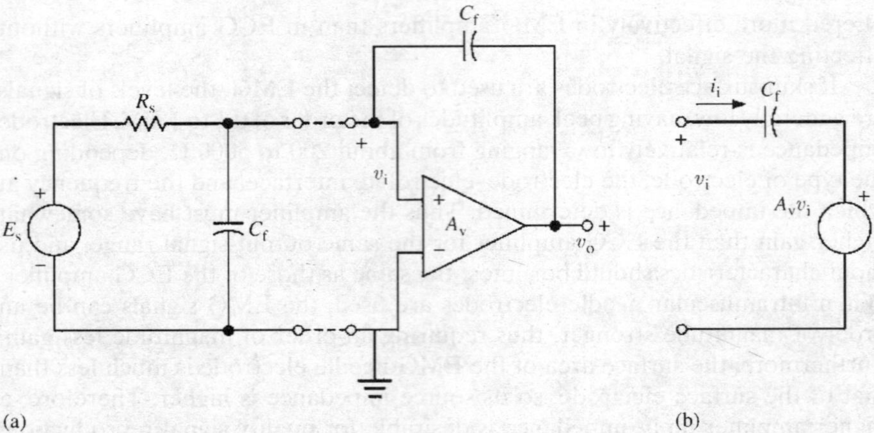


**Figure 6.17** (a) Basic arrangement for negative-input-capacitance amplifier. Basic amplifier is on the right-hand side; equivalent source with lumped series resistance $R_s$ and shunt capacitance $C_s$ is on the left. (b) Equivalent circuit of basic negative-input-capacitance amplifier.

where $A_v$ is the amplifier gain, provided the op amp itself draws no current. This equation can be rearranged as follows:

$$v_i = \frac{1}{(1 - A_v)C_f} \int i_i \, dt \tag{6.12}$$

Thus the equivalent capacitance at the amplifier input is $(1 - A_v)C_f$. If $A_v$ is greater than unity, this equivalent capacitance is negative. The amplifier is connected to the microelectrode, with its high source resistance $R_s$. The shunt capacitance from the electrode and cable is $C_s$. The total circuit capacitance is

$$C = C_s + (1 - A_v)C_f \tag{6.13}$$

which is zero when

$$C_s = (A_v - 1)C_f \tag{6.14}$$

This condition can be met by adjusting either the amplifier gain $A_v$ or the feedback capacitance $C_f$.

In practical negative-input-capacitance amplifiers, the idealized condition of (6.14) cannot be met, because the gain of any amplifier has some frequency dependence. There are thus frequencies where the input capacitance of the amplifier does not cancel the source capacitance, and the circuit does not have an ideal transient response. The amplifier employs positive feedback and does not have an ideal frequency response, so it is possible for the conditions of oscillation to be met at some frequency, and the amplifier will then become unstable. Thus it is important that the amplifier be carefully adjusted to meet the condition of (6.14) as closely as possible without becoming unstable. Another consequence of the positive feedback is that the amplifier tends to be noisy. This is not a serious problem, however, because the voltages from microelectrodes are usually relatively high. A noninverting amplifier with adjustable gain greater than one can be used to drive a shield around the wire leading to the + input. Then the stray capacitance between the wire and the shield can serve as $C_f$ and the shield minimizes interference.

## ELECTROENCEPHALOGRAPH AMPLIFIERS

Figure 6.16 shows that the electroencephalograph (EEG) requires an amplifier with a frequency response of from 0.1 to 100 Hz. When surface electrodes are used, as in clinical electroencephalography, amplitudes of signals range from 25 to 100 μV. Thus amplifiers with relatively high gain are required. These electrodes are smaller than those used for the ECG, so they have somewhat higher source impedances, and a high input impedance is essential in the EEG amplifier. Because the signal levels are so small, common-mode voltages can have more serious effects. Therefore, more stringent efforts must be made to reduce common-mode interference, as well as to use amplifiers with higher CMRRs and low noise.

**EXAMPLE 6.5** A small rural hospital would like to purchase an electroencephalograph but cannot afford to build a shielded room in which to measure patients' EEGs. A clinical engineer has determined that there can be common-mode noise on their patients with amplitudes as large as 100 mV. What must the minimum CMRR of their electroencephalograph be so that an EEG signal of 25 μV amplitude has no more than 1% common-mode noise?

**ANSWER** The SNR at the amplifier input can be as low as

$$\mathrm{SNR} = \frac{25 \times 10^{-6}\ \mathrm{V}}{10^{-1}\ \mathrm{V}} = 2.5 \times 10^{-4} \tag{E6.15}$$

The SNR at the output or display of the electroencephalograph must be at least

$$\mathrm{SNR} = (1\%)^{-1} = 100 \tag{E6.16}$$

The CMRR then must be the ratio of the output SNR to that at the input

$$\mathrm{CMRR} = \frac{100}{2.5 \times 10^{-4}} = 4 \times 10^5 \tag{E6.17}$$

or $20 \log_{10}(4 \times 10^5)\ \mathrm{dB} = 112\ \mathrm{dB}$.

This is within the range of CMRR available in high-quality differential amplifiers. (Pallás-Areny and Webster, 1990).

## 6.7 EXAMPLE OF A BIOPOTENTIAL PREAMPLIFIER

As we have seen, biopotential amplifiers can be used for a variety of signals. The gain and frequency response are two important variables that relate the amplifier to the particular signal. An important factor common to all amplifiers is the first stage, or preamplifier. This stage must have low noise, because its output must be amplified through the remaining stages of the amplifier, and any noise is amplified along with the signal. It must also be coupled directly to the electrodes (no series capacitors) to provide optimal low-frequency response as well as to minimize charging effects on coupling capacitors from input bias current. Of course, every attempt should be made to minimize this current. Even without coupling capacitors it can polarize the electrodes, resulting in polarization overpotentials that produce a large dc offset voltage at the amplifiers' input. This is why preamplifiers often have relatively low voltage gains. The offset potential is coupled directly to the input, so it could saturate high-gain preamplifiers, cutting out the signal altogether. To eliminate the saturating effects of this dc potential, the preamplifier can be capacitor-coupled to the remaining amplifier stages. A final consideration is that the preamplifier must have a very high input impedance, because it represents the load on the electrodes (Thakor, 1988).

Often, for safety reasons, the preamplifier either is electrically isolated from the remaining amplifier stages (and hence from the power lines) (Section 14.9) or is located near the signal source to minimize interference pickup on the high-impedance lead wires. In the latter case, we can use a battery-powered preamplifier with low power consumption or a power supply that is electrically isolated with this circuit.

Figure 6.18 shows the circuit of an ECG amplifier. The instrumentation amplifier of Figure 3.5 is used to provide very high input impedance. High common-mode rejection is achieved by adjusting the potentiometer to about 47 kΩ. Electrodes may produce an offset potential of up to 0.3 V. Thus, to prevent saturation, the dc-coupled stages have a gain of only 25. Coupling capacitors are not placed at the input because this would block the op-amp bias current. Adding resistors to supply the bias current would lower the $Z_{in}$. Coupling capacitors placed after the first op amps would have to be impractically large. Therefore, the single 1 μF coupling capacitor and the 3.3 MΩ resistor form a high-pass filter. The resulting 3.3 s time constant passes all frequencies above 0.05 Hz. The output stage is a noninverting amplifier that has a gain of 32 (Section 3.3).

A second 3.3 MΩ resistor is added to balance bias-current source impedances. The 150 kΩ and 0.01 μF low-pass filter attenuates frequencies above 106 Hz. Switch $S_1$ may be momentarily closed to decrease the discharge time constant when the output saturates. This is required after defibrillation or lead switching to charge the 1 μF capacitor rapidly to the new value and return the output to the linear region. We do *not* discharge the capacitor voltage to zero. Rather, we want the right end to be at 0 V when the left end is at the dc voltage determined by the electrode offset voltage. Switch closure may be automatic, via a circuit that detects when the output is in saturation, or it may be manual.

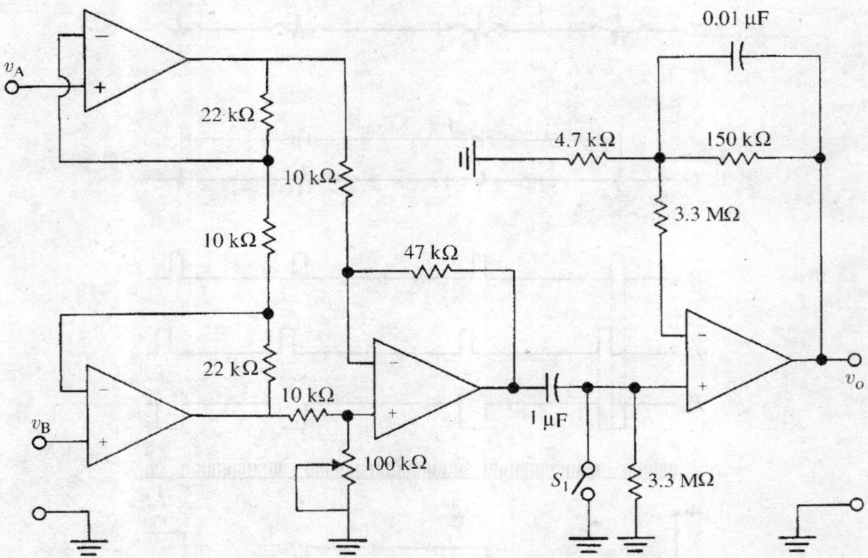


**Figure 6.18** This ECG amplifier has a gain of 25 in the dc-coupled stages. The high-pass filter feeds a noninverting-amplifier stage that has a gain of 32. The total gain is $25 \times 32 = 800$. When μA 776 op amps were used, the circuit was found to have a CMRR of 86 dB at 100 Hz and a noise level of 40 mV peak to peak at the output. The frequency response was 0.05 to 106 Hz for ±3 dB and was flat over 4 to 40 Hz. A single op-amp chip, the LM 324, that contains four individual op amps could also be used in this circuit reducing the total parts count.

Although any general-purpose op amp such as the 741, 301, and 358 is satisfactory in this circuit, an op amp such as the 411, which has lower bias current, may be preferred.

Spinelli *et al.* (2004) developed an ECG amplifier based on standard low-power op amps and a single 5 V power supply. It accepts input offset voltages up to ±500 mV, yields a CMRR of 102 dB at 50 Hz, and provides a reset behavior for recovering from overloads or artifacts. Dobrev *et al.* (2008) describe a circuit that measures the ECG using two electrodes instead of the usual three.

## 6.8 OTHER BIOPOTENTIAL SIGNAL PROCESSORS

### CARDIOTACHOMETERS

A cardiotachometer is a device for determining heart rate. The signal most frequently used is the ECG. However, software for deriving heart rate from signals such as the arterial pressure waveform, pulse oximeter pulse waves, or heart sounds has also been developed.

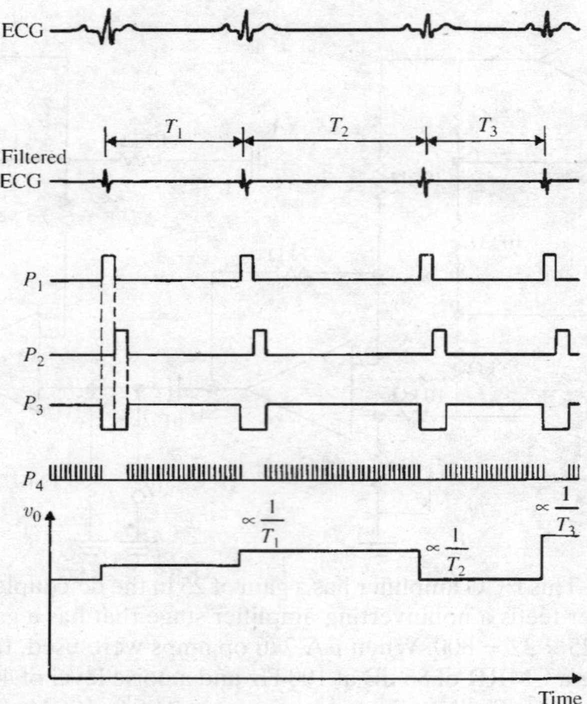


**Figure 6.19 Timing diagram for beat-to-beat cardiotachometer**

The beat-to-beat cardiotachometer determines the reciprocal of the time interval between heartbeats for each beat and presents it as the heart rate for that particular interval. Any slight variability in the interval between beats shows up as a variation in the instantaneous heart rate determined by this method.

Figure 6.19 shows the timing diagram beat-to-beat cardiotachometer. In software, the ECG initially passes through a bandpass filter, which passes QRS complexes while reducing artifact and most of the P and T waves. In one example, a threshold detector triggers the pulse $P_1$.

A 1 kHz clock signal enters a counting register whenever $P_3$ is high. Because $P_3$ is high during the interval between QRS complexes, the 1 ms pulses coming from the clock ($P_4$) accumulate in register 1 during this period. If the register is initially at zero, the number of pulses in the register by the time the next QRS complex arrives equals the number of milliseconds in the interval between this QRS complex and the previous one. Once the gate prohibits additional clock pulses from entering register 1, pulse $P_1$ enables the signal in this register to be stored in a second register, which serves as a memory. Software calculates $v_o$ using

$$v_o = \frac{k}{T_R} \tag{6.15}$$

where $k$ is a constant and $T_R$ is the interval between QRS complexes. We see that $v_o$ is proportional to the reciprocal of the beat-to-beat time interval of the original ECG; in other words, it is proportional to the heart rate. Note that this voltage shifts with each heart beat and that its amplitude is calculated from the duration of the previous beat-to-beat interval.

Alarm circuits can also be used with this type of cardiotachometer. These compare the signal in register 1 to determine whether an interval of longer than a preset value has occurred (this could happen if the heart rate were too low). Software can monitor the signal in register 2 to determine whether it is less than a preset value, a situation that would occur if the heart rate were too high. In either case, the software can then be used to activate appropriate alarms.

## ELECTROMYOGRAM INTEGRATORS

It is frequently of interest to quantify the amount of EMG activity measured by a particular system of electrodes. Such quantification often assumes the form of taking the absolute value of the EMG and integrating it.

The raw EMG, amplified appropriately $v_1$, is fed to software, which in one example takes the absolute value. As indicated in the waveform of Figure 6.20, only positive-going signals $v_2$ result following this. The negative-going portions of the signal have been inverted, making them positive. Software then integrates the signal. Once the integrator output has exceeded a preset threshold level $v_t$, a comparator then reinitiates integration of the EMG until the cycle repeats itself.

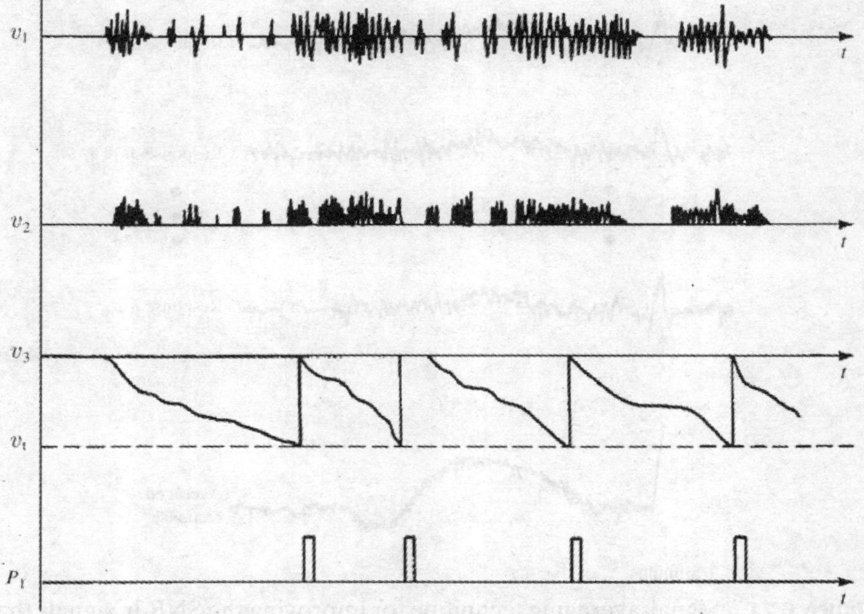


**Figure 6.20** The various waveforms for the EMG integrator

We can view the output from the integrator in two ways. The actual voltage output from the integrator can be recorded on a conventional recorder or computer to give the actual integral at any instant. The total integral necessary to reset the integrator is known, so at any instant the integral equals the number of times the integrator has been reset, multiplied by this calibration constant, plus whatever is recorded as being in the integrator at that time. Another way to view the output of the integrator is to count the number of reset pulses $P_t$. We then determine the approximate integral by determining the number of resets over a specific time interval and calculating total activity.

## EVOKED POTENTIALS AND SIGNAL AVERAGERS

Often in neurophysiology we are interested in looking at the neurological response to a particular stimulus. This response is electric in nature, and it frequently represents a very weak signal with a very poor signal-to-noise ratio (SNR). When the stimulus is repeated, the same or a very similar response is repeatedly elicited. This is the basis for biopotential signal processors that can obtain an enhanced response by means of repeated application of the stimulus (Childers, 1988).

Figure 6.21 shows how signal averaging works. The response to each stimulus is recorded. The time at which each stimulus occurs is considered the

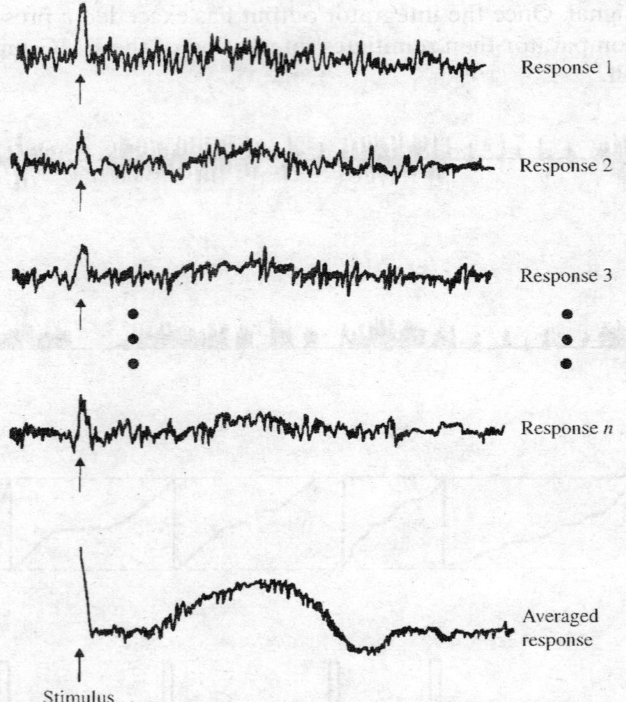


**Figure 6.21** Signal-averaging technique for improving the SNR in signals that are repetitive or respond to a known stimulus.

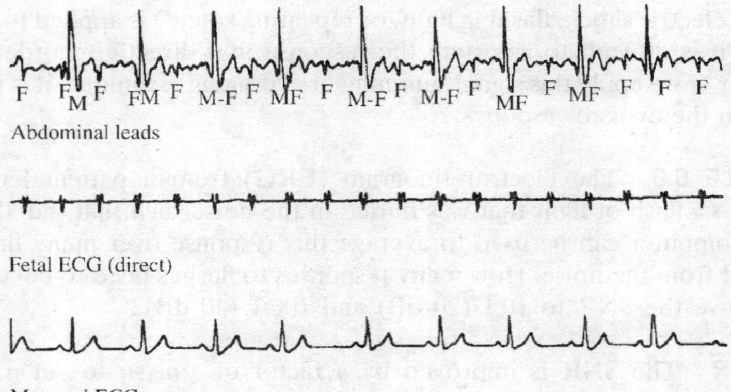


**Figure 6.22 Typical fetal ECG obtained from the maternal abdomen** F represents fetal QRS complexes; M represents maternal QRS complexes. Maternal ECG and fetal ECG (recorded directly from the fetus) are included for comparison. (From J. F. Roux, M. R. Neuman, and R. C. Goodlin, "Monitoring of intrapartum phenomena." In *CRC Critical Reviews in Bioengineering*, 2, January 1975, pp. 119–158 Copyright CRC Press. Used by permission of CRC Press, Inc.)

reference time, and the values for each response at this reference time are summed to get the total response at the reference time. This process is repeated for the values of the responses sampled immediately after the reference time, and the sum is determined for this point in time after the stimulus. The process is then repeated for each sample point after the reference time so that a waveform that is the sum of the individual responses can be displayed, as shown at the bottom of Figure 6.22. The only limits on the number of samples that can be summed are the available memory for storing the responses and the time required to collect the data. Practical signal averaging algorithms can process more than 1000 repeated responses to extract the weak response waveform from the noise.

The noise on the individual responses is random with respect to the stimulus. This means that if a large enough sample is taken, some positive-going noise pulses at a particular instant after the stimulus partially cancel some negative-going noise spikes at the same instant. Thus the net sum of the noise at any instant following the stimulus increases as $\sqrt{n}$, where $n$ is the number of responses. The evoked response, on the other hand, follows the same time course after each stimulus. Thus there is no cancellation in this signal as the individual responses are summed. Instead, the amplitude of the evoked response increases in direct proportion to $n$. By repetitive summing, one is thus able to enhance the SNR by the factor $n/\sqrt{n} = \sqrt{n}$.

This technique is frequently used with the EEG and ERG. As stated earlier in this chapter, EEGs obtained from surface electrodes are very weak and consequently can have a high noise component. When a repetitive stimulus (such as electric shock, flashing light, or repeating sound) is applied to the test subject, it is difficult to ascertain the response in a directly recorded EEG. However, if we apply this signal summing or averaging technique, it is possible to obtain the evoked response.

**EXAMPLE 6.6** The electroretinogram (ERG) from a patient had a response to a flash of light that was buried in the noise such that the SNR was 1:1. A computer can be used to average this response over many flashes to extract it from the noise. How many responses to flashes need to be averaged to improve the SNR to 10:1 (20 dB) and 100:1 (40 dB)?

**ANSWER** The SNR is improved by a factor of $\sqrt{n}$, so to get a 10-fold improvement we need

$$\begin{aligned} 10 &= \sqrt{n} \\ n &= (10)^2 = 100 \text{ samples averaged.} \end{aligned} \tag{E6.18}$$

For a 100-fold improvement we need

$$\begin{aligned} 100 &= \sqrt{n} \\ (100)^2 &= n = 10{,}000 \text{ samples averaged} \end{aligned} \tag{E6.19}$$

Signal averaging is usually performed on a computer. The basic scheme involves digitizing the signal and then locating the stimulus. The response is stored in memory. After the second application of the stimulus, the signal is digitized and stored, and the stimulus is located. The first sample of the response after the stimulus is added to the first sample of the response to the first stimulus, and the sum remains in memory. The second samples taken of each response are added, and so on. The summed signal can be displayed on an oscilloscope, a chart recorder or printer. The operator of the system can look at the sum after each application of the stimulus to determine how many stimuli are necessary to extract the signal from the noise adequately.

This technique can be used without applying the external stimulus. One example of its use is the recording of the ECG of a fetus. Although it is possible to record the fetal R waves from electrodes placed on the abdomen of the mother, artifacts generated by the ECG of the mother and other biopotentials, as well as by electrode noise, obscure the finer details of the fetal ECG. A signal-averaging technique similar to that we have described can be applied by using the fetal R wave in the same capacity as the stimulus. In this case the computer locates the R wave and averages several hundred milliseconds of the signal prior to it and several hundred milliseconds of the signal following it, in order to recover the complete P-QRS-T configuration of the fetal ECG. Such averaging techniques do not always work, however, because the various intervals of the fetal ECG, as well as the waveforms themselves, may change slightly from one beat to the next. The sum is an average of all the recorded

ECG configurations and might provide a waveform that does not indicate the single-beat ECG of the fetal heart.

## FETAL ECG

As we have said, physicians can determine the ECG of a fetus from a pair of biopotential-sensing electrodes placed on the abdomen of the mother. Often it is necessary to try several different placements to get the best signal. Once the best placement is determined, we obtain a recording such as that shown in the top trace of Figure 6.22. For comparison, Figure 6.22 also shows a direct ECG of the same fetus and a direct ECG of the same mother. The fetal ECG signal is usually quite weak; it generally has an amplitude of around 50 μV or less. This makes it extremely difficult to record the heartbeat of the fetus by using electrodes attached to the abdomen of the mother during labor, when the mother is restless and motion artifact as well as EMG interfere. There is also considerable interference from the ECG of the mother (Neuman, 2006).

Note that the QRS complexes of the mother are much stronger than those of the fetus, which makes it difficult to determine the fetal heart rate electronically from recordings of this type. This information can be obtained manually, however, by measuring the fetal R–R interval on the chart and converting it to heart rate.

Several methods have been devised for improving the quality of fetal ECGs obtained by attaching electrodes to the mother's abdomen. In addition to the signal-averaging technique, physicians have applied various forms of anticoincidence detectors to eliminate the maternal QRS complexes (Offnet and Moisand, 1966). This method, as shown in the block diagram of Figure 6.23, uses at least three electrodes: one on the mother's chest, one at the upper part or fundus of the uterus, and one over the lower part of the uterus. The ECG of the mother is obtained from the top two electrodes, and the fetal-plus-maternal signal is obtained from the bottom two. The center

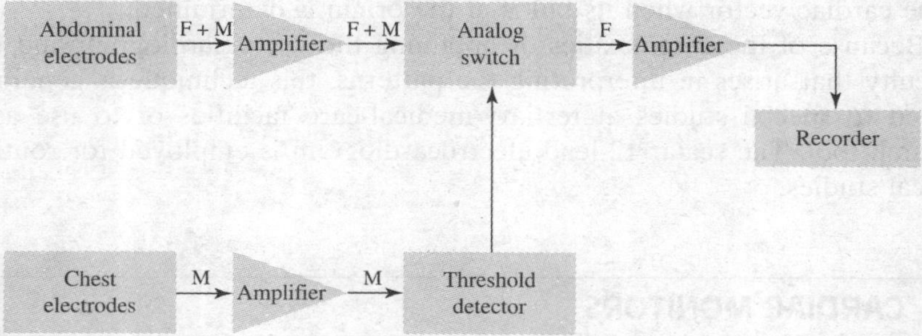


**Figure 6.23** Block diagram of a scheme for isolating fetal ECG from an abdominal signal that contains both fetal and maternal ECGs. (From J. F. Roux, M. R. Neuman, and R. C. Goodlin, "Monitoring of intrapartum phenomena." In *CRC Critical Reviews in Bioengineering*, 2, January 1975, pp. 119–158 Copyright CRC Press. Used by permission of CRC Press, Inc.)

electrode is common to both. A threshold detector determines the mother's QRS complexes and uses this information to turn off an analog switch between the electrodes recording the fetal ECG and the recording apparatus. Therefore, whenever a maternal QRS complex is detected, the signal from the abdominal leads is temporarily blocked until the end of the QRS complex, thereby eliminating it from the abdominal recording. Note that this technique also eliminates any fetal QRS complexes that occur simultaneously with the maternal ones. Modern systems incorporate computing circuits to recognize the absence of this fetal signal and to compensate for it when determining the fetal heart rate. One must always be cautious in using such a system since it can anticipate a fetal beat during a maternal QRS complex, but, in fact, the beat did not occur during the maternal QRS.

### THE VECTORCARDIOGRAPH

In Section 6.2 we looked at the basis of the ECG and defined the cardiac vector. The ensuing description of the electrocardiograph showed how a particular component of the cardiac vector could be recorded. Such scalar ECGs are the type that are usually taken. However, we can obtain more information from a *vectorcardiogram* (VCG). A VCG shows a three-dimensional—or at least a two-dimensional—picture of the orientation and magnitude of the cardiac vector throughout the cardiac cycle. It is difficult for practical machines to display the VCG in three dimensions, but it is relatively simple to display it in two dimensions—or, in other words, its component in a particular plane of the body.

Special lead systems have been developed that can provide the $x$, $y$, and $z$ components of the ECG. Any two of these can be fed into a vectorcardiograph to arrive at the VCG for the plane defined by the axes. The signal from the lead for one axis is connected to input 1, and that for the other enters input 2. These signals are then plotted one versus the other on the readout screen and/or they are printed. For each heartbeat, a vector loop representing the locus of the tip of the cardiac vector when its tail is at the origin is determined.

Because of the complexities of obtaining the vectorcardiogram and the difficulty that arises in interpreting the patterns, this technique is generally limited to special studies at tertiary-medical-care facilities or to use as a research tool. The scalar 12-lead electrocardiogram is employed for routine clinical studies.

## 6.9 CARDIAC MONITORS

There are several clinical situations in which continuous observation of the ECG and heart rate is important to the care of the patient. Continuous observation of the ECG during the administration of anesthesia helps doctors monitor the patient's condition while he or she is undergoing medical

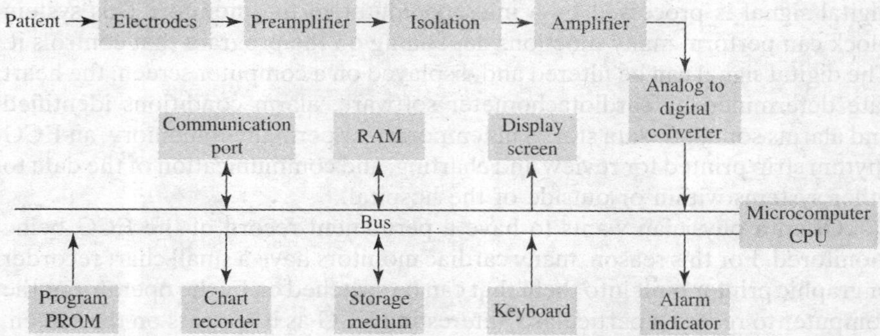


**Figure 6.24** The cardiac monitor displays a continuous electrocardiogram and heart rate and also identifies alarm conditions.

procedures and during recovery from anesthesia. Constant monitoring of the ECG and heart rate of the myocardial-infarction patient during the danger period of several days following the initial incident has made possible the early detection of life-threatening cardiac arrhythmias. Continuous monitoring of the fetal heart rate during labor may help in the early detection of complications.

These and other clinical applications of continuous monitoring of the ECG and heart rate are made possible by *cardiac monitors*. Figure 6.24 shows the basic cardiac monitor in block-diagram form. Its front-end circuitry is similar to that of the electrocardiograph. A pair of electrodes, usually located on the anterior part of the chest, pick up the ECG and are connected by lead wires to the input circuit of the monitor. The input circuit contains circuitry, as described in Section 6.4, to protect the monitor from high-voltage transients that can occur during defibrillation procedures.

The next stage of the monitor is a standard biopotential amplifier designed to amplify the ECG. Although it is best to have the frequency-response characteristics described in Section 6.2, cardiac monitors often have a slightly narrower frequency response than would be acceptable for a diagnostic electrocardiograph. The reason for this is that much of the motion-artifact signal seen during movement of the patient is at very low frequencies. By filtering out some of these low frequencies, we can obtain a vast improvement in SNR and recording stability without seriously affecting the information that pertains to cardiac rhythm in the ECG. Frequency response should be from 0.67 to 40 Hz (Anonymous, 1992). Cardiac monitors should not trigger on pacemaker spikes, which continue even when the heart has stopped. To avoid double counting, cardiac monitors should not trigger on tall T waves (Anonymous, 1990).

Patient isolation circuitry (Section 6.2) is usually found in the circuit following an ECG preamplifier. This is followed by an additional amplifier to raise the signal to levels appropriate for further processing.

In most modern cardiac monitors, the amplified ECG signal is digitized by an ADC, and the remaining processing is carried out by a computer. The digital signal is processed by a microcomputer in the monitor. This system block can perform many functions depending on the program that controls it. The digital signal can be filtered and displayed on a computer screen, the heart rate determined by cardiotachometer software, alarm conditions identified and alarms sounded, data stored in temporary or permanent memory, an ECG rhythm strip printed for review and charting, and communication of the data to other systems within or outside of the hospital.

Often a physician wants to have a permanent record of the ECG being monitored. For this reason, many cardiac monitors have a small chart recorder or graphic printer built into them that can be switched on by the operator or the computer to record a particularly interesting ECG as it appears on the screen.

It is often desirable to have a record of the events in the ECG that lead up to a serious arrhythmia. Such a record can be made if the digital signal is fed first to a memory loop, which delays the ECG signal by about 15 s. The output from the memory loop can then be fed to the printer or chart recorder where the hard copy is produced. Thus, when the operator of the monitor sees an interesting ECG waveform or the monitor itself detects a clinically significant arrhythmia, the information can be obtained from the memory loop to give a record of the events that led up to that particular pattern.

The heart rate is determined from the ECG using a computer algorithm that performs the function of a cardiotachometer. The output is displayed on a rate display so that the operator can immediately tell the patient's heart rate. Alarm circuitry to warn of high and low heart rate is also associated with this algorithm. The alarm system can also produce a hard copy of the events that led up to the alarm for analysis by clinicians. This can be a valuable aid to clinicians in selecting appropriate therapy for the alarm-producing event.

Most hospitals also utilize cardiac monitors in an organized system called an *intensive-care unit*. In such units, there are individual monitors at each patient's bedside that display the ECG in real time as well as the heart rate and any alarm conditions that have recently occurred. These individual monitors are connected to a central unit located at the nursing station that shows the ECGs for all patients being monitored, along with a heart-rate display and alarm indicator for each patient. A printer at the central station can be activated either locally or by remote control from the individual monitors at the patient's bedside.

Computer algorithms that can recognize cardiac arrhythmias and record the frequency of their occurrence are also included in cardiac monitors. The machines can also prepare hard-copy charts showing trends in the patient's monitored parameters and can keep records of various therapeutic measures taken by the clinical staff. The computer can also be a big help in the intensive-care unit by carrying out many observational and charting functions, thereby freeing the clinical staff to care for the patient (Nazeran, 2006).

The availability of microcomputers and high-capacity electronic memory has made it possible to monitor ambulatory patients with detection of cardiac arrhythmias. These monitors consist of an ECG amplifier that provides a signal to an ADC, where it is digitized and stored in memory for later download and analysis. Such devices can collect data from ambulatory patients, and these data are analyzed later by a computer (Jurgen, 1976).

Microcomputers in cardiac monitors perform two basic functions, data management and data analysis. In the former case, the microcomputer controls the various components of the system and directs the transport of data from one block to another along the bus. Carrying out the second function involves the actual analysis of the electrocardiogram. It includes filtering and artifact reduction, identification of the various components of the electrocardiogram, determination of the heart rate, and identification of arrhythmias. More than one microcomputer can be used in a monitor system to carry out these functions. The microcomputer is under the software control. This makes it possible to update the monitor by replacing the software rather than modifying any hardware of the instrument.

The microcomputer can temporarily store the data, and an alternative medium such as a separate hard drive is used to archive selected incidents or the entire monitored data. There is also a staff interface to the system that consists of a keyboard and a display monitor.

Computerized cardiac monitors can be integrated into other hospital information systems. Frequently these monitors also have a network connection that enables them to interact with other information systems or to transmit data to physicians' offices located away from the intensive-care unit.

Ambulatory cardiac monitors are often used in the diagnosis and treatment of heart disease. The most frequently applied ambulatory monitor—the Holter monitor—includes a miniature digital recorder with electronic memory that the patient wears. These devices consist of a battery-powered ECG amplifier and recorder that are connected to electrodes placed on the patient's chest. The instrument is sufficiently small to allow the patient to wear it like a necklace, and the recorder memory can hold from 24 to 48 h of continuous ECG recording. Some recorders can collect data from three leads simultaneously so that vectorcardiograms can be stored. Special computerized playback units rapidly analyze the data files for cardiac arrhythmias and display these portions of the electrocardiogram on a computer screen or generate a hard-copy printout of them. The playback units also summarize the total recording in a report that indicates variables such as heart rate, variability in heart rate, type and number of arrhythmias, and amount of artifact.

Holter monitors are used by physicians to detect cardiac arrhythmias that occur infrequently in patients and are usually not detected during office or hospital examinations. Microelectronics has made it possible to make these monitor–recorders so small that they can be surgically implanted under the skin of patients or incorporated into other implanted devices such as pacemakers. The Medtronic Corp. (2008) Reveal Insertable Loop Recorder has a mass of only 17 g and can store up to 42 min of ECG. It can monitor a patient for up to 14 months with built-in electrodes. The recorder can either be activated by the patient when they experience the symptoms or be programmed to recognize and record significant events. By being implantable, the problems of patient compliance or electrode detachment are avoided.

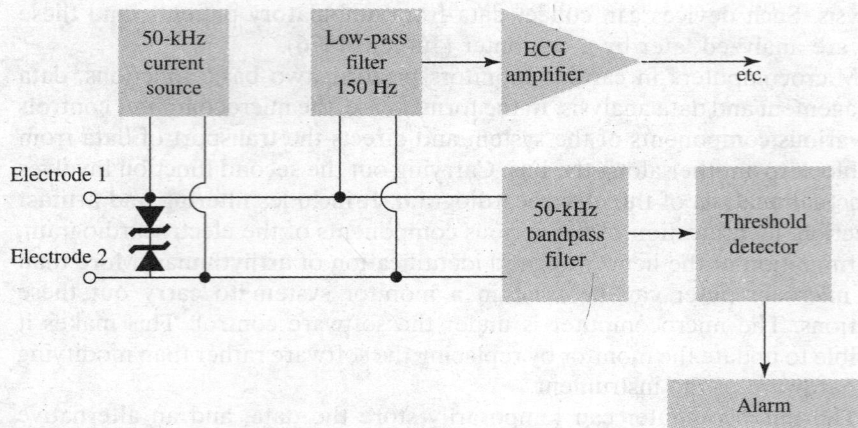


**Figure 6.25** Block diagram of a system used with cardiac monitors to detect increased electrode impedance, lead wire failure, or electrode falloff.

Farwell *et al.* (2006) have shown how this technology can impact clinical evaluation of patients with fainting spells that could be the result of infrequent life-threatening cardiac arrhythmias.

In situations in which cardiac monitors are used to observe a patient's ECG over a long period of time, artifact and failure of the monitor can occur as a result of a poor electrode–patient interface. The longer the electrodes remain on the patient, the more often this occurs. In intensive-care units, electrodes are routinely changed—sometimes once a shift, sometimes once a day—to ensure against this type of breakdown. Most cardiac monitors also have alarm circuits that indicate when electrodes fall off the patient or the electrode–patient connection degenerates.

Figure 6.25 is a block diagram of a typical lead fall-off alarm. A 50 kHz high-impedance source is connected across the electrodes. Peak amplitudes of the current can be as great as 100 to 200 μA without any risk to the patient, because the microshock hazard to excitable tissue decreases as the frequency increases above 1 kHz (Figure 14.3). The current passes through the body between the electrodes, and, as long as there is good electrode contact, the voltage drop is relatively small. If the electrode connections become poor, as can happen when the electrolyte gel begins to dry, or if one of the electrodes falls off or the wire breaks, the impedance between the electrodes increases considerably. This causes the voltage produced by the 50 kHz source to rise. The high-frequency signal is separated from the ECG by the filtering scheme, as shown. The ECG passes through a low-pass filter with approximately a 150 Hz corner frequency, and is processed in the usual way. A bandpass filter with a 50 kHz center frequency passes the voltage resulting from the current source to a threshold detector. This detector sets off an alarm when the voltage exceeds a certain threshold, which would correspond to poor electrode contact. When an electrode falls off the patient, the interelectrode impedance should increase to infinity, resulting in the possibility of 50 kHz voltages high enough to cause some damage to the electronic devices. For this reason, a high-voltage protection circuit, such as that described in Section 6.4, is frequently connected across the input terminals to the monitor. In the case shown in Figure 6.25, back-to-back zener diodes are used.

## 6.10 BIOTELEMETRY

Biopotential and other signals are often processed by radiotelemetry, a technique that provides a wireless link between the patient and the majority of the signal-processing components. By using a miniature radio transmitter attached to the patient to broadcast the information over a limited range, clinicians can monitor a patient or study a research animal while the subject has full mobility. This technique also provides the best method of isolating the patient from the recording equipment and power lines. For a single-channel system of biopotential radiotelemetry, a miniature battery-operated radio transmitter is connected to the electrodes on the patient. This transmitter broadcasts the biopotential over a limited range to a remotely located receiver, which detects the radio signals and recovers the signal for further processing. In this situation there is obviously negligible connection or stray capacitance between the electrode circuit connected to the radio transmitter and the rest of the instrumentation system. The receiving system can even be located in a room separate from the patient's. Hence the patient is completely isolated, and the only risk of electric shock that the patient runs is due to the battery-powered transmitter itself. Thus, if the transmitter power supply is kept at a low voltage, there is negligible risk to the patient.

Many types of radiotelemetry systems are used in biomedical instrumentation (Ziaie, 2006). The basic configuration of the system, however, is pretty much the same for all. A preamplifier amplifies the ECG signal to a level at which it can modulate the transmitter. Pulse-code modulation in the range of 100 to 500 MHz is the dominant method. The entire transmitter is powered by a small battery pack. It is carried by the patient and usually attached by means of a special harness. Ultraminiature radio transmitters can be attached by surgical tape directly to the patient's skin. In research with experimental animals, experimenters can surgically implant the tiny transmitters within the bodies of the animals so that no external connections or wires are required. Stuart Mackay of Boston University pioneered this technique many years ago (Mackay, 1970), and many applications from wildlife biology to clinical medicine followed. Today, the technique is routinely found in hospital intensive-care and step-down units for cardiac monitoring (Budinger, 2003).

In the receiving system, a pickup antenna receives the modulated signal. The signal is then demodulated to recover the original information from the carrier. The signal can be further amplified to provide a usable output. The receiver system is generally powered directly from the power line, because it is in a permanent location and is not attached to the patient in any way.

The bandwidth of the system is determined by the rate at which it is sampled. Theoretically, the rate of sampling should be at least twice that of the highest-frequency component to be transmitted, but in practical circuits the rate of sampling is usually at least five times that of the highest-frequency component.

It is important to note that, although radiotelemetry systems provide ideal isolation with no patient ground required, they are not completely immune to problems of electric noise. Because coupling is achieved by a radiated electromagnetic signal, other electromagnetic signals at similar frequencies can interfere and cause artifacts. In extreme cases, these other signals can even bring about complete loss of signal.

In addition, the relative orientation between transmitting and receiving antennas is important. There can be orientations in which none of the signals radiated from the transmitting antenna are picked up by the receiving antenna. In such cases, there is no transmission of signals. In high-quality radiotelemetry systems, it is therefore important to have a means of indicating when signal interference or signal dropout is occurring. Such a signal makes it possible to take steps to rectify this problem and informs the clinical staff that the information being received is noise and should be disregarded.

The advent of wireless computer communication systems has affected biotelemetry as well. Telemetry systems capable of two-way communication utilize the standardized wireless computer connection protocols such as WiFi, Bluetooth and ZigBee. Complete transceiver (transmitter and receiver) systems for these protocols are available on a single integrated circuit chip, so very small wireless devices can now be realized. These can be incorporated into wireless sensing networks that can either be implanted in the body or incorporated into clothing. Although systems such as Bluetooth and ZigBe are limited to short range, external transponders can extend coverage.

## PROBLEMS

**6.1** What position of the cardiac vector at the peak of the R wave of an electrocardiogram gives the greatest sum of voltages for leads I, II, and III?

**6.2** What position of the cardiac vector during the R wave gives identical signals in leads II and III? What does the ECG seen in lead I look like for this orientation of the vector?

**6.3** An ECG has a scalar magnitude of 1 mV on lead II and a scalar magnitude of 0.5 mV on lead III. *Calculate* the scalar magnitude on lead I.

**6.4** Design a system that has as inputs the *scalar* voltages of lead II and lead III and as output the *scalar* voltage of the cardiac vector **M**.

**6.5** Design the lead connections for the VF and aVF leads. For each, choose minimal resistor values that meet the requirements for input impedance given in Table 6.1.
**6.6** A student designs a new lead system by inverting Einthovens's triangle. She places one electrode on each hip and one on the neck. For this new system, design a resistor network (show the circuit and give resistor values) to yield conventional lead aVF (show polarity). Explain the reason for each resistor.
**6.7** Design an electrocardiograph with an input-switching system such that we can record the six frontal-plane leads by means of changing the switch.
**6.8** Discuss the factors that enter into choosing a resistance value for the three resistors used to establish the Wilson central terminal. Describe the advantages and disadvantages of having this resistance either very large or very small.
**6.9** The central terminal requirements for an electrocardiograph that meets the recommendations of Table 6.1 sets the minimal value of the resistances at 1.7 MΩ. Show that this value is a result of the specification given in Table 6.1.
**6.10** A student attempts to measure his own ECG on an oscilloscope having a differential input. For Figure 6.11, $Z_{in} = 1\,\text{M}\Omega$, $Z_1 = 20\,\text{k}\Omega$, $Z_2 = 10\,\text{k}\Omega$, $Z_G = 30\,\text{k}\Omega$, and $i_{db} = 0.5\,\mu\text{A}$. Calculate the power-line interference the student observes.
**6.11** Design a driven-right-leg circuit, and show all resistor values. For 1 μA of 60 Hz current flowing through the body, the common-mode voltage should be reduced to 2 mV. The circuit should supply no more than 5 μA when the amplifier is saturated at ±13 V.
**6.12** An engineer sees no purpose for $R/2$ in Figure 6.5(a) and replaces it with a wire in order to simplify the circuit. What is the result?
**6.13** An ECG lead is oriented such that its electrodes are placed on the body in positions that pick up an electromyogram from the chest muscles as well as the electrocardiogram. Design a circuit that separates these two signals as well as possible, and discuss the limitations of such a circuit.
**6.14** A cardiac monitor is found to have 1 mV p-p of 60 Hz interference. Describe a procedure that you could use to determine whether this is due to an electric field or a magnetic field pickup.
**6.15** Assume zero skin–electrode impedance, and design (give component values for) simple *filters* that will attenuate incoming 1 MHz radiofrequency interference to 0.001 of its former value. Sketch the placement of these filters (show all connections) to prevent interference from entering an ECG amplifier. Then calculate the 60 Hz interference that they cause for common-mode voltage of 10 mV and skin–electrode impedances of 50 kΩ and 40 kΩ.
**6.16** You design an ECG machine using FETs such that the $Z_{in}$ of Figure 6.11 exceeds 100 MΩ. Because of radiofrequency (RF) interference, you wish to add equal shunt capacitors at the two $Z_{in}$ locations. For $v_{cm} = 10\,\text{mV}$, $Z_2 = 100\,\text{k}\Omega$, and $Z_1 = 80\,\text{k}\Omega$, calculate the maximal capacitance so 60 Hz $|v_A - v_B| = 10\,\mu\text{V}$. Calculate the result using (6.19).
**6.17** Silicon diodes having a forward resistance of 2 Ω are to be used as voltage-limiting devices in the protection circuit of an electrocardiograph. They are connected as shown in Figure 6.14(b). The protection circuit is shown

in Figure 6.13. If voltage transients as high as 500 V can appear at the electrocardiograph input during defibrillation, what is the minimal value of $R$ that the designer can choose so that the voltage at the preamplifier input does not exceed 800 mV? Assume that the silicon diodes have a breakdown voltage of 600 mV.

**6.18** For Figure 6.15, assume $I_d = 500$ nA and RL skin impedance is 100 kΩ. Design (give component values for) a *driven-right-leg* circuit to achieve $v_{cm} = 10\ \mu$V.

**6.19** For Figure 6.17, assume $C_s = 10$ pF and $C_f = 20$ pF. Design the amplifier circuit to replace the triangle containing $A_v$. Use an op amp and passive components to achieve an ideal negative-input capacitance amplifier. Show the circuit diagram and connections to other components that appear in Figure 6.17.

**6.20** Design a technique for automatically calibrating an electrocardiograph at the beginning of each recording. The calibration can consist of a 1 mV standardizing pulse.

**6.21** A student decides to remove the switch across the 3.3 MΩ resistor in Figure 6.18 and place it across the 1 μF capacitor to "discharge the capacitor after defibrillation." Sketch what the typical output looks like before, during, and after defibrillation and switch closure, and explain why it looks that way.

**6.22** Redesign Figure 6.18 by placing a capacitor in series with the 10 kΩ resistor between the two inverting inputs. Eliminate the last op amp, and adjust other components to keep the same gain, corner frequencies, and ability to use a switch to return the output to the linear region.

**6.23** Design a biopotential preamplifier that is battery-powered and isolated in such a way that there is less than 0.5 pF coupling capacitance between the input and output terminals. The amplifier should have a nominal gain of 10 and an input impedance greater than 10 MΩ differentially and greater than 10 GΩ with respect to ground. The output impedance should be less than 100 Ω and single ended.

**6.24** Design a circuit that uses one op amp plus other passive components that will detect QRS complexes of the ECG even when the amplitude of the T wave exceeds that of the QRS complex and provides output signals suitable for counting these complexes on a counter.

**6.25** Design an automatic reset circuit for an electrocardiograph.

**6.26** Design an arrhythmia-detection system for detecting and counting the PVCs shown in Figure 4.18. Note that PVCs occur earlier than expected, but the following beat occurs at the normal time, because it is generated by the SA node. Show a block diagram, and describe the operation of the system.

**6.27** In an evoked-response experiment in which the EEG is studied after a patient is given the stimulus of a flashing light, the experimenter finds that the response has approximately the same amplitude as the random noise of the signal. If a signal averager is used, how many samples must be averaged to get an SNR of 10:1? If we wanted an SNR of 100:1, would it be practical to use this technique?

**6.28** A physician wishes to obtain two simultaneous ECGs in the frontal plane from leads that have lead vectors at right angles. The signal will be used

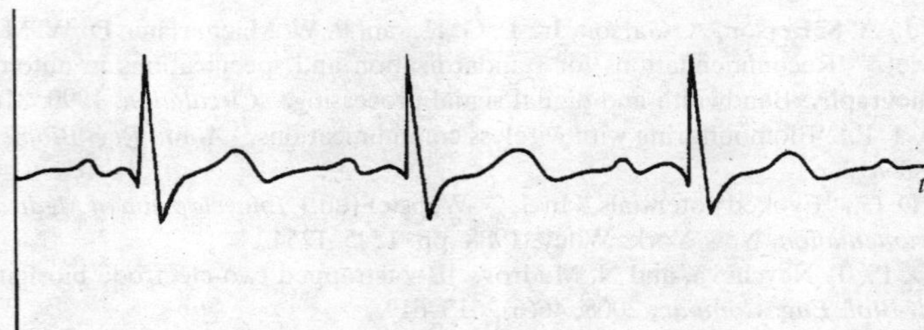


**Figure P6.1**

to generate a VCG. Describe how you would go about obtaining these two signals, and suggest a test to determine whether the leads are truly orthogonal.

**6.29** The ECG shown in Figure P6.1 is distorted as a result of an instrumentation problem. Discuss possible causes of this distortion, and suggest means of correcting the problem.

**6.30** Figure P6.2 shows ECGs from simultaneous leads I and II. Sketch the vector loop for this QRS complex in the frontal plane.

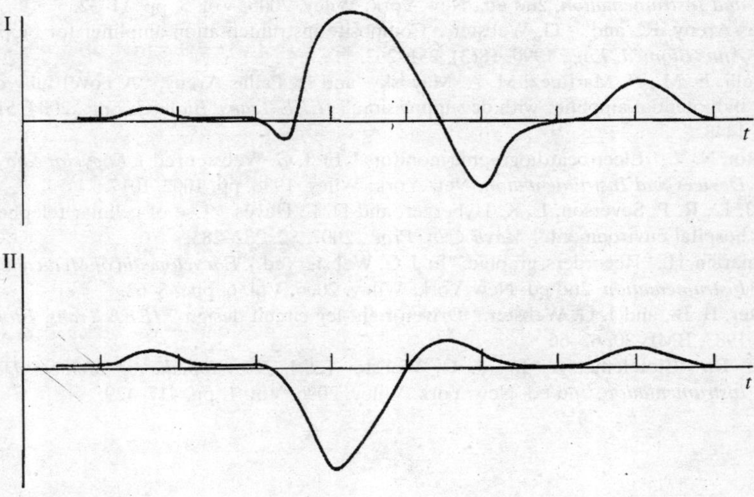


**Figure P6.2**

## REFERENCES

Anonymous, "Ambulatory ECG monitors." *Health Devices*, 1989, 18, 295–321.

Anonymous, "Diagnostic electrocardiographic devices" ANSI/AAMI EC11–1991. Arlington, VA: Association for the Advancement of Medical Instrumentation, 1991.

Anonymous, "Cardiac monitors, heart rate meters and alarms." ANSI/AAMI EC13–1992. Arlington, VA: Association for the Advancement of Medical Instrumentation, 1992.

Bailey, J. J., A. S. Berson, A. Garson, Jr., L. G. Horan, P. W. MacFarlane, D. W. Mortara, and C. Zywietz, "Recommendations for standardization and specifications in automated electrocardiography: Bandwidth and digital signal processing." *Circulation*, 1990, 81(2), 730–739.

Budinger, T. F., "Biomonitoring with wireless communications," *Annu. Rev. Biomed. Eng.*, 2003, 5, 383–412.

Childers, D. G., "Evoked potentials." In J. G. Webster (ed.), *Encyclopedia of Medical Devices and Instrumentation*. New York: Wiley, 1988, pp. 1245–1254.

Dobrev D. P., T. Neycheva, and N. Mudrov, "Bootstrapped two-electrode biosignal amplifier." *Med. Biol. Eng. Comput.*, 2008, 46(6), 613–619.

Farwell, D J, N Freemantle, and N Sulke, "The clinical impact of implantable loop recorders in patients with syncope." *Eur. Heart J.*, February 2006, 27(3), 351–356.

Grobstein, S. R., and R. D. Gatzke, "A battery-powered ECG monitor for emergency and operating room environments." *Hewlett-Packard J.*, September 1977, 29(1), 26–32.

Huhta, J. C., and J. G. Webster, "60-Hz interference in electrocardiography." *IEEE Trans. Biomed. Eng.*, 1973, BME-20, 91–101.

Jurgen, R. K., "Software (and hardware) for the 'medics." *IEEE Spectrum*, April 1976, 13(4), 40–43.

Mackay, R. S., *Biomedical Telemetry*, 2nd ed. New York: Wiley, 1970.

Medtronic Corp., Reveal Insertable Loop Recorder, 2008. http://www.medtronic.com/physician/reveal/index.html.

Nazeran, H., "Electrocardiography, computers in." In J. G. Webster (ed.), *Encyclopedia of Medical Devices and Instrumentation*, 2nd ed. New York: Wiley, 2006, Vol. 3, pp. 34–53.

Neuman, M. R., "Neonatal monitoring" In J. G. Webster (ed.), *Encyclopedia of Medical Devices and Instrumentation*, 2nd ed., New York: Wiley, 2006, Vol. 5, pp. 11–32.

Pallás-Areny, R., and J. G. Webster, "Composite instrumentation amplifier for biopotentials." *Ann. Biomed. Eng.*, 1990, 18(3), 251–262.

Spinelli, E. M., N. Martínez, M. A. Mayosky, and R. Pallàs-Areny, "A novel fully differential biopotential amplifier with dc suppression." *IEEE Trans. Biomed. Eng.*, 2004, 51(8), 1444–1448.

Thakor, N. V., "Electrocardiographic monitors." In J. G. Webster (ed.), *Encyclopedia of Medical Devices and Instrumentation*. New York: Wiley, 1988, pp. 1002–1017.

Tri, J. L., R. P. Severson, L. K. Hyberger, and D. L. Hayes, "Use of cellular telephones in the hospital environment." *Mayo Clin. Proc.*, 2007, 82, 282–285.

Vermariën, H., "Recorders, graphic." In J. G. Webster (ed.), *Encyclopedia of Medical Devices and Instrumentation*, 2nd ed. New York: Wiley, 2006, Vol. 6, pp. 48–62.

Winter, B. B., and J. G. Webster, "Driven-right-leg circuit design." *IEEE Trans. Biomed. Eng.*, 1983, BME-30, 62–66.

Ziaie, B., "Biotelemetry." In J. G. Webster (ed.), *Encyclopedia of Medical Devices and Instrumentation*, 2nd ed. New York: Wiley, 2006, Vol. 1, pp. 417–429.

# 7

# BLOOD PRESSURE AND SOUND

Robert A. Peura

Determining an individual's blood pressure is a standard clinical measurement, whether taken in a physician's office or in the hospital during a specialized surgical procedure. Blood-pressure values in the various chambers of the heart and in the peripheral vascular system help the physician determine the functional integrity of the cardiovascular system. A number of direct (invasive) and indirect (noninvasive) techniques are being used to measure blood pressure in the human. The accuracy of each should be established, as well as its suitability for a particular clinical situation.

Fluctuations in pressure recorded over the frequency range of hearing are called *sounds*. The sources of heart sounds are the vibrations set up by the accelerations and decelerations of blood.

The function of the blood circulation is to transport oxygen and other nutrients to the tissues of the body and to carry metabolic waste products away from the cells. In Section 4.6 we pointed out that the heart serves as a four-chambered pump for the circulatory system. This is illustrated in Figure 4.12. The heart is divided into two pumping systems, the right side of the heart and the left side of the heart. The pulmonary circulation and the systemic circulation separate these two pumps and their associated valves. Each pump has a filling chamber, the atrium, which helps to fill the ventricle, the stronger pump. Figure 7.15 is a diagram that shows how the electric and mechanical events are related during the cardiac cycle. The four heart sounds are also indicated in this diagram.

Figure 7.1 is a schematic diagram of the circulatory system. The left ventricle ejects blood through the aortic valve into the aorta, and the blood is then distributed through the branching network of arteries, arterioles, and capillaries. The resistance to blood flow is regulated by the arterioles, which are under local, neural, and endocrine control. The exchange of the nutrient material takes place at the capillary level. The blood then returns to the right side of the heart via the venous system. Blood fills the right atrium, the filling chamber of the right heart, and flows through the tricuspid valve into the right ventricle. The blood is pumped from the right ventricle into the pulmonary artery through the pulmonary valve. It next flows through the pulmonary arteries, arterioles, capillaries, and veins to the left atrium. At the pulmonary capillaries, $O_2$ diffuses from the lung alveoli to the blood,

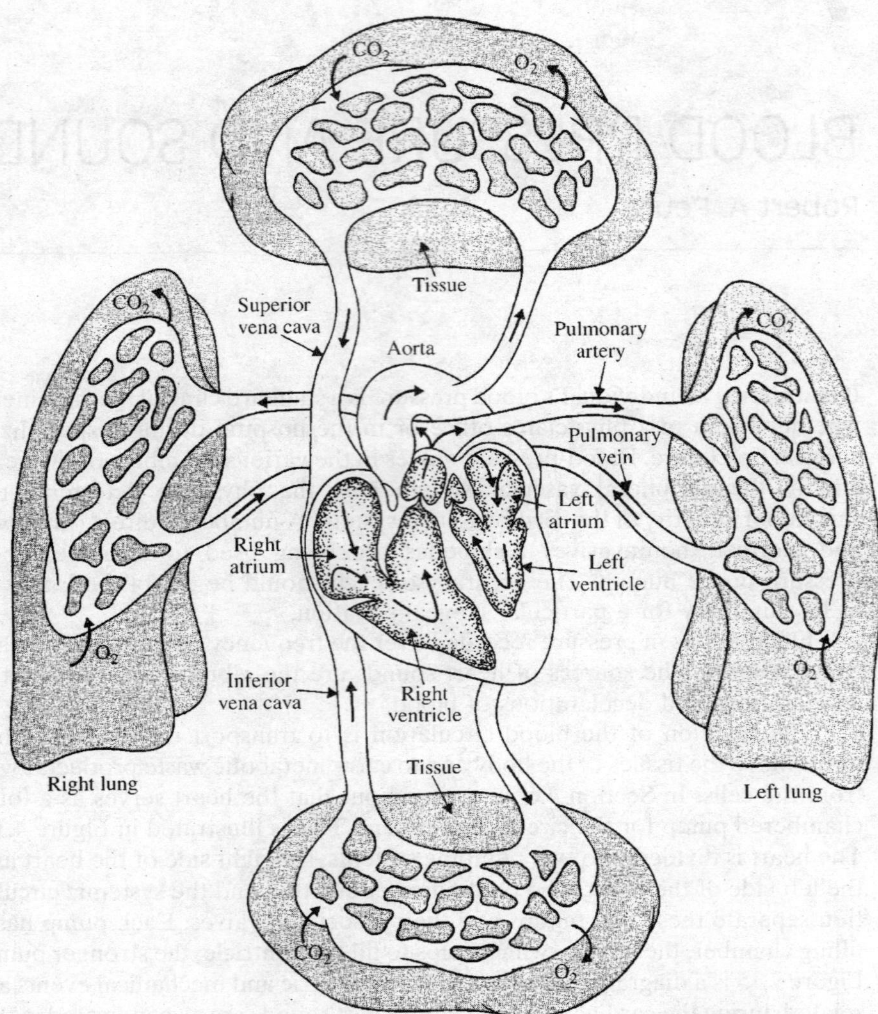


**Figure 7.1** The left ventricle ejects blood into the systemic circulatory system. The right ventricle ejects blood into the pulmonary circulatory system.

and $CO_2$ diffuses from the blood to the alveoli. The blood flows from the left atrium, the filling chamber of the left heart, through the mitral valve into the left ventricle. When the left ventricle contracts in response to the electric stimulation of the myocardium (discussed in detail in Section 4.6), blood is pumped through the aortic valve into the aorta.

The pressures generated by the right and left sides of the heart differ somewhat in shape and in amplitude (see Figure 7.2). As we noted in Section 4.6, cardiac contraction is caused by electric stimulation of the cardiac muscle. An electric impulse is generated by specialized cells located in the sino-atrial node of the right atrium. This electric impulse quickly spreads over both atria.

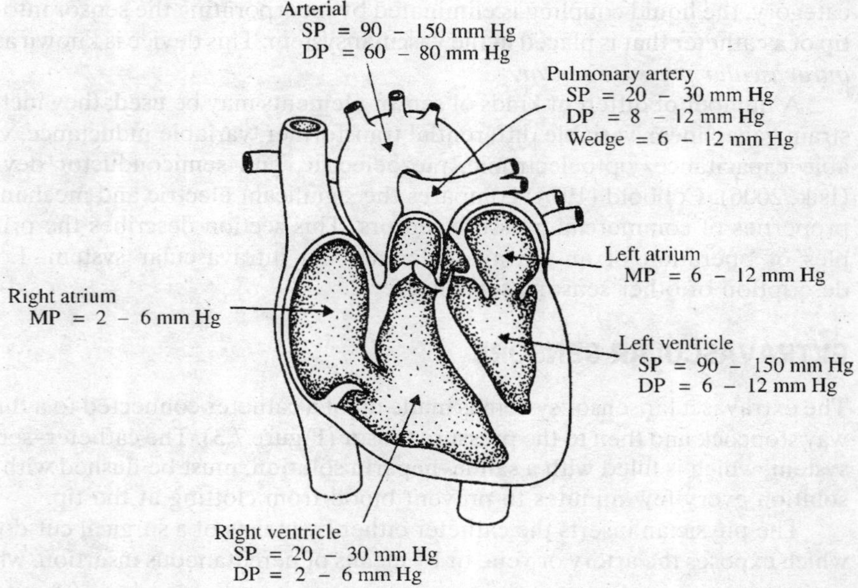


**Figure 7.2 Typical values of circulatory pressures** SP is the systolic pressure, DP is the diastolic pressure, and MP is the mean pressure. The wedge pressure is defined in Section 7.13.

At the junction of the atria and ventricles, the electric impulse is conducted after a short delay at the atrioventricular node. Conduction quickly spreads over the interior of both ventricles by means of a specialized conduction system, the His bundle, and the Purkinje system. Conduction then propagates throughout both ventricles. This impulse causes mechanical contraction of both ventricles. Mechanical contraction of the ventricular muscle generates ventricular pressures that force blood through the pulmonary and aortic valves into the pulmonary circulation and the systemic circulation, causing pressures in each. Section 7.9 describes the correlation of the four heart sounds with the electric and mechanical events of the cardiac cycle. Briefly, the heart sounds are associated with the movement of blood during the cardiac cycle. Murmurs are vibrations caused by the turbulence in the blood moving rapidly through the heart.

## 7.1 DIRECT MEASUREMENTS

Blood-pressure sensor systems can be divided into two general categories according to the location of the sensor element. The most common clinical method for directly measuring pressure is to couple the vascular pressure to an external sensor element via a liquid-filled catheter. In the second general category, the liquid coupling is eliminated by incorporating the sensor into the tip of a catheter that is placed in the vascular system. This device is known as an *intravascular pressure sensor*.

A number of different kinds of sensor elements may be used; they include strain gage, linear-variable differential transformer, variable inductance, variable capacitance, optoelectronic, piezoelectric, and semiconductor devices (Isik, 2006). Cobbold (1974) compares the significant electric and mechanical properties of commercial pressure sensors. This section describes the principles of operation of an extravascular and an intravascular system. For a description of other sensors, see Chapter 2.

## EXTRAVASCULAR SENSORS

The extravascular sensor system is made up of a catheter connected to a three-way stopcock and then to the pressure sensor (Figure 7.3). The catheter–sensor system, which is filled with a saline–heparin solution, must be flushed with the solution every few minutes to prevent blood from clotting at the tip.

The physician inserts the catheter either by means of a surgical cut-down, which exposes the artery or vein, or by means of percutaneous insertion, which

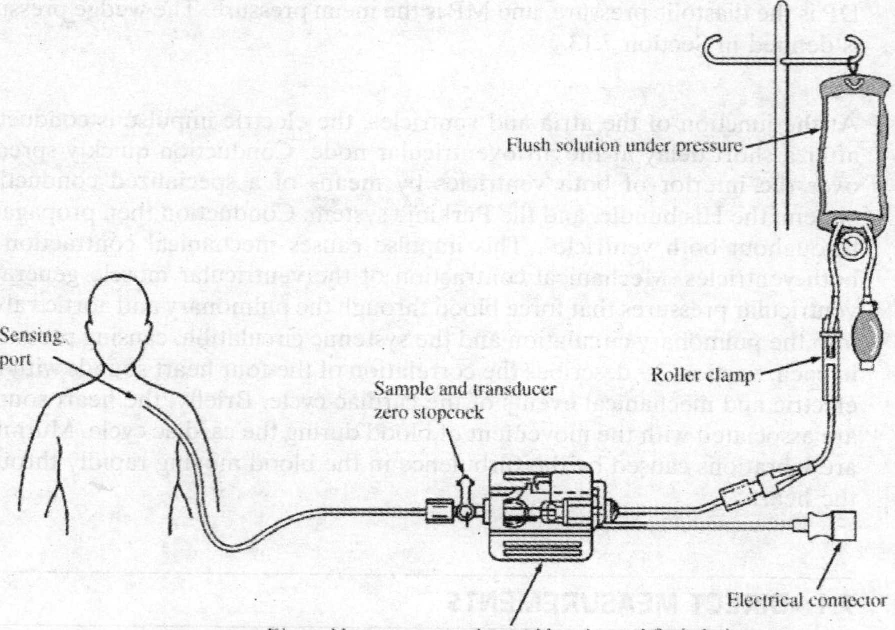


**Figure 7.3 Extravascular pressure-sensor system** A catheter couples a flush solution (heparinized saline) through a disposable pressure sensor with an integral flush device to the sensing port. The three-way stopcock is used to take blood samples and zero the pressure sensor.

involves the use of a special needle or guide-wire technique. Blood pressure is transmitted via the catheter liquid column to the sensor and, finally, to the diaphragm, which is deflected. Figure 2.2(a) shows an early pressure sensor, in which the displacement of the diaphragm is transmitted to a system composed of a moving armature and an unbonded strain gage. Figure 2.5 shows a modern disposable blood-pressure sensor.

## INTRAVASCULAR SENSORS

Catheter-tip sensors have the advantage that the hydraulic connection via the catheter, between the source of pressure and the sensor element, is eliminated. The frequency response of the catheter–sensor system is limited by the hydraulic properties of the system. Detection of pressures at the tip of the catheter without the use of a liquid-coupling system can thus enable the physician to obtain a high frequency response and eliminate the time delay encountered when the pressure pulse is transmitted in a catheter–sensor system.

A number of basic types of sensors are being used commercially for the detection of pressure in the catheter tip. These include various types of strain-gage systems bonded onto a flexible diaphragm at the catheter tip. Gages of this type are available in the F 5 catheter [1.67 mm outer diameter (OD)] size. In the French scale (F), used to denote the diameter of catheters, each unit is approximately equal to 0.33 mm. Smaller-sized catheters may become available as the technology improves and the problems of temperature and electric drift, fragility, and nondestructive sterilization are solved more satisfactorily. A disadvantage of the catheter-tip pressure sensor is that it is more expensive than others and may break after only a few uses, further increasing its cost per use.

The fiber-optic intravascular pressure sensor can be made in sizes comparable to those described above, but at a lower cost. The fiber-optic device measures the displacement of the diaphragm optically by the varying reflection of light from the back of the deflecting diaphragm. (Recall that Section 2.14 detailed the principles of transmission of light along a fiber bundle.) These devices are inherently safer electrically, but unfortunately they lack a convenient way to measure relative pressure without an additional lumen either connected to a second pressure sensor or vented to the atmosphere.

A fiber-optic microtip sensor for *in vivo* measurements inside the human body is shown in Figure 7.4 (a) in which one leg of a bifurcated fiber bundle is connected to a light-emitting diode (LED) source and the other to a photodetector (Hansen, 1983). The pressure-sensor tip consists of a thin metal membrane mounted at the common end of the mixed fiber bundle. External pressure causes membrane deflection, varying the coupling between the LED source and the photodetector. Figure 7.4(b) shows the output signal versus membrane deflection. Optical fibers have the property of emitting and accepting light within a cone defined by the acceptance angle $\theta_A$, which is equal to the fiber numerical aperture, $N_A$ (Section 2.14). The coupling between LED source and detector is a function of the overlap of the two acceptance angles

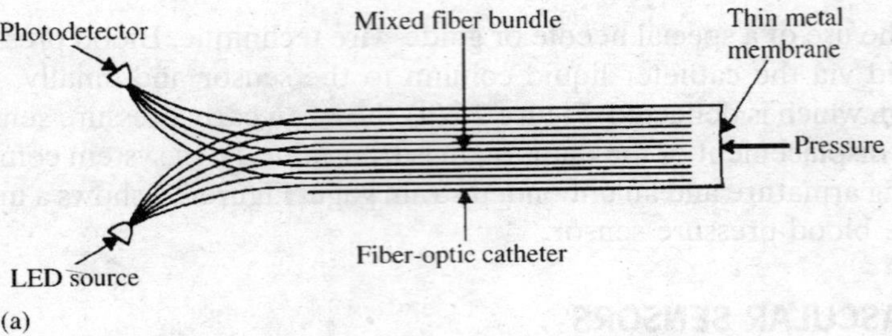


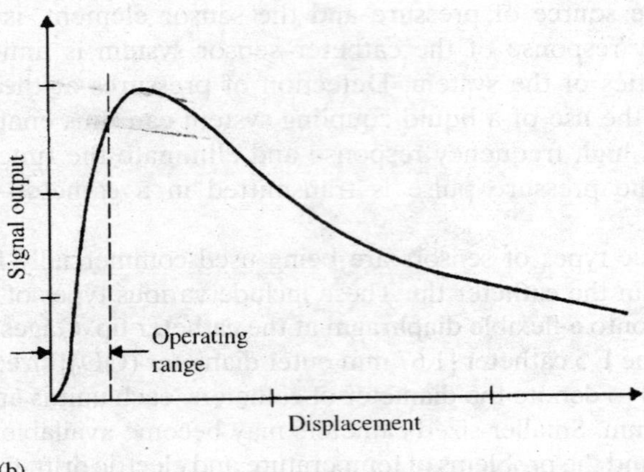


**Figure 7.4** (a) Schematic diagram of an intravascular fiber-optic pressure sensor. Pressure causes deflection in a thin metal membrane that modulates the coupling between the source and detector fibers. (b) Characteristic curve for the fiber-optic pressure sensor.

on the pressure-sensor membrane. The operating portion of the curve is the left slope region where the characteristic is steepest.

Roos and Carroll (1985) describe a fiber-optic pressure sensor for use in magnetic resonance imaging (MRI) fields in which a plastic shutter assembly modulates the light transversing a channel between source and detector. Neuman (2006) described a fiber-optic pressure sensor for intracranial pressure measurements in the newborn. Figure 7.5 shows a schematic of the device, which is applied to the anterior fontanel. Pressure is applied with the sensor such that the curvature of the skin surface is flattened. When this applanation occurs, equal pressure exists on both sides of the membrane, which consists of soft tissue between the scalp surface and the dura. Monitoring of the probe pressure determines the dura pressure. Pressure bends the membrane, which moves a reflector. This varies the amount of light coupling between the source and detector fibers.

Air pressure from a pneumatic servo system controls the air pressure within the pressure sensor, which is adjusted such that diaphragm—and thus

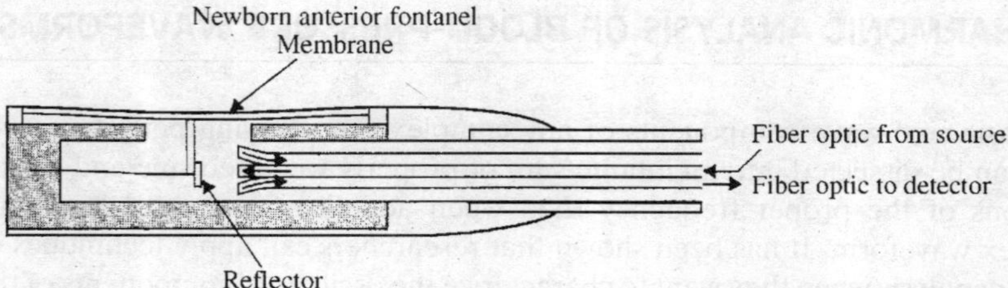


**Figure 7.5** Fiber-optic pressure sensor for intracranial pressure measurements in the newborn. The sensor membrane is placed in contact with the anterior fontanel of the newborn.

the fontanel tissue—is flat, indicating that the sensor air pressure and the fontanel or intracranial pressure are equal.

Similar pressure-unloading techniques are used in thin, compliant sensors that measure interface pressures between the skin and support structures such as seat cushions (Webster, 1991).

Silicon fusion bonding is used to fabricate micro silicon pressure-sensor chips (Howe *et al.*, 1990). A wedge-shaped cavity is etched in a silicon wafer to form a diaphragm. Piezoresistive strain gages are implanted and a metal connection is made in order to create a sensor for a catheter tip micropressure sensor.

## DISPOSABLE PRESSURE SENSORS

Traditionally, physiological pressure sensors have been reusable devices, but most modern hospitals have adopted inexpensive, disposable pressure sensors in order to lower the risk of patient cross-contamination and reduce the amount of handling of pressure sensors by hospital personnel. Because reusable pressure sensors are subject to the abuses of reprocessing and repeated user handling, they tend to be less reliable than disposable sensors.

By micromachining silicon, a pressure diaphragm is etched and piezoresistive strain gages are diffused into the diaphragm for measuring its displacement. This process results in a small, integrated, sensitive, and relatively inexpensive pressure sensor. This silicon chip is incorporated into a disposable pressure-monitoring tubing system. The disposable pressure sensor system also contains a thick-film resistor network that is laser trimmed to remove offset voltages and set the same sensitivity for similar disposable sensors. In addition, a thick-film thermistor network is usually incorporated for temperature compensation. The resistance of the bridge elements is usually high in order to reduce self-heating, which may cause erroneous results. This results in high output impedance for the device. Thus, a high-input impedance monitor must be used with disposable pressure sensors.

Pressure sensors can monitor blood pressure in postsurgical patients as part of a closed-loop feedback system. Such a system injects controlled amounts of the drug nitroprusside to stabilize the blood pressure (Yu, 2006).

## 7.2 HARMONIC ANALYSIS OF BLOOD-PRESSURE WAVEFORMS

The basic sine-wave components of any complex time-varying periodic waveform can be dissected into an infinite sum of properly weighted sine and cosine functions of the proper frequency that, when added, reproduce the original complex waveform. It has been shown that researchers can apply techniques of Fourier analysis when they want to characterize the oscillatory components of the circulatory and respiratory systems, because two basic postulates for Fourier analysis—periodicity and linearity—are usually satisfied (Attinger *et al.*, 1970).

Cardiovascular physiologists and some clinicians have been employing Fourier-analysis techniques in the quantification of pressure and flow since this method was established in the 1950s. Early Fourier analysis used bandpass filters. More recent analysts have used computer techniques to obviate the need for special hardware. The advantage of the technique is that it allows for a quantitative representation of a physiological waveform; thus it is quite easy to compare corresponding harmonic components of pulses.

O'Rourke (1971) points out that the physician who turns to a standard medical textbook for assistance in interpreting the arterial pulse is likely to be confused, misled, and disappointed. He further indicates that in recent years, analysis of the frequency components of the pulse appears to have yielded more information on arterial properties than any other approach. He proposes that the arterial pulse be represented in terms of its frequency components.

The blood-pressure pulse can be divided into its fundamental component (of the same frequency as the blood-pressure wave) and its significant harmonics. Figure 7.6 shows the first six harmonic components of the blood-pressure wave

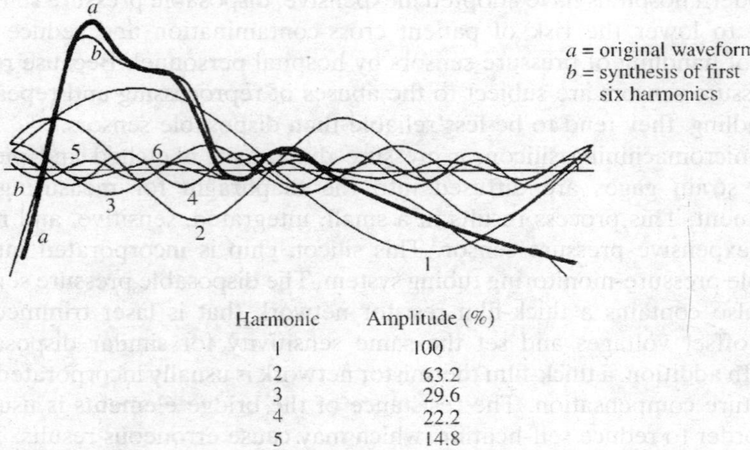


| Harmonic | Amplitude (%) |
|---|---|
| 1 | 100 |
| 2 | 63.2 |
| 3 | 29.6 |
| 4 | 22.2 |
| 5 | 14.8 |
| 6 | 11.8 |

**Figure 7.6 The first six harmonics of the blood-pressure waveform** The table gives relative values for amplitudes. (From T. A. Hansen, "pressure measurement in the human organism." *Acta Physiologica Scandinavica*, 1949, 19, Suppl. 68, 1–227. Used with permission.)

and the resultant sum. When we compare the original waveform and the waveform reconstructed from the Fourier components, we find that they agree quite well, indicating that the first six harmonics give a fairly good reproduction. Note that the amplitude of the sixth harmonic is approximately 12% of the fundamental. We can achieve more faithful reproduction of the original waveform by adding higher harmonic components.

## 7.3 DYNAMIC PROPERTIES OF PRESSURE-MEASUREMENT SYSTEMS

An understanding of the dynamic properties of a pressure-measurement system is important if we wish to preserve the dynamic accuracy of the measured pressure. Errors in measurement of dynamic pressure can have serious consequences in the clinical situation. For instance, an underdamped system can lead to overestimation of pressure gradients across stenotic (narrowed) heart valves. The liquid-filled catheter sensor is a hydraulic system that can be represented by either distributed- or lumped-parameter models. Distributed-parameter models are described in the literature (Fry, 1960), which gives an accurate description of the dynamic behavior of the catheter-sensor system. However, distributed-parameter models are not normally employed, because the single-degree-of-freedom (lumped-parameter) model is easier to work with, and the accuracy of the results obtained by using these models is acceptable for the clinical situation.

### ANALOGOUS ELECTRIC SYSTEMS

The modeling approach taken here develops a lumped-parameter model for the catheter and sensor separately and shows how, with appropriate approximations, it reduces to the lumped-parameter model for a second-order system. Figure 7.7 shows the physical model of a catheter–sensor system. An increase in pressure at the input of the catheter causes a flow of liquid to the right from the catheter tip, through the catheter, and into the sensor. This liquid shift causes a deflection of the sensor diaphragm, which is sensed by an electromechanical system. The subsequent electric signal is then amplified.

A liquid catheter has inertial, frictional, and elastic properties represented by inertance, resistance, and compliance, respectively. Similarly, the sensor has these same properties, in addition to the compliance of the diaphragm. Figure 7.7(b) shows an electric analog of the pressure-measuring system, wherein the analogous elements for hydraulic inertance, resistance, and compliance are electric inductance, resistance, and capacitance, respectively.

The analogous circuit in Figure 7.7(b) can be simplified to that shown in Figure 7.8(a). The compliance of the sensor diaphragm is much larger than that of the liquid-filled catheter or sensor cavity, provided that the saline solution is bubble-free and the catheter material is relatively noncompliant. The resistance and inertance of the liquid in the sensor can be neglected compared to

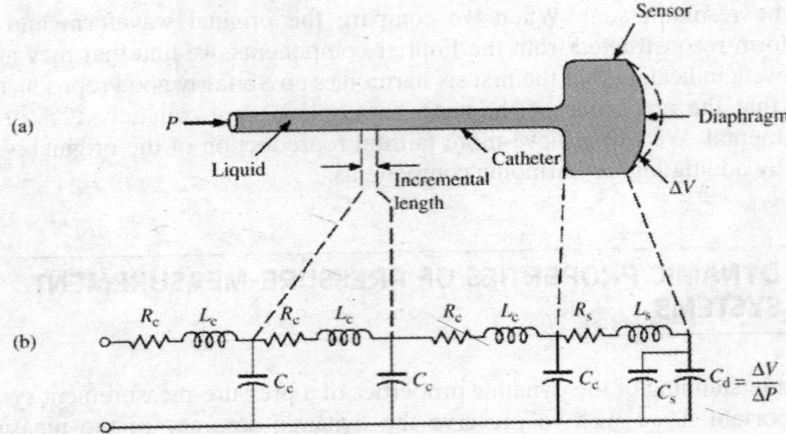


**Figure 7.7** (a) Physical model of a catheter–sensor system. (b) Analogous electric system for this catheter–sensor system. Each segment of the catheter has its own resistance $R_c$, inertance $L_c$, and compliance $C_c$. In addition, the sensor has resistance $R_s$, inertance, $L_s$, and compliance $C_s$. The compliance of the diaphragm is $C_d$.

those of the liquid in the catheter. Let us now derive equations relating the resistance and inductance to the properties of the system.

The liquid resistance $R_c$ of the catheter is due to friction between shearing molecules flowing through the catheter. It can be represented by the equation

$$R_c = \frac{\Delta P}{F} \ (\mathrm{Pa \cdot s/m^3}) \tag{7.1}$$

or

$$R_c = \frac{\Delta P}{\bar{u} A}$$

where

$p$ = pressure difference across the segment in Pa (pascal = $\mathrm{N/m^2}$)
$F$ = flow rate, $\mathrm{m^3/s}$
$\bar{u}$ = average velocity, m/s
$A$ = cross-section area, $\mathrm{m^2}$

Poiseuille's equation enables us to calculate $R_c$ when we are given the values of catheter length $L$, in meters; radius $r$, in meters; and liquid viscosity $\eta$, in pascal-seconds. The equation applies for laminar or Poiseuille flow. It is

$$R_c = \frac{8 \eta L}{\pi r^4} \tag{7.2}$$

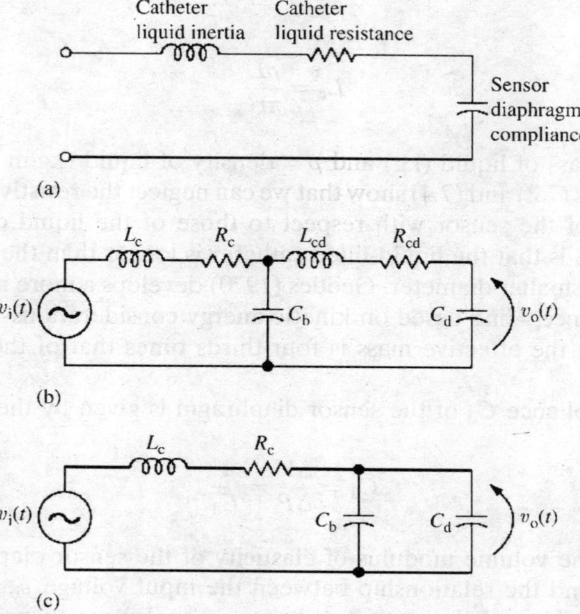


**Figure 7.8** (a) Simplified analogous circuit. Compliance of the sensor diaphragm is larger than compliance of catheter or sensor cavity for a bubble-free, noncompliant catheter. The resistance and inertance of the catheter are larger than those of the sensor, because the catheter has longer length and smaller diameter. (b) Analogous circuit for catheter–sensor system with a bubble in the catheter. Catheter properties proximal to the bubble are inertance $L_c$ and resistance $R_c$. Catheter properties distal to the bubble are $L_{cd}$ and $R_{tf}$. Compliance of the diaphragm is $C_d$; compliance of the bubble is $C_b$. (c) Simplified analogous circuit for catheter–sensor system with a bubble in the catheter, assuming that $L_{cd}$ and $R_{cd}$ are negligible with respect to $R_c$ and $L_c$.

The liquid inertance $L_c$ of the catheter is due primarily to the mass of the liquid. It can be represented by the equation

$$L_c = \frac{\Delta P}{dF/dt}\,(\mathrm{Pa \cdot s^2/m^3}) \tag{7.3}$$

or

$$L_c = \frac{\Delta P}{aA}$$

where $a$ = acceleration, m/s$^2$.

This equation reduces further to

$$L_c = \frac{m}{A^2}$$

or

$$L_c = \frac{\rho L}{\pi r^2} \tag{7.4}$$

where $m$ = mass of liquid (kg) and $\rho$ = density of liquid ($kg/m^3$).

Equations (7.2) and (7.4) show that we can neglect the resistive and inertial components of the sensor with respect to those of the liquid catheter. The reason for this is that the liquid-filled catheter is longer than the cavity of the sensor and of smaller diameter. Geddes (1970) develops a more refined model of fluid inertance—one based on kinetic-energy considerations—in which he considers that the effective mass is four-thirds times that of the fluid in the catheter.

The compliance $C_d$ of the sensor diaphragm is given by the equation

$$C_d = \frac{\Delta V}{\Delta P} = \frac{1}{E_d}$$

where $E_d$ is the volume modulus of elasticity of the sensor diaphragm.

We can find the relationship between the input voltage $v_i$, analogous to applied pressure, and the output voltage $v_o$, analogous to pressure at the diaphragm, by using Kirchhoff's voltage law. Thus,

$$v_i(t) = \frac{L_c C_d d^2 v_o(t)}{dt^2} + \frac{R_c C_d d v_o(t)}{dt} + v_o(t) \tag{7.5}$$

Using the general form of a second-order system equation derived in Section 1.10, we can show that the natural undamped frequency $\omega_n$ is $1/(L_c C_d)^{1/2}$ and that the damping ratio $\zeta$ is $(R_c/2)(C_d/L_c)^{1/2}$. For the hydraulic system under study, by substituting (7.2) and (7.4) into the expressions for $\omega_n$ and $\zeta$, we can show that

$$f_n = \frac{r}{2}\left(\frac{1}{\pi \rho L}\frac{\Delta P}{\Delta V}\right)^{1/2} \tag{7.6}$$

and

$$\zeta = \frac{4\eta}{r^3}\left(\frac{L(\Delta V/\Delta P)}{\pi \rho}\right)^{1/2} \tag{7.7}$$

Table 7.1 lists a number of useful relationships and pertinent constants.

We can study the transient response and the frequency response of the catheter–sensor system by means of the analogous electric circuit. In addition, we can study the effects of changes in the hydraulic system by adding appropriate elements to the circuit. For example, an air bubble in the liquid makes the system more compliant. Thus its effect on the system is the same as

**Table 7.1 Mechanical Characteristics of Fluids**

| Parameter | Substance | Temperature | Value |
|---|---|---|---|
| $\eta$ | Water | 20 °C | 0.001 Pa·s |
| $\eta$ | Water | 37 °C | 0.0007 Pa·s |
| $\eta$ | Air | 20 °C | 0.000018 Pa·s |
| $\rho$ | Air | 20 °C | 1.21 kg/m$^3$ |
| $\Delta V/\Delta P$ | Water | 20 °C | $0.53 \times 10^{-15}$m$^5$/N per ml volume |
| $\eta$ | Blood | All | $\cong 4 \times \eta$ for water |

that caused by connecting an additional capacitor in parallel to that representing the diaphragm compliance. Example 7.1 illustrates how the analogous circuit is used.

**EXAMPLE 7.1** A 5 mm-long air bubble has formed in the rigid-walled catheter connected to a Statham P23Dd sensor. The catheter is 1 m long, 6 French diameter, and filled with water at 20 °C. (The isothermal compression of air $\Delta V/\Delta P$ is 1 ml/cm of water pressure per liter of volume.) Plot the frequency-response curve of the system with and without the bubble. (Internal radius of the catheter is 0.46 mm; volume modulus of elasticity of the diaphragm is $0.49 \times 10^{15}$ N/m$^5$.)

**ANSWER** The analogous circuit for the hydraulic system with and without the bubble is shown in Figure 7.8(b) and (c). We can calculate the values of the natural frequency $f_n$ and the damping ratio $\zeta$ without the bubble by using (7.6) and (7.7). That is,

$$f_n = \frac{r}{2}\left(\frac{1}{\pi L}\frac{\Delta P}{\rho \Delta V}\right)^{1/2}$$
$$= \frac{0.046 \times 10^{-2}}{2}\left(\frac{1}{\pi(1)}\frac{0.49 \times 10^{15}}{1 \times 10^3}\right)^{1/2} = 91 \text{ Hz}$$
$$\zeta = \frac{4\eta}{r^3}\left(\frac{L}{\pi\rho}\frac{\Delta V}{\Delta P}\right)^{1/2}$$
$$= \frac{4(0.001)}{(0.046 \times 10^{-2})^3}\left(\frac{1}{\pi}\frac{1}{(1 \times 10^3)(0.49 \times 10^{15})}\right)^{1/2} = 0.033$$

The frequency response for the catheter–sensor system is shown in Figure 7.9.

The next step is to calculate the new values of $\zeta$ and $f_n$, for the case in which a bubble is present. Because the two capacitors are in parallel, the total capacitance for the circuit is equal to the sum of these two. That is,

$$C_t = C_d + C_b \tag{7.8}$$

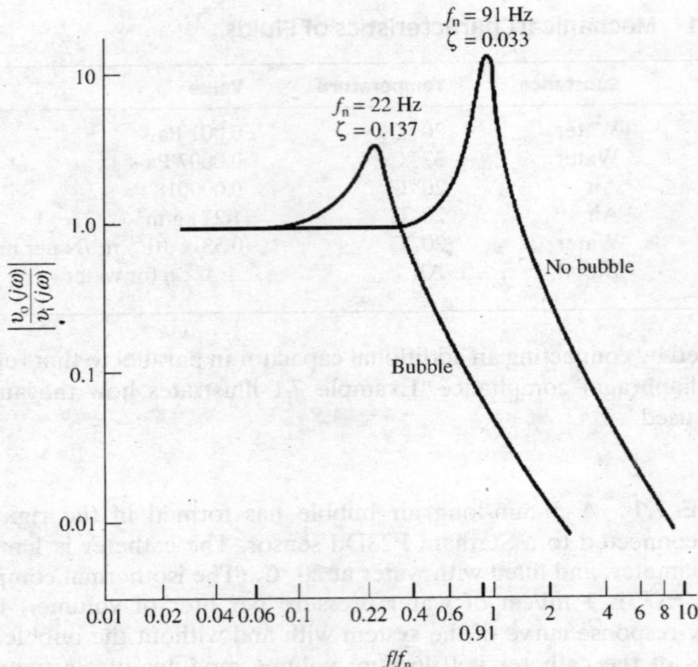


**Figure 7.9** Frequency-response curves for catheter–sensor system with and without bubbles. Natural frequency decreases from 91 to 22 Hz and damping ratio increases from 0.033 to 0.137 with the bubble present.

or

$$C_t = \frac{\Delta V}{\Delta P_d} + \frac{\Delta V}{\Delta P_b}$$

The value of $\Delta V/\Delta P_d = 1/E_d = 2.04 \times 10^{-15}\ \mathrm{m^5/N}$. The volume of the bubble is

$$\pi r^2 l = 3.33 \times 10^{-9}\ \mathrm{m^3} = 3.33 \times 10^{-6}\ \text{liter}$$

One centimeter of water pressure is 98.5 N/m². Thus

$$\Delta V/\Delta P_b = \frac{3.33 \times 10^{-9} 1 \times (1 \times 10^{-3} \mathrm{m^3/1})}{98.5\ \mathrm{N/m^2}} = 3.38 \times 10^{-14}\ \mathrm{m^5/N}$$

Consequently, $C_t = 3.38 \times 10^{-14}\ \mathrm{m^5/N}$. We can find the new values for $f_n$ and $\zeta$ by referring to (7.6) and (7.7) and assuming that the only parameter that changes is the value of $\Delta V/\Delta P$. Thus

$$f_{n,\,\text{bubble}} = f_{n,\,\text{no bubble}} \left( \frac{\Delta P \Delta V_{\text{total}}}{\Delta P/\Delta V_{\text{no bubble}}} \right)^{1/2}$$

or

$$f_{n,\,\text{bubble}} = 92\left(\frac{2.04 \times 10^{-15}}{3.38 \times 10^{-14}}\right)^{1/2} = 22\,\text{Hz}$$

and

$$\zeta_{\text{bubble}} = \zeta_{\text{no bubble}}\left(\frac{\Delta V/\Delta P_{\text{total}}}{\Delta V/\Delta P_{\text{no bubble}}}\right)^{1/2} = 0.137$$

The frequency response for the system with the bubble present is shown in Figure 7.9. Note that the bubble lowers $f_n$ and increases $\zeta$. This lowering of $f_n$ may cause distortion problems with the higher harmonics of the blood-pressure waveform.

**EXAMPLE 7.2** By changing only the radius of the catheter, redesign the (no-bubble) catheter of Figure 7.9 to achieve the damping ratio $\zeta = 1$. Calculate the resulting natural frequency $f_n$.

**ANSWER** From Eq. (7.7), $r^3/r_0^3 = \zeta/\zeta_0$.

$$r^3 = (1.0/0.033)(0.46\,\text{mm})^3 = 0.0032 \quad r = 0.147\,\text{mm}$$

From Eq. (7.6), $f_n/f_{n0} = r/r_0$,

$$f_n = 91(0.147)/(0.5) = 29\,\text{Hz}$$

**EXAMPLE 7.3** Water is not a perfect liquid because it has a finite volume modulus of elasticity. Therefore, a theoretical upper limit of high-frequency response exists for a water-filled sensor–catheter system. Find the maximal $f_n$ for a sensor that has a 0.50 ml liquid chamber and that is connected to the pressure source by means of a #20 ($r = 0.29\,\text{mm}$) 50 mm-long steel needle.

**ANSWER** A steel needle is used for the catheter, so the volume modulus of elasticity of the catheter is assumed to be zero. We do not consider the volume modulus of elasticity of the diaphragm because we want the theoretical upper limit of frequency response. Thus $\Delta V/\Delta P$ for this example is that of water, $0.53 \times 10^{-15}\,\text{m}^5/\text{N}$ per milliliter volume. The total volume of the water is equal to the volume of the liquid chamber of the sensor plus the volume of the cylindrical needle.

$$V_t = 0.5 + \pi(0.029)^2(5)\,\text{ml} = 0.513\,\text{ml}$$

$$\left(\frac{\Delta V}{\Delta P}\right)_{\text{water}} = (0.53 \times 10^{-15})(0.513) = 0.272 \times 10^{-15}\,\text{m}^5/\text{N}$$

$$f_n = \frac{0.029 \times 10^{-2}}{2}\left(\frac{1}{\pi(0.05)(1000)(0.27 \times 10^{-15})}\right)^{1/2} = 700\,\text{Hz}$$

## 7.4 MEASUREMENT OF SYSTEM RESPONSE

The response characteristics of a catheter–sensor system can be determined by two methods. The simplest and most straightforward technique involves measuring the transient step response for the system. A potentially more accurate method—but a more complicated one because it requires special equipment—involves measuring the frequency response of the system.

### TRANSIENT STEP RESPONSE

The basis of the transient-response method is to apply a sudden step input to the pressure catheter and record the resultant damped oscillations of the system. This is also called the *pop* technique, for reasons that will become evident in the following discussion. The transient response can be found by the method shown in Figure 7.10.

The catheter, or needle, is sealed in a tube by a screw adaptor that compresses a rubber washer against the insert. Flushing of the system is accomplished by passing excess liquid out of the three-way stopcock. The test is performed by securing a rubber membrane over the tube by means of an O-ring. Surgical-glove material is an excellent choice for the membrane. The technician pressurizes the system by squeezing the sphygmomanometer bulb, punctures the balloon with a burning match or hot soldering iron, and observes the response. The response should be observed on a recorder running at a speed that makes it possible to distinguish the individual oscillations. However, if the frequency bandwidth of the recorder is inadequate, the technician can use a storage oscilloscope or data acquisition system.

Figure 7.11 shows an example of the transient response. In this case the response represents a second-order system. The technician can measure the

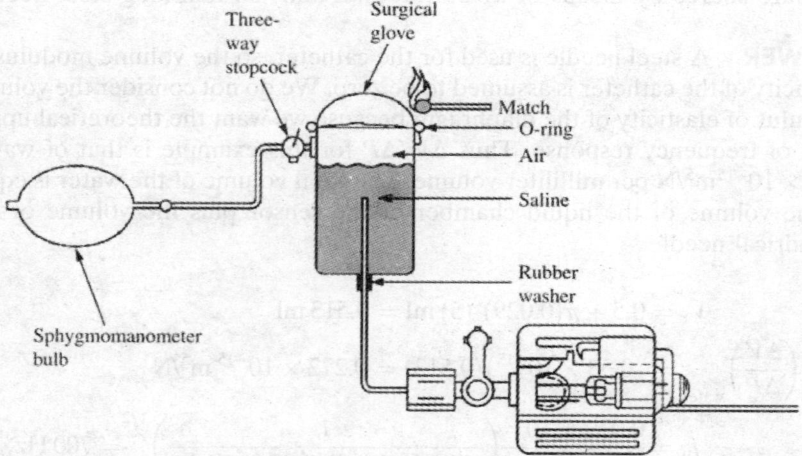


**Figure 7.10** Transient-response technique for testing a pressure-sensor–catheter-sensor system.

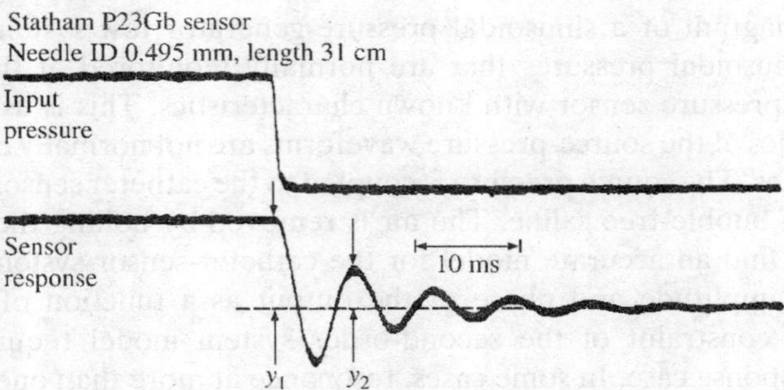


**Figure 7.11 Pressure-sensor transient response** Negative-step input pressure is recorded on the top channel; the bottom channel is sensor response for a Statham P23Gb sensor connected to a 31 cm needle (0.495 mm ID). (From I. T. Gabe, "Pressure measurement in experimental physiology," In D. H. Bergel (ed.), I, Vol. I, New York: Academic Press, 1972.)

amplitude ratio of successive positive peaks and determine the logarithmic decrement Λ. Equation (1.38) yields the damping ratio $\zeta$. The observer can measure $T$, the time between successive positive peaks, and determine the undamped natural frequency from $\omega_n = 2\pi/\left[T(1-\zeta^2)^{1/2}\right]$.

## SINUSOIDAL FREQUENCY RESPONSE

As we noted before, the sinusoidal frequency-response method is more complex because it requires more specialized equipment. Figure 7.12 is a

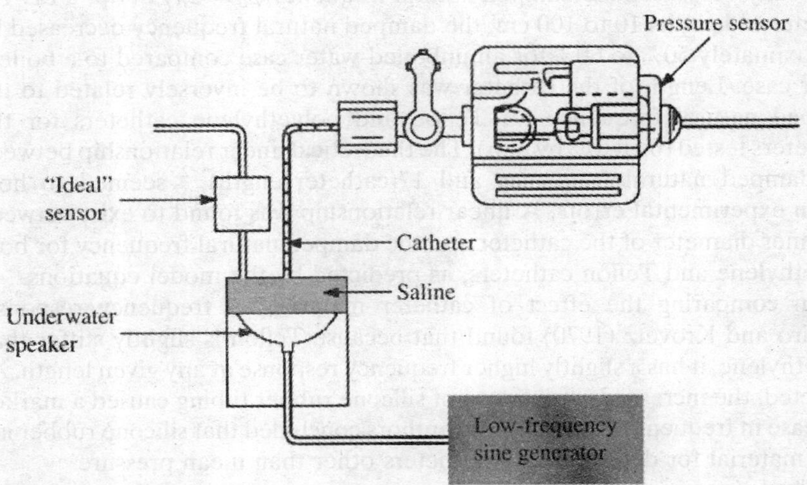


**Figure 7.12 A sinusoidal pressure-generator test system** A low-frequency sine generator drives an underwater-speaker system that is coupled to the catheter of the pressure sensor under test. An "ideal" pressure sensor, with a frequency response from 0 to 100 Hz, is connected directly to the test chamber housing and monitors input pressure.

schematic diagram of a sinusoidal pressure-generator test system. A pump produces sinusoidal pressures that are normally monitored at the pressure source by a pressure sensor with known characteristics. This is used because the amplitudes of the source-pressure waveforms are not normally constant for all frequencies. The source pressure is coupled to the catheter sensor under test by means of bubble-free saline. The air is removed by boiling the liquid.

We can find an accurate model for the catheter-sensor system by determining the amplitude and phase of the output as a function of frequency without the constraint of the second-order system model required in the transient-response case. In some cases, resonance at more than one frequency may be present.

## 7.5 EFFECTS OF SYSTEM PARAMETERS ON RESPONSE

We have shown in our discussion of the model of the catheter–sensor system that the values of the damping ratio $\zeta$ and natural frequency $\omega_n$ are functions of the various system parameters. This section reports on experimental verification of these theoretical derivations (Shapiro and Krovetz, 1970). By using step transient-response and sinusoidal pressure-generation techniques similar to those described above, these investigators determined the effects on the performance of the catheter–sensor system of de-aerating water and of using various catheter materials and connectors. They found that even minute air bubbles, which increase the compliance of the catheter manometer system, drastically decreased the damped natural frequency $\omega_d = 2\pi/T$. For a PE-190 catheter of lengths 10 to 100 cm, the damped natural frequency decreased by approximately 50% to 60% for an unboiled-water case compared to a boiled-water case. Length of the catheter was shown to be inversely related to the damped natural frequency for Teflon and polyethylene catheters for the diameters tested (0.58 to 2.69 mm). The theoretical linear relationship between the damped natural frequency and $1/(\text{catheter length})^{1/2}$ seemed to hold within experimental errors. A linear relationship was found to exist between the inner diameter of the catheter and the damped natural frequency for both polyethylene and Teflon catheters, as predicted by the model equations.

In comparing the effect of catheter material on frequency response, Shapiro and Krovetz (1970) found that because Teflon is slightly stiffer than polyethylene, it has a slightly higher frequency response at any given length. As expected, the increased compliance of silicone rubber tubing caused a marked decrease in frequency response. The authors concluded that silicone rubber is a poor material for determining parameters other than mean pressure.

They examined the effect of connectors on the system response by inserting—in series with the catheter—various connecting needles that added little to the overall length of the system. They found that the damped natural frequency was linearly related to the needle bore for needles of the same length. The connector serves as a simple series hydraulic damper that decreases the frequency response. They suggested that the fewest possible number of connectors be used and that all connectors be tight fitting and have a water seal. In further tests, they found that coils and bends in the catheter cause changes in the resonant frequency. However, the magnitude of these changes was insignificant compared with changes caused by factors that affected compliance.

## 7.6 BANDWIDTH REQUIREMENTS FOR MEASURING BLOOD PRESSURE

When we know the representative harmonic components of the blood-pressure waveform—or, for that matter, any periodic waveform—we can specify the bandwidth requirements for the instrumentation system. As with all biomedical measurements, bandwidth requirements are a function of the investigation.

For example, if the mean blood pressure is the only parameter of interest, it is of little value to try to achieve a wide bandwidth system. It is generally accepted that harmonics of the blood-pressure waveform higher than the tenth may be ignored. As an example, the bandwidth requirements for a heart rate of 120 bpm (or 2 Hz) would be 20 Hz.

For a perfect reproduction of the original waveform, there should be no distortion in the amplitude or phase characteristics. The waveshape can be preserved, however, even if the phase characteristics are not ideal. This is the case if the relative amplitudes of the frequency components are preserved but their phases are displaced in proportion to their frequency. Then the synthesized waveform gives the original waveshape, except that it is delayed in time, depending on the phase shift.

Measurements of the derivative of the pressure signal increase the bandwidth requirements, because the differentiation of a sinusoidal harmonic increases the amplitude of that component by a factor proportional to its frequency. As with the original blood-pressure waveform, a Fourier analysis of the derivative signal can estimate the bandwidth requirements for the derivative of the blood pressure. The amplitude-versus-frequency characteristics of any catheter–manometer system used for the measurement of ventricular pressures that are subsequently differentiated must remain flat to within 5%, up to the 20th harmonic (Gersh *et al.*, 1971).

## 7.7 TYPICAL PRESSURE-WAVEFORM DISTORTION

Accurate measurements of blood pressure are important in both clinical and physiological research. This section gives examples of typical types of distortion of blood-pressure waveform that are due to an inadequate frequency response of the catheter-sensor system.

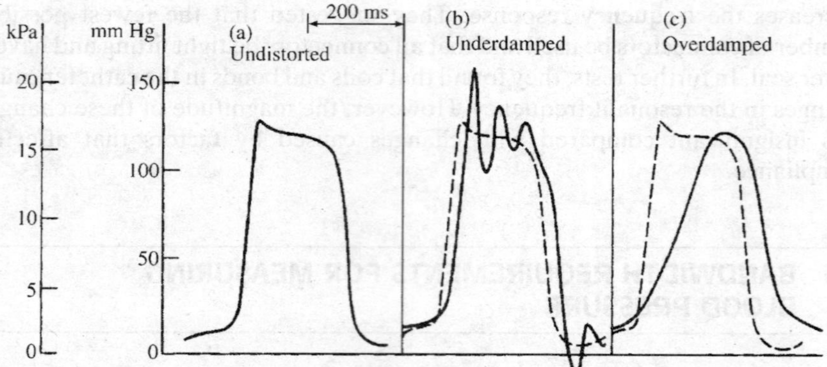


**Figure 7.13 Pressure-waveform distortion** (a) Recording of an undistorted left-ventricular pressure waveform via a pressure sensor with bandwidth dc to 100 Hz. (b) Underdamped response, where peak value is increased. A time delay is also evident in this recording. (c) Overdamped response that shows a significant time delay and an attenuated amplitude response.

There may be serious consequences when an underdamped system leads to overestimation of the pressure gradients across a stenotic (narrowed) heart valve. Figure 7.13 shows examples of distortion of pressure waveform. The actual blood-pressure waveform [Figure 7.13(a)] was recorded with a high-quality pressure sensor with a bandwidth from dc to 100 Hz. Note that in the underdamped case, the amplitude of the higher-frequency components of the pressure wave are amplified, whereas for the overdamped case these higher-frequency components are attenuated. The actual peak pressure [Figure 7.13(a)] is approximately 130 mm Hg (17.3 kPa). The underdamped response [Figure 7.13(b)] has a peak pressure of about 165 mm Hg (22 kPa), which may lead to a serious clinical error if this peak pressure is used to assess the severity of aortic-valve stenosis. The minimal pressure is in error, too; it is $-15$ mm Hg($-2$ kPa) and the actual value is 5 mm Hg (0.7 kPa). There is also a time delay of approximately 30 ms in the underdamped case.

The overdamped case [Figure 7.13(c)] shows a significant time delay of approximately 150 ms and an attenuated amplitude of 120 mm Hg (16 kPa); the actual value is 130 mm Hg (17.3 kPa). This type of response can occur in the presence of a large air bubble or a blood clot at the tip of the catheter.

An underdamped catheter–sensor system can be transformed to an overdamped system by pinching the catheter. This procedure increases the damping ratio $\zeta$ and has little effect on the natural frequency. (See Problem 7.6.)

Another example of distortion in blood-pressure measurements is known as *catheter whip*. Figure 7.14 shows these low-frequency oscillations that appear in the blood-pressure recording. This may occur when an aortic ventricular catheter, in a region of high pulsatile flow, is bent and whipped about by the accelerating blood. This type of distortion can be minimized by

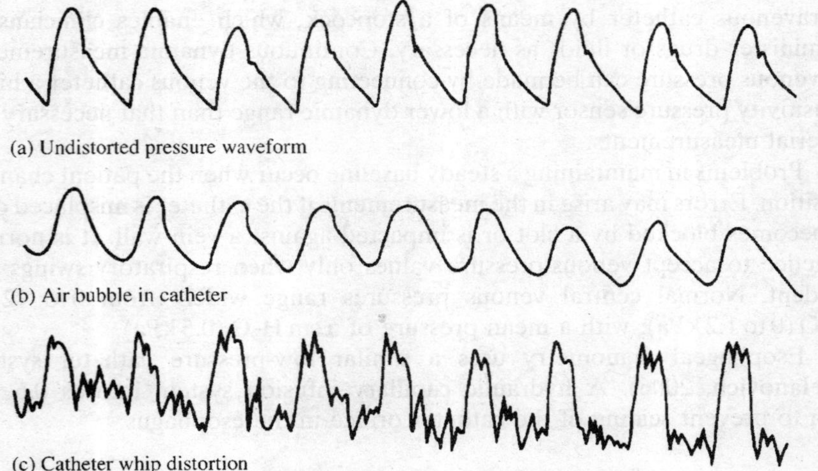


**Figure 7.14 Distortion during the recording of arterial pressure** The bottom trace is the response when the pressure catheter is bent and whipped by accelerating blood in regions of high pulsatile flow.

the use of stiff catheters or by careful placement of catheters in regions of low flow velocity.

## 7.8 SYSTEMS FOR MEASURING VENOUS PRESSURE

Measurements of venous pressure are an important aid to the physician for determining the function of the capillary bed and the right side of the heart. The pressure in the small veins is lower than the capillary pressure and reflects the value of the capillary pressure. The intrathoracic venous pressure determines the diastolic filling pressure of the right ventricle (Rushmer, 1970). The central venous pressure is measured in a central vein or in the right atrium. It fluctuates above and below atmospheric pressure as the subject breathes, whereas the extrathoracic venous pressure is 2 to 5 cm $H_2O$ (0.2 to 0.5 kPa) above atmospheric. The reference level for venous pressure is at the right atrium.

Central venous pressure is an important indicator of myocardial performance. It is normally monitored on surgical and medical patients to assess proper therapy in cases of heart dysfunction, shock, hypovolemic or hypervolemic states, or circulatory failure. It is used as a guide to determine the amount of liquid a patient should receive.

Physicians usually measure steady state or mean venous pressure by making a percutaneous venous puncture with a large-bore needle, inserting a catheter through the needle into the vein, and advancing it to the desired position. The needle is then removed. A plastic tube is attached to the intravenous catheter by means of a stopcock, which enables clinicians to administer drugs or fluids as necessary. Continuous dynamic measurements of venous pressure can be made by connecting to the venous catheter a high-sensitivity pressure sensor with a lower dynamic range than that necessary for arterial measurements.

Problems in maintaining a steady baseline occur when the patient changes position. Errors may arise in the measurements if the catheter is misplaced or if it becomes blocked by a clot or is impacted against a vein wall. It is normal practice to accept venous-pressure values only when respiratory swings are evident. Normal central venous pressures range widely from 0 to 12 cm $H_2O$ (0 to 1.2 kPa), with a mean pressure of 5 cm $H_2O$ (0.5 kPa).

Esophageal manometry uses a similar low-pressure catheter system (Velanovich, 2006). A hydraulic capillary infusion system infuses 0.6 ml/min to prevent sealing of the catheter orifice in the esophagus.

## 7.9 HEART SOUNDS

The auscultation of the heart gives the clinician valuable information about the functional integrity of the heart. More information becomes available when clinicians compare the temporal relationships between the heart sounds and the mechanical and electric events of the cardiac cycle. This latter approach is known as *phonocardiography*.

There is a wide diversity of opinion concerning the theories that attempt to explain the origin of heart sounds and murmurs. More than 40 different mechanisms have been proposed to explain the first heart sound. A basic definition shows the difference between heart sounds and murmurs (Rushmer, 1970). Heart sounds are vibrations or sounds due to the acceleration or deceleration of blood, whereas murmurs are vibrations or sounds due to blood turbulence.

### MECHANISM AND ORIGIN

Figure 7.15 shows how the four heart sounds are related to the electric and mechanical events of the cardiac cycle. The first heart sound is associated with the movement of blood during ventricular systole (Rushmer, 1970). As the ventricles contract, blood shifts toward the atria, closing the atrioventricular valves with a consequential oscillation of blood. The first heart sound further originates from oscillations of blood between the descending root of the aorta and ventricle and from vibrations due to blood turbulence at the aortic and pulmonary valves. Splitting of the first heart sound is defined as an asynchronous closure of the tricuspid and mitral valves. The second heart sound is a low-frequency vibration associated with the deceleration and reversal of flow in the aorta and pulmonary artery and with the closure of the semilunar valves (the valves situated between the ventricles and the aorta or the pulmonary trunk).

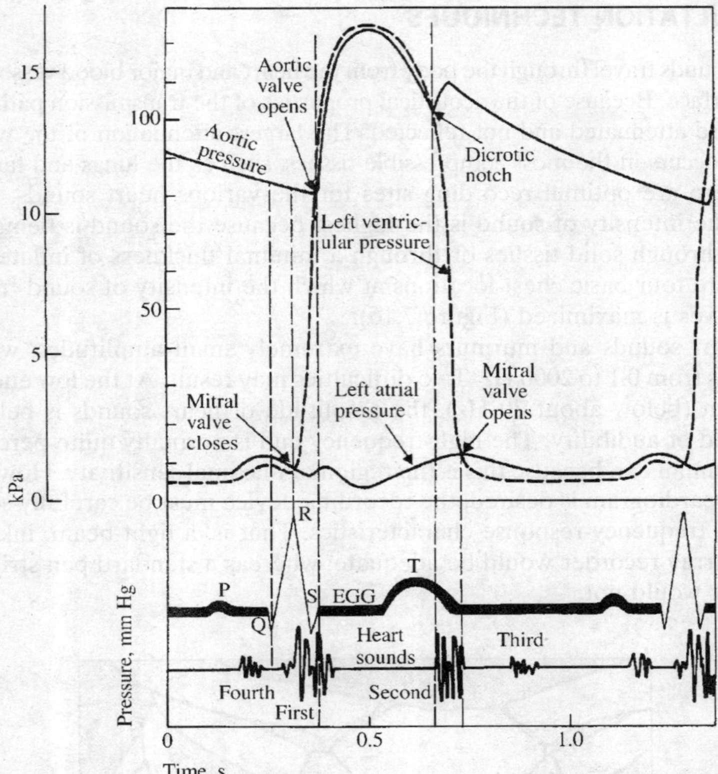


**Figure 7.15** Correlation of the four heart sounds with electric and mechanical events of the cardiac cycle.

This second heart sound is coincident with the completion of the T wave of the ECG.

The third heart sound is attributed to the sudden termination of the rapid-filling phase of the ventricles from the atria and the associated vibration of the ventricular muscle walls, which are relaxed. This low-amplitude, low-frequency vibration is audible in children and in some adults.

The fourth or atrial heart sound—which is not audible but can be recorded by the phonocardiogram—occurs when the atria contract and propel blood into the ventricles.

The sources of most murmurs, developed by turbulence in rapidly moving blood, are known. Murmurs during the early systolic phase are common in children, and they are normally heard in nearly all adults after exercise. Abnormal murmurs may be caused by stenoses and insufficiencies (leaks) at the aortic, pulmonary, and mitral valves. They are detected by noting the time of their occurrence in the cardiac cycle and their location at the time of measurement.

## AUSCULTATION TECHNIQUES

Heart sounds travel through the body from the heart and major blood vessels to the body surface. Because of the acoustical properties of the transmission path, sound waves are attenuated and not reflected. The largest attenuation of the wavelike motion occurs in the most compressible tissues, such as the lungs and fat layers.

There are optimal recording sites for the various heart sounds, sites at which the intensity of sound is the highest because the sound is being transmitted through solid tissues or through a minimal thickness of inflated lung. There are four basic chest locations at which the intensity of sound from the four valves is maximized (Figure 7.16).

Heart sounds and murmurs have extremely small amplitudes, with frequencies from 0.1 to 2000 Hz. Two difficulties may result. At the low end of the spectrum (below about 20 Hz), the amplitude of heart sounds is below the threshold of audibility. The high-frequency end is normally quite perceptible to the human ear, because this is the region of maximal sensitivity. However, if a phonocardiogram is desired, the recording device must be carefully selected for high frequency-response characteristics. That is, a light-beam, ink-jet, or digital-array recorder would be adequate, whereas a standard pen strip-chart recorder would not.

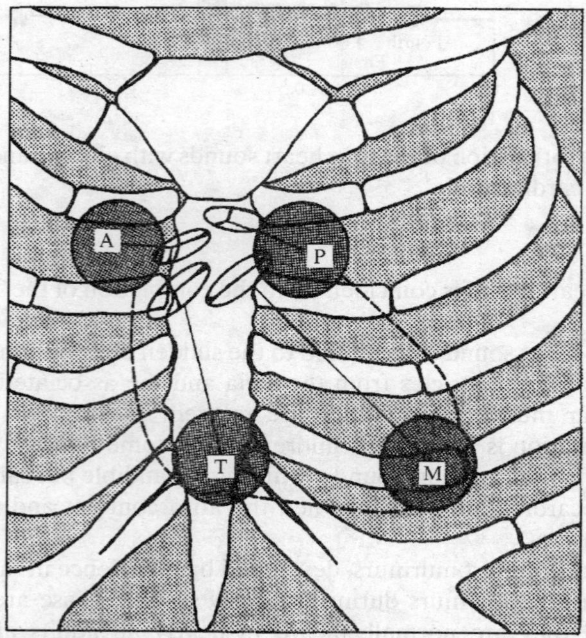


**Figure 7.16 Auscultatory areas on the chest** A, aortic; P, pulmonary; T, tricuspid; and M, mitral areas. (From A. C. Burton, *Physiology and Biophysics of the Circulation*, 2nd ed. Copyright © 1972 by Year Book Medical Publishers, Inc., Chicago. Used by permission.)

Because heart sounds and murmurs are of low amplitude, extraneous noises must be minimized in the vicinity of the patient. It is standard procedure to record the phonocardiogram for nonbedridden patients in a specially designed, acoustically quiet room. Artifacts from movements of the patient appear as baseline wandering.

## STETHOSCOPES

Stethoscopes are used to transmit heart sounds from the chest wall to the human ear. Some variability in interpretation of the sounds stems from the user's auditory acuity and training. Moreover, the technique used to apply the stethoscope can greatly affect the sounds perceived.

Ertel *et al.* (1966a; 1966b) have investigated the acoustics of stethoscope transmission and the acoustical interactions of human ears with stethoscopes. They found that stethoscope acoustics reflected the acoustics of the human ear. Younger individuals revealed slightly better responses to a stethoscope than their elders. The mechanical stethoscope amplifies sound because of a standing-wave phenomenon that occurs at quarter wavelengths of the sound. Figure 7.17 is a typical frequency-response curve for a stethoscope; it shows that the mechanical stethoscope has an uneven frequency response, with many resonance peaks.

These investigators emphasized that the critical area of the performance of a stethoscope (the clinically significant sounds near the listener's threshold of hearing) may be totally lost if the stethoscope attenuates them as little 3 dB.

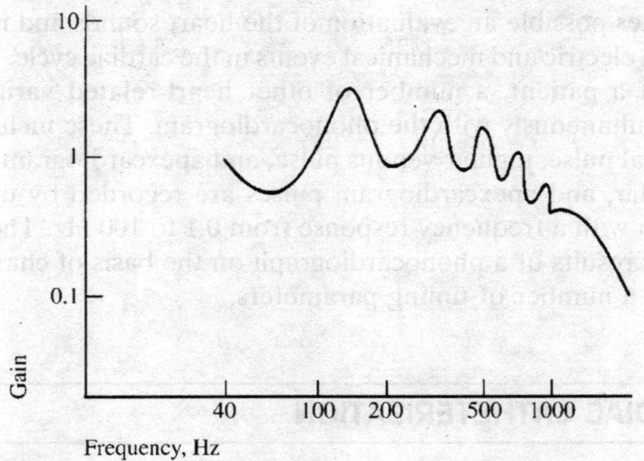


**Figure 7.17** The typical frequency-response curve for a stethoscope can be found by applying a known audio-frequency signal to the bell of a stethoscope by means of a headphone-coupler arrangement. The audio output of the stethoscope earpiece was monitored by means of a coupler microphone system. (From Ertel *et al.* (1966); by permission of American Heart Association.)

A physician may miss, with one instrument, sounds that can be heard with another.

When the stethoscope chest piece is firmly applied, low frequencies are attenuated more than high frequencies. The stethoscope housing is in the shape of a bell. It makes contact with the skin, which serves as the diaphragm at the bell rim. The diaphragm becomes taut with pressure, thereby causing an attenuation of low frequencies.

Loose-fitting earpieces cause additional problems, because the leak that develops reduces the coupling between the chest wall and the ear, with a consequent decrease in the listener's perception of heart sounds and murmurs.

Stethoscopes are also useful for listening to the sounds caused by airflow obstruction or lung collapse (Loudon and Murphy, 2006).

Engineers have proposed many types of electronic stethoscopes. These devices have selectable frequency-response characteristics ranging from the "ideal" flat-response case and selected bandpasses to typical mechanical-stethoscope responses. Physicians, however, have not generally accepted these electronic stethoscopes, mainly because they are unfamiliar with the sounds heard with them. Their size, portability, convenience, and resemblance to the mechanical stethoscope are other important considerations.

## 7.10 PHONOCARDIOGRAPHY

A phonocardiogram is a recording of the heart sounds and murmurs (Vermariën, 2006). It eliminates the subjective interpretation of these sounds and also makes possible an evaluation of the heart sounds and murmurs with respect to the electric and mechanical events in the cardiac cycle. In the clinical evaluation of a patient, a number of other heart-related variables may be recorded simultaneously with the phonocardiogram. These include the ECG, carotid arterial pulse, jugular venous pulse, and apexcardiogram. The indirect carotid, jugular, and apexcardiogram pulses are recorded by using a microphone system with a frequency response from 0.1 to 100 Hz. The cardiologist evaluates the results of a phonocardiograph on the basis of changes in waveshape and in a number of timing parameters.

## 7.11 CARDIAC CATHETERIZATION

The cardiac-catheterization procedure is a combination of several techniques that are used to assess hemodynamic function and cardiovascular structure. Cardiac catheterization is performed in virtually all patients in whom heart surgery is contemplated. This procedure yields information that may be crucial in defining the timing, risks, and anticipated benefit for a given patient (Grossman, 1974). Catheterization procedures are performed in specialized laboratories outfitted with x-ray equipment for visualizing heart structures and the position of various pressure catheters. In addition, measurements are made of cardiac output, blood and respiratory gases, blood-oxygen saturation, and metabolic products. The injection of radiopaque dyes into the ventricles or aorta makes it possible for the clinician to assess ventricular or aortic function. In a similar fashion, injection of radiopaque dyes into the coronary arteries makes possible a clinical evaluation of coronary-artery disease. In the following paragraphs, we shall discuss a number of specific procedures carried out in a catheter laboratory.

Clinicians can measure pressures in all four chambers of the heart and in the great vessels by positioning catheters, during fluoroscopy, in such a way that they can recognize the characteristic pressure waveforms. They measure pressures across the four valves to determine the valves' pressure gradients.

An example of a patient with aortic stenosis will help illustrate the procedure. Figure 7.18(a) shows the pressures of the stenotic patient before the operation: Note the pressures in the left ventricle and in the aorta and the systolic pressure gradient. Figure 7.18(b) reflects the situation after the operation: Note the marked decrease in the pressure gradient brought about by the insertion of a ball-valve aortic prosthesis. These pressures may be measured by using a two-lumen catheter positioned such that the valve is located between the two catheter openings. The clinician can find the various time indices that describe the injection and filling periods of the heart directly from the recordings of blood pressure in the heart.

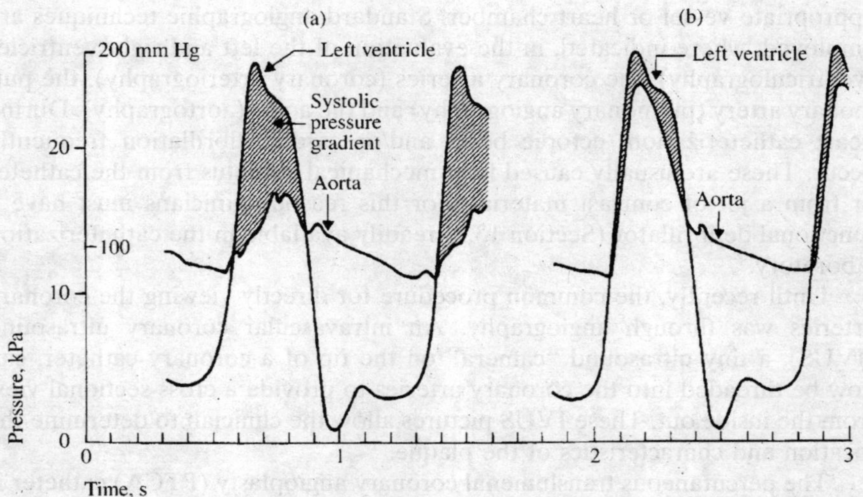


**Figure 7.18** (a) Systolic pressure gradient (left ventricular aortic pressure) across a stenotic aortic valve. (b) Marked decrease in systolic pressure gradient with insertion of an aortic ball valve.

Clinicians can also use balloon-tipped, flow-directed catheters without fluoroscopy (Ganz and Swan, 1974). An inflated balloon at the catheter tip is carried by the bloodstream from the intrathoracic veins through the right atrium, ventricle, and pulmonary artery and into a small pulmonary artery—where it is wedged, blocking the local flow. The wedge pressure in this pulmonary artery reflects the mean pressure in the left atrium, because a column of stagnant blood on the right side of the heart joins the free-flowing blood beyond the capillary bed.

This catheter is also commonly used to measure cardiac output using the principle of thermodilution. Cardiac output is valuable for assessing the pumping function of the heart and can also be measured using dye dilution, the Fick method, and impedance cardiography (Sections 8.1, 8.2 and 8.7).

Blood samples can be drawn from within the various heart chambers and vessels where the catheter tip is positioned. These blood samples are important in determining the presence of shunts between the heart chambers or great vessels. For example, a shunt from the left to the right side of the heart is indicated by a higher-than-normal $O_2$ content in the blood in the right heart in the vicinity of the shunt. The $O_2$ content is normally determined by an oximeter (Section 10.3). Cardiac blood samples are also used to assess such metabolic end products as lactate, pyruvate, $CO_2$, and such injected substances as radioactive materials and colored dyes.

Angiographic visualization is an essential tool used to evaluate cardiac structure. Radiopaque dye is injected rapidly into a cardiac chamber or blood vessel, and the hemodynamics are viewed and recorded on x-ray film, movie film, or videotape. (In Section 12.6 we will discuss the principles of radiography and fluoroscopy.) Specially designed catheters and power injectors are used in order that a bolus of contrast material can be delivered rapidly into the appropriate vessel or heart chamber. Standard angiographic techniques are employed, where indicated, in the evaluation of the left and right ventricles (ventriculography), the coronary arteries (coronary arteriography), the pulmonary artery (pulmonary angiography) and the aorta (aortography). During heart catheterization, ectopic beats and/or cardiac fibrillation frequently occur. These are usually caused by a mechanical stimulus from the catheter or from a jet of contrast material. For this reason, clinicians must have a functional defibrillator (Section 13.2) readily available in the catheterization laboratory.

Until recently, the common procedure for directly viewing the coronary arteries was through angiography. An intravascular coronary ultrasound (IVUS), a tiny ultrasound "camera" on the tip of a coronary catheter, can now be threaded into the coronary arteries to provide a cross-sectional view from the inside out. These IVUS pictures allow the clinician to determine the location and characteristics of the plaque.

The percutaneous translumenal coronary angioplasty (PTCA) catheter is used to enlarge the lumen of stenotic coronary arteries, thereby improving distal flow and relieving symptoms of ischemia and signs of myocardial hypoperfusion. After initial coronary angiography is performed and the coronary lesions are adequately visualized, a guiding catheter is introduced and passed around the aortic arch. The PTCA catheter is then placed over the guide wire and connected to a manifold (for pressure recording and injections) and to the inflation device. The guide wire is generally advanced into the coronary artery, across from and distal to the lesion to be dilated. A balloon catheter is advanced over the wire and placed across the stenosis. The pressure gradient across the stenosis is measured by using the pressure lumens on the PTCA catheter. This measurement is done to determine the severity of the stenosis. The balloon is repeatedly inflated—usually for 30 to 60 s each time—until the stenosis is fully expanded. Test injections are performed to determine whether the coronary artery flow has been improved. (Clinicians observe the distal runoff by using a radiopaque dye.)

A successful PTCA is an alternative to coronary by-pass surgery for a large proportion of patients with coronary artery disease. It avoids the morbidity associated with thoracotomy, cardiopulmonary by-pass, and general anesthesia. In addition, the hospital stay is much shorter. The patient can be discharged about a day after the procedure. Restenosis following coronary angioplasty has been shown to recur in 15% to 35% of cases. In order to help prevent restenosis a stent is commonly inserted. The stent, an expandable metal mesh tube, acts as a scaffold at the site of the blockage. It pushes against the intima of the artery to keep it open. Stenting has helped to reduce the stenosis reclosure rate. However, restenosis still occurs within a year of angioplasty or even longer because of cell regrowth. The use of drug-eluding stents, which release a drug over time directly to the artery intima most likely to reblock have been shown to significantly reduce the restenosis rate to low single digits.

Areas of a valve orifice can be calculated from basic fluid-mechanics equations (Herman *et al.*, 1974). Physicians can assess valvular stenosis by measuring the pressure gradient across the valve of interest and the flow through it.

Bernoulli's equation for frictionless flow (Burton, 1972) is

$$P_t = P + \rho g h + \frac{\rho u^2}{2} \tag{7.9}$$

where

$P_t$ = fluid total pressure

$P$ = local fluid static pressure

$\rho$ = fluid density

$g$ = acceleration of gravity (Appendix A.1)

$h$ = height above reference level

$u$ = fluid velocity

We first assume frictionless flow for the model shown in Figure 7.19 and equate total pressures at locations 1 and 2. We assume that the difference in

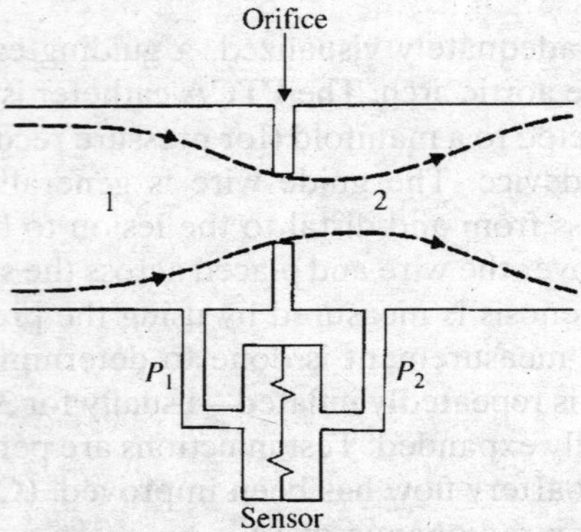


**Figure 7.19 Model for deriving equation for heart-valve orifice area** $P_1$ and $P_2$ are upstream and downstream static pressures. Velocity $u$ is calculated for minimal flow area $A$ at location 2.

heights is negligible and that the velocity at location 1 is negligible compared with $u$, the velocity at location 2. Then (7.9) reduces to

$$P_1 - P_2 = \frac{\rho u^2}{2} \tag{7.10}$$

from which

$$u = \left(\frac{2(P_1 - P_2)}{\rho}\right)^{1/2}$$

At location 2, the flow $F = Au$, where $A$ is the area. Hence

$$A = \frac{F}{u} = F\left(\frac{\rho}{2(P_1 - P_2)}\right)^{1/2} \tag{7.11}$$

In practice, there are losses due to friction, and the minimal flow area is smaller than the orifice area. Hence (7.10) becomes

$$A = \frac{F}{c_\mathrm{d}}\left(\frac{\rho}{2(P_1 - P_2)}\right)^{1/2} \tag{7.12}$$

where $c_\mathrm{d}$ is a discharge coefficient. It has been found empirically that for semilunar valves, septal defects, and patent ductus, $c_\mathrm{d} = 0.85$, whereas for mitral valves, $c_\mathrm{d} = 0.6$ (Yellin *et al.*, 1975).

**EXAMPLE 7.4** Calculate the approximate area of the aortic valve for the patient with the aortic and left-ventricular pressures shown in Figure 7.18(a). The patient's cardiac output was measured by thermodilution as 6400 ml/min and the heart rate as 78 bpm. Blood density is 1060 kg/m$^3$.

**ANSWER** From Figure 7.18(a), the ejection period is 0.31 s, and the average pressure drop is 7.33 kPa. During the ejection period, the flow (in SI units) is

$$\begin{aligned} F &= (6.4 \times 10^{-3}\ \mathrm{m^3/min})(1/78\ \mathrm{min/beat})(1/0.31\ \mathrm{beats/s}) \\ &= 264 \times 10^{-6}\ \mathrm{m^3/s} \end{aligned}$$

From (12) we have

$$\begin{aligned} A &= \frac{264 \times 10^{-6}}{0.85}\left(\frac{1060}{2(7330)}\right)^{1/2} \\ &= 83 \times 10^{-6}\ \mathrm{m^2} = 83\ \mathrm{mm^2} \end{aligned}$$

## 7.12 EFFECTS OF POTENTIAL AND KINETIC ENERGY ON PRESSURE MEASUREMENTS

In certain situations, the effects of potential- and kinetic-energy terms in the measurement of blood pressure may yield inaccurate results.

Bernoulli's equation (7.9) shows that the total pressure of a fluid remains constant in the absence of dissipative effects. The static pressure $P$ of the fluid is the desired pressure; it is measured in a blood vessel when the potential- and kinetic-energy terms are zero.

We first examine the effect of the potential-energy term on the static pressure of the fluid. When measurements of blood pressure are taken with the patient in a supine (on-the-back) position and with the sensor so placed that it is at heart level, no corrections need be made for the potential-energy term. However, when the patient is sitting or standing, the long columns of blood in the arterial and venous pressure systems contribute a hydrostatic pressure, $\rho gh$.

For a patient in the erect position, the arterial and venous pressure both increase to approximately 85 mm Hg (11.3 kPa) at the ankle. When the arm is held above the head, the pressure in the wrist becomes about 40 mm Hg (5.3 kPa). The sensor diaphragm should be placed at the same level as the pressure source. If this is not possible, the difference in height must be accounted for. For each 1.3 cm increase in height of the source, 1.0 mm Hg (133 Pa) must be added to the sensor reading.

The kinetic-energy term $\rho u^2/2$ becomes important when the velocity of blood flow is high. When a blood-pressure catheter is inserted into a blood vessel or into the heart, two types of pressures can be determined—side (static) and end (total) pressures. "Side pressure" implies that the end of the catheter has openings at right angles to the flow. In this case, the pressure reading is accurate because the kinetic-energy term is minimal. However, if the catheter pressure port is in line with the flow stream, then the kinetic energy of the fluid

**Table 7.2 Relative Importance of the Kinetic-Energy Term in Different Parts of the Circulation**

| Vessel | Vel (cm/s) | KE (mm Hg) | Systolic (mm Hg) | Systolic (kPa) | % KE of Total |
|---|---|---|---|---|---|
| Aorta (systolic) | | | | | |
| At rest | 100 | 4 | 120 | (16) | 3 |
| Cardiac output at 3 × rest | 300 | 36 | 180 | (24) | 17 |
| Brachial artery | | | | | |
| At rest | 30 | 0.35 | 110 | (14.7) | 0.3 |
| Cardiac output at 3 × rest | 90 | 4 | 120 | (16) | 3 |
| Venae cavae | | | | | |
| At rest | 30 | 0.35 | 2 | (0.3) | 12 |
| Cardiac output at 3 × rest | 90 | 3.2 | 3 | (0.4) | 52 |
| Pulmonary artery | | | | | |
| At rest | 90 | 3 | 20 | (2.7) | 13 |
| Cardiac output at 3 × rest | 270 | 27 | 25 | (3.3) | 52 |

SOURCE: From A. C. Burton, *Physiology and Biophysics of the Circulation*. Copyright 1972 by Year Book Medical Publishers, Inc., Chicago. Used by permission.

at that point is transformed into pressure. If the catheter pressure port faces upstream, the recorded pressure is the side pressure plus the additional kinetic-energy term $\rho u^2/2$. On the other hand, if the catheter pressure port faces downstream, the value is approximately $\rho u^2/2$ less than the side pressure. When the catheter is not positioned correctly, artifacts may develop in the pressure reading.

The data given in Table 7.2 demonstrate the relative importance of the kinetic-energy term in different parts of the circulation (Burton, 1972). As Table 7.2 shows, there are situations in the aorta, venae cavae, and pulmonary artery in which the kinetic-energy term is a substantial part of the total pressure. For the laminar-flow case, this error decreases as the catheter pressure port is moved from the center of the vessel to the vessel wall, where the average velocity of flow is less. The kinetic-energy term could also be important in a disease situation in which an artery becomes narrowed.

**EXAMPLE 7.5** Determine whether the kinetic-energy term is significant for measurements of pressure in the human descending aorta. Assume that the peak velocity of flow in the center of the aorta is approximately 1.5 m/s and that the density of the blood $\rho$ is 1060 kg/m$^3$.

**ANSWER** The kinetic energy (K.E.) term is $(1/2)\rho V^2$

$$\text{K.E.} = \frac{1}{2}(1050\,\text{kg/m}^3)(1.5\,\text{m/s})^2 = 1181\,\text{Pa}$$

or in terms of mm Hg,

$$\text{K.E.} = 1181/133 = 9\,\text{mm Hg}$$

The orientation of the pressure catheter can significantly affect the measured aortic pressure. Under laminar flow conditions, this error may be decreased by moving the tip to wall where the average flow velocity is less.

## 7.13 INDIRECT MEASUREMENTS OF BLOOD PRESSURE

Indirect measurement of blood pressure is an attempt to measure intra-arterial pressures noninvasively. The most standard manual techniques employ either the palpation or the auditory detection of the pulse distal to an occlusive cuff. Figure 7.20 shows a typical system for indirect measurement of blood pressure. It employs a sphygmomanometer consisting of an inflatable cuff for occlusion of the blood vessel, a rubber bulb for inflation of the cuff, and either a mercury or an aneroid manometer for detection of pressure.

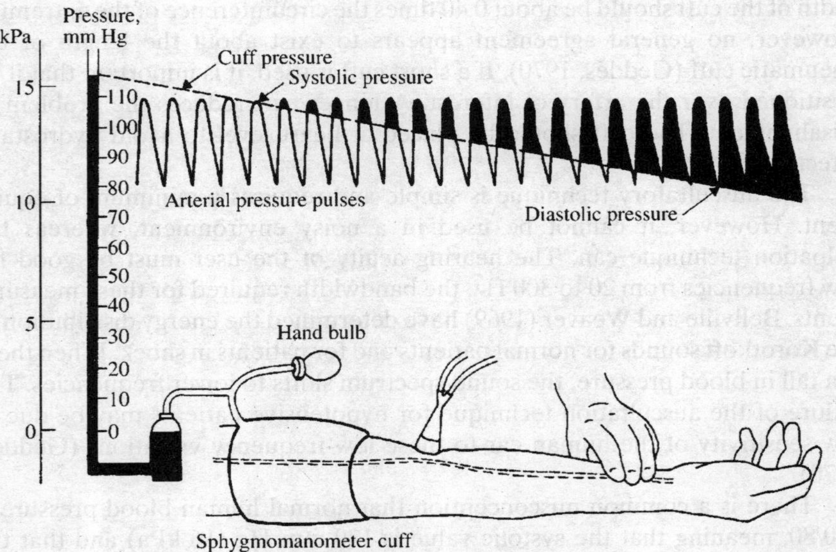


**Figure 7.20 Typical indirect blood-pressure measurement system** The sphygmomanometer cuff is inflated by a hand bulb to pressure above the systolic level. Pressure is then slowly released, and blood flow under the cuff is monitored by a microphone or stethoscope placed over a downstream artery. The first Korotkoff sound detected indicated systolic pressure, whereas the transition from muffling to silence brackets diastolic pressure. (From R.F. Rushmer, *Cardiovascular Dynamics*, 3rd ed., 1970. Philadelphia: W.B. Saunders Co. Used with permission.)

Blood pressure is measured in the following way. The occlusive cuff is inflated until the pressure is above systolic pressure and then is slowly bled off (2 to 3 mm Hg/s) (0.3 to 0.4 kPa/s). When the systolic peaks are higher than the occlusive pressure, the blood spurts under the cuff and causes a palpable pulse in the wrist (Riva–Rocci method). Audible sounds (Korotkoff sounds) generated by the flow of blood and vibrations of the vessel under the cuff are heard through a stethoscope. The manometer pressure at the first detection of the pulse indicates the systolic pressure. As the pressure in the cuff is decreased, the audible Korotkoff sounds pass through five phases (Geddes, 1970). The period of transition from muffling (phase IV) to silence (phase V) brackets the diastolic pressure.

In employing the palpation and auscultatory techniques, you should take several measurements, because normal respiration and vasomotor waves modulate the normal blood-pressure levels. These techniques also suffer from the disadvantage of failing to give accurate pressures for infants and hypotensive patients.

Using an occlusive cuff of the correct size is important if the clinician is to obtain accurate results. The pressure applied to the artery wall is assumed to be equal to that of the external cuff. However, the cuff pressure is transmitted via interposed tissue. With a cuff of sufficient width and length, the cuff pressure is evenly transmitted to the underlying artery. It is generally accepted that the width of the cuff should be about 0.40 times the circumference of the extremity. However, no general agreement appears to exist about the length of the pneumatic cuff (Geddes, 1970). If a short cuff is used, it is important that it be positioned over the artery of interest. A longer cuff reduces the problem of misalignment. The cuff should be placed at heart level to avoid hydrostatic effects.

The auscultatory technique is simple and requires a minimum of equipment. However, it cannot be used in a noisy environment, whereas the palpation technique can. The hearing acuity of the user must be good for low frequencies from 20 to 300 Hz, the bandwidth required for these measurements. Bellville and Weaver (1969) have determined the energy distribution of the Korotkoff sounds for normal patients and for patients in shock. When there is a fall in blood pressure, the sound spectrum shifts to lower frequencies. The failure of the auscultation technique for hypotensive patients may be due to low sensitivity of the human ear to these low-frequency vibrations (Geddes, 1970).

There is a common misconception that normal human blood pressure is 120/80, meaning that the systolic value is 120 mm Hg (16 kPa) and that the diastolic value is 80 mm Hg (10.7 kPa). This is not the case. A careful study (by Master *et al.*, 1952) showed that the age and sex of an individual determine the "normal value" of blood pressure.

A number of techniques have been proposed to measure automatically and indirectly the systolic and diastolic blood pressure in humans (Cobbold, 1974). The basic technique involves an automatic sphygmomanometer that inflates and deflates an occlusive cuff at a predetermined rate. A sensitive detector is used to measure the distal pulse or cuff pressure. A number of kinds of detectors have been employed, including ultrasonic, piezoelectric, photoelectric, electroacoustic, thermometric, electrocardiographic, rheographic, and tissue-impedance devices (Greatorex, 1971; Visser and Muntinga, 1990). Three of the commonly used automatic techniques are described in the following paragraphs.

The first technique employs an automated auscultatory device wherein a microphone replaces the stethoscope. The cycle of events that takes place begins with a rapid (20 to 30 mm Hg/s) (2.7 to 4 kPa/s) inflation of the occlusive cuff to a preset pressure about 30 mm Hg higher than the suspected systolic level. The flow of blood beneath the cuff is stopped by the collapse of the vessel. Cuff pressure is then reduced slowly (2 to 3 mm Hg/s) (0.3 to 0.4 kPa/s). The first Korotkoff sound is detected by the microphone, at which time the level of the cuff pressure is stored. The muffling and silent period of the Korotkoff sounds is detected, and the value of the diastolic pressure is also stored. After a few minutes, the instrument displays the systolic and diastolic pressures and recycles the operation. Design considerations for various types of automatic indirect methods of measurement of blood pressure can be found in the literature (Greatorex, 1971).

The ultrasonic determination of blood pressure employs a transcutaneous Doppler sensor that detects the motion of the blood-vessel walls in various states of occlusion. Figure 7.21 shows the placement of the compression cuff over two small transmitting and receiving ultrasound crystals (8 MHz) on the arm (Stegall *et al.*, 1968). The Doppler ultrasonic transmitted signal is focused on the vessel wall and the blood. The reflected signal (shifted in frequency) is detected by the receiving crystal and decoded (Section 8.4). The difference in frequency, in the range of 40 to 500 Hz, between the transmitted and received signals is proportional to the velocity of the wall motion and the blood velocity. As the cuff pressure is increased above diastolic but below systolic, the vessel opens and closes with each heartbeat, because the pressure in the artery oscillates above and below the applied external pressure in the cuff. The opening and closing of the vessel are detected by the ultrasonic system.

As the applied pressure is further increased, the time between the opening and closing decreases until they coincide. The reading at this point is the systolic pressure. Conversely, when the pressure in the cuff is reduced, the time between opening and closing increases until the closing signal from one pulse coincides with the opening signal from the next. The reading at this point is the diastolic pressure, which prevails when the vessel is open for the complete pulse.

The advantages of the ultrasonic technique are that it can be used with infants and hypotensive individuals and in high-noise environments. A disadvantage is that movements of the subject's body cause changes in the ultrasonic path between the sensor and the blood vessel. Complete reconstruction of the arterial-pulse waveform is also possible via the ultrasonic method. A timing pulse from the ECG signal is used as a reference. The clinician uses the pressure in the cuff when the artery opens versus the time

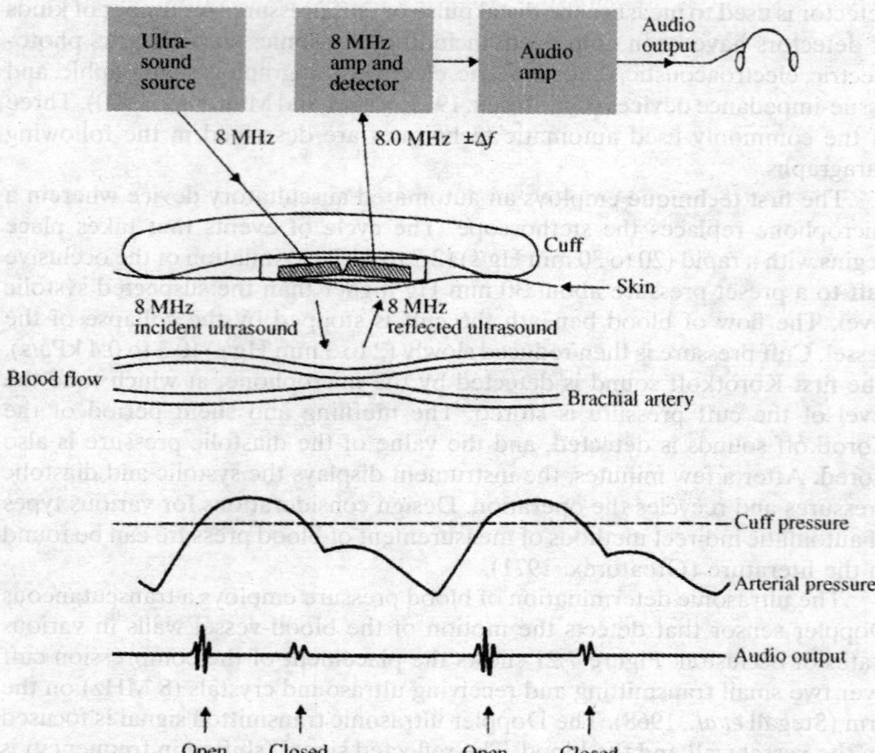


**Figure 7.21** **Ultrasonic determination of blood pressure** A compression cuff is placed over the transmitting (8 MHz) and receiving (8 MHz $\pm \Delta f$) crystals. The opening and closing of the blood vessel are detected as the applied cuff pressure is varied. (From H. F. Stegall, M. B. Kardon, and W. T. Kemmerer, "Indirect measurement of arterial blood pressure by Doppler ultrasonic sphygmomanometry." *J. Appl. Physiol.*, 1968, 25, 793–798. Used with permission.)

from the ECG R wave to plot the rising portion of the arterial pulse. Conversely, the clinician uses the cuff pressure when the artery closes versus the time from the ECG R wave to plot the falling portion of the arterial pulse.

The oscillometric method, a noninvasive blood pressure technique, measures the amplitude of oscillations that appear in the cuff pressure signal which are created by expansion of the arterial wall each time blood is forced through the artery. The uniqueness of the oscillometric method, a blood-pressure cuff technique, is that specific characteristics of the compression cuff's entrained air volume are used to identify and sense blood-pressure values. The cuff-pressure signal increases in strength in the systolic pressure region, reaching a maximum when the cuff pressure is equal to mean arterial pressure. As the cuff pressure drops below this point, the signal strength decreases proportionally to the cuff air pressure bled rate. There is no clear transition in cuff-pressure oscillations to identify diastolic pressure since arterial wall expansion continues to happen below diastolic pressure while blood is forced through the artery (Geddes, 1984). Thus, oscillometric monitors employ proprietary algorithms to estimate the diastolic pressure.

Ramsey (1991) has indicated that, using the oscillometric method, the mean arterial pressure is the single blood-pressure parameter, which is the most robust measurement, as compared with systolic and diastolic pressure, because it is measured when the oscillations of cuff pressure reach the greatest amplitude. This property usually allows mean arterial pressure to be measured reliably even in case of hypotension with vasoconstriction and diminished pulse pressure.

When the cuff pressure is raised quickly to pressures higher than systolic pressure it is observed that the radial pulse disappears. Cuff pressures above systolic cause the underlying artery to be completely occluded. However, at suprasystolic cuff pressures, small amplitude pressure oscillations occur in the cuff pressure due to artery pulsations under the upper edge of the cuff, which are communicated to the cuff through the adjacent tissues. With slow cuff-pressure reductions, when the cuff pressure is just below systolic pressure, blood spurts through the artery and the cuff-pressure oscillations become larger. Figure 7.22 illustrates the ideal case in which the cuff pressure is monitored by a pressure sensor connected to a strip chart recorder. A pressure slightly above systolic pressure is detected by determining the shift from small-amplitude oscillations at cuff pressure slightly above systolic pressure and when the cuff pressure begins to increase amplitude (point 1). As the cuff

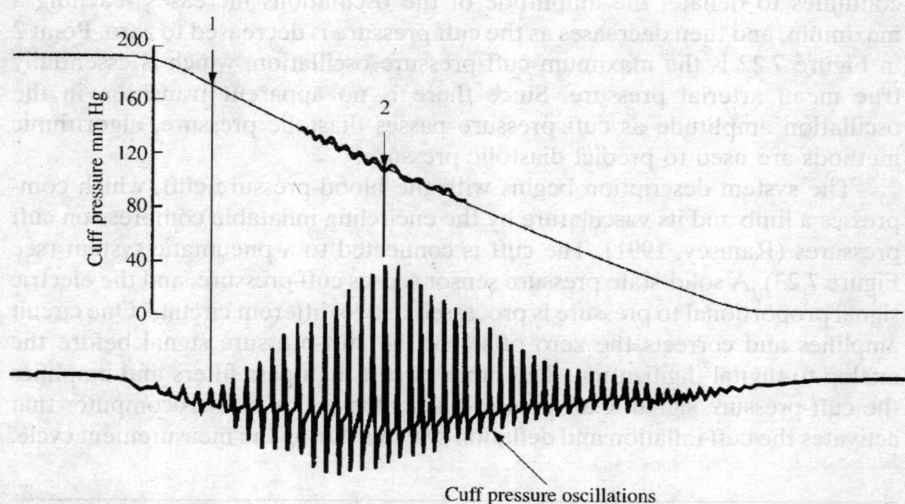


**Figure 7.22 The oscillometric method** A compression cuff is inflated above systolic pressure and slowly deflated. Systolic pressure is detected (point 1) where there is a transition from small amplitude oscillations (above systolic pressure) to increasing cuff-pressure amplitude. The cuff-pressure oscillations increase to a maximum (point 2) at the mean arterial pressure.

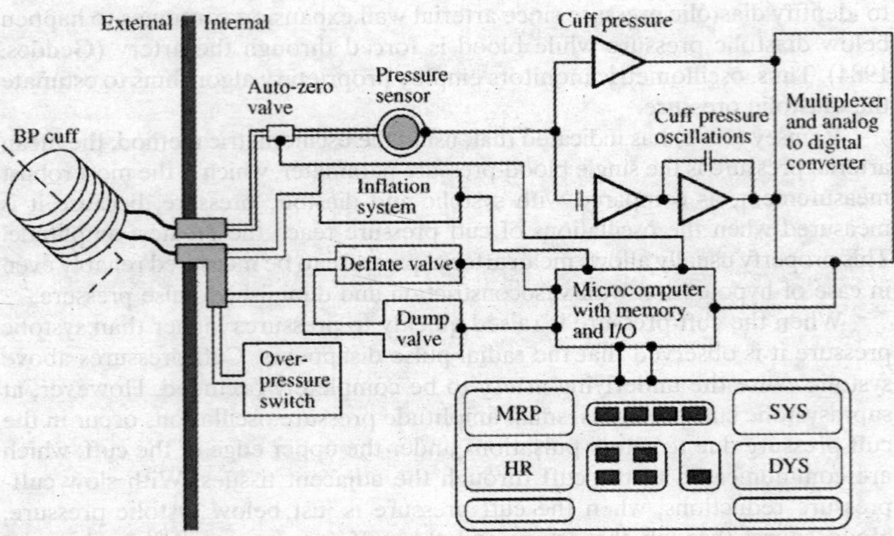


**Figure 7.23** Block diagram of the major components and subsystems of an oscillometric blood-pressure monitoring device, based on the Dinamap unit, I/O = input/output; MAP = mean arterial pressure; HR = heart rate; SYS = systolic pressure; DYS = diastolic pressure. [From Ramsey M III. Blood Pressure monitoring: automated oscillometric devices, *J. Clin. Monit.* 1991, 7, 56–67]

continues to deflate, the amplitude of the oscillations increases reaching a maximum, and then decreases as the cuff pressure is decreased to zero. Point 2 in Figure 7.22 is the maximum cuff-pressure oscillation, which is essentially true mean arterial pressure. Since there is no apparent transition in the oscillation amplitude as cuff pressure passes diastolic pressure, algorithmic methods are used to predict diastolic pressure.

The system description begins with the blood-pressure cuff, which compresses a limb and its vasculature by the encircling inflatable compression cuff pressures (Ramsey, 1991). The cuff is connected to a pneumatic system (see Figure 7.23). A solid-state pressure sensor senses cuff pressure, and the electric signal proportional to pressure is processed in two different circuits. One circuit amplifies and corrects the zero offset of the cuff-pressure signal before the analog-to-digital digitization. The other circuit high-pass filters and amplifies the cuff-pressure signal. Cuff pressure is controlled by a microcomputer that activates the cuff inflation and deflation systems during the measurement cycle.

## 7.14 TONOMETRY

The basic principle of tonometry is that, when a pressurized vessel is partly collapsed by an external object, the circumferential stresses in the vessel wall are removed and the internal and external pressures are equal. This approach has been used quite successfully to measure intra-ocular pressure and has been used with limited success to determine intraluminal arterial pressure.

The force-balance technique can be used to measure intra-ocular pressure. Based on the Imbert–Fick law, the technique enables the clinician to find intra-ocular pressure by dividing the applanation force by the area of applanation. Goldmann (1957) developed an applanation tonometer, which is the currently accepted clinical standard. With this technique, the investigator measures the force required to flatten a specific optically determined area. Mackay and Marg (1960) developed a sensor probe that is applied to the corneal surface; the cornea is flattened as the probe is advanced. The intra-ocular pressure is detected by a force sensor in the center of an annular ring, which unloads the bending forces of the cornea from the sensor.

Forbes *et al.* (1974) developed an applanation tonometer that measures intra-ocular pressure without touching the eye. An air pulse of linearly increasing force deforms and flattens the central area of the cornea, and it does so within a few milliseconds. The instrument consists of three major components. The first is a pneumatic system that delivers an air pulse the force of which increases linearly with time. As the air pulse decays, it causes a progressive reduction of the convexity of the cornea and, finally, a return to its original shape.

The second component, the system that monitors the applanation, determines the occurrence of applanation with microsecond resolution by continuously monitoring the status of the curvature of the cornea. Figure 7.24 (a) and (b) shows the systems of optical transmission and detection and the light rays reflected from an undisturbed and an applanated cornea, respectively.

Two obliquely oriented tubes are used to detect applanation. Transmitter tube T directs a collimated beam of light at the corneal vertex; a telecentric receiver R observes the same area. The light reflected from the cornea passes through the aperture A and is sensed by the detector D. In the case of the undisturbed cornea, the detector receives little or no light. As the cornea's

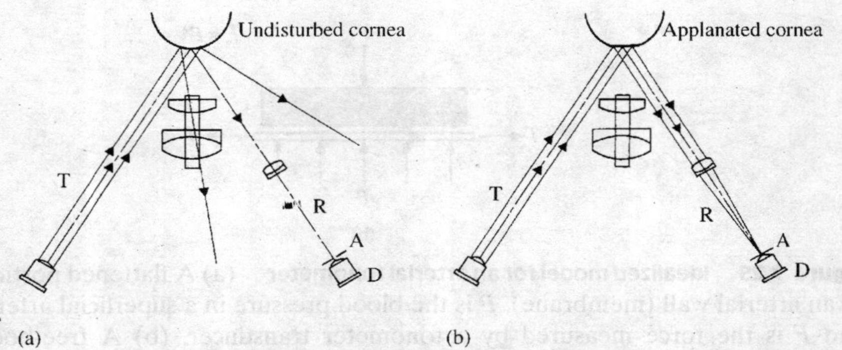


**Figure 7.24 Monitoring system for noncontact applanation tonometer** [From M. Forbes, G. Pico, Jr., and B. Grolman, "A Noncontact Applanation Tonometer, Description and Clinical Evaluation," *J. Arch. Ophthalmology*, 1975, 91, 134-140. Copyright © 1975, American Medical Association. Used with permission.]

convexity is progressively reduced to the flattened condition, the amount of light detected is increased. When the cornea is applanated, it acts like a plano-mirror with a resulting maximal detected signal. When the cornea becomes concave, a sharp reduction in light detection occurs. The current source for the pneumatic solenoid is immediately shut off when applanation is detected in order to minimize further air-pulse force impinging on the cornea. A direct linear relationship has been found between the intra-ocular pressure and the time interval to applanation.

The principles of operation of the arterial tonometry are very similar to those for the ocular tonometry, discussed above. The arterial tonometer measures dynamic arterial blood pressure, i.e., it furnishes continuous measurements of arterial pressure throughout the total heart cycle (Eckerle, 2006). The instrument sensor is placed over a superficial artery that is supported from below by bone. The radial artery at the wrist is a convenient site for arterial tonometer measurements. The arterial tonometer suffers from relatively high cost when compared to a conventional sphygmomanometer. One significant advantage of the arterial tonometer is its ability to make noninvasive, non-painful, continuous measurements for long periods of time.

Figure 7.25 shows an arterial tonometer model that depicts system operation in which the arterial blood pressure, $P$, from a superficial artery and the

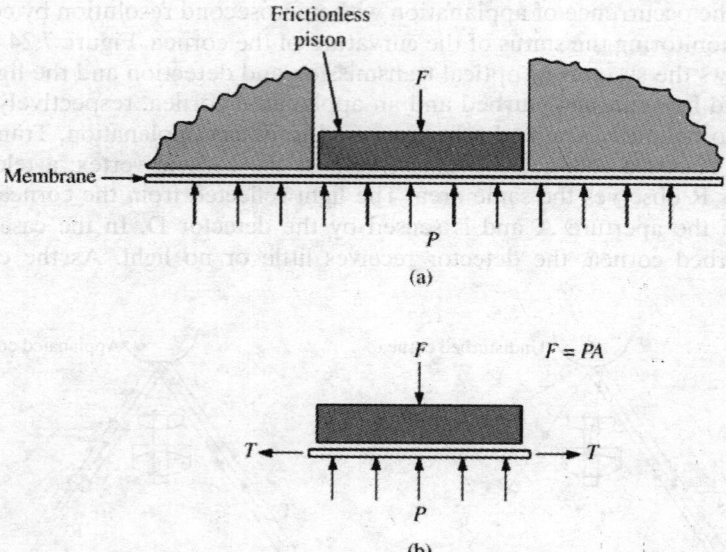


**Figure 7.25 Idealized model for an arterial tonometer** (a) A flattened portion of an arterial wall (membrane). $P$ is the blood pressure in a superficial artery, and $F$ is the force measured by a tonometer transducer. (b) A free-body diagram for the idealized model of (a) in which $T$ is the membrane tensile force perpendicular to both $F$ and $P$. [From Eckerle, J. D., "Tonometry, arterial." In J. G. Webster (ed.), *Encyclopedia of Medical Devices and Instrumentation*, 2nd ed. New York: Wiley, 2006, Vol. 6, pp. 402–410.]

force, $F$, is measured by a tonometer sensor. The artery wall is represented by a flat ideal membrane, M. A free-body diagram is used to describe the force balances. The ideal membrane only transmits a tensile force, $T$, without any bending moment. Vertical force balance shows that the tension vector, $T$, is perpendicular to the pressure vector. Thus, the force, $F$, is in quadrature to and independent of $T$ and only depends on the blood pressure and the area of the frictionless piston, $A$. Thus, measurement of the force, $F$, permits direct measurement of the intra-arterial pressure.

Eckerle (2006) indicates that several conditions must be met by the tonometer sensor and an appropriate superficial artery for proper system operation:

1. A bone provides support for the artery, opposite to the applied force.
2. The hold-down force flattens the artery wall at the measurement site without occluding the artery.
3. Compared to artery diameter, the skin thickness over the artery is insignificant.
4. The artery wall has the properties of an ideal membrane.
5. The arterial rider, positioned over the flattened area of the artery, is smaller than the artery.
6. The force transducer spring constant $K_T$ is larger than the effective spring constant of the artery.

When all these conditions hold, it has been shown on a theoretical basis that the electrical output signal of the force sensor is directly proportional to the intra-arterial blood pressure (Pressman and Newgard, 1963). However, a major practical problem with the above approach, using a single arterial tonometer, is that the arterial rider must be precisely located over the superficial artery. A solution to this problem is the use of an arterial tonometer with multiple element sensors. Figure 7.26 shows a linear array of force sensors and arterial riders positioned such that at least one element of the array is centered over the artery. A computer algorithm is used to automatically select from the multiple sensors, the sensor element which is positioned over the artery. One approach is to use two pressure distribution characteristics in the vicinity of the artery in which an element-selection algorithm searches for a (spatial) local minimum in diastolic pressure in a region near the maximum pulse amplitude (Eckerle, 2006). The sensor with these characteristics is assumed to be centered over the artery, and the blood pressure from this sensor is measured with this element.

In addition to positioning the sensor over the artery, the degree of arterial flattening is another important factor for accurate tonometric pressure measurements. The hold-down force $F_1$, (in Figure 7.26), which causes arterial flattening, is a function of the interaction of anatomical factors. The hold-down force for each subject must be determined before tonometric readings can be taken. The hold-down force is gradually increased (or decreased) while recording the tonometer sensor output.

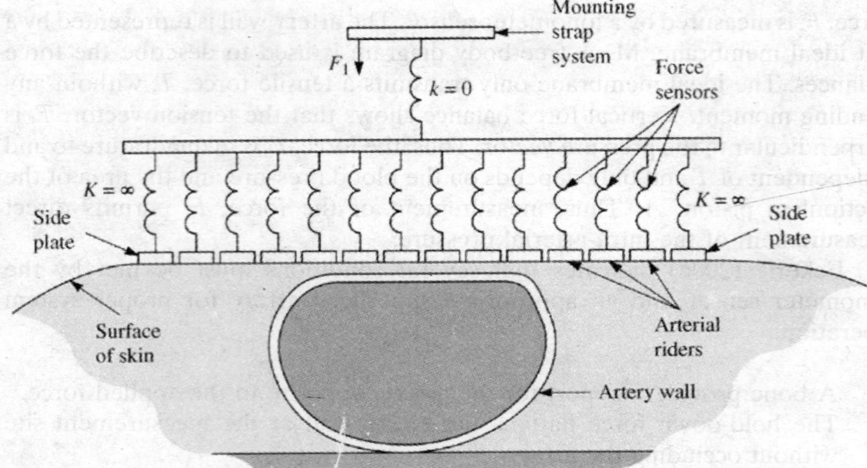


**Figure 7.26 Multiple-element arterial tonometer** The multiple element linear array of force sensors and arterial riders are used to position the system such that some element of the array is centered over the artery. [From Eckerle, J. D., "Tonometry, arterial," in J. G. Webster (ed.), *Encyclopedia of Medical Devices and Instrumentation.* 2nd ed. New York: Wiley, 2006, vol. 6, pp. 402–410.]

Multiple-element tonometer sensors have been manufactured from a monolithic silicon substrate using anisotropic etching to define pressure-sensing diaphragms (10 μm thick in the silicon). Piezoresistive strain gages in the diaphragms are fabricated using integrated-circuit (IC) processing techniques. The strain gage's resistance is used to determine the pressure exerted on each sensor element.

Note that the radial artery is not the only measurement site at which a tonometer may be applied. Other possible sites for tonometric measurements include the brachial artery at the inner elbow (the antecubital fossa), the temporal artery in front of the ear, and the dorsalis pedis artery on the upper foot (Eckerle, 2006). Arterial tonometers have not been commercially successful because of inaccuracy caused by wrist movement, tendons overlying arteries, etc.

Gizdulich and Wesseling (1990) measure the arterial pressure in the finger continuously and indirectly by using the Peñás method. They apply counter-pressure just sufficient to hold the arteries under a pressure cuff at their unstressed diameter at zero transmural pressure monitored by an infrared plethysmograph. Because the method occludes the veins, continuous use for more than 20 min causes discomfort and swelling. Thus, the pressure must be relieved periodically.

**EXAMPLE 7.6** Design a noninvasive (no breaks in the skin) system for measuring the velocity of propagation of a blood-pressure wave from the aortic valve in the heart to the radial artery on the wrist. Name and describe the sensors required, their placement, the expected waveforms, and indicate the times required to measure velocity of propagation.

**ANSWER** Place a piezoelectric pressure sensor on the neck to measure carotid pulse. Place a similar sensor on the wrist to measure radial pulse. Use a digital storage oscilloscope to display both waveforms and measure the difference in timing of pulse upstroke $t$ for the two waveforms. Measure distance from the aortic root to neck $d_n$. Measure distance from aortic root to wrist $d_w$.

$$\text{Velocity} = \text{distance/time} = (d_w - d_n)/t$$

## PROBLEMS

**7.1** Compare the transient-step and sinusoidal-frequency methods for determining the response characteristics of a catheter-sensor system.

**7.2** Find (a) the damping ratio, (b) the undamped frequency, and (c) the frequency-response curve of the pressure sensor for which the transient response to a step change in pressure is shown in Figure 7.11.

**7.3** Find the frequency-response curve of the sensor in Problem 7.2, given that its chamber is filled with the whole blood at body temperature (37 °C). The original data in Problem 7.2 were obtained with water at 20 °C.

**7.4** What happens to the frequency response of a P23Dd sensor, 6 F, 1 m, water-filled catheter system (at 20 °C) when a tiny pinhole leak occurs at the junction of the catheter and sensor? The leak allows a 0.40 ml/min flow for a pressure head of 100 mm Hg (13.3 kPa). Plot frequency-response curves for the system with and without the leak. (An intentional leak is often desirable to permit constant flushing of the catheter and thus inhibit the formation of clots.)

**7.5** A low-pass filter is added to the catheter of a pressure-sensor–catheter-sensor system by pinching the catheter. The system consists of a Statham P23Dd sensor and a 1 m, 6 F, polyethylene catheter. The pinch effectively reduces the diameter of the catheter to 25% of its original diameter.

**a.** How long must the pinch be for the system's damping factor to be equal to 0.7?

**b.** Sketch the frequency response for the system with and without the pinch.

**c.** Sketch the time response for the system with and without the pinch when it is excited by a 100 mm-Hg step input.

**d.** Discuss how faithfully the two systems will reproduce the blood-pressure waveform for humans, dogs, and shrews with heart-rate variations of 1 to 3.3 beats/s, 1.5 to 5 beats/s, and 12 to 22 beats/s, respectively.

**7.6** A heart murmur has a frequency of 300 Hz. Give the block diagram and sketch waveforms for the special instrumentation that enables us to show the occurrence of this murmur on a 0 to 80 Hz pen recorder.

**7.7** Name the two basic causes of abnormal heart murmurs. For each type, give an example and show on a sketch when it occurs relative to systole and diastole.

**7.8** In block-diagram form, show the elements required for an automatic indirect system for measuring blood pressure.

**7.9** Design a portable system for indirectly measuring blood pressure every 5 min on ambulatory subjects. It should operate without attention from the subject for 24 h. Show a block diagram and describe the system's operation, including power source, sensor, storage, and algorithm.

**7.10** A patient who has been vomiting for several days is dehydrated. Liquid is infused through a venous catheter at the rate of 250 ml/h. Sketch the resulting central venous pressure versus time, and explain any large change in the slope of the curve. How does the jugular venous pulse change during this procedure?

**7.11** One of the problems of tonometers is that each operator pushes with a different force. Sketch the block diagram of a system that would apply a ramp input of force from low to high and pick out the maximal pulse pressure (systolic minus diastolic). Sketch the expected output versus time.

## REFERENCES

Attinger, E. O., A. Anne, and D. A. McDonald, "Use of Fourier series for the analysis of biological systems." *Biophys. J.*, 1970, 6, 291–304.

Bellville, J. W., and C. S. Weaver, *Techniques in Clinical Physiology*. New York: Macmillan, 1969.

Burton, A. C., *Physiology and Biophysics of the Circulation*, 2nd ed. Chicago: Year Book, 1972.

Cobbold, R. S. C., *Transducers for Biomedical Measurements: Principles and Applications*. New York: Wiley, 1974.

Eckerle, J. S., "Tonometry, arterial." In J. G. Webster (ed.), *Encyclopedia of Medical Devices and Instrumentation*, 2nd ed. New York: Wiley, 2006, Vol. 6, pp. 402–410.

Ertel, P. Y., M. Lawrence, R. K. Brown, and A. M. Stern, "Stethoscope acoustics I. The doctor and his stethoscope." *Circulation*, 1966a, 34, 889–898.

Ertel, P. Y., M. Lawrence, R. K. Brown, and A. M. Stern, "Stethoscope acoustics II. Transmission and filtration patterns." *Circulation*, 1966b, 34, 899–908.

Forbes, M., G. Pico, Jr., and B. Grolman, "A noncontact applanation tonometer, description and clinical evaluation." *J. Arch. Ophthal.*, 1974, 91, 134–140.

Fry, D. L., "Physiologic recording by modern instruments with particular reference to pressure recording." *Physiol. Rev.*, 1960, 40, 753–788.

Ganz, W., and H. J. C. Swan, "Balloon-tipped flow-directed catheters." In W. Grossman (ed.), *Cardiac Catheterization and Angiography*. Philadelphia: Lea & Febiger, 1974.

Geddes, L. A., *Cardiovascular Devices and Their Applications*. New York: Wiley, 1984.

Geddes, L. A., *The Direct and Indirect Measurement of Blood Pressure*. Chicago: Year Book, 1970.

Gersh, B. J., C. E. W. Hahn, and C. P. Roberts, "Physical criteria for measurement of left ventricular pressure and its first derivative." *Cardiovasc. Res.*, 1971, 5, 32–40.

Gizdulich, P., and K. H. Wesseling, "Reconstruction of brachial arterial pulsation from finger arterial pressure." *Proc. Annu. Int. Conf. IEEE Eng. Med. Biol. Soc.*, 1990, 12, 1046–1047.

Goldmann, H., "Applanation tonometry." In F. W. Newell (ed.), *Glaucoma: Transactions of the Second Conference,* December 1956, Princeton, NJ. Madison, NJ: Madison Printing, 1957, pp. 167–220.

Greatorex, C. A., "Indirect methods of blood-pressure measurement." In B. W. Watson (ed.), *IEE Medical Electronics Monographs 1–6*. London: Peter Peregrinus, 1971.

Grossman, W., *Cardiac Catheterization and Angiography*. Philadelphia: Lea & Febiger, 1974.

Hansen, A. T., "Fiber-optic pressure transducers for medical application." *Sensors and Actuators*, 1983, 4, 545–554.

Herman, M. V., P. F. Cohn, and R. Gorlin, "Resistance to blood flow by stenotic valves: Calculation of orifice area." In W. Grossman (ed.), *Cardiac Catheterization and Angiography*. Philadelphia: Lea & Febiger, 1974.

Howe, R. T., R. S. Muller, K. J. Gabriel, and W. S. N. Trimmer, "Silicon micromechanics: Sensors and actuators on a chip." *IEEE Spectrum*, 1990, 27(7), 29–35.

Isik, C., "Blood pressure measurement." In J. G. Webster (ed.), *Encyclopedia of Medical Devices and Instrumentation*, 2nd ed., New York: Wiley, 2006, Vol. 1, pp. 485–490.

Loudon, R. G., and R. L. H. Murphy, "Lung sounds." In J. G. Webster (ed.), *Encyclopedia of Medical Devices and Instrumentation*, 2nd ed., New York: Wiley, 2006, pp. 277–282.

Mackay, R. S., and E. Marg, "Fast automatic ocular pressure measurement based on an exact theory." *IRE Trans. Med. Electron.*, 1960, ME-7, 61–67.

Master, A. M., C. I. Garfield, and M. B. Walters, *Normal Blood Pressure and Hypertension*. Philadelphia: Lea & Febiger, 1952.

Neuman, M. R., "Neonatal monitoring." In J. G. Webster (ed.), *Encyclopedia of Medical Devices and Instrumentation*, 2nd ed. New York: Wiley, 2006, Vol. 5, pp. 11–32.

O'Rourke, P. L., "The arterial pulse in health and disease." *Amer. Heart J.*, 1971, 82, 687–702.

Pressman, G. L., and P. M. Newgard, "A transducer for the continuous external measurement of arterial blood pressure." *IEEE Trans. Biomed. Electron.*, 1963, 10, 73–81.

Ramsey, M., III, "Blood pressure monitoring: automated oscillometric devices." *J. Clin. Monit.*, 1991, 7, 56–67.

Roos, C. F., and F. E. Carroll, Jr., "Fiber-optic pressure transducer for use near MR magnetic fields." *Radiology*, 1985, 156, 548.

Rushmer, R. F., *Cardiovascular Dynamics*, 3rd ed. Philadelphia: Saunders, 1970.

Shapiro, G. G., and L. J. Krovetz, "Damped and undamped frequency responses of underdamped catheter manometer systems." *Amer. Heart J.*, 1970, 80, 226–236.

Stegall, H. F., M. B. Kardon, and W. T. Kemmerer, "Indirect measurement of arterial blood pressure by Doppler ultrasonic sphygmomanometry." *J. Appl. Physiol.*, 1968, 25, 793–798.

Velanovich, V., "Esophageal manometry." In J. G. Webster (ed.), *Encyclopedia of Medical Devices and Instrumentation*, 2nd ed. New York: Wiley, 2006, Vol. 3, pp. 229–233.

Vermariën, H., "Phonocardiography." In J. G. Webster (ed.), *Encyclopedia of Medical Devices and Instrumentation*, 2nd ed., New York: Wiley, 2006, Vol. 5, pp. 278–290.

Visser, K. R., and J. H. J. Muntinga, "Blood pressure estimation investigated by electric impedance measurement." *Proc. Annu. Int. Conf. IEEE Eng. Med. Biol. Soc.*, 1990, 12, 691–692.

Webster, J. G. (ed.), *Prevention of Pressure Sores: Engineering and Clinical Aspects*. Bristol, England: Adam Hilger, 1991.

Yellin, E. L., R. W. M. Prater, and C. S. Peskin, "The application of the Gorlin equation to the stenotic mitral valve." In A. C. Bell and R. M. Nerem (eds.), *1975 Advances in Bioengineering*. New York: Am. Soc. Mech. Engr., 1975.

Yu, Y.-C., "Blood pressure, automatic control of." In J. G. Webster (ed.), *Encyclopedia of Medical Devices and Instrumentation*, 2nd ed., New York: Wiley, 2006, Vol. 1, pp. 490–500.

# 8

# MEASUREMENT OF FLOW AND VOLUME OF BLOOD

John G. Webster

One of the primary measurements the physician would like to acquire from a patient is that of the concentration of $O_2$ and other nutrients in the cells. Such quantities are normally so difficult to measure that the doctor is forced to accept the second-class measurements of blood flow and changes in blood volume, which usually correlate with concentration of nutrients. If blood *flow* is difficult to measure, the physician may settle for the third-class measurement of blood *pressure*, which usually correlates adequately with blood flow. If blood pressure cannot be measured, the physician may fall back on the fourth-class measurement of the ECG, which usually correlates adequately with blood pressure.

Note that the measurement of blood flow—the main subject of this chapter—is the one that most closely reflects the primary measurement of concentration of $O_2$ in the cells. However, measurement of blood flow is usually more difficult to make and more invasive than measurement of blood pressure or of the ECG.

Commonly used flowmeters, such as the orifice or turbine flowmeters, are unsuitable for measuring blood flow because they require cutting the vessel and can cause formation of clots. The specialized techniques described in this chapter have therefore been developed.

## 8.1 INDICATOR-DILUTION METHOD THAT USES CONTINUOUS INFUSION

The indicator-dilution methods described in this chapter do not measure instantaneous pulsatile flow but, rather, flow averaged over a number of heartbeats.

### CONCENTRATION

When a given quantity $m_0$ of an indicator is added to a volume $V$, the resulting concentration $C$ of the indicator is given by $C = m_0/V$. When an additional quantity $m$ of indicator is then added, the incremental increase in concentration is $\Delta C = m/V$. When the fluid volume in the measured space is continuously removed and replaced, as in a flowing stream, then in order to maintain a fixed change in concentration, the clinician must continuously add a fixed quantity of indicator per unit time. That is, $\Delta C = (dm/dt)/(dV/dt)$. From this equation, we can calculate flow (Donovan and Taylor, 2006).

$$F = \frac{dV}{dt} = \frac{dm/dt}{\Delta C} \tag{8.1}$$

**EXAMPLE 8.1** Derive (8.1) using principles of mass transport.

**ANSWER** The rate at which indicator enters the vessel is equal to the indicator's input concentration $C_i$, times the flow $F$. The rate at which indicator is injected into the vessel is equal to the quantity per unit time, $dm/dt$. The rate at which indicator leaves the vessel is equal to the indicator's output concentration $C_o$ times $F$. For steady state, $C_iF + dm/dt = C_oF$ or $F = (dm/dt)/(C_o - C_i)$.

## FICK TECHNIQUE

We can use (8.1) to measure *cardiac output* (blood flow from the heart) as follows (Capek and Roy, 1988):

$$F = \frac{dm/dt}{C_a - C_v} \tag{8.2}$$

where

$F$ = blood flow, liters/min
$dm/dt$ = consumption of $O_2$, liters/min
$C_a$ = arterial concentration of $O_2$, liters/liter
$C_v$ = venous concentration of $O_2$, liters/liter

Figure 8.1 shows the measurements required. The blood returning to the heart from the upper half of the body has a different concentration of $O_2$ from the blood returning from the lower half, because the amount of $O_2$ extracted by the brain is different from that extracted by the kidneys, muscles, and so forth. Therefore, we cannot accurately measure $C_v$ in the right atrium. We must measure it in the pulmonary artery after it has been mixed by the pumping action of the right ventricle. The physician may float the catheter into place by temporarily inflating a small balloon surrounding the tip. This is done through a second lumen in the catheter.

As the blood flows through the lung capillaries, the subject adds the indicator (the $O_2$) by breathing in pure $O_2$ from a spirometer (see Figure 9.6).

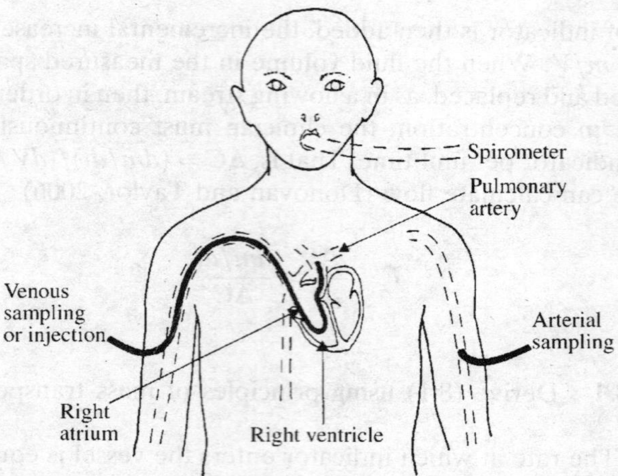


**Figure 8.1 Several methods of measuring cardiac output** In the Fick method, the indicator is $O_2$; consumption is measured by a spirometer. The arterial-venous concentration difference is measured by drawing samples through catheters placed in an artery and in the pulmonary artery. In the dye-dilution method, dye is injected into the pulmonary artery and samples are taken from an artery. In the thermodilution method, cold saline is injected into the right atrium and temperature is measured in the pulmonary artery.

The exhaled $CO_2$ is absorbed in a soda-lime canister, so the consumption of $O_2$ is indicated directly by the net gas-flow rate.

The clinician can measure the concentration of the oxygenated blood $C_a$ in any artery, because blood from the lung capillaries is well mixed by the left ventricle and there is no consumption of $O_2$ in the arteries. An arm or leg artery is generally used.

**EXAMPLE 8.2** Calculate the cardiac output, given the following data: spirometer $O_2$ consumption 250 ml/min; arterial $O_2$ content, 0.20 ml/ml; venous $O_2$ content, 0.15 ml/ml.

**ANSWER** From (8.2),

$$F = \frac{dm/dt}{C_a - C_v}$$

$$= \frac{0.25 \text{ liter/min}}{(0.20 \text{ liter/liter}) - (0.15 \text{ liter/liter})}$$

$$= 5 \text{ liters/min} \tag{8.3}$$

The units for the concentrations of $O_2$ represent the volume of $O_2$ that can be extracted from a volume of blood. This concentration is very high for blood, because large quantities of oxygen can be bound to hemoglobin. It would be very low if water were flowing through the vessels, even if the $PO_2$ were identical in both cases.

The Fick technique is nontoxic, because the indicator ($O_2$) is a normal metabolite that is partially removed as blood passes through the systemic capillaries. The cardiac output must be constant over several minutes so that the investigator can obtain the slope of the curve for $O_2$ consumption. The presence of the catheter causes a negligible change in cardiac output.

## 8.2 INDICATOR-DILUTION METHOD THAT USES RAPID INJECTION

### EQUATION

The continuous-infusion method has been largely replaced by the rapid-injection method, which is more convenient. A bolus of indicator is rapidly injected into the vessel, and the variation in downstream concentration of the indicator versus time is measured until the bolus has passed. The solid line in Figure 8.2 shows the fluctuations in concentration of the indicator that occur after the injection. The dotted-line extension of the exponential decay shows the curve that would result if there were no recirculation. For this case we can calculate the flow as outlined in the following paragraphs.

An increment of blood of volume $dV$ passes the sampling site in time $dt$. The quantity of indicator $dm$ contained in $dV$ is the concentration $C(t)$ times the incremental volume. Hence $dm = C(t)dV$. Dividing by $dt$, we obtain $dm/dt = C(t)dV/dt$. But $dV/dt = F_i$, the instantaneous flow; therefore

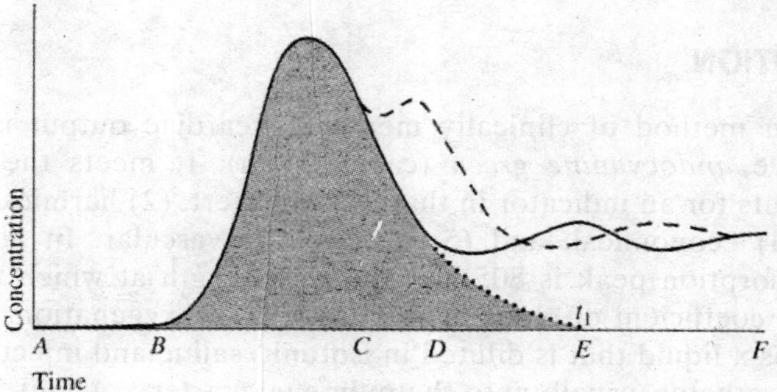


**Figure 8.2 Rapid-injection indicator-dilution curve** After the bolus is injected at time $A$, there is a transportation delay before the concentration begins rising at time $B$. After the peak is passed, the curve enters an exponential decay region between $C$ and $D$, which would continue decaying along the dotted curve to $t_1$ if there were no recirculation. However, recirculation causes a second peak at $E$ before the indicator becomes thoroughly mixed in the blood at $F$. The dashed curve indicates the rapid recirculation that occurs when there is a hole between the left and right sides of the heart.

$dm = F_i C(t)dt$. Integrating over time through $t_1$, when the bolus has passed the downstream sampling point, we obtain

$$m = \int_0^{t_1} F_i C(t)dt \quad (8.4)$$

where $t_1$ is the time at which all effects of the first pass of the bolus have died out (point $E$ in Figure 8.2). The mixing of the bolus and the blood within the heart chambers and the lungs smooths out minor variations in the instantaneous flow $F_i$ produced by the heartbeat. Thus we can obtain the average flow $F$ from

$$F = \frac{m}{\int_0^{t_1} C(t)dt} \quad (8.5)$$

The integrated quantity in (8.5) is equal to the shaded area in Figure 8.2, and we can obtain it by counting squares or using a planimeter. A computer can extrapolate the dotted line in real time and compute the flow.

If the initial concentration of indicator is not zero—as may be the case when there is residual indicator left over from previous injections—then (8.5) becomes

$$F = \frac{m}{\int_0^{t_1} [\Delta C(t)]\, dt} \quad (8.6)$$

## DYE DILUTION

A common method of clinically measuring cardiac output is to use a colored dye, *indocyanine green* (cardiogreen). It meets the necessary requirements for an indicator in that it is (1) inert, (2) harmless, (3) measurable, (4) economical, and (5) always intravascular. In addition, its optical absorption peak is 805 nm, the wavelength at which the optical absorption coefficient of blood is independent of oxygenation. The dye is available as a liquid that is diluted in isotonic saline and injected directly through a catheter, usually into the pulmonary artery. About 50% of the dye is excreted by the kidneys in the first 10 min, so repeat determinations are possible.

The plot of the curve for concentration versus time is obtained from a constant-flow pump, which draws blood from a catheter placed in the femoral or brachial artery. Blood is drawn through a colorimeter cuvette (Figure 2.17), which continuously measures the concentration of dye, using the principle of absorption photometry (Section 11.1). The 805 nm channel of a two-channel blood oximeter can be used for measuring dye-dilution curves. The clinician calibrates the colorimeter by mixing known amounts of dye and blood and drawing them through the cuvette.

The shape of the curve can provide additional diagnostic information. The dashed curve in Figure 8.2 shows the result when a left-right shunt (a hole between the left and right sides of the heart) is present. Blood recirculates faster than normal, resulting in an earlier recirculation peak. When a right-left shunt is present, the delay in transport is abnormally short, because some dye reaches the sampling site without passing through the lung vessels.

## THERMODILUTION

The most common method of measuring cardiac output is that of injecting a bolus of cold saline as an indicator. A special four-lumen catheter (Trautman and D'ambra, 2006) is floated through the brachial vein into place in the pulmonary artery. A syringe forces a gas through one lumen; the gas inflates a small, doughnut-shaped balloon at the tip. The force of the flowing blood carries the tip into the pulmonary artery. The cooled saline indicator is injected through the second lumen into the right atrium. The indicator is mixed with blood in the right ventricle. The resulting drop in temperature of the blood is detected by a thermistor located near the catheter tip in the pulmonary artery. The third lumen carries the thermistor wires. The fourth lumen, which is not used for the measurement of thermodilution, can be used for withdrawing blood samples. The catheter can be left in place for about 24 h, during which time many determinations of cardiac output can be made, something that would not be possible if dye were being used as the indicator. Also, it is not necessary to puncture an artery.

We can derive the following equation, which is analogous to (8.6).

$$F = \frac{Q}{\rho_b C_b \int_0^{t_1} \Delta T_b(t)\, dt} \; (\mathrm{m^3/s}) \tag{8.7}$$

where

$Q$ = heat content of injectate, J($= V_i \Delta T_i \rho_i c_i$)

$\rho_b$ = density of blood, kg/m$^3$

$c_b$ = specific heat of blood, J/(kg·K)

When an investigator uses the thermodilution method, there are a number of problems that cause errors. (1) There may be inadequate mixing between the injection site and the sampling site. (2) There may be an exchange of heat between the blood and the walls of the heart chamber. (3) There is heat exchange through the catheter walls before, during, and after injection. However, the instrument can be calibrated by simultaneously performing dye-dilution determinations and applying a correction factor that corrects for several of the errors.

## 8.3 ELECTROMAGNETIC FLOWMETERS

The electromagnetic flowmeter measures instantaneous pulsatile flow of blood and thus has a greater capability than indicator-dilution methods, which measure only average flow. It operates with any conductive liquid, such as saline or blood.

### PRINCIPLE

The electric generator in a car generates electricity by induction. Copper wires move through a magnetic field, cutting the lines of magnetic flux and inducing an emf in the wire. This same principle is exploited in a commonly used blood flowmeter, shown in Figure 8.3. Instead of copper wires, the flowmeter depends on the movement of blood, which has a conductance similar to that of saline. Faraday's law of induction gives the formula for the induced emf.

$$e = \int_0^{L_1} \mathbf{u} \times \mathbf{B} \cdot d\mathbf{L}$$

where

$\mathbf{B}$ = magnetic flux density, T

$\mathbf{L}$ = length between electrodes, m

$\mathbf{u}$ = instaneous velocity of blood, m/s

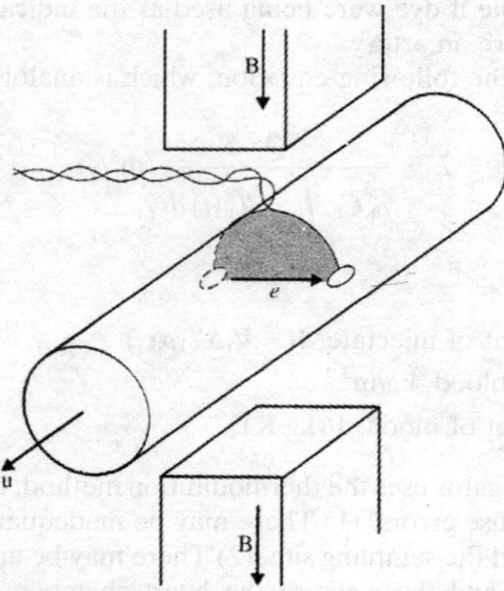


**Figure 8.3 Electromagnetic flowmeter** When blood flows in the vessel with velocity $\mathbf{u}$ and passes through the magnetic field $\mathbf{B}$, the induced emf $e$ is measured at the electrodes shown. When an ac magnetic field is used, any flux lines cutting the shaded loop induce an undesired transformer voltage.

For a uniform magnetic field $B$ and a uniform velocity profile $u$, the induced emf is

$$e = BLu \tag{8.8}$$

where these three components are orthogonal.

Let us now consider real flowmeters, several of which exhibit a number of divergences from this ideal case. If the vessel's cross section were square and the electrodes extended the full length of two opposite sides, the flowmeter would measure the correct average flow for any flow profile. The electrodes are small, however, so velocities near them contribute more to the signal than do velocities farther away.

Figure 8.4 shows the weighting function that characterizes this effect for circular geometry. It shows that the problem is less when the electrodes are located outside the vessel wall. The instrument measures correctly for a uniform flow profile. For axisymmetric nonuniform flow profiles, such as the parabolic flow profile resulting from laminar flow, the instrument measurement is correct if $u$ is replaced by $\overline{u}$, the average flow velocity. Because we usually know the cross-sectional area $A$ of the lumen of the vessel, we can multiply $A$ by $\overline{u}$ to obtain $F$, the volumetric flow. However, in many locations of

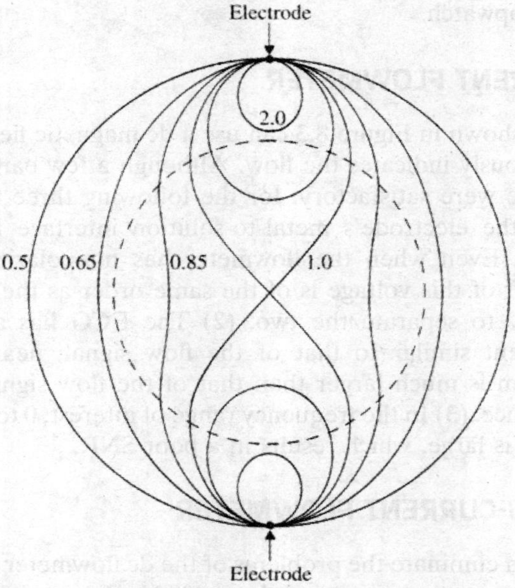


**Figure 8.4** Solid lines show the weighting function that represents relative velocity contributions (indicated by numbers) to the total induced voltage for electrodes at the top and bottom of the circular cross section. If the vessel wall extends from the outside circle to the dashed line, the range of the weighting function is reduced. (Adapted from J. A. Shercliff, *The Theory of Electromagnetic Flow Measurement*, © 1962, Cambridge University Press.)

blood vessels in the body, such as around the curve of the aorta and near its branches, the velocity profile is asymmetric, so errors result.

Other factors can also cause error.

1. Regions of high velocity generate higher incremental emfs than regions of low velocity, so circulating currents flow in the transverse plane. These currents cause varying drops in resistance within the conductive blood and surrounding tissues.
2. The ratio of the conductivity of the wall of the blood vessel to that of the blood varies with the *hematocrit* (percentage of cell volume to blood volume), so the shunting effects of the wall cause a variable error.
3. Fluid outside the wall of the vessel has a greater conductivity than the wall, so it shunts the flow signal.
4. The magnetic-flux density is not uniform in the transverse plane; this accentuates the problem of circulating current.
5. The magnetic-flux density is not uniform along the axis, which causes circulating currents to flow in the axial direction.

To minimize these errors, most workers recommend calibration for animal work by using blood from the animal—and, where possible, the animal's own vessels also. Blood or saline is usually collected in a graduated cylinder and timed with a stopwatch.

## DIRECT-CURRENT FLOWMETER

The flowmeter shown in Figure 8.3 can use a dc magnetic field, so the output voltage continuously indicates the flow. Although a few early dc flowmeters were built, none were satisfactory, for the following three reasons. (1) The voltage across the electrode's metal-to-solution interface is in series with the flow signal. Even when the flowmeter has nonpolarizable electrodes, the random drift of this voltage is of the same order as the flow signal, and there is no way to separate the two. (2) The ECG has a waveform and frequency content similar to that of the flow signal; near the heart, the ECG's waveform is much larger than that of the flow signal and therefore causes interference. (3) In the frequency range of interest, 0 to 30 Hz, $1/f$ noise in the amplifier is large, which results in a poor SNR.

## ALTERNATING-CURRENT FLOWMETER

The clinician can eliminate the problems of the dc flowmeter by operating the system with an ac magnet current of about 400 Hz. Lower frequencies require bulky sensors, whereas higher frequencies cause problems due to stray capacitance. The operation of this carrier system results in the ac flow voltage shown in Figure 8.5. When the flow reverses direction, the voltage changes phase by 180°, so the phase-sensitive demodulator (described in Section 3.15) is required to yield directional output.

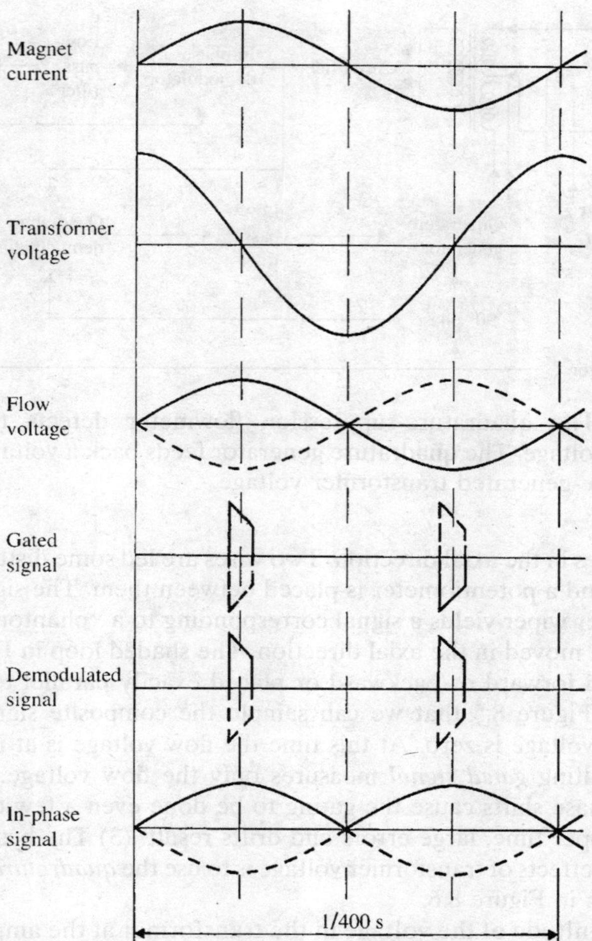


**Figure 8.5 Electromagnetic flowmeter waveforms** The transformer voltage is 90° out of phase with the magnet current. Other waveforms are shown solid for forward flow and dashed for reverse flow. The gated signal from the gated-sine-wave flowmeter includes less area than the in-phase signal from the quadrature-suppression flowmeter.

Although ac operation is superior to dc operation, the new problem of *transformer voltage* arises. If the shaded loop shown in Figure 8.3 is not exactly parallel to the $B$ field, some ac magnetic flux intersects the loop and induces a transformer voltage proportional to $dB/dt$ in the output voltage. Even when the electrodes and wires are carefully positioned, the transformer voltage is usually many times larger than the flow voltage, as indicated in Figure 8.5. The amplifier voltage is the sum of the transformer voltage and the flow voltage.

There are several solutions to this problem. (1) It may be eliminated at the source by use of a *phantom electrode*. One of the electrodes is separated into

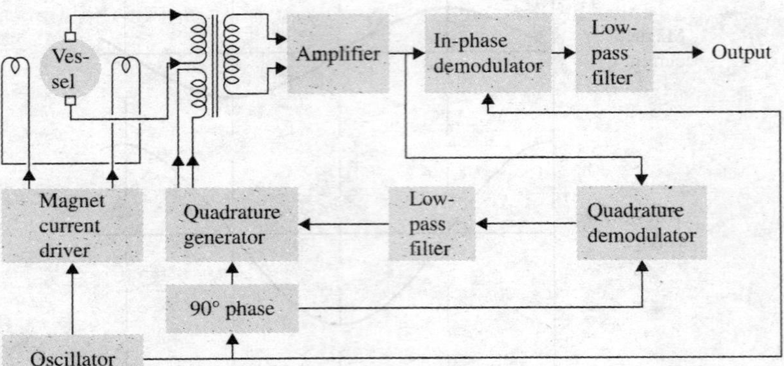


**Figure 8.6** The quadrature-suppression flowmeter detects the amplifier quadrature voltage. The quadrature generator feeds back a voltage to balance out the probe-generated transformer voltage.

two electrodes in the axial direction. Two wires are led some distance from the electrodes, and a potentiometer is placed between them. The signal from the potentiometer wiper yields a signal corresponding to a "phantom" electrode, which can be moved in the axial direction. The shaded loop in Figure 8.3 can thus be tilted forward or backward or placed exactly parallel to the $B$ field. (2) Note in Figure 8.5 that we can sample the composite signal when the transformer voltage is zero. At this time the flow voltage is at its maximum, and the resulting *gated signal* measures only the flow voltage. However, if undesired phase shifts cause the gating to be done even a few degrees away from the proper time, large errors and drifts result. (3) The best method for reducing the effects of transformer voltage is to use the *quadrature-suppression* circuit shown in Figure 8.6.

The magnitude of the voltage in the transformer at the amplifier output is detected by the quadrature demodulator, which has a full-wave-rectified output. This is low-pass-filtered to yield a dc voltage, which is then modulated by the quadrature generator to produce a signal proportional to the transformer voltage. The signal is fed to a balancing coil on the input transformer, thus balancing out the transformer voltage at the input. With enough gain in this negative-feedback loop, the transformer voltage at the amplifier output is reduced by a factor of 50. This low transformer voltage prevents overloading of the in-phase demodulator, which extracts the desired in-phase flow signal shown in Figure 8.5. By choosing low-noise FETs for the amplifier input stage, the proper turns ratio on the step-up transformer (Section 3.13), and full-wave demodulators, we can obtain an excellent SNR.

Some flowmeters, unlike the sine-wave flowmeters described previously, use *square-wave excitation*. In this case the transformer voltage appears as a very large spike, which overloads the amplifier for a short time. After the amplifier recovers, the circuit samples the square-wave flow voltage and processes it to obtain the flow signal. To prevent overload of the amplifier, *trapezoidal excitation* has also been used.

**EXAMPLE 8.3** On a common time scale, sketch the waveforms for the magnet current, flow signal, and transformer voltage for the following electromagnetic flowmeters: (1) gated sine wave, (2) square wave, and (3) trapezoidal. Indicate the best time for sampling each flow signal.

**ANSWER** For gated sine wave, waveforms are exactly like those in Figure 8.5. Sample the composite signal when the transformer voltage is zero. Transformer voltage is proportional to $dB/dt$. Taking the derivative of square wave $B$ yields spikes at transitions. Because the amplifier is not perfect, these take time to decay. Best time to sample is near the end of transformer voltage $= 0$. Trapezoidal $B$ yields reasonable $dB/dt$, so sample during time transformer voltage $= 0$.

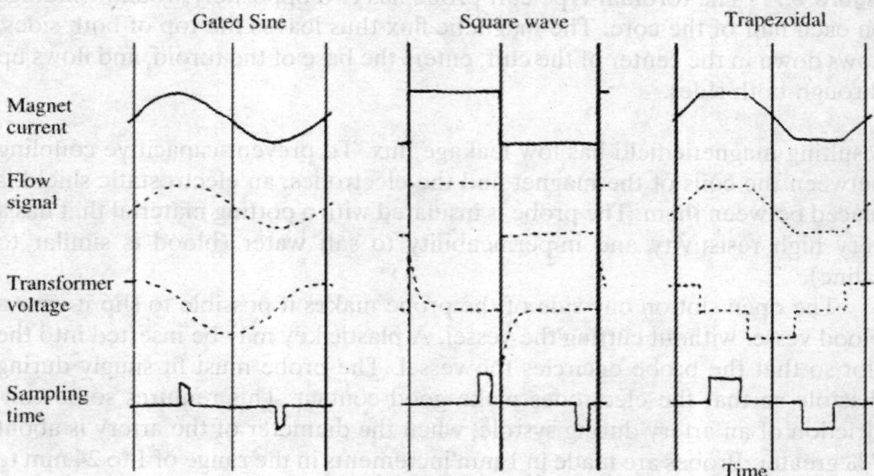


## PROBE DESIGN

A variety of probes to measure blood flow have been used (Cobbold, 1974). The electrodes for these probes are usually made of platinum. Best results are obtained when the electrodes are platinized (electrolytically coated with platinum) to provide low impedance and are recessed in a cavity to minimize the flow of circulating currents through the metal. When the electrodes must be exposed, bright platinum is used, because the platinized coating wears off anyway. Bright platinum electrodes have a higher impedance and a higher noise level than platinized ones.

Some probes do not use a magnetic core, but they have lower sensitivity. A common *perivascular probe* is shown in Figure 8.7, in which a toroidal laminated Permalloy core is wound with two oppositely wound coils. The

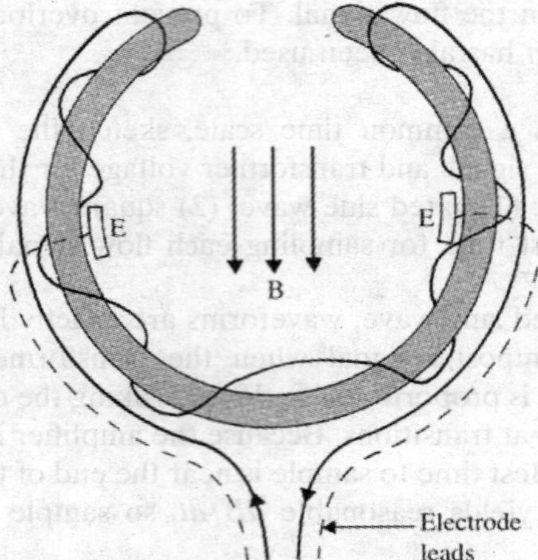


**Figure 8.7** The toroidal-type cuff probe has two oppositely wound windings on each half of the core. The magnetic flux thus leaves the top of both sides, flows down in the center of the cuff, enters the base of the toroid, and flows up through both sides.

resulting magnetic field has low leakage flux. To prevent capacitive coupling between the coils of the magnet and the electrodes, an electrostatic shield is placed between them. The probe is insulated with a potting material that has a very high resistivity and impermeability to salt water (blood is similar to saline).

The open slot on one side of the probe makes it possible to slip it over a blood vessel without cutting the vessel. A plastic key may be inserted into the slot so that the probe encircles the vessel. The probe must fit snugly during diastole so that the electrodes make good contact. This requires some constriction of an artery during systole, when the diameter of the artery is about 7% greater. Probes are made in 1 mm increments in the range of 1 to 24 mm to ensure a snug fit on a variety of sizes of arteries. To be able to measure any size of artery requires a considerable expenditure for probes: Individual probes typically cost $500 each. The probes do not operate satisfactorily on veins, because the electrodes do not make good contact when the vein collapses. Special flow-through probes are used outside the body for measuring the output of cardiac-bypass pumps.

## 8.4 ULTRASONIC FLOWMETERS

The ultrasonic flowmeter, like the electromagnetic flowmeter, can measure instantaneous flow of blood. The ultrasound can be beamed through the skin, thus making transcutaneous flowmeters practical. Advanced types of ultrasonic flowmeters can also measure flow profiles. These advantages are making the ultrasonic flowmeter the subject of intensive development. Let us examine some aspects of this development.

## TRANSDUCERS

For the transducer to be used in an ultrasonic flowmeter, we select a piezoelectric material (Section 2.6) that converts power from electric to acoustic form (Christensen, 1988). Lead zirconate titanate is a crystal that has the highest conversion efficiency. It can be molded into any shape by melting. As it is cooled through the Curie temperature, it is placed in a strong electric field to polarize the material. It is usually formed into disks that are coated on opposite faces with metal electrodes and driven by an electronic oscillator. The resulting electric field in the crystal causes mechanical constriction. The pistonlike movements generate longitudinal plane waves, which propagate into the tissue. For maximal efficiency, the crystal is one-half wavelength thick. Any cavities between the crystal and the tissue must be filled with a fluid or watery gel in order to prevent the high reflective losses associated with liquid–gas interfaces.

Because the transducer has a finite diameter, it will produce diffraction patterns, just as an aperture does in optics. Figure 8.8 shows the outline of the beam patterns for several transducer diameters and frequencies. In the *near field*, the beam is largely contained within a cylindrical outline and there is little spreading. The intensity is not uniform, however: There are multiple maximums and minimums within this region, caused by interference. The near field extends a distance $d_{nf}$ given by

$$d_{nf} = \frac{D^2}{4\lambda} \tag{8.9}$$

where $D$ = transducer diameter and $\lambda$ = wavelength.

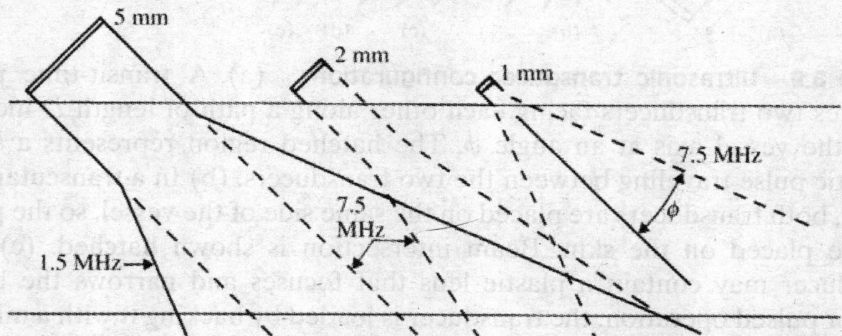


**Figure 8.8** Near and far fields for various transducer diameters and frequencies. Beams are drawn to scale, passing through a 10 mm-diameter vessel. Transducer diameters are 5, 2, and 1 mm. Solid lines are for 1.5 MHz, dashed lines for 7.5 MHz.

In the *far field* the beam diverges, and the intensity is inversely proportional to the square of the distance from the transducer. The angle of beam divergence $\phi$, shown in Figure 8.8, is given by

$$\sin \phi = \frac{1.2\lambda}{D} \tag{8.10}$$

Figure 8.8 indicates that we should avoid the far field because of its lower spatial resolution. To achieve near-field operation, we must use higher frequencies and larger transducers.

To select the operating frequency, we must consider several factors. For a beam of constant cross section, the power decays exponentially because of absorption of heat in the tissue. The absorption coefficient is approximately proportional to frequency, so this suggests a low operating frequency. However, most ultrasonic flowmeters depend on the power scattered back from moving red blood cells. The backscattered power is proportional to $f^4$, which suggests a high operating frequency. The usual compromise dictates a frequency between 2 and 10 MHz.

## TRANSIT-TIME FLOWMETER

Figure 8.9(a) shows the transducer arrangement used in the transit-time ultrasonic flowmeter (Christensen, 1988). The effective velocity of sound in the vessel is equal to the velocity of sound, $c$, plus a component due to $\hat{u}$, the

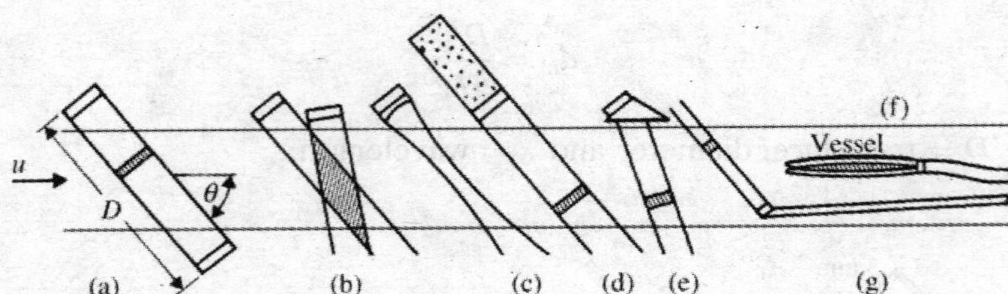


**Figure 8.9 Ultrasonic transducer configurations** (a) A transit-time probe requires two transducers facing each other along a path of length $D$ inclined from the vessel axis at an angle $\phi$. The hatched region represents a single acoustic pulse traveling between the two transducers. (b) In a transcutaneous probe, both transducers are placed on the same side of the vessel, so the probe can be placed on the skin. Beam intersection is shown hatched. (c) Any transducer may contain a plastic lens that focuses and narrows the beam. (d) For pulsed operation, the transducer is loaded by backing it with a mixture of tungsten powder in epoxy. This increases losses and lowers $Q$. Shaded region is shown for a single time of range gating. (e) A shaped piece of Lucite on the front loads the transducer and also refracts the beam. (f) A transducer placed on the end of a catheter beams ultrasound down the vessel. (g) For pulsed operation, the transducer is placed at an angle.

velocity of flow of blood averaged along the path of the ultrasound. For laminar flow, $\hat{u} = 1.33\,\overline{u}$, and for turbulent flow, $\hat{u} = 1.07\,\overline{u}$, where $\overline{u}$ is the velocity of the flow of blood averaged over the cross-sectional area. Because the ultrasonic path is along a single line rather than averaged over the cross-sectional area, $\hat{u}$ differs from $\overline{u}$. The transit time in the downstream (+) and upstream (−) directions is

$$t = \frac{\text{distance}}{\text{conduction velocity}} = \frac{D}{c \pm \hat{u}\cos\theta} \tag{8.11}$$

The difference between upstream and downstream transit times is

$$\Delta t = \frac{2\,D\hat{u}\cos\theta}{(c^2 - \hat{u}^2\cos^2\theta)} \cong \frac{2\,D\hat{u}\cos\theta}{c^2} \tag{8.12}$$

and thus the average velocity $\hat{u}$ is proportional to $\Delta t$. A short acoustic pulse is transmitted alternately in the upstream and downstream directions. Unfortunately, the resulting $\Delta t$ is in the nanosecond range, and complex electronics are required to achieve adequate stability. Like the electromagnetic flowmeter, the transit-time flowmeter and similar flowmeters using a phase-shift principle can operate with either saline or blood as a fluid, because they do not require particulate matter for scattering. However, they do require invasive surgery to expose the vessel.

## CONTINUOUS-WAVE DOPPLER FLOWMETER

When a target recedes from a fixed source that transmits sound, the frequency of the received sound is lowered because of the Doppler effect. For small changes, the fractional change in frequency equals the fractional change in velocity.

$$\frac{f_d}{f_0} = \frac{u}{c} \tag{8.13}$$

where

$f_d$ = Doppler frequency shift
$f_0$ = source frequency
$u$ = target velocity
$c$ = velocity of sound

The flowmeter shown in Figure 8.10 requires particulate matter such as blood cells to form reflecting targets. The frequency is lowered twice. One shift occurs between the transmitting source and the moving cell that receives the

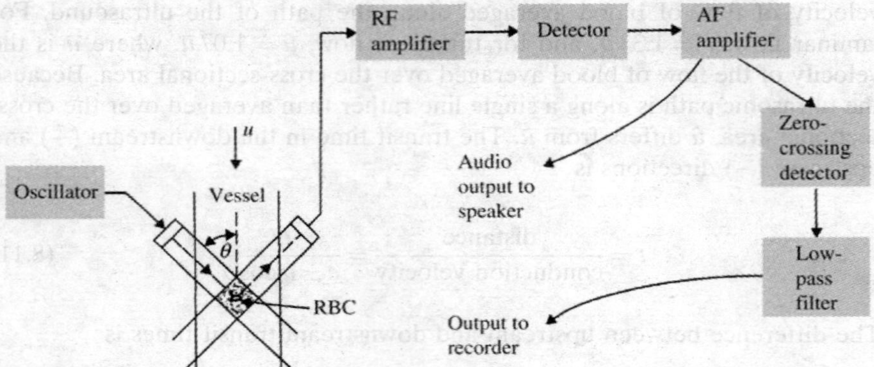


**Figure 8.10 Doppler ultrasonic blood flowmeter** In the simplest instrument, ultrasound is beamed through the vessel walls, backscattered by the red blood cells, and received by a piezoelectric crystal.

signal. The other shift occurs between the transmitting cell and the receiving transducer.

$$\frac{f_d}{f_0} = \frac{2u}{c+u} \cong \frac{2u}{c} \tag{8.14}$$

The approximation is valid, because $c \cong 1500$ m/s and $u \cong 1.5$ m/s. The velocities do not all act along the same straight line, so we add an angle factor

$$f_d = \frac{2\, f_0 u \cos\theta}{c} \tag{8.15}$$

where $\theta$ is the angle between the beam of sound and the axis of the blood vessel, as shown in Figure 8.10. If the flow is not axial, or the transducers do not lie at the same angle, such as in Figure 8.9(b), we must include additional trigonometric factors.

Figure 8.10 shows the block diagram of a simple continuous-wave flowmeter. The oscillator must have a low output impedance to drive the low-impedance crystal. Although at most frequencies the crystal transducer has a high impedance, it is operated at mechanical resonance, where the impedance drops to about 100 Ω. The ultrasonic waves are transmitted to the moving cells, which reflect the Doppler-shifted waves to the receiving transducer. The receiving transducer is identical to the transmitting transducer. The amplified radio-frequency (RF) signal plus carrier signal is detected to produce an audio-frequency (AF) signal at a frequency given by (8.15).

Listening to the audio output using a speaker, we get much useful qualitative information. A simple *frequency-to-voltage converter* provides a quantitative output to a recorder. The *zero-crossing detector* emits a fixed-area pulse each time the audio signal crosses the zero axis. These pulses are low-pass-filtered to produce an output proportional to the velocity of the blood cells.

Although the electromagnetic blood flowmeter is capable of measuring both forward and reverse flow, the simple ultrasonic-type flowmeter full-wave rectifies the output, and the sense of direction of flow is lost. This results because—for either an increase or a decrease in the Doppler-shifted frequency—the beat frequency is the same. Examination of the field intersections shown in Figure 8.10 suggests that the only received frequency is the Doppler-shifted one. However, the received carrier signal is very much larger than the desired Doppler-shifted signal. Some of the RF carrier is coupled to the receiver by the electric field from the transmitter. Because of side lobes in the transducer apertures, some of the carrier signal travels a direct acoustic path to the receiver. Other power at the carrier frequency reaches the receiver after one or more reflections from fixed interfaces. The resulting received signal is composed of a large-amplitude signal at the carrier frequency plus the very low (approximately 0.1%) amplitude Doppler-shifted signal.

The Doppler-shifted signal is not at a single frequency, as implied by (8.15), for several reasons.

1. Velocity profiles are rarely blunt, with all cells moving at the same velocity. Rather, cells move at different velocities, producing different shifts of the Doppler frequency.
2. A given cell remains within the beam-intersection volume for a short time. Thus the signal received from one cell is a pure frequency multiplied by some time-gate function, yielding a band of frequencies.
3. Acoustic energy traveling within the main beam, but at angles to the beam axis, plus energy in the side lobes, causes different Doppler-frequency shifts due to an effective change in $\theta$.
4. Tumbling of cells and local velocities resulting from turbulence cause different Doppler-frequency shifts.

All these factors combine to produce a band of frequencies. The resulting spectrum is similar to band-limited random noise, and from this we must extract flow information.

We would like to have high gain in the RF amplifier in order to boost the low-amplitude Doppler-frequency components. But the carrier is large, so the gain cannot be too high or saturation will occur. The RF bandwidth need not be wide, because the frequency deviation is only about 0.001 of the carrier frequency. However, RF-amplifier bandwidths are sometimes much wider than required, to permit tuning to different transducers.

The detector can be a simple square-law device such as a diode. The output spectrum contains the desired difference (beat) frequencies, which lie in the audio range, plus other undesired frequencies.

**EXAMPLE 8.4** Calculate the maximal audio frequency of a Doppler ultrasonic blood flowmeter that has a carrier frequency of 7 MHz, a transducer angle of 45°, a blood velocity of 150 cm/s, and an acoustic velocity of 1500 m/s.

**ANSWER** Substitute these data into (8.15).

$$f_d = \frac{2(7 \times 10^6\ \text{Hz})(1.5\ \text{m/s})\cos 45^\circ}{1500\ \text{m/s}} \cong 10\ \text{kHz} \tag{8.16}$$

The dc component must be removed with a high-pass filter in the AF amplifier. We require a corner frequency of about 100 Hz in order to reject large Doppler signals due to motion of vessel walls. Unfortunately, this high-pass filter also keeps us from measuring slow cell velocities (less than 1.5 cm/s), such as occur near the vessel wall. A low-pass filter removes high frequencies and also noise. The corner frequency is at about 15 kHz, which includes all frequencies that could result from cell motion, plus an allowance for spectral spreading.

In the simplest instruments, the AF output drives a power amplifier and speaker or earphones. The output is a band of frequencies, so it has a whooshing sound that for steady flows sounds like random noise. Venous flow sounds like a low-frequency rumble and may be modulated when the subject breathes. Arterial flow, being pulsatile, rises to a high pitch once each beat and may be followed by one or more smaller, easily heard waves caused by the under-damped flow characteristics of arteries. Thus this simple instrument can be used to trace and qualitatively evaluate blood vessels within 1 cm of the skin in locations in the legs, arms, and neck. We can also plot the spectrum of the AF signal versus time to obtain a more quantitative indication of velocities in the vessel.

The function of the *zero-crossing detector* is to convert the AF input frequency to a proportional analog output signal. It does this by emitting a constant-area pulse for each crossing of the zero axis. The detector contains a comparator (a Schmitt trigger), so we must determine the amount of hysteresis for the comparator. If the input were a single sine wave, the *signal-to-hysteresis ratio* (SHR) could be varied over wide limits, and the output would indicate the correct value. But the input is band-limited random noise. If the SHR is low, many zero crossings are missed. As the SHR increases, the indicated frequency of the output increases. A SHR of 7 is a good choice because the output does not vary significantly with changes in SHR. Automatic gain control can be used to maintain this ratio. Very high SHRs are not desirable; noise may trigger the comparator. The signal increases and decreases with time because of the beating of the signal components at the various frequencies. Thus the short-term SHR fluctuates, and for a small portion of the time the signal is too low to exceed the hysteresis band.

**EXAMPLE 8.5** Design a comparator with a SHR of 7, as required for the Doppler zero-crossing detector.

**ANSWER** Assume that the signal has been amplified so that its input p–p value equals the $\pm 10$ V linear range for an op amp. Then our thresholds should be $\pm 10/7 = \pm 1.4$ V. Use the circuit shown in Figure 3.6(a). Because the input is symmetric about zero, $v_{\text{ref}} = 0$ V. Assume the op amp output saturates at $\pm 12$ V. The p–p width of the hysteresis loop is four times the voltage across $R_3$, or $2.8/4 = 0.7$. Assume $R_3 = 1\ \text{k}\Omega$. Then

$$\frac{R_2 + R_3}{R_3} = \frac{R_2 + 1\ \text{k}\Omega}{1\ \text{k}\Omega} = \frac{12}{0.7}$$

$$R_2 = 16.1\ \text{k}\Omega.\ \text{Choose}\ R_1 = 10\ \text{k}\Omega.$$

The output of the zero-crossing detector is a series of pulses. These pulses are passed through a low-pass filter to remove as many of the high-frequency components as possible. The filter must pass frequencies from 0 to 25 Hz in order to reproduce the frequencies of interest in the flow pulse. However, the signal is similar to band-limited random noise. Thus the pulses are not at uniform intervals, even for a fixed flow velocity, but are more like a Poisson process. Hence the output contains objectionable noise. The low-pass filter must therefore be chosen as a compromise between the high corner frequency desired to reproduce the flow pulse and the low corner frequency desired for good filtering of noise.

A major defect of the detector used in simple flowmeters is that it cannot detect the direction of flow. The recorded output looks as it would if the true velocity had been full-wave rectified. Compared with the electromagnetic flowmeter, this is a real disadvantage, because reverse flow occurs frequently in the body. A first thought might be to translate the Doppler-shifted frequencies not to the region about dc, but to the region about 20 kHz. Forward flow might thus be 30 kHz, and reverse flow 10 kHz. The difficulty with this approach is that the high-amplitude carrier signal is translated to 20 kHz. The Doppler signals are so small that considerable effort is required to build any reasonable frequency-to-voltage converter that is not dominated by the 20 kHz signal.

A better approach is to borrow a technique from radar technology, which is used to determine not only the speed at which an aircraft is flying but also its direction. This is the *quadrature-phase detector*.

Figure 8.11(a) shows the analog portion of the quadrature-phase detector (McLeon, 1967). A phase-shift network splits the carrier into two components that are in quadrature, which means that they are 90° apart. These reference cosine and sine waves must be several times larger than the RF-amplifier output, as shown in Figure 8.12(a). The reference waves and the RF-amplifier output are linearly summed to produce the RF envelope shown in Figure 8.12(b). We assume temporarily that the RF-amplifier output contains no carrier.

If the flow of blood is in the same direction as the ultrasonic beam, we consider the blood to be flowing away from the transducer, as shown in Figure 8.11(a). For this direction, the Doppler-shift frequency is lower than that of the carrier. The phase of the Doppler wave lags behind that of the reference

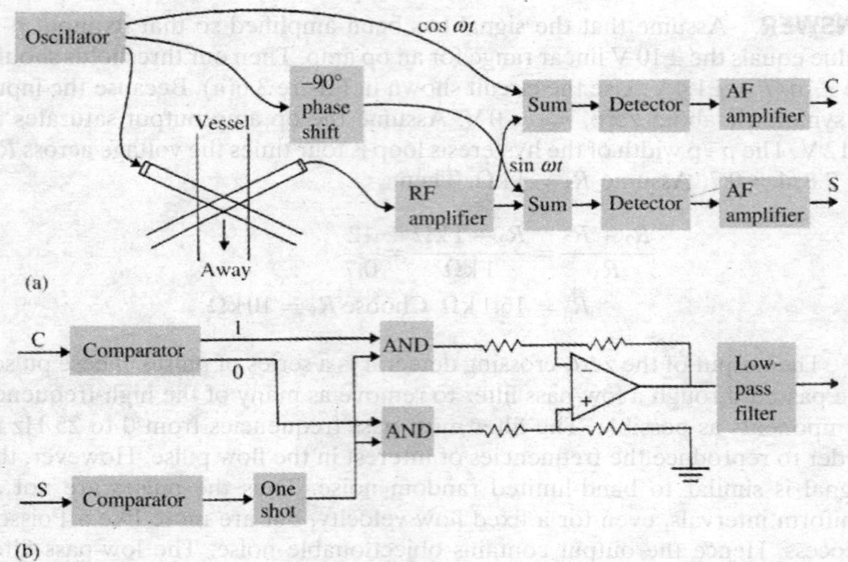


**Figure 8.11 Directional Doppler block diagram** (a) Quadrature-phase detector: Sine and cosine signals at the carrier frequency are summed with the RF output before detection. The output C from the cosine channel then leads (or lags) the output S from the sine channel if the flow is away from (or toward) the transducer. (b) Logic circuits route one-shot pulses through the top (or bottom) AND gate when the flow is away from (or toward) the transducer. The differential amplifier provides bidirectional output pulses that are then filtered.

carrier, and the Doppler vector [see Figure 8.12(a)] rotates clockwise. In Figure 8.12(b), for time 1, the carrier and the Doppler add, producing a larger sum in the cosine channel. The sine channel is unchanged. For time 2, the carrier and the Doppler add, producing a larger sum in the sine channel. Similar reasoning produces the rest of the wave for times 3 and 4. Note that the sine channel lags behind the cosine channel.

If the flow of blood is toward the transducer, the Doppler frequency is higher than the carrier frequency, and the Doppler vector rotates counterclockwise. This produces the dashed waves shown in Figure 8.12(b), and the phase relation between the cosine and sine channels is reversed. Thus, by examining the sign of the phase, we measure direction of flow. The detector produces AF waves that have the same shape as the RF envelope.

Figure 8.11(b) shows the logic that detects the sign of the phase. The cosine channel drives a comparator, the digital output of which, shown in Figure 8.12(b), is used for gating and does not change with direction of flow of blood. The sine channel triggers a one-shot the width of which must be short. Depending on the direction of flow, this one-shot is triggered either at the beginning of or halfway through the period, as shown in Figure 8.12(b). The

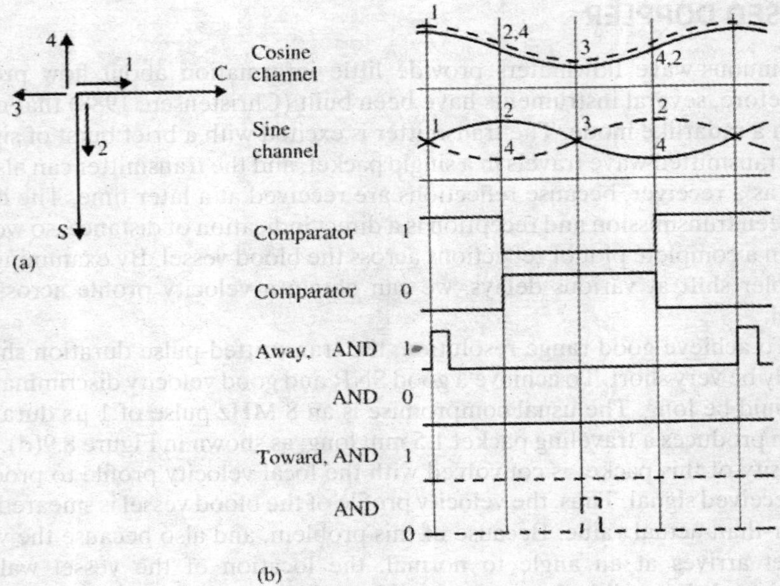


**Figure 8.12 Directional Doppler signal waveforms** (a) Vector diagram: The sine wave at the carrier frequency lags the cosine wave by 90°. If flow is away from the transducer, the Doppler frequency is lower than the carrier. The short vector represents the Doppler signal and rotates clockwise, as shown by the numbers 1, 2, 3, and 4. (b) Timing diagram: The top two waves represent the single-peak envelope of the carrier plus the Doppler before detection. Comparator outputs respond to the cosine channel audio signal after detection. One-shot pulses are derived from the sine channel and are gated through the correct AND gate by comparator outputs. The dashed lines indicate flow toward the transducer.

AND gates then gate it into the top or bottom input of the differential amplifier, thus producing a bidirectional output.

The preceding discussion is correct for a sinusoidal RF signal. Our RF signal is like band-limited random noise, however, so there is some time shifting of the relations shown in Figure 8.12(b). Also, a large fixed component at the carrier frequency is present, which displaces the Doppler vectors away from the position shown. As long as the reference cosine and sine waves are more than twice the amplitude of the total RF output, time shifting of the gating relations is not excessive. These time shifts are not problems in practice; a short one-shot pulse can shift almost ±90° before passing out of the correct comparator gate.

It is possible to add another one-shot and several logic blocks to obtain pulse outputs on both positive and negative zero crossings. This doubles the frequency of the pulse train and reduces the fluctuations in the output to 0.707 of their former value.

## PULSED DOPPLER

Continuous-wave flowmeters provide little information about flow profile. Therefore, several instruments have been built (Christensen, 1988) that operate in a radarlike mode. The transmitter is excited with a brief burst of signal. The transmitted wave travels in a single packet, and the transmitter can also be used as a receiver, because reflections are received at a later time. The delay between transmission and reception is a direct indication of distance, so we can obtain a complete plot of reflections across the blood vessel. By examining the Doppler shift at various delays, we can obtain a velocity profile across the vessel.

To achieve good range resolution, the transmitted-pulse duration should ideally be very short. To achieve a good SNR and good velocity discrimination, it should be long. The usual compromise is an 8 MHz pulse of 1 μs duration, which produces a traveling packet 1.5 mm long, as shown in Figure 8.9(d). The intensity of this packet is convolved with the local velocity profile to produce the received signal. Thus, the velocity profile of the blood vessel is smeared to a larger-than-actual value. Because of this problem, and also because the wave packet arrives at an angle to normal, the location of the vessel walls is indistinct. It is possible, however, to mathematically "deconvolve" the instrument output to obtain a less smeared representation of the velocity profile.

There are two constraints on pulse repetition rate $f_r$. First, to avoid *range ambiguities*, we must analyze the return from one pulse before sending out the next. Thus

$$f_r < \frac{c}{2R_m} \tag{8.17}$$

where $R_m$ is the maximal useful range. Second, we must satisfy the *sampling theorem*, which requires that

$$f_r > 2f_d \tag{8.18}$$

Combining (8.17) and (8.18) with (8.15) yields

$$u_m(\cos\theta)R_{max} < \frac{c^2}{8f_0} \tag{8.19}$$

which shows that the product of the range and the maximal velocity along the transducer axis is limited. In practice, measurements are constrained even more than indicated by (8.19) because of (1) spectral spreading, which produces some frequencies higher than those expected, and (2) imperfect cutoff characteristics of the low-pass filters used to prevent *aliasing* (generation of fictitious frequencies by the sampling process).

Because we cannot easily start and stop an oscillator in 1 μs, the first stage of the oscillator operates continuously. The transmitter and the receiver both use a common piezoelectric transducer, so a *gate* is required to turn off the signal from the transmitter during reception. A one-stage gate is not sufficient to isolate the large transmitter signals from the very small received signals. Therefore, two gates in series are used to turn off the transmitter.

The optimal transmitted signal is a pulse-modulated sine-wave carrier. Although it is easy to generate this burst electrically, it is difficult to transduce this electric burst to a similar acoustic burst. The crystal transducer has a high $Q$ (narrow bandwidth) and therefore rings at its resonant frequency long after the electric signal stops. Therefore, the transducer is modified to achieve a lower $Q$ (wider bandwidth) by adding mass to the back [Figure 8.9(d)] or to the front [Figure 8.9(e)]. The $Q$ is not lowered to a desirable value of about 2 to 5, because this would greatly decrease both the efficiency of the transmission and the sensitivity of the reception. The $Q$ is generally 5 to 15, so some ringing still exists.

When we generate a short sine-wave burst, we no longer have a single frequency. Rather, the pulse train of the repetition rate is multiplied by the carrier in time, producing carrier sidebands in the frequency domain. This spectrum excites the transducer, producing a field that is more complex than that for continuous-wave excitation. This causes spectral spreading of the received signal.

### LASER DOPPLER BLOOD FLOWMETER

In a laser Doppler blood flowmeter, a 5 mW He–Ne laser beams 632.8 nm light through fiber optics into the skin (Khaodhiar and Veves, 2006). Moving red blood cells in the skin frequency shift the light and cause spectral broadening. Reflected light is carried by fiber optics to a photodiode. Filtering, weighting, squaring, and dividing are necessary for signal processing. Capillary blood flow has been studied in the skin and many other organs.

## 8.5 THERMAL-CONVECTION VELOCITY SENSORS

### PRINCIPLE

The thermodilution methods described in Sections 8.1 and 8.2 depend on the mixing of the heat indicator into the entire flow stream. In contrast, thermal velocity sensors depend on convective cooling of a heated sensor and are therefore sensitive only to local velocity.

Figure 8.13(a) shows a simple probe. The thermistor $R_u$ is heated to a temperature difference $\Delta T$ above blood temperature by the power $W$ dissipated by current passing through $R_u$. Experimental observations (Grahn *et al.*, 1969) show that these quantities are related to the blood velocity $u$ by

$$\frac{W}{\Delta T} = a + b \log u \tag{8.20}$$

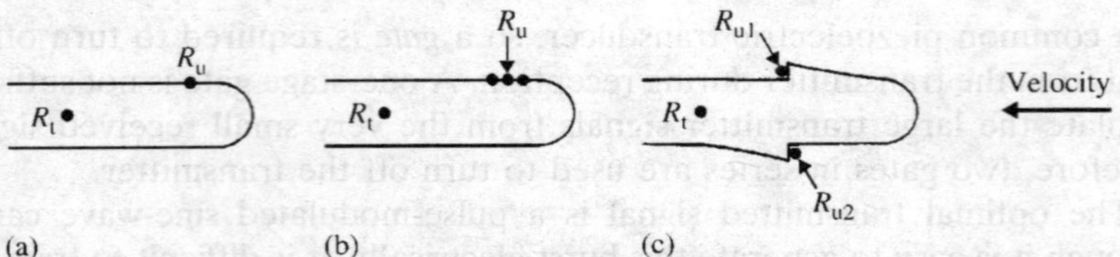


**Figure 8.13 Thermal velocity probes** (a) Velocity-sensitive thermistor $R_u$ is exposed to the velocity stream. Temperature-compensating thermistor $R_t$ is placed within the probe. (b) Thermistors placed down- and upstream from $R_u$ are heated or not heated by $R_u$, thus indicating velocity direction. (c) Thermistors exposed to and shielded from flow can also indicate velocity direction.

where $a$ and $b$ are constants. Thus the method is nonlinear, with a large sensitivity at low velocities and a small sensitivity at high velocities.

## PROBES

Catheter-tip probes are designed with two types of sensors (Cobbold, 1974). The first type uses the thermistors shown in Figure 8.13 and provides a high sensitivity and reasonable resistance values. Because the thermistor shown in Figure 8.13(a) is cooled equally for both directions of velocity, the output of the instrument is a full-wave-rectified replica of the true velocity. To overcome this limitation, the probe shown in Figure 8.13(b) has two additional thermistors located a few tenths of a millimeter downstream and upstream from $R_u$. Depending on the direction of velocity, one or the other is heated by the heat carried through the blood from the thermistor $R_u$. These two additional thermistors are placed in a bridge that is balanced for zero velocity. A comparator detects the bridge unbalance and switches the output from positive to negative. The probe shown in Figure 8.13(c) uses two velocity sensors arranged so that one is exposed to the fluid velocity while the other is shielded from the fluid velocity.

The second type of sensor uses a glass bead with a thin strip of platinum deposited on its surface. The platinum may be painted on and then fired in a furnace, or it may be *sputtered* (deposited by electric discharge in a vacuum). A disadvantage of platinum-film sensors is their low resistance (a few ohms) and low sensitivity.

A real question arises about what is actually being measured. When a catheter is inserted into a blood vessel, the sensor may be centered and thus measure maximal velocity, or it may be against the wall of the vessel and thus measure a low velocity. One way of ensuring that the sensor is not against the wall is to rotate the catheter, searching for the maximal output. Catheters are also sensitive to radial velocity of blood, as well as to radial vibrations of the catheter (catheter whip). Thus, in addition to any errors due to measuring velocity, errors in trying to estimate flow can arise from lack of knowledge about location of the sensor. Either type of probe (if it is made sufficiently small) can be placed at the end of a hypodermic needle and inserted perpendicular to the vessel for measuring velocity profiles.

## CIRCUIT

A *constant-current* sensor circuit cannot be used for two reasons. First, the time constant of the sensor embedded in the probe is a few tenths of a second—much too long to achieve the desired frequency response of 0 to 25 Hz. Second, to achieve a reasonable sensitivity at high velocities, the sensor current must be so high that when the flow stops, lack of convection cooling increases the sensor temperature more than 5 °C above the blood temperature and fibrin coats the sensor.

The *constant-temperature* sensor circuit shown in Figure 8.14 overcomes both of these problems. The circuit is initially unbalanced by adjusting $R_1$. The unbalance is amplified by the high-gain op amp, and its output is fed back to power the resistance bridge. Operation of the circuit is as follows: Assume that thermistor $R_u$ is 5 °C higher than blood temperature because of self-heating. If the velocity increases, $R_u$ cools and its resistance increases. A more positive voltage enters the noninverting op-amp terminal, so $v_b$ increases. This increases bridge power and $R_u$ heats up, thus counteracting the original cooling. The system uses high-gain negative feedback to keep the bridge always in balance. Thus $R_u$ remains nearly constant, and therefore its temperature remains nearly constant. The high-gain negative feedback divides the sensor time constant by a factor equal to the loop gain, so frequency response is greatly improved. In effect, if the sensor becomes slightly cooled, the op amp can provide a large quantity of power to rapidly heat it back to the desired temperature.

The circuit operates satisfactorily with only one sensor, $R_u$, provided that the blood temperature is constant. Should the blood temperature vary, a temperature–compensating thermistor $R_t$ is added to keep the bridge in balance. So that its rise in temperature is very small, $R_t$ must have a much lower resistance–temperature coefficient than $R_u$, to ensure that $R_t$ is a sensor of temperature and not of velocity. The thermal resistance of $R_t$ can be lowered by making it large in size, by using a heat sink, or by placing it within the probe so that the effective cooling area is much larger. Another solution is to increase

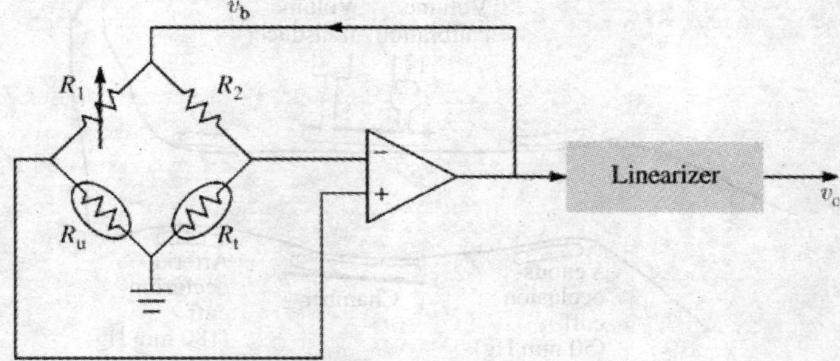


**Figure 8.14 Thermal velocity meter circuit** A velocity increase cools $R_u$, the velocity-measuring thermistor. This increases voltage to the noninverting op-amp input, which increases bridge voltage $v_b$ and heats $R_u$. $R_t$ provides temperature compensation.

the resistance values for $R_2$ and $R_t$ so that their power dissipation is much lower.

A linearizer is required to solve (8.20). We may square $v_b$ to obtain $W$ and then use an antilog converter to obtain $v_o$. For the directional probe shown in Figure 8.17(b), a unity-gain inverting amplifier and switch may be used to yield the direction of flow.

Calibration can be accomplished by using a sinusoidal-flow pump or a cylindrical pan of liquid rotating on a turntable.

The main use of thermal-velocity sensors is to measure the velocity of blood and to compile velocity profiles in studies of animals, although such sensors have also been regularly used to measure velocity and acceleration of blood at the aortic root in human patients undergoing diagnostic catheterization. The same principle has also been applied to the measurement of the flow of air in lungs and ventilators by installing a heated platinum wire in a breathing tube.

## 8.6 CHAMBER PLETHYSMOGRAPHY

Plethysmographs measure changes in volume. The only accurate way to measure changes in volume of blood in the extremities noninvasively is to use a chamber plethysmograph. By timing these volume changes, we can measure flow by computing $F = dV/dt$. A cuff is used to prevent venous blood from leaving the limb—hence the name *venous-occlusion plethysmography* (Seagar *et al.*, 1984).

### EQUIPMENT

Figure 8.15 shows the equipment used in a venous-occlusion plethysmograph. The chamber has a rigid cylindrical outer container and is placed around the leg.

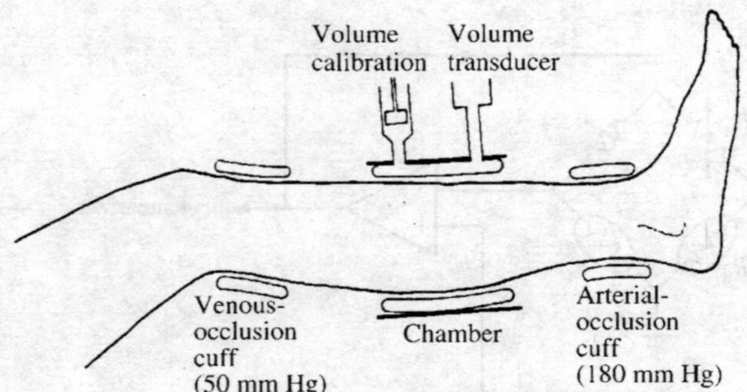


**Figure 8.15** In chamber plethysmography, the venous-occlusion cuff is inflated to 50 mm Hg (6.7 kPa), stopping venous return. Arterial flow causes an increase in volume of the leg segment, which the chamber measures. The text explains the purpose of the arterial-occlusion cuff.

As the volume of the leg increases, the leg squeezes some type of bladder and decreases its volume. If the bladder is filled with water, the change in volume may be measured by observing the water rising in a calibrated tube. For recording purposes, some air may be introduced above the water and the change in air pressure measured. Water-filled plethysmographs are temperature controlled to prevent thermal drifts. Because of their hydrostatic pressure, they may constrict the vessels in the limb and cause undesirable physiological changes.

Air may be used in the bladder and the resulting changes in pressure measured directly. Some systems do not use a bladder. They attempt to seal the ends of a rigid chamber to the limb, but then leaks may be a problem. One device uses a pneumotachometer to measure the flow of air into and out of the chamber. This flow is then integrated to yield changes in volume. This equipment is designed to accommodate a variety of limb sizes, so the chambers and bladders are made in a family of sizes. Alternatively, a single chamber may be used for several sizes of limb. Devices that are capable of doing this are made with iris diaphragms that form the ends of the chamber and close down on the limb.

## METHOD

Figure 8.16 shows the sequence of operations that yields a measurement of flow (Raines and Darling, 1976). A calibration may be marked on the record by injecting into the chamber a known volume of fluid, using the volume-calibration syringe. The venous-occlusion cuff is then applied to a limb and pressurized to 50 mm Hg (6.7 kPa), which prevents venous blood from leaving the limb. Arterial flow is not hindered by this cuff pressure, and the increase in volume of blood in the limb per unit time is equal to the arterial inflow. If the chamber completely encloses the limb distal to the cuff, the arterial flow into the limb is measured. If the chamber encloses only a segment of a limb, as shown in Figure 8.15, an arterial-occlusion cuff distal to the chamber must be inflated to 180 mm Hg (24 kPa) to ensure that the changes in chamber volume measure only arterial flow entering the segment of the limb.

A few seconds after the cuffs are occluded, the venous pressure exceeds 50 mm Hg (6.7 kPa), venous return commences, and the volume of blood in the

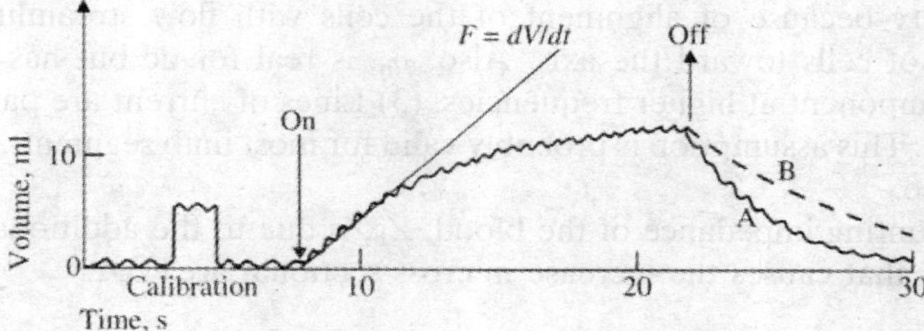


**Figure 8.16** After venous-occlusion cuff pressure is turned on, the initial volume-versus-time slope is caused by arterial inflow. After the cuff is released, segment volume rapidly returns to normal (A). If a venous thrombosis blocks the vein, return to normal is slower (B).

limb segment plateaus. When the clinician releases the pressure of the venous-occlusion cuff, the volume of blood in the limb segment rapidly returns to normal (Figure 8.16, curve A). If a venous thrombosis (vein clot) partially blocks the return of venous blood, the volume of blood in the veins returns to normal more slowly (Figure 8.16, curve B). This technique is a useful non-invasive test for venous thrombosis.

Brunswig Newring *et al.* (2006) note that the measurement of erection, or penile tumescence, is the only physiological response that reliably differentiates male sexual arousal from other emotional states. Early water- or air-filled chamber plethysmographs for measuring tumescence have been replaced by less bulky circular metal bands and elastic strain gages.

## 8.7 ELECTRICAL-IMPEDANCE PLETHYSMOGRAPHY

It is simple to attach electrodes to a segment of tissue and measure the resulting impedance of the tissue. As the volume of the tissue changes in response to pulsations of blood (as happens in a limb) or the resistivity changes in response to increased air in the tissue (as happens in the lung), the impedance of the tissue changes (Hutten, 2006).

Electrical-impedance plethysmography has been used to measure a wide variety of variables, but in many cases the accuracy of the method is poor or unknown.

### PRINCIPLE

In the early 1950s, Nyboer (1970) developed the equations used in impedance plethysmography. However, we shall follow Swanson's (1976) derivation, which is conceptually and mathematically simpler. Figure 8.17 shows Swanson's model of a cylindrical limb. The derivation requires three assumptions: (1) The expansion of the arteries is uniform. This assumption is probably valid in healthy vessels, but it may not be valid in diseased ones. (2) The resistivity of blood, $\rho_b$, does not change. In fact, $\rho_b$, decreases with velocity because of alignment of the cells with flow streamlines and movement of cells toward the axis. Also, $\rho_b$, is real for dc but has a small reactive component at higher frequencies. (3) Lines of current are parallel to the arteries. This assumption is probably valid for most limb segments, but not for the knee.

The shunting impedance of the blood, $Z_b$, is due to the additional blood volume $\Delta V$ that causes the increase in cross-sectional area $\Delta A$.

$$Z_b = \frac{\rho_b L}{\Delta A} \tag{8.21}$$

$$\Delta V = L\,\Delta A = \frac{\rho_b L^2}{Z_b} \tag{8.22}$$

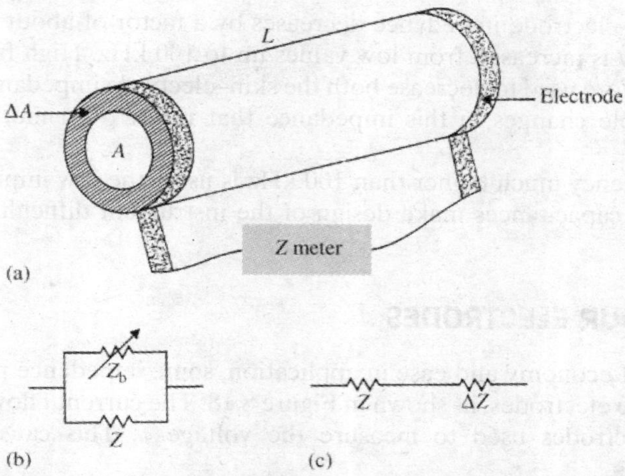


**Figure 8.17** (a) A model for impedance plethysmography. A cylindrical limb has length $L$ and cross-sectional area $A$. With each pressure pulse, $A$ increases by the shaded area $\Delta A$. (b) This causes impedance of the blood, $Z_b$, to be added in parallel to $Z$. (c) Usually $\Delta Z$ is measured instead of $Z_b$.

But we must replace the $Z_b$ of Figure 8.17(b) in terms of the normally measured $\Delta Z = [(Z_b \| Z) - Z]$ of Figure 8.17(c). Now

$$\Delta Z = \frac{ZZ_b}{Z + Z_b} - Z = \frac{-Z^2}{Z + Z_b} \tag{8.23}$$

and because $Z \ll Z_b$,

$$\frac{1}{Z_b} \cong \frac{-\Delta Z}{Z^2} \tag{8.24}$$

Substituting (8.24) in (8.22) yields

$$\Delta V = \frac{-\rho_b L^2 \Delta Z}{Z^2} \tag{8.25}$$

If the assumptions are valid, (8.25) shows that we can calculate $\Delta V$ from $\rho_b$ (Geddes and Baker, 1989) and from other quantities that are easily measured.

Although (8.25) is valid at any frequency, there are several considerations that suggest the use of a frequency of about 100 kHz.

1. It is desirable to use a current greater than 1 mA in order to achieve adequate SNR. At low frequencies this current causes an unpleasant shock. However, the current required for perception increases with frequency (Section 14.2). Therefore, frequencies above 20 kHz are used to avoid perception of the current.

2. The skin–electrode impedance decreases by a factor of about 100 as the frequency is increased from low values up to 100 kHz. High frequencies are therefore used to decrease both the skin–electrode impedance and the undesirable changes in this impedance that result from motion of the patient.
3. If a frequency much higher than 100 kHz is used, the low impedances of the stray capacitances make design of the instrument difficult.

## TWO OR FOUR ELECTRODES

For reasons of economy and ease in application, some impedance plethysmographs use two electrodes, as shown in Figure 8.18. The current $i$ flows through the same electrodes used to measure the voltage $v$. This causes several problems.

1. The current density is higher near the electrodes than elsewhere in the tissue. This causes the measured impedance, $Z = v/i$, to weight impedance of the tissue more heavily near the electrodes than elsewhere in the tissue.
2. Pulsations of blood in the tissue cause artifactual changes in the skin–electrode impedance, as well as changes in the desired tissue impedance. Because the skin–electrode impedance is in series with the desired tissue

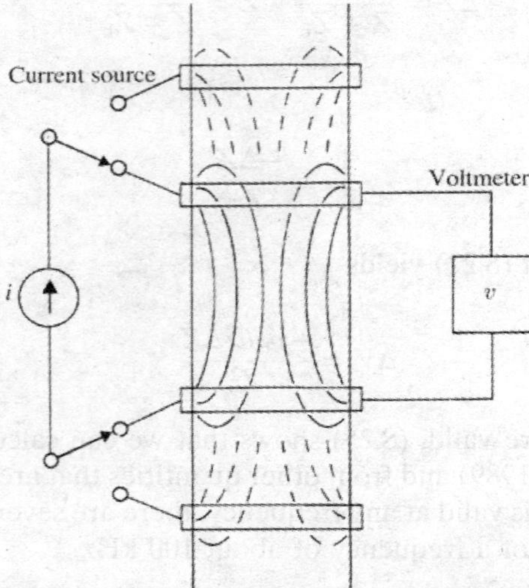


**Figure 8.18** In two-electrode impedance plethysmography, switches are in the position shown, resulting in a high current density (solid lines) under voltage-sensing electrodes. In four-electrode impedance plethysmography, switches are thrown to the other position, resulting in a more uniform current density (dashed lines) under voltage-sensing electrodes.

impedance, it is impossible to separate the two and determine the actual change in impedance of the tissue.

3. The current density is not uniform in the region of interest, so (8.25) cannot be used.

To solve these problems, clinicians use the four-electrode impedance plethysmograph shown in Figure 8.18. The current flows through the two outer electrodes, so the current density is more uniform in the region sensed by the two inner voltage electrodes. Variations in skin–electrode impedance cause only a second-order error.

## CONSTANT-CURRENT SOURCE

Figure 8.19 shows the circuit of a four-electrode impedance plethysmograph. Ideally, the current source $i$ causes a constant current to flow through $Z$, regardless of changes in $\Delta Z$ or other impedances. In practice, however, a shunting impedance $Z_i$ results from stray and cable capacitance. At 100 kHz, 15 pF of stray capacitance causes an impedance of about 100 kΩ. Thus changes in $Z_1$, $\Delta Z$, and $Z_4$ cause the constant current to divide between $Z$ and $Z_i$ in a changing manner. In practice this is not a problem, because changes in $Z_1$, $\Delta Z$, and $Z_4$ are small, and careful design can keep $Z_i$ large enough. Also, $Z$ and $Z_i$; are close to 90° out of phase, which reduces the effects of the problem.

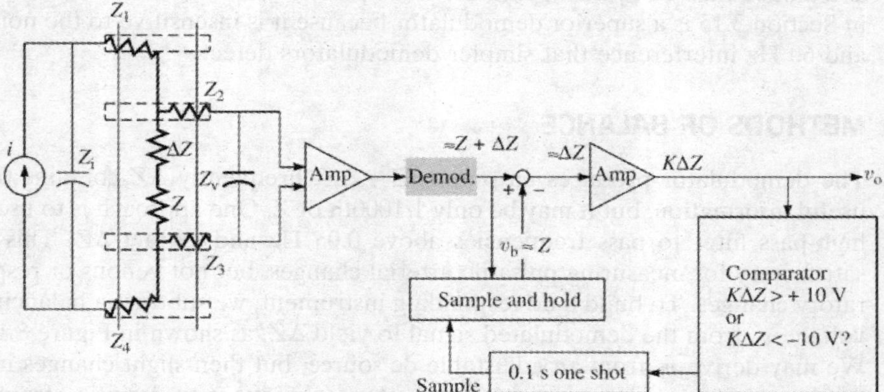


**Figure 8.19** In four-electrode impedance plethysmography, current is injected through two outer electrodes, and voltage is sensed between two inner electrodes. Amplification and demodulation yield $Z + \Delta Z$. Normally, a balancing voltage $v_b$ is applied to produce the desired $\Delta Z$. In the automatic-reset system, when saturation of $v_o$ occurs, the comparator commands the sample and hold to sample $Z + \Delta Z$ and hold it as $v_b$. This resets the input to the final amplifier and $v_o$ to zero. Further changes in $\Delta Z$ cause changes in $v_o$ without saturation.

Frequently the constant current is supplied through a low-capacity transformer to prevent ground-loop problems.

## VOLTAGE-SENSING AMPLIFIER

Figure 8.19 shows that electrodes $Z_2$ and $Z_3$ are used to sense the voltage. Ideally, the voltage amplifier has an input impedance sufficiently high that no current flows through $Z_2$ and $Z_3$. In practice, however, a shunting impedance $Z_v$ results from stray, cable, and amplifier capacitance. Thus changes in $Z_2$ and $Z_3$ cause the desired voltage to be attenuated in a changing manner. In practice this is not a problem, because changes in $Z_2$ and $Z_3$ are small, and careful design can keep $Z_v$ large enough. Also, $Z_2$ and $Z_3$ are 90° out of phase with $Z_v$, which reduces the effects of the problem. Not shown in Figure 8.19 are common-mode impedances from each amplifier input to ground. These impedances can convert common-mode voltages to erroneous differential voltages unless the instrument is carefully designed. Frequently, the voltage is sensed through a low-capacity transformer, which greatly reduces common-mode and ground-loop problems. The amplifier requires only modest gain, because a typical voltage sensed is $v = iZ = (0.004)(40) = 0.16\text{ V}$.

## DEMODULATION

The output of the amplifier is a large 100 kHz signal, amplitude-modulated a small amount by $i\Delta Z$. This $i\Delta Z$ may be demodulated by any AM detector, such as a diode followed by a low-pass filter. The phase-sensitive detector described in Section 3.15 is a superior demodulator because it is insensitive to the noise and 60 Hz interference that simpler demodulators detect.

## METHODS OF BALANCE

The demodulator produces an output $Z + \Delta Z$. Frequently $\Delta Z$ contains the useful information, but it may be only 1/1000th of $Z$. One approach is to use a high-pass filter to pass frequencies above 0.05 Hz and extract $\Delta Z$. This is satisfactory for measuring pulsatile arterial changes, but not venous or respiratory changes. To build a dc-responding instrument, we subtract a balancing voltage $v_b$ from the demodulated signal to yield $\Delta Z$, as shown in Figure 8.19. We may derive $v_b$ from an adjustable dc source, but then slight changes in $i$ produce artifactual changes in $\Delta Z$. A better technique is to derive $v_b$ from a rectified signal from the master oscillator that generates $i$. Then the system behaves like a Wheatstone bridge: A change in excitation voltage does not unbalance the bridge.

But still there is a problem. When the electrodes are first applied or when the patient moves, $Z$ changes by an amount much larger than $\Delta Z$. The operator must manually adjust $v_b$ to keep $\Delta Z$ small, which is necessary if the operator is to be able to amplify and display $\Delta Z$ adequately. An *automatic-reset system* has been developed to eliminate the bother of manual adjustment.

Whenever $\Delta Z$ saturates its amplifier, a sample-and-hold circuit makes $v_b = Z + \Delta Z$, which momentarily resets $\Delta Z$ to zero. The sudden vertical-reset trace is easily distinguished from the slower-changing physiological data. Shankar and Webster (1984) detail design of an automatically balancing electrical-impedance plethysmograph.

## APPLICATIONS

Electrical-impedance plethysmography is used to measure a wide variety of changes in the volume of tissue (Geddes and Baker, 1989). Electrodes placed on both legs provide an indication of whether pulsations of volume are normal (Shankar and Webster, 1991). If the pulsatile waveform in one leg is much smaller than that in the other, this indicates an obstruction in the first leg. If pulsatile waveforms are reduced in both legs, this indicates an obstruction in their common supply. A clinically useful noninvasive method for detecting venous thrombosis in the leg is venous-occlusion plethysmography. When impedance plethysmography measures the changes in volume shown in Figure 8.16, this approach replaces the cumbersome chamber shown in Figure 8.15.

Electrodes on each side of the thorax provide an excellent indication of rate of ventilation, but they give a less accurate indication of volume of ventilation. Such transthoracic electrical impedance monitoring is widely used for infant apnea monitoring to prevent sudden infant death syndrome (SIDS). Computer algorithms use pattern recognition techniques such as threshold crossing, adaptive threshold, and peak detection to reject cardiogenic and movement artifacts (Neuman, 2006).

Electrodes around the neck and around the waist cause current to flow through the major vessels connected to the heart. The resulting changes in impedance provide a rough estimate of beat-by-beat changes in cardiac output (Kubicek *et al.*, 1970). Mohapatra (1988) provides an extensive review of this *impedance cardiography*. The impedance-cardiographic outputs from the neck, upper thorax, and lower thorax during supine, sitting, and bicycle exercise have been measured (Patterson *et al.*, 1991). Arrangements of spot electrodes do not duplicate band electrodes and do not yield good estimates of cardiac output but estimate only regional flow. Band electrodes yield good estimates of cardiac output for normals, but they may fail to give reasonable predictions on very sick patients.

Although Nyboer (1970) and others claim that flow of blood in the limbs can be measured, Swanson (1976) shows their techniques to be poor predictors of flow.

An eight-electrode catheter in the left ventricle injects current through band electrodes 1 and 8 and measures voltages from all the electrodes in between (Valentinuzzi and Spinelli, 1989). The change in impedance yields change in ventricular volume and, from this, cardiac output. Plots of pressure-volume diagrams and their area yield stroke work.

Some systems claim to measure body water and body fat by measuring the electric impedance between the limbs. However, a wrist-to-ankle measurement is influenced mostly by the impedance of the arm and leg and less than 5% of the total impedance is contributed by the trunk, which has half the body mass. Separate measurements of the arms, legs, and trunk might improve the prediction (Patterson, 1989).

The number of independent measurements from $N$ electrodes is equal to $N(N - 1)/2$. If we place 16 electrodes around the thorax, we can obtain 120 independent measurements and can use these data to compute a two-dimensional image of resistivity distribution within the thorax. A review describes methods of injecting current patterns, measuring electrode voltages, and optimizing reconstruction algorithms to create these images (Webster, 1990). The spatial resolution is only about 10%, but this *electrical-impedance tomography* may be useful for monitoring the development of pneumonia, measuring stomach emptying, or monitoring ventilation.

The advantages of electrical-impedance plethysmography are that it is noninvasive and that it is relatively simple to use. The disadvantages are that it is not sufficiently accurate for many of the attempted applications and that even the cause of the changes in impedance is not clear in some cases.

## 8.8 PHOTOPLETHYSMOGRAPHY

Light can be transmitted through a capillary bed. As arterial pulsations fill the capillary bed, the changes in volume of the vessels modify the absorption, reflection, and scattering of the light. Although photoplethysmography is simple and indicates the timing of events such as heart rate, it provides a poor measure of changes in volume, and it is very sensitive to motion artifact.

### LIGHT SOURCES

Figure 8.20 shows two photoplethysmographic methods, in which sources generate light that is transmitted through the tissue (Geddes and Baker, 1989). A miniature tungsten lamp may be used as the light source, but the

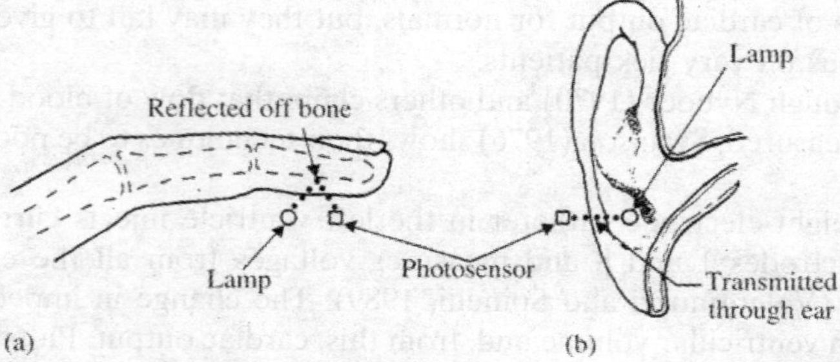


**Figure 8.20** (a) Light transmitted into the finger pad is reflected off bone and detected by a photosensor. (b) Light transmitted through the aural pinna is detected by a photosensor.

heat generated causes vasodilation, which alters the system being measured. This may be considered desirable, however, because a larger pulse is produced. A less bulky unit may be formed using a GaAs LED (Lee *et al.*, 1975), which produces a narrow-band source with a peak spectral emission at a wavelength of 940 nm [Figure 2.18(a)].

## PHOTOSENSORS

Photoconductive cells have been used as sensors, but they are bulky and present a problem in that prior exposure to light changes the sensitivity of the cell. In addition, a filter is required to restrict the sensitivity of the sensor to the near-infrared region so that changes in blood $O_2$ content that are prominent in the visible-light region will not cause changes in sensitivity. A less bulky unit can be formed using an Si phototransistor. A filter that passes only infrared light is helpful for all types of sensors to prevent 120 Hz signals from fluorescent lights from being detected. This does not prevent dc light from tungsten lights or daylight from causing baseline shifts, so lightproof enclosures are usually provided for these devices.

## CIRCUITS

The output from the sensor represents a large value of transmittance, modulated by very small changes due to pulsations of blood. To eliminate the large baseline value, frequencies above 0.05 Hz are passed through a high-pass filter. The resulting signal is greatly amplified to yield a sufficiently large waveform. Any movement of the photoplethysmograph relative to the tissue causes a change in the baseline transmittance that is many times larger than the pulsation signal. These large artifacts due to motion saturate the amplifier; thus it is a good thing to have a means of quickly restoring the output trace.

**EXAMPLE 8.6** Design the complete circuit for a solid-state photoplethysmograph.

**ANSWER** A typical LED requires a forward current of 15 mA. Using a 15 V supply would require a series resistor of $R_L = v/i = 15/0.015 = 1\,\text{k}\Omega$. A typical phototransistor passes a maximum of 150 μA. To avoid saturation, choose a series resistor $R_\text{p} = v/i = 15/0.00015 = 100\,\text{k}\Omega$. The largest convenient paper capacitor is 2 μF. The output resistor $R_\text{o} = 1/(2\pi f_0 C) = 1/[2\pi(0.05)(2 \times 10^{-6})] = 1.6\,\text{M}\Omega$. Figure 8.21 shows the circuit.

## APPLICATIONS

For a patient who remains quiet, the photoplethysmograph can measure heart rate. It offers an advantage in that it responds to the pumping action of the heart and not to the ECG. When properly shielded, it is unaffected by the use of electrosurgery, which usually disables the ECG. However, when the patient is in a

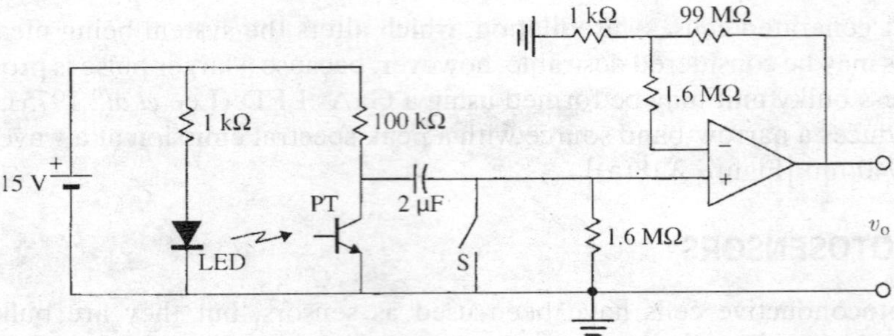


**Figure 8.21** In this photoplethysmograph, the output of a light-emitting diode is altered by tissue absorption to modulate the phototransistor. The dc level is blocked by the capacitor, and switch S restores the trace. A

state of shock, vasoconstriction causes peripheral flow to be greatly reduced, and the resulting small output may make the device unusable. To prevent this problem, the device has been used to transmit light through the nasal septum (Groveman *et al.*, 1966). This technique monitors terminal branches of the internal carotid artery and yields an output that correlates with cerebral blood flow.

## PROBLEMS

**8.1** *Clearance* is defined as the minimal volume of blood entering an organ per unit time required to supply the amount of indicator removed from the blood per unit time during the blood's passage through the organ. Derive a formula for renal clearance, given the arterial concentration of the indicator para amino hippuric acid (PAH), all of which is excreted by the kidneys into the urine. Give units.

**8.2** In Figure 8.2, the final concentration at time *F* is higher than the initial concentration at time *A*. Write a formula that yields the circulating blood volume from the information obtained during an indicator dilution test. Give units.

**8.3** In the decaying exponential portion of Figure 8.2, the concentrations at times *C* and *D* are given. Calculate the shaded area under the dotted curve between times *C* and *E*. Give units.

**8.4** A physician is using the rapid-injection thermodilution method of finding a patient's cardiac output. Calculate the cardiac output (in milliliters per second and in liters per minute) from the following data:

$$V_i = 10\,\text{ml},\ \Delta T_i = -30\,\text{K}$$

$$\rho_i = 1005\,\text{kg/m}^3,\ c_i = 4170\,\text{J/(kg}\cdot\text{K)}$$

$$\rho_b = 1060\,\text{kg/m}^3,\ c_b = 3640\,\text{J/(kg}\cdot\text{K)}$$

$$\int_0^{t_1} \Delta T_b dt = -5.0\,\text{s}\cdot\text{K}$$

**8.5** Name the indicator-dilution technique for measuring cardiac output that does *not* require arterial puncture. Give the equation for calculating cardiac output, and define all terms.
**8.6** For cardiac catheterization, describe the characteristics of the dye used to improve *visualization*. Describe the characteristics of the dye used for measuring *cardiac output*.
**8.7** The maximal average velocity of blood in a dog, 1 m/s, occurs in the dog's aorta, which is 0.015 m in diameter. The magnetic flux density in an electromagnetic blood flowmeter is 0.03 T. Calculate the voltage at the electrodes.
**8.8** In order to determine the frequency response of an electromagnetic flowmeter, the clinician can transiently short-circuit the magnet current by using a microswitch. For steady flow, sketch the resulting output of the flowmeter. Describe the mathematical steps you could implement on a computer in order to convert the resulting transient wave to the flowmeter's frequency response.
**8.9** For Figure 8.6, design a simpler electromagnetic flowmeter without quadrature suppression. Show the block diagram and show all connections for a ring demodulator.
**8.10** For the Doppler ultrasonic flowmeter shown in Figure 8.9(b), suppose that the two transducers are inclined at angles $\theta$ and $\phi$ to the axis. Derive a formula for $f_d$, the Doppler frequency shift.
**8.11** For Figure 8.11, show how to add another one-shot block and several logic blocks to obtain pulse outputs on both positive and negative zero crossings.
**8.12** A pulsed Doppler flowmeter has $f_r = 15\,\text{kHz}$, $f_0 = 8\,\text{MHz}$, and $\theta = 45°$. Calculate $R_m$ and $u_m$.
**8.13** Expand Figures 8.14 and 8.13(b) to show a complete block diagram of a directionally sensitive thermal velocity meter and probe.
**8.14** The chamber plethysmograph shown in Figure 8.15 has a volume of 200 ml. Calculate the rapid change in tissue volume that produces a 120 Pa change in chamber pressure. Assume an adiabatic process: $P(V)^{1.4} = \text{constant}$.
**8.15** Calculate the arterial inflow for the test shown in Figure 8.16.
**8.16** For Figure 8.19, assume $Z + \Delta Z = Z_2 = Z_3 = 100\,\Omega$ and $Z_V = -j2000\,\Omega$ (capacitive). How large is the error caused by a 5 Ω change in $Z_2$? Is an error of this magnitude important?
**8.17** Design a circuit that uses the same two electrodes (plus one ground electrode) to monitor ventilation by impedance and the conventional ECG, with no cross interference.

## REFERENCES

Brunswig Newring, K. A., C. Draper, and W. O'Donohue, "Sexual instrumentation." In J. G. Webster (ed.), *Encyclopedia of Medical Devices and Instrumentation*, 2nd ed., New York: Wiley, 2006, Vol. 6, pp. 149–163.

Capek, J. M., and R. J. Roy, "Fick techniques." In J. G. Webster (ed.), *Encyclopedia of Medical Devices and Instrumentation*. New York: Wiley, 1988, pp. 1302–1314.

Christensen, D. A., *Ultrasonic Bioinstrumentation*. New York: Wiley, 1988.

Cobbold, R. S. C., *Transducers for Biomedical Measurements: Principles and Applications*. New York: Wiley, 1974.

Donovan, F. M, and B. C. Taylor, "Cardiac output, indicator dilution measurement of." In J. G. Webster (ed.), *Encyclopedia of Medical Devices and Instrumentation*, 2nd ed., New York: Wiley, 2006, Vol. 2, pp. 21–25.

Geddes, L. A., and L. E. Baker, *Principles of Applied Biomedical Instrumentation*, 3rd ed., New York: Wiley, 1989.

Grahn, A. R., M. H. Paul, and H. U. Wessel, "A new direction-sensitive probe for catheter-tip thermal velocity measurements." *J. Appl. Physiol.*, 1969, 27, 407–412.

Groveman, J., D. D. Cohen, and J. B. Dillon, "Rhinoplethysmography: Pulse monitoring at the nasal septum." *Anesth. Analg.*, 1966, 45, 63.

Hutten, H., "Impedance plethysmography." In J. G. Webster (ed.), *Encyclopedia of Medical Devices and Instrumentation*, 2nd ed., New York: Wiley, 2006, Vol. 4, pp. 120–132.

Khaodhiar, L., and A. Veves, "Cutaneous blood flow, Doppler measurement of." In J. G. Webster (ed.), *Encyclopedia of Medical Devices and Instrumentation*, 2nd ed., New York: Wiley, 2006, Vol. 2, pp. 378–384.

Kubicek, W. G., A. H. L. From, R. P. Patterson, D. A. Witsoe, A. Castenda, R. G. Lilleki, and R. Ersek, "Impedance cardiography as a noninvasive means to monitor cardiac function." *J. Assoc. Adv. Med. Instrum.*, 1970, 4, 79–84.

Lee, A. L., A. J. Tahmoush, and J. R. Jennings, "An LED-transistor photoplethysmograph." *IEEE Trans. Biomed. Eng.*, 1975, BME-22, 243–250.

McLeod, F. D., "A directional Doppler flowmeter." *Dig. Int. Conf. Med. Biol. Eng.*, Stockholm, 1967, 213.

Mohapatra, S. N., "Impedance cardiography," In J. G. Webster (ed.), *Encyclopedia of Medical Devices and Instrumentation*. New York: Wiley, 1988, pp. 1622–1632.

Neuman, M. R., "Neonatal monitoring," In J. G. Webster (ed.), *Encyclopedia of Medical Devices and Instrumentation*, 2nd ed., New York: Wiley, 2006, Vol. 5, pp. 11–32.

Nyboer, J., *Electrical Impedance Plethysmography*, 2nd ed. Springfield, IL: C. C. Thomas, 1970.

Patterson, R. P., L. Wang, and B. Raza, "Impedance cardiography using band and regional electrodes in supine, sitting, and during exercise." *IEEE Trans. Biomed. Eng.*, 1991, 38, 393–400.

Patterson, R., "Body fluid determinations using multiple impedance measurements." *IEEE Eng. Med. Biol. Magazine*, 1989, 8 (1), 16–18.

Raines, J., and R. C. Darling, "Clinical vascular laboratory: Criteria, procedures, instrumentation." *Med. Electronics Data*, 1976, 7 (1), 33–52.

Seagar, A. D., J. M. Gibbs, and F. M. David, "Interpretation of venous occlusion plethsmographic measurements using a simple model.", *Med. Biol. Eng. Comput.*, 1984, 22, 12–18.

Shankar, R., and J. G. Webster, "Noninvasive measurement of compliance in leg arteries." *IEEE Trans. Biomed. Eng.*, 1991, 38, 62–67.

Shankar, T. M. R., and J. G. Webster, "Design of an automatically balancing electrical impedance plethysmography." *J. Clin. Eng.*, 1984, 9, 129–134.

Shercliff, J. A., *The Theory of Electromagnetic Flow Measurement*. Cambridge: Cambridge University Press, 1962.

Swanson, D. K., "Measurement errors and origin of electrical impedance changes in the limbs." Ph.D. dissertation, Department of Electrical and Computer Engineering, University of Wisconsin, Madison, Wisconsin, 1976.

Trautman, E. D., and M. N. D'ambra, "Cardiac output, thermodilution measurement of." In J. G. Webster (ed.), *Encyclopedia of Medical Devices and Instrumentation*, 2nd ed., New York; Wiley, Vol. 2, 2006, pp. 25–35.

Valentinuzzi, M. E., and J. C. Spinelli, "Intracardiac measurements with the impedance technique." *IEEE Eng. Med. Biol. Magazine*, 1989, 8 (1), 27–34.

Webster, J. G. (ed.), *Electrical Impedance Tomography*. Bristol, England: Adam Hilger, 1990.

# 9

# MEASUREMENTS OF THE RESPIRATORY SYSTEM

Frank P. Primiano, Jr.

This chapter deals with the processes in the lungs that are involved in the exchange of gases between the blood and the atmosphere. Measurement of variables associated with these processes enables the physician to perform two clinically relevant tasks: assess the functional status of the respiratory system (lungs, airways, and chest wall) and intervene in its function.

The objective assessment of respiratory function is performed clinically on two time scales. One is relatively long, involving discrete observations, usually in the form of *pulmonary function tests* (PFT), at intervals on the order of days to years. In pulmonary function testing, a subject's parameter values are compared to those expected from specific populations—either normal populations or those with documented diseases (Primiano, 1981). The required parameters of respiratory function are evaluated using well-defined computational procedures operating on variables measured under specified experimental conditions. Tests of pulmonary function are used to (1) screen the general population for disease; (2) serve as part of periodic physical examinations, especially of individuals with chronic pulmonary conditions; (3) evaluate acute changes during episodes of disease; and (4) follow up after treatment.

The second time scale on which respiratory function is assessed is very short; observations are made either continuously or at intervals on the order of minutes to hours. This activity comes under the heading of *patient monitoring* and is performed in a hospital setting, usually in an intensive care unit (ICU). It is warranted in crisis situations such as might result from trauma, drug overdose, major surgery, or disease. (See Section 13.6.)

Therapeutic modification of respiratory function can be achieved through surgery, the use of drugs, or physical intervention with respiratory-assist devices. Except for extreme, acute circumstances—such as cardiac surgery, in which the lungs are completely by-passed and blood is arterialized in an extracorporeal oxygenator (Section 13.3)—these approaches attempt to control arterial blood gases by manipulating the composition and distribution of pulmonary gas and the distribution of the flow of pulmonary blood. The same variables used to evaluate lung function can be monitored to provide objective feedback information for this external control of the system.

There is a myriad of instruments that have been used to measure variables associated with respiration. Consequently, we shall limit our discussion to clinically applicable devices that yield accurate, quantitative measures suitable for the computation of parameters routinely evaluated for pulmonary function tests and for pulmonary status assessment during mechanical ventilation. This eliminates from detailed discussion those devices that have primary applications as patient-monitoring or physical-diagnosis tools. Examples include devices used in imaging techniques (x-ray films, CT, MRI, PET) and a large group of instruments used to estimate or detect lung-volume change (see the review by Sackner, 1980), such as fluoroscopes; magnetometers; various electrical, mechanical and pneumatic devices placed on or around the torso; nasal temperature sensors; and force plates to detect body movements associated with breathing.

The literature in respiratory physiology suffers from a very poor system of notation (Primiano and Chatburn, 2006). This system evolved, to some extent, from an effort to accommodate the clinically oriented audience. The symbols used in this chapter are a compromise between those found in the respiratory literature (Macklem, 1986; Miller *et al.,* 1987) and those found in the physical sciences literature. For example, in the respiratory literature, $V$ represents the "gas volume" (Miller *et al.* 1987) within a container, such as the lungs, and $\dot{V}$ represents "flow of gas" (Macklem, 1986). However, because the gas in the lungs can be expanded and compressed, the rate of change of lung volume is not necessarily equal to the volume flow of gas entering the lungs through the nose and mouth, although, in many circumstances, it is well approximated by this flow. Nevertheless, to emphasize the distinction between these two physical entities, we will use $\dot{V}$ for the rate of change of volume of a container having volume $V$ and $Q$ for the flow of a fluid (gas or liquid) into it, as is commonly done in physics and fluid mechanics. We could not use $F$ for flow, as is done in the rest of this book, because $F$ is routinely used in respiratory physiology to denote molar fraction (fractional concentration) of a gas species in a mixture. Other symbols will be defined as they are introduced.

## 9.1 MODELING THE RESPIRATORY SYSTEM

Which of the many respiratory variables is to be measured depends on the type of behavior under study as well as on a concept of how the system functions. Ideas about how the respiratory system functions are usually formalized in abstract (that is, verbal or mathematical) models. Not only are the variables that are to be measured specified by models of the respiratory system, but such models also define characteristic parameters of respiratory function and are the basis for the design of experiments to evaluate these parameters. In addition, they motivate control strategies and devices that are used to produce effective respiratory assistance. The definitions and discussions of lung physiology are based on models of the lungs (Primiano and Chatburn, 1988).

Therefore, before we attempt measurements, we should understand the essential features of the respiratory system and some approaches to modeling that we can use not only for the respiratory system but also for the measurement devices themselves.

Because it is the respiratory function of living individuals that is to be evaluated, measurements must be minimally invasive, cause minimal discomfort, and be acceptable for use in a clinical environment. This greatly limits the number and types of measurements that can be made and leads to the use of lumped-parameter models. For the sake of discussion, it is convenient to divide respiratory function into two categories: (1) *gas transport* in the lungs (including extrapulmonary airways and pulmonary capillaries) and (2) *mechanics* of the lungs and chest wall. The models describing gas transport deal primarily with changes in concentrations of gas species and volume flow of gas, whereas the models dealing with mechanics primarily relate pressure, lung volume, and rate of change of lung volume. Bear in mind that these two categories are highly interrelated, and the models and measurements from one complement those from the other (Ligas, 2006).

## GAS TRANSPORT

Models of gas transport, both in the gas phase and across the alveolar-capillary membrane into the blood, are developed from mass balances for the pulmonary system depicted as a set of compartments. What can be considered as a basic gas-transport unit of the lungs is shown in Figure 9.1(a). It consists of a variable-volume alveolar compartment, with its contents well mixed by diffusion; a well-mixed, flow-through blood compartment that exchanges gases with the alveolar compartment by diffusion; and a constant volume dead space. Gas moves by convection through the dead space, which acts only as a time-delay conduit between its outer opening and its associated alveolar volume. A *pair* of normal lungs during quiet breathing may be represented satisfactorily by the system shown in Figure 9.1(a). Lungs undergoing maximal volume changes, subjected to very high ($\gg 1$ Hz) ventilatory frequencies, or afflicted with diseases that produce abnormal gas transport may require more complicated models comprising combinations of such units, in parallel or in series or both.

A dynamic mass balance can be written for any chemical species X or set of species in the breathed gas mixture. If the production of X by chemical reaction in a system were negligible, a species mass balance could be written as

$$\begin{matrix}\text{Rate of mass}\\ \text{accumulation}\\ \text{of X in the}\\ \text{system}\end{matrix} = \sum_{i=1}^{n} \begin{matrix}\text{Rate of mass}\\ \text{convection}\\ \text{of X through}\\ \text{port } i\end{matrix} - \begin{matrix}\text{Net rate of}\\ \text{diffusion out}\\ \text{of the system}\end{matrix} \qquad (9.1)$$

This can also be written as a molar balance, because the number of moles $N$ is the ratio of the mass of X to its molecular weight (in mass units). Define $\rho_{\text{AWO}}\text{X}$

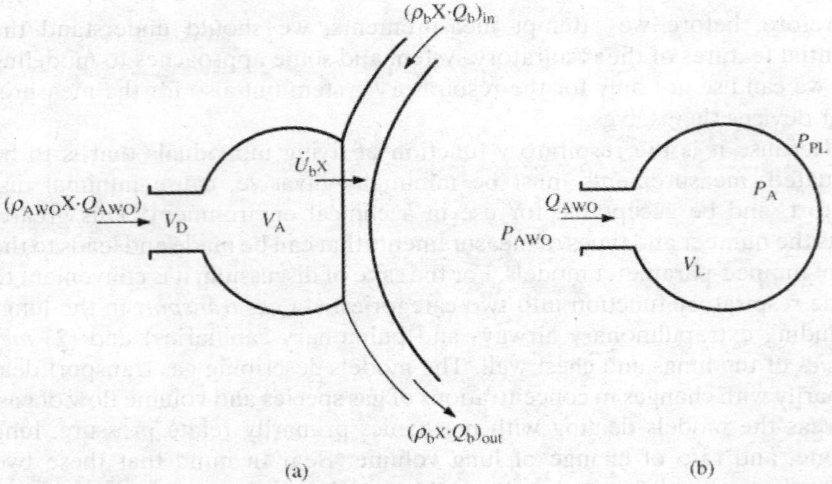


**Figure 9.1 Models of the lungs** (a) Basic gas-transport unit of the pulmonary system. Here $(\rho x \cdot Q)$ is the molar flow of X through the airway opening (AWO) and the pulmonary capillary blood network, b. $\dot{U}_b x$ is the net rate of molar uptake—that is, the net rate of diffusion of X into the blood. $V_D$ and $V_A$ are the dead-space volume and alveolar volume, respectively. (b) A basic mechanical unit of the pulmonary system. $P_A$ is the pressure inside the lung—that is, in the alveolar compartment. $P_{PL}$ and $P_{AWO}$ are the pressures on the pleural surface of the lungs and at the AWO, respectively. $V_L$ is the volume of the gas space within the lungs, including the airways; $Q_{AWO}$ is the volume flow of gas into the lungs measured at the AWO.

as the mole density (moles per unit volume) of species X and $Q_{AWO}$ as its volume flow (volume per unit time), each measured at the airway opening (AWO). Then a molar balance for X in the gas phase in the model of the lungs in Figure 9.1 (a) would be

$$\frac{d(N_L x)}{dt} = (\rho_{AWO} x \cdot Q_{AWO}) - \dot{U}_b x \tag{9.2}$$

in which $\dot{U}_b x$ is the net molar rate of uptake of X by the blood. The number of moles of X in the lungs, $N_L x$, is the sum of the moles in the dead-space volume, $N_D x$, and the alveolar compartment, $N_A x$.

## MECHANICS

We can conveniently model the mechanical behavior of the respiratory system as a combination of pneumatic and mechanical elements (Chatburn and Primiano, 1988). Figure 9.1(b) shows an idealized mechanical unit of the lungs. It consists of a deformable pressure vessel made of a material that exhibits both viscoelastic and plastic behavior and a nonrigid airway that has a

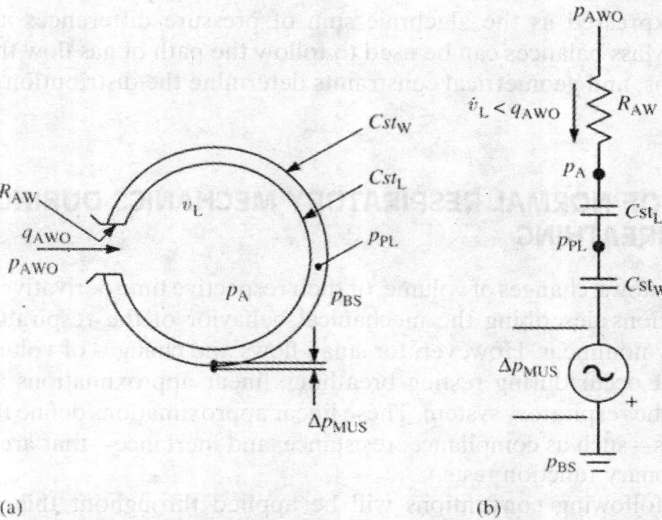


**Figure 9.2 Models of normal ventilatory mechanics for small-amplitude, low-frequency (normal lungs, resting) breathing** (a) Lung mechanical unit enclosed by chest wall. (b) Equivalent circuit for model in Figure 9.2(a).

variable resistance to convective flow. The system contains a mixture of ideal gases and saturated water vapor that exhibits inertia during acceleration through the airway and that undergoes an isothermal process during changes of state.

Even though each of the millions of alveoli and terminal airways potentially could act as a separate mechanical unit, it has been found that the mechanics of a *pair* of normal lungs during quiet breathing can be represented by the single unit of Figure 9.1(b). However, at high rates of breathing, normal and abnormal pulmonary systems may require models containing combinations of such units. Note that only in rare instances, such as when there is only a single gas space in each model, do compartments of the gas-transport units [Figure 9.1(a)] correspond one-to-one to mechanical units [Figure 9.1(b)] in the same lungs.

An additional deformable pressure vessel representing the chest wall surrounding the lungs has been added to the system in Figure 9.2(a). The chest wall includes all extrapulmonary structures, such as ribs, respiratory muscles, and abdominal contents that can undergo motions as a result of breathing. The gap between the lung unit and the chest wall represents the liquid-filled interpleural space.

The mechanics of the respiratory system are described by the relationships between pressure differences across the various subsystems and the changes in volume and flow of gas through them. The subsystems are defined between points in the system at which representative pressures can be computed or measured. Consequently, the difference in pressure across the entire system can be expressed as the algebraic sum of pressure differences across subsystems. Mass balances can be used to follow the path of gas flow through the subsystems, and geometrical constraints determine the distribution of volume changes.

## MODEL OF NORMAL RESPIRATORY MECHANICS DURING QUIET BREATHING

When the flows, changes of volume, or their respective time derivatives are large, the equations describing the mechanical behavior of the respiratory system are highly nonlinear. However, for small flows and changes of volume such as those that occur during resting breathing, linear approximations adequately describe the respiratory system. These linear approximations define the familiar properties—such as compliance, resistance, and inertance—that are evaluated for pulmonary function tests.

The following conventions will be applied throughout this chapter to facilitate writing linearized equations. Lowercase letters for a variable will indicate small changes of that variable about an operating point or reference level.

$$y = Y - \hat{Y}$$

where $\hat{Y}$ indicates some fixed reference value for $Y$. All linearized equations, therefore, are written in lowercase variables. A delta, $\Delta$, will indicate differences between two spatial points.

$$\Delta Y = Y_i - Y_j$$

where $i$ and $j$ indicate different positions, such as AWO and PL. Therefore, the change in the pressure difference across the lungs (the transpulmonary pressure difference) would be

$$(P_{\mathrm{AWO}} - P_{\mathrm{PL}}) - (\hat{P}_{\mathrm{AWO}} - \hat{P}_{\mathrm{PL}}) = \Delta P_{\mathrm{L}} - \Delta \hat{P}_{\mathrm{L}} = \Delta p_{\mathrm{L}}$$

If the alveoli and chest wall exhibit predominantly elastic behavior, the following set of linear equations can be used as a simple model of the mechanics of the respiratory system for normal tidal breathing in the atmosphere [Figure 9.2(a)].

$$p_{\mathrm{AWO}} - p_{\mathrm{A}} = R_{\mathrm{AW}} q_{\mathrm{AWO}} \quad (9.3a)$$

$$p_{\mathrm{A}} - p_{\mathrm{PL}} = \frac{1}{\mathrm{Cst_L}} v_{\mathrm{L}} \quad (9.3b)$$

$$\Delta p_{\mathrm{MUS}} + (p_{\mathrm{PL}} - p_{\mathrm{BS}}) = \frac{1}{\mathrm{Cst_W}} v_{\mathrm{L}} \quad (9.3c)$$

in which lowercase letters are used to designate changes in the following variables with respect to an operating point:

$P_{AWO}$ = hydrostatic pressure at the airway opening

$P_A$ = representative pressure within the lungs (alveolar pressure)

$P_{PL}$ = representation of the average force per unit area acting on the pleural surfaces (interpleural pressure)

$\Delta P_{MUS}$ = representation of the average force per unit area on the chest wall that would cause the same movements produced by the active contraction of the respiratory muscles during breathing (muscle pressure difference)

$P_{BS}$ = hydrostatic pressure acting on the body surface, except at the airway opening

$Q_{AWO}$ = volume flow of gas at the airway opening

$V_L$ = volume of the gas space in the system, assumed to be entirely within the lungs and airways

Three mechanical properties are included in (9.3): airway resistance $R_{AW}$, pulmonary static compliance $Cst_L$, and chest-wall static compliance $Cst_W$. We can evaluate these parameters by applying general definitions of flow resistance through a conduit and compliance of a deformable structure. The resistance to flow of a gas through a conduit is the ratio of the change in pressure drop along the conduit to the change of flow through it while the change in volume of the conduit is zero.

$$R = \frac{\partial(\Delta P)}{\partial Q} \tag{9.4}$$

The "static" compliance of a structure is the ratio of the change in volume of the structure to the change in pressure difference across it while all flows and derivatives of volume are zero.

$$Cst = \frac{\partial V}{\partial(\Delta P)} \tag{9.5}$$

In (9.4) and (9.5), $\Delta P$ is the pressure difference across the system under study. Therefore, for the airway,

$$R_{AW} = \frac{\partial(P_{AWO} - P_A)}{\partial Q_{AWO}} \tag{9.6}$$

The partial derivatives in (9.4) through (9.6) are used to indicate that all other variables must be constant when these parameters are evaluated. In particular, $Cst$ can be evaluated experimentally only when the system is at static equilibrium—that is, when all flows and rates of change of volume and pressure in the system are zero. In this situation $P_{AWO} - P_A = 0$, and

$(P_A - P_{PL})$ can be measured as $(P_{AWO} - P_{PL})$. Thus pulmonary static compliance can be evaluated as

$$Cst_L = \frac{V_L(t_2) - V_L(t_1)}{\Delta P_L(t_2) - \Delta P_L(t_1)} \tag{9.7}$$

in which

$$\Delta P_L = (P_{AWO} - P_{PL}) \tag{9.8}$$

is the *transpulmonary* pressure difference, and $t_1$ and $t_2$ are two instants in time at which the system is completely motionless and at two different volumes.

It is impossible to measure the muscle pressure difference, $\Delta P_{MUS}$, directly. Consequently, chest-wall static compliance can be evaluated only when $\Delta P_{MUS} = 0$. This occurs, by definition, when the respiratory muscles are completely relaxed. Defining the difference in pressure across the chest wall as

$$\Delta P_W = P_{PL} - P_{BS} \tag{9.9}$$

we obtain chest-wall static compliance from

$$Cst_W = \frac{V_L(t_4) - V_L(t_3)}{\Delta P_W(t_4) - \Delta P_W(t_3)} \tag{9.10}$$

in which $t_4$ and $t_3$ are two instants at which the system is static and at two different volumes, *and* the respiratory muscles are completely relaxed.

As the lungs change volume and lose or gain gas through the airway opening, the gas inside is compressed or expanded transiently. During fast changes in volume, this can produce an inequality between the instantaneous rate of volume change, $\dot{V}_L$, and the volume flow of gas at the mouth, $Q_{AWO}$. However, for normal, tidal breathing, this effect can be neglected and $Q_{AWO}$ can be taken as a good approximation to $\dot{V}_L$. Therefore, (9.3a) and (9.3b) can be combined and rewritten as

$$P_{AWO} - P_{PL} = \frac{1}{Cst_L} v_L + R_{AW} \dot{v}_L \tag{9.11}$$

Equations (9.3c) and (9.11), which describe Figure 9.2(a), can also be represented by the analogous equivalent circuit in Figure 9.2(b).

**EXAMPLE 9.1** You are to design a "volume-controlled" positive pressure ventilator that produces a constant (rectangular wave shape) flow ($\dot{v}_L = \dot{V}_L$) at the airway opening during inspiration of duration, $T_I$, until a set tidal volume, $V_T$, is achieved. Then it can maintain that $V_T$ for a set hold time, $T_H$, before permitting a passive, unimpeded exhalation over the exhalation interval, $T_E$. Assuming the patient is sedated and paralyzed and has normal lungs, write an expression for (a) the peak inspiratory pressure (PIP) difference that must be produced by the ventilator at the airway opening to achieve $V_T$ and (b) the inspiratory pressure difference that the ventilator must maintain to hold the lung volume at $V_T$ during $T_H$.

**ANSWER**

**a.** As a first approximation model of a normal respiratory system, combine (9.3c) (chest wall) and (9.11) (lungs): $p_{AWO} - p_{BS} + \Delta p_{MUS} = (1/Cst_W + 1/Cst_L)v_L + R_{AW}\dot{v}_L = v_L/Cst_{TR} + R_{AW}\dot{v}_L$ in which the "total respiratory" compliance is given by $Cst_{TR} = Cst_L Cst_W/(Cst_L + Cst_W)$. A positive pressure ventilator produces inspiration by increasing the pressure ($p_{VENT}$) at the airway opening (rather than by reducing the pressure on the body surface), usually at the inlet to an endotracheal tube (ET) inserted into the patient's airway. For a paralyzed patient, $\Delta p_{MUS}$ is, by definition, zero. When the patient's body surface is exposed to atmospheric pressure, changes in body surface pressure can be neglected. If the flow into the patient during inhalation is constant, then the volume change is a ramp, $v_L = \dot{V}_L t$, that will reach its maximum value when $v_L$ reaches $V_T$ at $T_I$. Therefore, $p_{VENT} = v_L/Cst_{TR} + R_{AW}\dot{v}_L$ and $PIP = (1/Cst_{TR} + R_{AW}/T_I)\,V_T$, where $R_{AW}$ includes the resistance of the ET.

**b.** During the inspiratory breath hold, flow is zero, and $v_L = V_T$. Therefore, $p_{VENT} = V_T/Cst_{TR}$

## MEASURABLE VARIABLES IN THE RESPIRATORY SYSTEM

Even though a number of variables are included in the simple models of gas transport and mechanics shown in Figures 9.1 and 9.2, only a very limited subset can be measured directly. These include volume flow of gas through the mouth and nose (and, equivalently, a measure of its integral, the volume of gas breathed); pressure at the mouth and nose and body surface; partial pressures or concentrations of various gases in gas mixtures passing through the mouth and nose, and in discrete samples of blood *in vitro;* and temperature, including body-core temperature. The values of all other variables in the preceding equations cannot be measured directly but must be inferred from measurements of other variables. A notable example is change in lung volume, which is routinely obtained from gas flow or gas volume change measured at the mouth and nose, i.e., the airway opening.

# 9.2 MEASUREMENT OF PRESSURE

Two noteworthy characteristics of respiratory pressure measurements are the manner in which pressure is measured and the fact that most of the measurements involve pressure differences. All the pressures included in the respiratory models given in Section 9.1 are described in the respiratory literature as "lateral pressure" or "side pressure"; that is, the pressure is measured at the wall of a vessel with the plane of the measurement port parallel to the direction of any flow that might exist. This defines the static or hydrostatic pressure of the fluid dynamicist. The total, or stagnation, pressure and the dynamic pressure at a point are never used in these models even though they may be used in instruments to measure flow (Hänninen, 1991). Confusion can arise, however, because of the way in which the terms *static* and *dynamic* are used with respect to pressure in the respiratory literature. It is standard practice to express the difference in hydrostatic pressure between two points as the sum of two time-varying components, the static component and the dynamic component. For example, the transpulmonary pressure difference can be written as

$$\Delta P_{\mathrm{L}} = (\Delta P_{\mathrm{L}})\mathrm{st} + (\Delta P_{\mathrm{L}})\mathrm{dyn} \tag{9.12}$$

The static component is defined as a function of only the volume change in the system. [For example, in (9.11), the first term on the right-hand side has been referred to as the static component of the transpulmonary pressure difference.] The dynamic component, which is the hydrostatic pressure difference minus its static component, is related only to flows, rates of change of volume, and their derivatives. The static component of a pressure difference, therefore, can be measured as the hydrostatic pressure difference when all flows, rates of volume change, and their derivatives are zero, that is, when the system is static.

## PRESSURE SENSORS

We can conveniently perform dynamic measurements of respiratory pressures using an electronic strain-gage pressure sensor with a tube or catheter as a probe. Section 7.3 described the characteristics of such systems for the circulatory system in which the catheter and sensor are filled with liquid. The same type of analysis can be used for gas-filled systems, except that the acoustic compliance of the gas may be of the same order of magnitude as—or even high than—the compliance of the sensor diaphragm. Therefore, an appropriate shunt capacitor must be included in the equivalent circuit for the device [Figure 7.8(a)].

An additional point must be considered, however, when a pressure difference is measured. Such measurements are usually accomplished with differential pressure sensors that have two chambers separated by a diaphragm connected to strain-sensitive elements. Gas is introduced into each chamber through a catheter. Therefore, the circuit of Figure 7.8(a) represents the mechanical or pneumatic transfer function for only one side of a differential pressure sensor. Note that the time-varying pressures that exist in the chambers on each side of the diaphragm are influenced by the transfer characteristics of the mechanical–pneumatic circuits between their respective pressure sources and the strain-sensing diaphragm. Thus it is extremely important that the frequency response of the transmission pathways on both sides of the sensor be matched over the frequency range of interest. This becomes critical when high-frequency changes in pressure are to be measured with sensors having chambers of unequal volumes on each side of the diaphragm.

## INTRAESOPHAGEAL PRESSURE

Computing pulmonary mechanical properties—for instance, pulmonary static compliance—from (9.7) and (9.8) requires a measure of the spatially averaged pressure acting on the pleural surfaces. Direct measurements of the pressure on the visceral pleural surface made by puncturing the thoracic wall and introducing a catheter into the interpleural space are not clinically applicable. Such measurements have shown, however, that a gravity-related pressure gradient exists in the thin liquid film in the interpleural space surrounding the lungs. This nonuniform pressure, which is lowest in the uppermost part of the chest, makes the point at which a representative pressure can be measured uncertain. Fortunately, the determination of mechanical properties from linearized equations such as (9.3) involves only changes in pressure about an operating point. This relaxes the requirement on the measurement of the absolute pressure.

A significant advance in clinical testing of pulmonary function was the development of a method of estimating changes in the average pressure on the visceral pleural surface from measurements of changes in the pressure in a bolus of fluid introduced into the esophagus. The most commonly used technique involves passing an air-filled catheter with a small latex balloon on its end through the nose into the esophagus (Macklem, 1974).

The esophagus, which is normally a flaccid, collapsed tube, is subjected to the pressure in the interpleural space (acting through the parietal pleura) and to the weight of other thoracic structures, primarily the heart. The pressure in the air trapped in a small balloon situated within the thoracic esophagus depends on the compression or expansion caused by these sources. Although the mean intraesophageal pressure does not equal the mean pressure on the pleural surface measured directly by catheter in the interpleural space, under certain conditions the *changes* in the pressure in the esophageal balloon reflect the *changes* in pressure on the pleural surface. The mechanical properties of the balloon and esophagus have minimal effect on the changes in pressure in the balloon if the amount of air in the balloon is sufficiently small that the balloon remains unstressed and the esophageal wall does not undergo motions large enough to influence the transmission of pressure into the balloon.

The balloon should be so located that pressure changes due to motions of other organs competing for space in the thoracic cavity are minimized. The largest noise signal comes from the heartbeat, which usually has a fundamental frequency (on the order of 1 Hz) much higher than that of resting breathing. A region below the upper third of the thoracic esophagus gives low cardiac interference and provides pressure variations that correspond well in magnitude and phase with directly measured representative changes in pleural pressure. The correspondence decreases as lung volume approaches the minimum achievable (the residual) volume. The frequency response of an esophageal balloon pressure-measurement system depends on the mechanical properties and dimensions of the pressure sensor, the catheter, the balloon, and the gas within the system. The use of helium instead of air can extend the usable frequency range of these systems.

## 9.3 MEASUREMENT OF GAS FLOW

When the lungs change volume during breathing, a mass of gas is transported through the airway opening by convective flow. Measurement of variables associated with the movement of this gas is of major importance in studies of the respiratory system. The volume flow and the time integral of volume flow are used to estimate rate of change of lung volume and changes of lung volume, respectively. Even though the devices we will describe here are calibrated and are used to measure volume flow or to estimate its time integral, the primary physical process involved is mass flow. Volume flow equals the mass flow divided by the density of the gas at the measurement site. The instruments used to measure volume flow are referred to as *volume flowmeters.* The volume occupied by a given mass (number of moles) of gas under known conditions of temperature and pressure is usually determined by using a spirometer (Section 9.4).

Even though breathing movements are cyclic by nature and involve alternating (bidirectional) gas flow, some tests of pulmonary function—such as those involving the single-breath washout, the forced expiratory vital-capacity maneuver, and the maximal voluntary ventilation—require the measurement of flow in only one direction. In addition, the precision and accuracy demanded of flow measurements vary greatly, depending on the settings in which the measurements are performed, from physiology and clinical function laboratories to mass screening centers to intensive care units. Consequently, there are a variety of instruments that can produce measurements useful in particular applications.

### REQUIREMENTS FOR RESPIRATORY GAS-FLOW MEASUREMENTS

Measurement of the motion of material passing through a system requires that the sensor be placed at a position traversed by a known fraction of the material. In respiratory experiments, especially those involving measurement of breathed gas, the usual practice is to have the entire flow stream pass through or into the instrument. This produces several potential problems. Any pressure imposed at the airway during measurements at the airway opening—for example, by a mechanical ventilator—must be withstood by the sensor without damage, distortion, or leakage. In addition, the device should not obstruct breathing or produce a back pressure during flow that might affect respiratory performance. For example, the American Thoracic Society recommends that volume-flow measuring devices used for maximal expiratory efforts have a resistance to flow of less than 1.5 cm $H_2O$/(liter/s) (Anonymous, 1995a).

As with any instrument, the gas-flow-measuring sensor must have a stable baseline (reference output) and sensitivity so that measurements are accurate. However, changes in composition and temperature of gas can affect the calibration factors of various flowmeters. These changes occur between inspired and expired gas and during expiration. Furthermore, inspired particles of dust, dirt, and medication and expired aerosolized organic particles from the respiratory system can deposit on sensitive parts of the sensors and contaminate them. This not only affects calibration but can also transmit disease. Therefore, the sensor must be either sterilizable or disposable.

One of the major sensor contaminants in expired gas is water. Unless the sensor is heated to near or above body temperature, it can act as a condenser for the saturated water vapor in the expirate. The resulting liquid can foul delicate sensors and change the effective cross-sectional area through which the gas must pass.

The measurement procedure must not alter inspired air by adding excessive heat or toxic substances. Such techniques as laser anemometry (which requires reflecting particles in the stream) and ion anemometry (which produces ozone) are not suitable for measurements at the airway opening. If the sensor is to monitor breathing continuously for a number of breaths, then its dead space becomes important. Carbon dioxide must be flushed out and $O_2$ replenished if the conduit tubing in the system is of such a volume that the patient will experience excessive rebreathing of expired gas.

The performance characteristics required of respiratory flowmeters depend upon the specific measurements to be made. These can be as different as the flow during quiet breathing of an infant to that during a maximal, forced expiration by an adult athlete. The amplitude ranges, measurement accuracies, and frequency responses necessary for several clinical applications have been presented by Sullivan *et al.* (1984).

Commonly used respiratory volume flowmeters fall into one of four categories: rotating-vane, ultrasonic, thermal-convection, and differential pressure flowmeters.

## ROTATING-VANE FLOWMETERS

This type of sensor has a small turbine in the flow path. The rotation of the turbine can be related to the volume flow of gas. Mechanical linkages have been used to display parameters of the flow (such as peak flow and integral over an expiration) on indicator dials on the instrument. Interruption of a light beam by the turbine has also been sensed and converted to voltages proportional to flow and/or its integral, to be recorded or displayed continuously. In devices such as this, the mass of the moving parts and the friction between them combine to prevent high-frequency motions of the turbine in response to accelerating flows. This precludes their use in the measurement of alternating bidirectional flows and makes them primarily suitable for clinical screening.

## ULTRASONIC FLOWMETERS

Section 8.4 described the operation and application of ultrasonic sensors in the measurement of blood flow. For respiratory measurements, investigators measure the effect of the flowing gas on the transit time of the ultrasonic signal. The transmitter–receiver crystal pair is mounted either externally and obliquely to the axis of the tube through which the gas flows or internally and coaxially with the flow. The transit time between the transmitter and receiver depends not only on the velocity of the gas between them but also on the composition and temperature of the gas.

In another approach, a rod is placed in the flow stream to produce a pattern of vortices. An ultrasonic transmitter and receiver are mounted diametrically opposite each other in the walls of the tube. The intensity of the ultrasonic signals passing perpendicular to the flow is modulated by the vortices. The modulating frequency is detected and calibrated in units of volume flow. Ultrasonic flowmeters measure unidirectional flows and are suitable for clinical monitoring.

## THERMAL-CONVECTION FLOWMETERS

Thermal-convection flowmeters employ sensing elements such as metal wires, metal films, and thermistors, the electrical resistances of which change with temperature. When operated in the self-heated mode, in which sufficient current is passed through them to maintain an average temperature above that of the surrounding fluid, these elements lose heat at a rate that depends on the local mass flow, temperature, specific heat, kinematic viscosity, and thermal conductivity of the fluid. If a feedback circuit is used to operate the primary sensing element at a constant temperature, then a second, unheated element can be included in the circuit to compensate for heat loss due to local, ambient temperature changes. (The thermal response time of the unheated element can be affected by condensation of water vapor from humid gas mixtures.) The details and operation of such devices and circuits are described in Section 8.5.

For situations in which gas properties are sufficiently constant, the output voltage from these circuits is a nonlinear function of mass flow only. Analog and digital implementations of piecewise-linear or polynomial approximations of this function have been developed to provide a linear mass-flow–voltage relationship.

Flowmeters using a single, temperature-compensated, heated wire (hot-wire anemometer) with a linearizing circuit provide unidirectional flow measurements that are satisfactory for testing pulmonary function. If a single hot wire is to be used to obtain volume flow continuously, several conditions must be fulfilled. For a gas of constant density, volume flow through a cross section is proportional to the average mass flow (averaged over the cross section). The mass-flow-sensing wire is very small (on the order of 5 μm in diameter and 1 to 2 mm in length) to satisfy heat-transfer and frequency-response requirements. Consequently, mass-flow is measured only locally in a correspondingly small region of the flow stream. The duct in which the sensor is located must be designed so that the position at which the measurement is made yields a value representative of the average mass flow through the entire cross section of the duct at every instant of time. At the low Mach numbers involved in respiratory flows, this requires that the velocity profile be well defined at all flows of interest. The variations in cross-sectional area upstream and downstream from the sensor can be optimized for this condition.

Although a single hot-wire sensor provides an output of the same polarity independent of the direction of flow, limiting its use to unidirectional flow, multiple sensors located at separate points along the flow path can be used with the appropriate circuitry to provide directional sensitivity, as described in Section 8.5. However, respiratory measurements involve a changing mixture of gases in the flow stream that affects the heat transfer from the heated wire. The significant variations in composition that occur between inspiration and expiration could invalidate the use of a single calibration factor. During a multibreath $N_2$ washout (Section 9.4), the $N_2$–$O_2$ ratio in the lung changes from approximately 4 to 1 on the first breath to nearly zero at the end of the test. Fortunately, the differences in thermal properties and densities of $N_2$ and $O_2$ offset each other sufficiently well that a linearized, temperature-compensated hot-wire anemometer can be used with a constant calibration factor for volume flow measurements during the successive expirations of a multibreath $N_2$ washout. In general, however, the sensor should be calibrated for the particular gas mixture to which it is exposed.

The hot-wire anemometer has a number of features that are advantageous in respiratory applications. It has an appropriate frequency response (the sensor itself can respond to frequencies into the kilohertz range). Moreover, because the sensing element in the flow stream is extremely small, the only back pressure produced is that caused by the flow through the duct. In unidirectional applications rebreathing does not occur, so dead space is irrelevant. Accurate readings can be made at low as well as high flow rates if the output is adequately linearized. Special circuits can be provided to overheat the sensor to burn off contaminants as necessary. The main disadvantage is the limitation to unidirectional flow. The relatively high cost of overcoming this with a paired hot-wire system may not be justified.

## DIFFERENTIAL PRESSURE FLOWMETERS

Convective flow occurs as a result of a difference in pressure between two points. From the relationship between pressure difference and volume flow through a system, measurement of the difference in pressure yields an estimate of flow. Flowmeters based on this idea have incorporated several mechanisms to establish the relationship between pressure drop and flow. These include the venturi, orifice, and flow resistors of various types. A flowmeter based on a modified pitot tube has also been developed.

***Venturis and Orifices*** Venturis and orifices with fixed-sized openings have inherently nonlinear pressure–flow relationships and require calibration charts, special circuitry, or digitally implemented algorithms to be useful as flow sensors. A passive, mechanically linearized orifice flowmeter has been produced in which an elastic flap moved by the pressure of the flowing gas impinging on it increases or decreases the orifice size (Sullivan *et al.*, 1984). However, sensors with computer-controlled orifices that can measure and/or control flow are also in use.

A two-stage, fixed-orifice system has been used to measure flow during forced expiratory vital-capacity maneuvers (Jones, 1990). At high flows, the gas stream passes through a large orifice. When the sensed pressure drop indicates that the flow has decreased to below 2 liter/s, a solenoid is activated, producing a step decrease in the opening and thus increasing the sensor's sensitivity to low flows. Parameters of the measured waveshape are presented on a digital readout.

***Pneumotachometers*** The flow sensors that historically have been, and continue to be, the mainstay of the respiratory laboratory utilize flow resistors with approximately linear pressure–flow relationships. These devices are usually referred to as *pneumotachometers* (Macia, 2006). (In general, the term *pneumotachometer* is synonymous with *gas volume flowmeter.)* Flow-resistance pneumotachometers are easy to use and can distinguish the directions of alternating flows. They also have sufficient accuracy, sensitivity, linearity, and frequency response for most clinical applications. In addition, they use the same differential pressure sensors and amplifiers required for other respiratory measurements. The following discussion primarily concerns these instruments.

Even though other flow-resistance elements have been incorporated in pneumotachometers, those most commonly used consist of either one (Silverman and Whittenberger, 1950) or more (Sullivan *et al.*, 1984) fine mesh screens [Figure 9.3(a)] placed perpendicular to flow, or a tightly packed bundle of capillary tubes or channels [Figure 9.3(b)] with its axis parallel to flow (Fleisch, 1925). These physical devices exhibit, for a wide range of unsteady flows, a nearly linear pressure-drop–flow relationship, with pressure drop approximately in phase with flow.

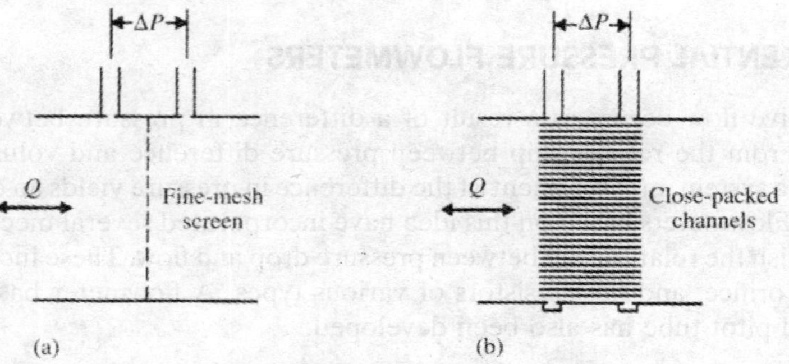


**Figure 9.3 Pneumotachometer flow-resistance elements** (a) screen and (b) capillary tubes or channels.

In practice, the element is mounted in a conduit of circular cross section. The pressure drop is measured across the resistance element at the wall of the conduit (within the boundary layer of the flow). The pressure tap on each side of the resistance is either a single hole through the conduit wall or multiple holes from a circumferential channel within the wall, which is connected to a common external tap.

Because the pressure drop is measured at a single radial distance from the center of the conduit, it is assumed that this pressure drop is representative of the pressure drop governing the total flow through the entire conduit cross section. Thus these flowmeters rely on the flow-resistive element to establish a consistent—though not uniform—velocity profile on each side of the element in the neighborhood of the pressure measurement. This, however, cannot be achieved independent of the ductwork in which the pneumotachometer is placed (Kreit and Sciurba, 1996). Therefore, the placement of the pressure ports and the configuration of the tubing that leads from the subject to the pneumotachometer and from the pneumotachometer to the remainder of the system are critical in determining the pressure-drop–flow relationship. This is especially important when alternating and/or high-frequency flow patterns are involved.

A number of trade-offs exist in the design and use of these sensors. The $\Delta P$–$Q$ relationship may be more linear for steady flow when there is a large axial separation between pressure ports than when there is a smaller separation. But during unsteady flow with high-frequency content, the pressure drop for a larger separation may be more influenced by inertial forces. If the sensor is to avoid excessive formation of vortices at high flow rates, the cross-sectional area of the conduit at the flow-resistance element must be large enough to reduce the velocity through the element. This area may be several times that of the mouth of the subject from which the gas originates, requiring an adapter or diffuser between the mouthpiece and the resistance element. If flow separation and turbulence are to be avoided as the cross-sectional area changes, the adapter should have a shallow internal angle, $\theta$, [Figure 9.4(a)] not

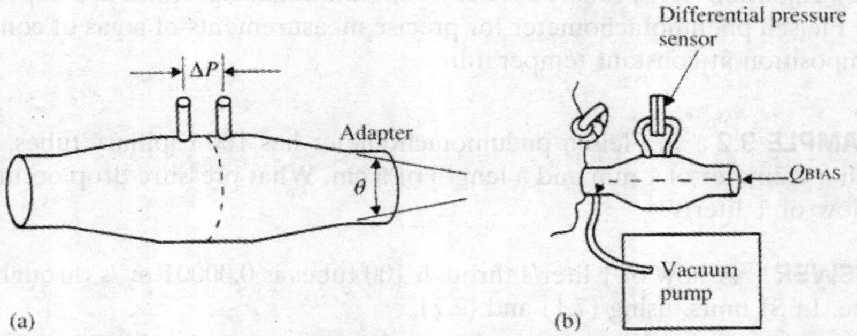


**Figure 9.4 Pneumotachometer for measurements at the mouth** (a) Diameter adapter that acts as a diffuser. (b) An application in which a constant flow is used to clear the dead space.

exceeding 15°. The shallower the angle, however, the greater is the distance between the mouth and the flow-resistance element. Symmetric drops in pressure for the same flow rate in either direction require that the geometries of the conduit on both sides of the resistance element be matched. The volume within the adapters and conduit represents a dead space for cyclic breathing. The designer, when designing the sensor, must balance the effects of decreased angle of the diffuser against the tolerable volume of dead space.

A bias flow can be used to clear this dead space. Air is drawn through the pneumotachometer from a side hole [Figure 9.4(b)] through a long tube connected to a vacuum pump. This causes a constant bias pressure drop across the pneumotachometer if the bias flow created is constant during the breathing of the patient. This approach can work well when high-frequency breathing patterns are of interest. But for low frequencies, such as those of tidal breathing, a regulating device may be required to prevent variation of the bias flow as the patient breathes.

The usable frequency range for capillary pneumotachometers is typically smaller than that for the screen type. Depending on its design, the screen-type pneumotachometer can exhibit a constant-amplitude ratio of pressure difference to flow, and zero phase shift up to as high as 70 Hz (Peslin *et al.,* 1972).

In air, the amplitude ratio of the Fleisch (capillary bundle) pneumotachometer is nearly constant at its steady-flow value up to approximately 10 Hz, increasing by 5% at 20 Hz. The phase angle between $\Delta P$ and $Q$ increases linearly with frequency to approximately 8.5° at 10 Hz, which corresponds to an approximate 2 ms time delay between flow and pressure difference. These values change with the kinematic viscosity of the gas (Finucane *et al.,* 1972). Peslin *et al.* (1972) modeled the Fleisch pneumotachometer for frequencies up to 70 Hz by an equation of the form

$$\Delta P = RQ + L\dot{Q} \tag{9.13}$$

where $L$ is the inertance (related to mass) of the gas in one capillary tube, defined by (7.4) and $R$ is the flow resistance for each capillary tube, defined by (7.2). Equation (9.13) can be used as a computational algorithm to compensate the Fleisch pneumotachometer for precise measurements of a gas of constant composition at constant temperature.

**EXAMPLE 9.2** A Fleisch pneumotachometer has 100 capillary tubes, each with a diameter of 1 mm and a length of 5 cm. What pressure drop occurs for a flow of 1 liter/s?

**ANSWER** A flow of 1 liter/s through 100 tubes is 0.00001 m$^3$/s through one tube. In SI units, using (7.1) and (7.2),

$$\Delta P = RF = \frac{8\eta LF}{\pi r^4} = \frac{8(0.000018)(0.05)(0.00001)}{\pi(0.0005)^4} = 367\ \text{Pa} = 3.74\ \text{cm}\ H_2O$$

An appropriately designed screen pneumotachometer may not require compensation provided by (9.13). However, it may instead be subject to equipment-generated, high-frequency noise in clinical applications. An additional point should be stressed: the frequency response of a pneumotachometer is no better than that of its associated differential pressure measurement system. It is essential that the pneumatic (acoustic) impedances, including those of the tubes and connectors between the pressure sensor and the pneumotachometer, on each side of the differential pressure sensor be balanced. This is most easily achieved by ensuring that the geometries and dimensions of the pneumatic pathways from the pneumotachometer to each side of the pressure sensor diaphragm are identical.

Equation (7.2) indicates that the resistance of the Fleisch pneumotachometer is proportional to the viscosity of the flowing gas mixture. The resistance of a screen pneumotachometer, though not computable from (7.2), is also proportional to the viscosity of the gas. The viscosity of a gas mixture depends on its composition and temperature (Turney and Blumenfeld, 1973). When inertance effects are negligible,

$$Q = \frac{\Delta P}{R(T, [Fx])} \tag{9.14}$$

where $Q$ is the flow measured by the pneumotachometer for a gas mixture with species molar fractions $[Fx] = [N_1/N, N_2/N, \ldots, Nx/N]$ at absolute temperature $T$. Pneumotachometers are routinely calibrated for steady flow with a single calibration factor being used during experiments. Instantaneous values of $T$ and $[Fx]$ are not constant during a single expiration, and their mean values change from expiration to inspiration. In particular, changes in viscosity of 10% to 15% occur from the beginning to the end of an experiment in which $N_2$ is washed out of the lungs by pure $O_2$. A continuous correction in calibration should be made when accurate results are desired.

The prevention of water-vapor condensation in a pneumotachometer is of particular importance. The capillary tubes and screen pores are easily blocked by liquid water, which decreases the effective cross-sectional area of the flow element and causes a change in resistance. Also, as water condenses, the composition of the gas mixture changes. To circumvent these problems, a common practice is to heat the pneumotachometer element, especially when more than a few consecutive breaths are to be studied. The Fleisch pneumotachometer is usually provided with an electrical resistance heater; the screen of the screen pneumotachometer can be heated by passing a current through it. In addition, heated wires can be placed inside, or heating tape or other electrical heat source can be wrapped around any conduit that carries expired gas.

***Pitot Tubes*** The difference between stagnation pressure (measured head-on into the flow) and static pressure (measured perpendicular to the flow) in a flowing gas is the dynamic pressure, and is related to the density and the square of the velocity of the gas. Pitot tubes are flow-measuring devices based on this relationship. A modified pitot instrument has been developed that uses two pressure ports, one facing upstream and the other, downstream (Hänninen, 1991). When flow is in one direction, one port measures stagnation pressure and the other assesses static pressure. When flow reverses, the roles of the ports also reverse permitting the alternating flows of breathing to be measured. During a breath, the inspired and expired gas compositions continuously change with concomitant changes in density. Simultaneous measurement of gas composition from the same location at which the pressure measurements are made permits compensation for variations in density. Flow resistance of 1.0 cm $H_2O$/(liter/s), dead space of 9.5 ml, volume accuracy (from the integral of flow) of ±6% and flow sensitivity of 0.07 liter/s have been reported.

## 9.4 LUNG VOLUME

The most commonly used indices of the mechanical status of the ventilatory system are the absolute volume and changes of volume of the gas space in the lungs achieved during various breathing maneuvers. Observe Figure 9.5 and assume that a subject's airway opening and body surface are exposed to atmospheric pressure. Then the largest volume to which the subject's lungs can be voluntarily expanded is defined as the *total lung capacity* (TLC). The smallest volume to which the subject can slowly deflate his or her lungs is the *residual volume* (RV). The volume of the lungs at the end of a quiet expiration when the respiratory muscles are relaxed is the *functional residual capacity* (FRC). The difference between TLC and RV is the *vital capacity* (VC), which defines the maximal change in volume the lungs can undergo

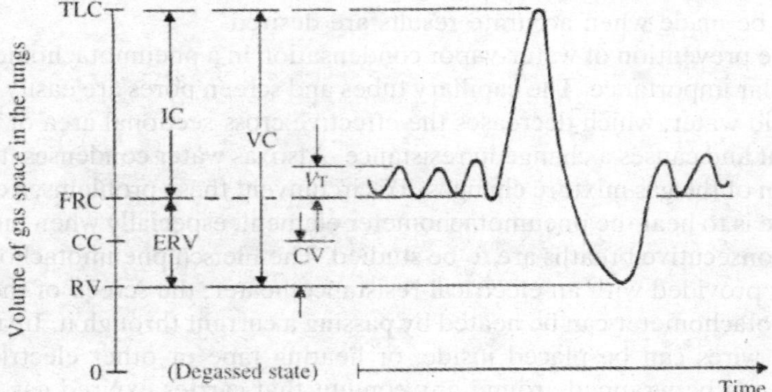


**Figure 9.5** Volume ranges of the intact ventilatory system (with no external loads applied). Total lung capacity, FRC, and RV are measured as absolute volumes. Vital capacity, IC, ERV, and $V_T$ are volume changes. Closing volume (CV) and closing capacity (CC) are obtained from a single-breath washout experiment.

during voluntary maneuvers. The vital capacity can be divided into the *inspiratory capacity* (IC = TLC – FRC) and the *expiratory reserve volume* (ERV = FRC – RV). The peak-to-peak volume change during a quiet breath is the *tidal volume* ($V_T$) (Petrini, 1988).

## CHANGES IN LUNG VOLUME: SPIROMETRY

The measurement of changes in lung volume has been approached in two ways. One is to measure the changes in the volume of the gas space within the body during breathing by using plethysmographic techniques (discussed in Section 9.5). The second approach, referred to as *spirometry,* involves measurements of the gas passing through the airway opening. The latter measurements can provide accurate, continuous estimates of changes in lung volume only when compression of the gas in the lungs is sufficiently small. The flow of moles of gas at the airway opening can be expressed as

$$\dot{N}_{AWO} = \rho_{AWO} Q_{AWO} \cong \rho_L \dot{V}_L \tag{9.15}$$

if we neglect the net rate of diffusion into the pulmonary capillary blood. This equation can be rearranged and, if the densities are essentially constant, integrated from some initial time $t_0$, as follows:

$$\frac{\rho_{AWO}}{\rho_L} \int_{t_0}^{t} Q_{AWO}\, dt \cong \int_{t_0}^{t} \dot{V}_L\, dt = V_L(t) - V_L(t_0) = v_L \tag{9.16}$$

in which $v_L$ is, according to the convention used here, the change in the volume of the lungs relative to the reference volume $V_L(t_0)$. The density ratio accounts for differences in mean temperature, pressure, and composition that may exist between the gas mixture inside the lungs and that in the measurement sensor external to the body.

For purposes of testing pulmonary function, (9.16) is frequently implemented directly by electronically integrating the output of a flowmeter placed at a subject's mouth (with the nose blocked). However, the most common procedure for estimating $v_L$—in use since the nineteenth century—is to continuously collect the gas passing through the airway opening and to compute the volume it occupied within the lungs. This represents a physical integration of the flow at the mouth; it is performed by a device called a *spirometer.* The widespread and historical use of this device has given rise to use of the term *spirometry* to mean the measurement of changes in lung volume for testing of pulmonary function, regardless of whether a spirometer, flowmeter plus integrator, or plethysmographic technique is used. Consequently, performance recommendations have been published by the American Thoracic Society (Anonymous, 1995a) for spirometry systems in general, regardless of the primary variable measured (volume change or flow) or the type of sensor used. The recommendations address volume range and accuracy, flow range, time interval for which data are to be collected, respiratory load imposed on

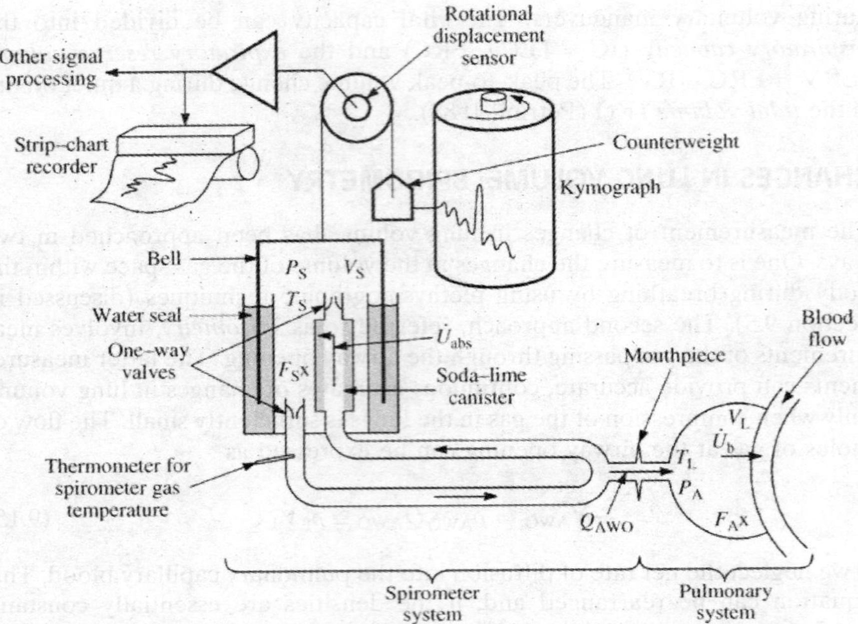


**Figure 9.6** A water-sealed spirometer set up to measure slow lung-volume changes. The soda-lime and one-way-valve arrangement prevent buildup of $CO_2$ during rebreathing.

the subject, and calibration standards to be met by such systems for various pulmonary function tests.

A spirometer is basically an expandable compartment consisting of a movable, statically counterbalanced, rigid chamber or "bell," a stationary base, and a dynamic seal between them (Figure 9.6). The seal is often water, but dry seals of various types have been used. Changes in internal volume of the spirometer, $V_S$, are proportional to the displacement of the bell. This motion is traditionally recorded on a rotating drum (kymograph) through direct mechanical linkage, but any displacement sensor can be used. A simple approach is to attach a single-turn, precision linear potentiometer to the shaft of the counterweight pulley and use it as a voltage divider. The electric output can then be processed or displayed.

The mouthpiece of the spirometer (Figure 9.6) is placed in the mouth of the subject, whose nose is blocked. As gas moves into and out of the spirometer, the pressure $P_S$ of the gas in the spirometer changes, causing the bell to move. Analysis of the dynamic mechanics of a spirometer indicates that these variations in pressure are reduced by minimizing (1) the mass of the bell and counterweight and the moment of inertia of the pulley, (2) the gas space in the spirometer and tubing, (3) the surface area of the liquid seal exposed to $P_S$, (4) the viscous and frictional losses by appropriate choice of lubricants and type of dynamic seal, and (5) the flow resistances of any inlet and outlet tubing and valves. During resting breathing, the pressure changes in the gas within the spirometer can be considered negligible. Therefore, only the temperature, average ambient pressure, and change in volume are needed to estimate the amount of gas exchanged with the spirometer. To use the spirometer for estimates of change in lung volume during breathing patterns of higher frequency ($>1$ Hz) requires, in addition to the variables just mentioned, knowledge of the acoustic compliance of the gas in the spirometer (see Problem 9.3) and continuous measurement of the change of the spirometer pressure relative to ambient pressure.

The system—lungs plus spirometer—can be modeled as two gas compartments connected such that the number of moles of gas lost by the lungs through the airway opening is equal and opposite to the number gained by the spirometer. For rebreathing experiments, most spirometer systems have a chemical absorber (soda lime) to prevent buildup of $CO_2$. When compression of gas in the lungs and in the spirometer is neglected, mass balances on the system yield

$$\rho_L \dot{V}_L + \dot{U}_b = -\rho_S \dot{V}_S - \dot{U}_{abs} \tag{9.17}$$

The net rates of uptake from the system by the pulmonary capillary blood, $\dot{U}_b$, and the absorber, $\dot{U}_{abs}$, can be assumed constant during steady breathing. Therefore, when (9.17) is integrated with respect to time, the combined effect of these uptakes is a change in volume essentially proportional to time. This can be approximated as a linear baseline drift easily separable from the breathing pattern. Consequently, rearrangement and integration of (9.17) yield

$$v_L \cong -\frac{\rho_S}{\rho_L}(v_S - \text{drift}) = -\frac{\rho_S}{\rho_L} v_{S'} \tag{9.18}$$

from which it can be seen that the change in lung volume is approximately proportional to $v_{S'}$, the volume change of the spirometer corrected for drift.

The constant of proportionality $(-\rho_S/\rho_L)$ can be expressed in terms of the measurable quantities, pressure and temperature, by applying an equation of state to the system. With the exception of saturated water vapor, all gases encountered during routine respiratory experiments obey the ideal-gas law during changes of state:

$$P = \frac{N}{V}\mathbf{R}T = \rho \mathbf{R}T \tag{9.19}$$

Where

$\mathbf{R}$ = universal gas constant

$T$ = absolute temperature

$\rho$ = mole density, which, for a well-mixed compartment, equals the ratio of moles of gas, $N$, in the compartment to the compartment volume, $V$

This relationship holds for an entire gas mixture and for an individual gas species X in the mixture. For the latter, the partial pressure $P_X$, number of moles $N_X$, and density $\rho_X = N_X/V$ are substituted into (9.19).

A difficulty in directly substituting (9.19) into (9.18) arises from the presence of water vapor in the system. The water vapor in the lungs is saturated at body-core temperature. The water vapor in the spirometer is also saturated, even in those with dry seals, after only a few exhalations from the warmer lungs into the cooler spirometer. Saturated water vapor does not follow (9.19) during changes of state. Instead, its partial pressure is primarily a function of temperature alone.

Processes in the lungs are approximately isothermal; the change in temperature in the spirometer during most pulmonary function tests is assumed small. Therefore, we can compute the partial pressure of the ideal dry gases—the total gas mixture excluding water vapor—as the mean total pressure (taken to be atmospheric pressure $P_{atm}$ for both the spirometer and the lungs) minus the partial pressure of saturated water vapor at the appropriate temperature. Equation (9.18) can then be evaluated as

$$v_L \cong -\left(\frac{(P_{atm} - P_{SH_2O})T_L}{(P_{atm} - P_{AH_2O})T_S}\right) v_{S'} \tag{9.20}$$

in which $P_{AH_2O}$ and $P_{SH_2O}$ are the partial pressures of saturated water vapor in the lung [47 mm Hg (6.27 kPa) at $T_L = 37$ °C] and in the spirometer (at the measured temperature in the spirometer, $T_S$), respectively.

## ABSOLUTE VOLUME OF THE LUNG

Because of the complex geometry and inaccessibility of the lungs, we cannot compute their volume accurately either from direct spatial measurements or from two- or three-dimensional pictures provided by various imaging techniques. Three procedures have been developed, however, that can give accurate estimates of the volume of gas in normal lungs. Two are based on static mass balances and involve the washout or dilution of a test gas in the lungs. The test gas must have low solubility in the lung tissue. That is, movement of the gas from the alveoli by diffusion into the parenchyma (tissue) and blood must be much less than that occurring by convection through the airways during the experiment. The third procedure is a total body plethysmographic technique employing dynamic mass balances and gas compression in the lungs (see Section 9.5). These estimates of lung volume provide a static baseline value of absolute lung volume that can be added to a continuous measure of the change of lung volume to provide a continuous estimate of absolute lung volume.

The computational formulas for the test-gas procedures described below are routinely derived in the literature in terms of a volume fraction of the test gas in a mixture. The volume fraction of a gas X is an alternative expression of, and is numerically equal to, its molar fraction, $F_X$. When the ideal-gas law (9.19) is applied to X alone and to the total mixture containing X, we can express $F_X$ in terms of the partial pressure of X, $P_X$.

$$F_X = \frac{N_X}{N} = \left(\frac{P_X V}{RT}\right)\left(\frac{RT}{PV}\right) = \frac{P_X}{P} \tag{9.21}$$

This follows from Dalton's law of partial pressures, for which all gases in a mixture are visualized as having the same temperature and occupying the same volume. On the other hand, the concept of volume fraction lends itself to the use of the spirometer to measure the volume occupied by a mass of gas at a given pressure and temperature. Assume that $N\text{x}$ moles of X at temperature $T$ occupy a volume $V\text{x}$ when subjected to a pressure $P$. These $N\text{x}$ moles of X are then added to an X-free gas mixture so that the total moles of mixture is $N$, and the mixture is allowed to occupy volume $V$ at pressure $P$. Applying the ideal-gas law to X before addition to the mixture and to the mixture after the addition of X, we can evaluate $F\text{x}$ for the final mixture as

$$F\text{x} = \frac{N\text{x}}{N} = \left(\frac{PV\text{x}}{\mathbf{R}T}\right)\left(\frac{\mathbf{R}T}{PV}\right) = \frac{V\text{x}}{V} \tag{9.22}$$

Thus the molar fraction $F\text{x}$ can be thought of either as a partial-pressure fraction (9.21), or as an equivalent-volume fraction (9.22) in which the volumes are those that the components of the gas or the gas mixture would occupy if all exhibited the *same* temperature and total pressure. However, in some experiments the temperature and/or total pressure changes from one measurement to another. Remember that in the mass balances describing such experiments, $F\text{x}$ represents molar fraction and must be evaluated as such to account for the observed changes in temperature and pressure. Instruments capable of measuring molar fractions and concentrations of gases in a mixture are described in Section 9.7.

## NITROGEN-WASHOUT ESTIMATE OF LUNG VOLUME

Figure 9.7 is a diagram of an apparatus that can be used during a multibreath $N_2$ washout. The subject inhales only an $N_2$-free gas mixture (for this example, $O_2$) because of the one-way valves, but she or he exhales $N_2$, $O_2$, $CO_2$, and water vapor. This experiment is routinely performed to measure FRC, so the subject is switched into the apparatus at the end of a quiet expiration following normal breathing of atmospheric air. He or she is allowed to breathe the $N_2$-free mixture in a relaxed manner around FRC with relatively constant tidal volumes for a fixed period of time (7 to 10 min) or until the $N_2$ molar fraction in the expirate is sufficiently near zero ($<2\%$).

A static mass (molar) balance on the $N_2$ in the lungs from before to after the washout yields an estimate of the lung volume at which the first inspiration of $O_2$ began. Assume that during the experiment, negligible amounts of $N_2$ diffuse into the alveolar gas from lung tissue and pulmonary capillary blood. Therefore, the change in the number of moles of $N_2$ in the lungs as a result of the washout is just the number lost during each expiration (and gained by the spirometer). Assuming that measurements of $N_2$ fraction are made on a

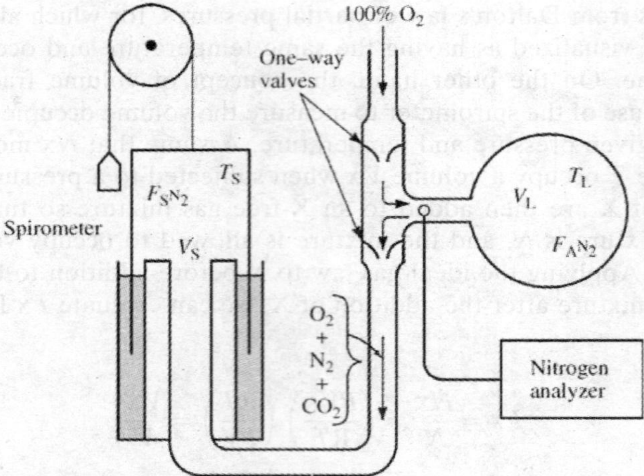


**Figure 9.7 Diagram of an $N_2$-washout experiment** The expired gas can be collected in a spirometer, as shown here, or in a rubberized-canvas or plastic Douglas bag. $N_2$ content is then determined off line. An alternative is to measure expiratory flow and nitrogen concentration continuously to determine the volume flow of expired nitrogen, which can be integrated to yield an estimate of the volume of nitrogen expired.

wet-gas basis and that the spirometer contained no $N_2$ at the start of the experiment, we find that a static mass balance yields

$$F_{AN_2}(t_1)\frac{V_L(t_1)}{T_L} - F_{AN_2}(t_2)\frac{V_L(t_2)}{T_L} = F_{SN_2}(t_2)\frac{V_S(t_2)}{T_S}$$

If the lung volume at the beginning of the washout, $t_1$, is the same as that at the finish, $t_2$, then the equation can be rearranged as follows:

$$V_L = \frac{T_L}{T_S}\left(\frac{F_{SN_2}(t_2)V_S(t_2)}{F_{AN_2}(t_1) - F_{AN_2}(t_2)}\right) \tag{9.23}$$

When this volume is that at the end of a quiet expiration, $V_L$ is the FRC.

All variables on the right-hand side of (9.23) are measurable. The numerator in the brackets in (9.23) represents the equivalent expired $N_2$ volume for the conditions in the measuring device (the spirometer in Figure 9.7). However, if the nitrogen molar fractions in (9.23) were to be measured on a dry-gas basis rather than on a wet basis as assumed here, the right-hand side would have to be multiplied by the dry-gas partial-pressure ratio $(P_{atm} - P_{SH_2O})/(P_{atm} - P_{AH_2O})$.

**EXAMPLE 9.3** In an $N_2$-washout experiment, the subject's cumulative expired volume into a spirometer is 5 liters. At the beginning of the experiment, the spirometer has a volume of 7 liters but contains no $N_2$. At the end of the experiment, the molar fraction of $N_2$ in the spirometer is 0.026 and the $F_{A}N_2$ of the subject has decreased by 0.1. The final temperature of the spirometer is 303 K. What was the lung volume at which the subject was breathing?

**ANSWER** $V_S(t_2) = 5$ liters + 7 liters, $F_SN_2(t_2) = 0.026$, $F_AN_2(t_1) - F_AN_2(t_2) = 0.1$, $T_S = 303\,\text{K}$, $T_L = 310\,\text{K}$

$$V_L = \frac{T_L}{T_S}\left(\frac{F_SN_2(t_2)V_S(t_2)}{F_AN_2(t_1) - F_AN_2(t_2)}\right) = \frac{310}{303}\left(\frac{0.026 \times 12}{0.1}\right) = 3.19\,\text{liter}$$

A washout experiment of this type gives an estimate of the volume of the gas space in the lungs that freely communicates with the airway opening. This is the entire alveolar volume in normal young, adult lungs. In diseased lungs, in which airways are totally or partially obstructed (by mucus, edema, bronchospasm, or tumors, for instance), this estimate of the gas volume in the lungs at FRC can be low.

## HELIUM-DILUTION ESTIMATE OF LUNG VOLUME

The procedure described in the previous paragraph involves the removal from the lungs of gas normally resident there in known concentration. An alternative approach is to add a measured amount of a nontoxic, insoluble *tracer* gas to the inspirate, and—after it is uniformly distributed in the lungs—determine its concentration and compute lung volume. Helium is often used as the tracer gas for this experiment, though argon and neon are also acceptable.

The lungs communicate directly with the spirometer, as shown in Figure 9.6. At the beginning of the experiment, a fixed amount of He is added to the spirometer. The amount of He added is routinely measured as an equivalent volume at the initial conditions in the spirometer. The change in volume of the spirometer due to addition of pure helium, $V_S\text{He}$, divided by the total spirometer volume after the addition of the helium, $V_S(t_1)$, is $F_S\text{He}(t_1)$, the molar fraction of helium on a wet-gas basis in the spirometer at the beginning of the experiment [see (9.22)].

The subject is typically allowed to begin rebreathing from the spirometer when the lung volume is at FRC. The subject breathes at his or her resting rate and tidal volume until the concentration of He in the lungs is in equilibrium with that in the spirometer—that is, until $F_A\text{He}(t_2) = F_S\text{He}(t_2)$. The tracer-gas molar fraction in the expirate is continuously measured by withdrawing a small stream of gas from the mouthpiece, passing it through a He analyzer, and returning it to the spirometer. Equilibration is judged to have occurred when the change in the He fraction from one breath to the next is arbitrarily small. As equilibration approaches, the mean spirometer volume is maintained at its original volume $V_S(t_1)$ by the addition of $O_2$ if required. The experiment is terminated at the end of a quiet expiration (FRC).

The He is redistributed between spirometer and lungs during rebreathing, but the total amount remains essentially constant because no appreciable quantities are lost by diffusion into the tissues. The average total number of moles of dry gas in the system is kept constant by chemically removing, via the soda-lime canister, the $CO_2$ added from the blood, and replenishing the $O_2$ taken up. Therefore, the system can be considered closed with respect to the test gas only, and a static mass (molar) balance for He may be written as

$$F_{S}\text{He}(t_1)\frac{V_S(t_1)}{T_S(t_1)} = F_{S}\text{He}(t_2)\frac{V_S(t_2)}{T_S(t_2)} + F_{A}\text{He}(t_2)\frac{V_L(t_2)}{T_L}$$

for molar fractions measured on a wet basis. This can be rearranged and evaluated when the He fractions in the lungs and spirometer are equal.

$$V_L = \frac{V_S(t_1)}{F_S\text{He}(t_2)}\left[\frac{T_L}{T_S(t_1)}F_S\text{He}(t_1) - \frac{T_L}{T_S(t_2)}F_S\text{He}(t_2)\right] \tag{9.24}$$

$V_L$ is an estimate of FRC for the experiment performed as we have described. Equation (9.24) is frequently rewritten in terms of the equivalent volume of He originally added to the system, $V_S\text{He}$.

$$V_L = \frac{T_L}{T_S(t_1)}\left(\frac{V_S\text{He}}{F_S\text{He}(t_2)}\right) - \frac{T_L}{T_S(t_2)}\left(\frac{V_S\text{He}}{F_S\text{He}(t_1)}\right) \tag{9.25}$$

If the molar fractions are measured on a dry basis, the temperature ratios in (9.24) and (9.25) must be multiplied by their corresponding dry-gas partial-pressure ratios: $[P_{atm} - P_S H_2O(t_1)]/(P_{atm} - P_A H_2O)$ and $[P_{atm} - P_S H_2O(t_2)]/(P_{atm} - P_A H_2O)$, respectively.

The volume computed from (9.24) and (9.25) is a measure of the volume of gas space in the lungs for which the final He molar fraction in the spirometer, $F_S\text{He}(t_2)$, is a representative value. If some parts of the lung do not communicate freely with the airway opening, as in obstructive lung disease, then these equations can provide a low estimate of the FRC.

## 9.5 RESPIRATORY PLETHYSMOGRAPHY

The term *plethysmography* refers, in general, to measurement of the volume or change in volume of a portion of the body. In respiratory applications, plethysmography has been approached in two ways: by inferring changes in thoracic-cavity volume from geometrical changes at discrete locations on the torso and by measuring the effects of changes in thoracic volume on variables associated with the gas within a total-body plethysmograph.

### THORACIC PLETHYSMOGRAPHY

Several devices have been used to measure continuously the kinematics (motions) of the chest wall that are associated with changes in thoracic volume

(Sackner, 1980). The electrical impedance of the thoracic cavity changes with breathing movements and can be sensed (Section 8.7) in order to monitor ventilatory activity. Impedance pneumographs are used for apnea detection and sleep studies in which the presence or absence (relative magnitude and frequency) of breathing movements rather than their actual volume changes are important. The application of magnetometers, strain gages, and variable-inductance sensors requires the simultaneous measurement of motion at two locations on the chest wall. During most breathing patterns, the chest wall behaves as though it has two predominant degrees of freedom corresponding to movements of the ribcage and the diaphragm. The weighted sum of the displacements of these two structures, with the movement of the abdomen taken as a measure of diaphragmatic motion, can yield an estimate of the volume change of the thoracic cavity.

*Magnetometers* and other linear-displacement sensors measure ribcage and abdominal diameters. *Strain gages* wrapped around the torso measure local perimeter changes during breathing. A small-diameter, mercury-filled, silicone rubber tube is often used as a ventilatory strain gage. The *respiratory inductive plethysmograph* employs a pair of wires, each attached in a *zigzag* pattern to its own highly compliant belt. One belt is placed around the ribcage and the other around the abdomen, so that each wire forms a single loop, and the pair is excited by a low-level radio-frequency signal. Changes in a loop's cross-sectional area produce corresponding changes in self-inductance. After demodulation, an output is obtained proportional to the local cross-sectional area of the segment of the chest wall that is encircled by the loop. Respiratory inductive plethysmographs are used in sleep laboratories to provide non-invasive, continuous (8 h or more) estimates of tidal volume and with other measures help to diagnose sleep apnea and disordered breathing during sleep (Broughton, 1993; Kryger, 2005).

Each of these devices measures a different primary geometrical variable (diameter, perimeter, or area), but each is used to estimate changes in thoracic volume as well as changes in relative volume between ribcage and diaphragm (via abdominal motion). The accuracy of these estimates varies among the techniques (there is generally a 5% to 10% error relative to spirometrically evaluated volume changes). Measurement artifacts are caused by body motion (changes in posture and torso shape) and extreme variations in breathing amplitude. However, with suitable calibration, the sensitivity of the inductive plethysmograph to such disturbances can be reduced (Verschakelen *et al.*, 1989).

## TOTAL-BODY PLETHYSMOGRAPHY

The *total-body plethysmograph* (TBP) is a rigid, constant-volume box in which the subject is completely enclosed. Clinically it is used primarily to evaluate the absolute volume of the lungs, and to provide a continuous estimate of alveolar pressure, from which airway resistance $R_{\mathrm{AW}}$ can be computed. There are three types or configurations of TBPs: pressure, volume-displacement, and flow-displacement TBPs. These names correspond to the primary plethysmographic variable that is measured and used to compute other variables associated with the lungs. Even though these names provide a means of identifying a particular configuration, they are misleading because a number of measurable plethysmographic variables change in all these systems in response to changes in respiratory variables (Primiano and Greber, 1975).

The pressure plethysmograph is a box that acts as though it were closed or gastight at the frequencies at which pressure changes are measured. The volume-displacement plethysmograph and the flow-displacement plethysmograph are referred to as *open* because each has an opening through which gas is intended to enter and leave. A spirometer or a volume flowmeter such as a pneumotachometer is placed at the opening, and pressure changes within these plethysmographs can be kept small by allowing movement of gas between the box and these measuring devices. Consequently, open boxes are suitable for maneuvers in which large changes in lung volume occur. For small-volume-amplitude maneuvers, such as panting, any of the boxes can be employed.

## GENERAL EQUATION FOR BREATHING WITHIN A TOTAL-BODY PLETHYSMOGRAPH

Absolute volume of the lungs and changes in alveolar pressure can be inferred from measurements in a TBP in which the subject can breathe within the box. The following analysis is restricted to the *pressure plethysmograph* (Figure 9.8), which is probably the most commonly used configuration. For simplicity, assume that the subject has a normal pulmonary system. Then a single mechanical unit [Figure 9.1(b)] can be used to model the lungs, and the representative alveolar pressure, $P_A$, is well defined as the pressure within the alveolar compartment (Figure 9.8). The airway exhibits a flow resistance so that, during breathing, $P_A$ does not equal the pressure at the airway opening, $P_{AWO}$. The gas space within the box outside the subject can be considered a single, well-mixed compartment containing a mixture of gas and unsaturated water vapor with its own variables, $P_B$, $V_B$, $N_B$, and $T_B$.

The volume of the plethysmograph $V_P$ is occupied by the tissues of the body $V_{TIS}$, the gas space in the lungs $V_L$, and the gas space in the box around the subject, $V_B$.

$$V_P = V_{TIS} + V_L + V_B \tag{9.26}$$

The tissues of the body, composed of liquids and solids, can be considered incompressible when compared with the gas in the lungs. During breathing movements, the tissues change shape, not volume. Also, because the volume of the plethysmograph is a constant (except during calibration procedures), changes in $V_P$ are zero. Consequently, the change in volume of the gas in the lungs is equal and opposite to the changes in volume of the gas space in the box.

$$dV_L = -dV_B \tag{9.27}$$

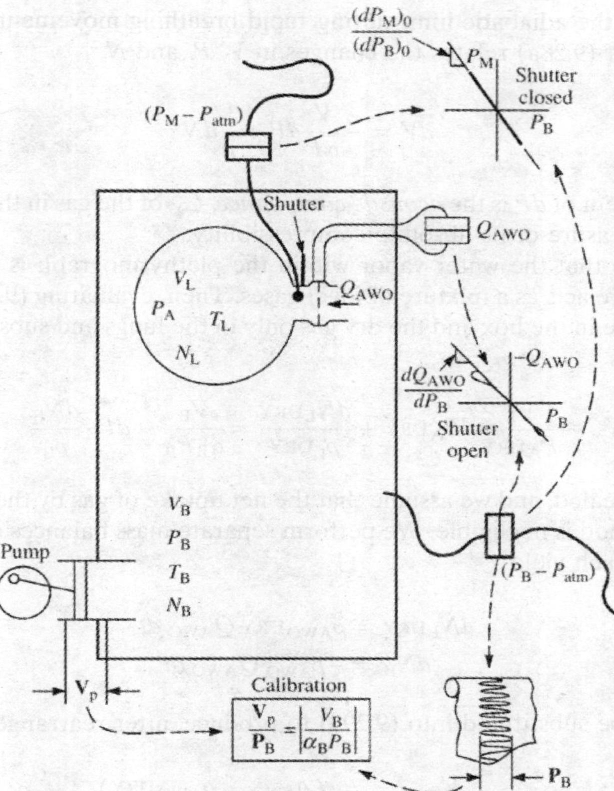


**Figure 9.8** A pressure-type total-body plethysmograph is used with the shutter closed to determine lung volume and with the shutter open to determine changes in alveolar pressure. Airway resistance can also be computed if volume flow of gas is measured at the airway opening. Because atmospheric pressure is constant, changes in the pressures of interest can be obtained from measurements made relative to atmospheric pressure.

These equal and opposite changes in volume produce changes in pressure within the lungs and within the gas space in the box as a result of thermodynamic processes. For the lungs and the box, each modeled as a well-mixed compartment, the volume, pressure, and number of moles of the ideal gases undergoing these processes can be related by a barotropic relation of the form

$$P\left(\frac{V}{N}\right)^{\alpha} = K \tag{9.28a}$$

in which $\alpha$ and $K$ are constants. For an isothermal process, such as occurs in the lungs, $\alpha = 1$; for an adiabatic process, $\alpha = 1.4$ (for a diatomic gas such as air). For any other process, $\alpha$ will be between these two limits. In the box, $\alpha$

approaches the adiabatic limit during rapid breathing movements. The total derivative of (9.28a) relates the changes in $V$, $P$, and $N$.

$$dV = -\frac{V}{\alpha P}dP + \frac{1}{\rho}dN \tag{9.28b}$$

The coefficient of $dP$ is the *acoustic compliance,* $C_g$, of the gas in the container. This is a measure of its absolute compressibility.

Assume that the water vapor within the plethysmograph is unsaturated and therefore acts as a mixture of ideal gases. Then, evaluating (9.28b) for the total mixture in the box and the dry gas only in the lungs and substituting into (9.27) yields

$$-\frac{V_L}{P_{A\,DRY}}dP_{A\,DRY} + \frac{dN_{L\,DRY}}{\rho_{L\,DRY}} = \frac{V_B}{\alpha_B P_B} - dP_B\frac{dN_B}{\rho_B} \tag{9.29a}$$

The box is sealed, and we assume that the net uptake of gas by the pulmonary capillary blood is negligible. We perform separate mass balances on the lungs and box, which yield

$$dN_{L\,DRY} = \rho_{AWO\,DRY}\, Q_{AWO}\, dt$$
$$dN_B = -\rho_{AWO}\, Q_{AWO}\, dt$$

These can be substituted into (9.29a) to produce, after rearrangement,

$$\frac{V_L}{P_{A\,DRY}}dP_{A\,DRY} = -\left[\frac{V_B}{\alpha_B P_B}dP_B + \left(\frac{\rho_{AWO}}{\rho_B} - \frac{\rho_{AWO\,DRY}}{\rho_{L\,DRY}}\right) Q_{AWO}\, dt\right] \tag{9.29b}$$

The ideal-gas law (9.19) can be used to express the densities in (9.29b) in terms of temperatures and pressures. The *mean* (hydrostatic) pressures of the total gas mixtures at the airway opening, within the lungs, and within the box are all equal to atmospheric pressure: $P_{AWO} = P_A = P_B = P_{atm}$. Because the partial pressure of saturated water vapor is primarily a function of temperature, and because the processes within the lungs are essentially isothermal, the changes in the total alveolar pressure are simply the changes in partial pressure of the dry gases within the lungs: $dP_A = dP_{A\,DRY}$. Consequently (9.29b) can be rewritten as

$$\frac{V_L}{(P_{atm} - P_{A\,H_2O})}dP_A$$
$$= -\left[\frac{V_B}{\alpha_B P_B}dP_B + \left(\frac{T_B}{T_{AWO}} - \frac{(P_{atm} - P_{AWO\,H_2O})\, T_L}{(P_{atm} - P_{A\,H_2O})\, T_{AWO}}\right) Q_{AWO}\, dt\right] \tag{9.30}$$

Equation (9.30) represents the governing equation for the total-body plethysmograph in which a subject breathes within the box. It may be used in separate experiments—one with the airway occluded, the other with it open—to compute an estimate of absolute volume of the lungs and a continuous estimate of alveolar pressure, respectively.

## VOLUME OF GAS WITHIN THE THORACIC CAVITY BY TOTAL-BODY PLETHYSMOGRAPH

If a subject were to attempt breathing movements within the TBP with his or her airway opening blocked, no gas would flow at that location and $Q_{AWO}$ would be equal to zero. Then (9.30) could be rewritten as

$$\frac{(dP_A)_0}{(dP_B)_0} = -\frac{(P_{atm} - P_{AH_2O})}{V_L}\frac{V_B}{\alpha_B P_B} \tag{9.31}$$

in which the subscript 0 designates zero flow at the airway opening. Equation (9.31) contains $V_L$, which represents the volume of the gas space within the thoracic cavity at the instant when the airway was blocked. We can compute this *volume of thoracic gas*, designated $V_{TG}$, from (9.31) if we know $V_B/\alpha_B P_B$, the acoustic compliance of the gas in the box, and if we know the changes in alveolar and box pressure during the blocked breathing movements. A two-step clinical procedure can be performed to evaluate these terms. One step involves a calibrating pump, and the other requires the subject to attempt to pant.

During airway occlusion, the lungs and the box can both be considered closed systems. Then $dN_B = 0$ and (9.28b) evaluated for the box indicates that $V_B/\alpha_B P_B$ can be computed as the ratio of a known change in volume in the gas space in the box to the change in box pressure it causes. The known change in volume is produced by a motor-driven, valveless piston pump mounted in the side of the box (Figure 9.8), which changes the volume $V_P$ of the plethysmograph itself. If the subject stops breathing and blocks his or her nose and mouth while the piston oscillates, the change in volume of the gas space in the box will be only the volume displacement of the pump, $\mathbf{V}_P$. The *amplitude* of the resulting box pressure change, $\mathbf{P}_B$, can be measured. If the frequency of the pump is approximately that of the breathing movements of the subject during the remainder of the experiment, then $\alpha_B$ will have essentially the same value in the two situations, and the ratio $\mathbf{V}_P/\mathbf{P}_B$ will yield the acoustic compliance of the gas in the box around the subject.

When the airway opening is blocked—by a shutter, for example (Figure 9.8)—we assume that, during attempted breathing movements, only compression and expansion of gas occur within the lungs and that no internal flows take place. Then the pressure at every point in the pulmonary gas space is in equilibrium, and a measurement at any accessible point in communication with the lungs (for instance, the mouth) reflects the changes in pressure occurring at every point in the pulmonary system. Therefore, changes in mouth pressure, $P_M$, behind the closed shutter during the subject's efforts to breathe are assumed equal to changes in pressure in the alveolar region resulting from the same maneuver; that is, $dP_M = dP_A$ when only compression and expansion of the gas occur.

For these conditions, (9.31) can be rearranged to yield $V_{TG}$ as an estimate of the absolute volume of the lungs,

$$V_{TG} = -(P_{atm} - P_{AH_2O}) \frac{\mathbf{V}_P}{\mathbf{P}_B} \frac{(dP_B)_0}{(dP_M)_0} \tag{9.32}$$

We can evaluate the ratio of change in box pressure to change in mouth pressure by displaying $P_M$ versus $P_B$ simultaneously on the two axes of an oscilloscope (Figure 9.8). Then $(dP_B)_0/(dP_M)_0$ represents the inverse of the average slope of the resulting curve, which for rapid panting movements against a closed shutter should be a straight line that retraces itself.

If the airway is occluded at the end of a quiet expiration, $V_{TG}$ can be used as an estimate of FRC. However, $V_{TG}$ is a measure of the total gas space within the body that is compressed and expanded during the closed-airway panting maneuver (DuBois *et al.*, 1956a). Normally this reflects just the gas space contained entirely within the nose, mouth, large airways, and thoracic cavity [plus any volume between the shutter and airway opening which must be subtracted from the volume obtained from (9.32)], because abdominal gas usually represents a negligible fraction of the gas space within the body. However, this approach cannot distinguish between gas within the lungs and any undissolved gas within the pleural space (pneumothorax). In a subject with no pneumothorax, $V_{TG}$ is an estimate of the total volume of all gas spaces in the pulmonary system, including those that may not communicate freely with the airway opening. Consequently, for normal subjects, $V_{TG}$ measured at the end of expiration corresponds closely to the FRC estimated by the gas-washout and dilution procedures described in Section 9.4. However, in subjects with obstructive lung disease, $V_{TG}$ is a more accurate estimate of FRC than the lower values calculated from the washout and dilution experiments.

## CHANGES IN ALVEOLAR PRESSURE BY TOTAL-BODY PLETHYSMOGRAPH

For the computation of a continuous estimate of changes in alveolar pressure during flow of gas through the airways, DuBois *et al.* (1965b) proposed making measurements during a voluntarily produced, high-frequency low-amplitude pant. This results in two primary advantages related to (9.30). First, it improves the validity of the assumption that the effects of gas exchange between the alveoli and pulmonary capillaries are negligible. Because the net uptake by the capillaries can be considered to occur at a nearly constant rate with only slight variation with breathing frequency, its major (low-frequency) component is easily separable from the changes in $P_B$ caused by respiratory movements. At panting frequencies the effects of nonzero net uptake can be assumed to appear primarily as a baseline drift.

Second, it reduces the size of the term involving $Q_{AWO}$. If low-volume amplitudes are produced even at high voluntary frequencies, $Q_{AWO}$ will not be large. The coefficient of $Q_{AWO}$ in (9.30) is the difference between two ratios; both of which are near unity. As the conditions at the airway opening approach either those of the gas space in the box or those in the lungs, the difference between these ratios departs from zero. The extent of this departure can limit the application of the procedure of breathing into the box for the estimation of alveolar pressure to small-volume-amplitude maneuvers unless the subject, during the measurements, breathes a gas mixture the density of which is very close to that of alveolar gas. During panting, the term involving $Q_{AWO}$ in (9.30) is routinely neglected.

High-frequency maneuvers also decrease the effects of leaks in the box. The combination of a small leak that has a high resistance to flow and the acoustic compliance of the gas in the large gas space in the box (about $10^3$ liters) acts as a high-pass filter to differences in pressure and as a low-pass filter to the flow between the inside and outside of the plethysmograph. Thus the higher the frequency of the changes in pressure in the box, the less degradation of the breathing-related signal due to leaks to the atmosphere. Note, however, that the high-pass-filter effects of small, controlled leaks in the box, or of leaky ballast chambers on the reference side of plethysmograph pressure sensors, are sometimes intentionally employed to eliminate slow drift in box-pressure readings. This drift can be related to increases in temperature of the gas in the box—increases produced by the subject—or to changes in ambient pressure such as those caused by the movement of elevators or the closing and opening of doors.

With these considerations in minds, we can simplify (9.30) to yield

$$dP_A \cong -\left(\frac{P_{atm} - P_{AH_2O}}{V_L}\right)\left(\frac{V_B}{\alpha_B P_B}\right) dP_B \tag{9.33}$$

This states that for high-frequency low-amplitude breathing, the change in alveolar pressure will be approximately proportional to changes in pressure in the box, given that the coefficient of $dP_B$ is constant. The dry partial pressure in the lungs, the pressure in the box, and the volume of the gas space in the box change very little for an individual as a result of breathing movements. However, $\alpha_B$ depends on the frequency of the maneuver, and it asymptotically approaches the adiabatic limit as frequency increases. Also the volume of the lung can change manyfold from RV to TLC, so a low-volume-amplitude maneuver is mandatory for $V_L$ to be nearly constant.

Note from the discussion of (9.31) that the coefficient of $dP_B$ in (9.33) can be evaluated from simultaneous measurements of mouth pressure and box pressure during an occluded-airway panting maneuver.

## 9.6 SOME TESTS OF RESPIRATORY MECHANICS

Pulmonary function tests can be divided into two groups: gas-transport tests, concerned with the movement of gas molecules between the atmosphere and blood (see Section 9.8), and mechanics tests that deal primarily with the relationships among lung volume, gas flow, and pressure differences. One of the ultimate objectives of mechanics tests is to determine whether the defect(s) that produce abnormal pressure–volume–flow relationships can be identified as intrinsic to the airways (lumen and/or walls), to the lung parenchyma surrounding and supporting the airways, or to extrapulmonary structures.

A distinction is often made, in pulmonary medicine, between obstructive and restrictive disease processes. This distinction is not, in general, equivalent to asking whether the defect is in the airways or not; it is based more on the functional impairment caused by a disease. *Obstruction* connotes dynamic mechanics, being associated with abnormal rates of change of volume or gas flows in the lungs during breathing movements. *Restriction,* on the other hand, connotes abnormal static mechanics. It is used to refer not only to the lungs but also to extrapulmonary structures (such as the chest wall, muscles, and the abdominal contents). This condition is indicated when the volume attained by the ventilatory system is inappropriate for the difference in pressure applied or when the differences in pressure that the respiratory muscles are capable of producing are abnormally low. Even though restriction and obstruction may not be completely separable in a given disease state, the presence of either or both can ideally be determined by making measurements on the respiratory system under two sets of conditions: static, when all flows and rates of change of all variables are zero, and dynamic, when some or all of these are nonzero.

## STATIC MECHANICS

When flows and rates of change of flow and volume are zero, the transpulmonary pressure difference, $\Delta P_L = P_{AWO} - P_{PL}$, as indicated by (9.3a) and (9.3b), reduces to a function of volume alone. Therefore, the static mechanical characteristics of the lungs can be obtained by measuring simultaneously the lung volume and the transpulmonary pressure difference, at various lung volumes, while no motions exist in the system. The pulmonary system exhibits a static, or plastic, hysteresis when cycled through a set of static lung volumes. Consequently, to define the $\Delta P$–$V$ relation for the lungs, we must standardize or note the initial volume and direction of change to subsequent volumes. In practice, the expiratory portion of the statically determined $\Delta P$–$V$ curve is routinely used to characterize the lungs.

***Static Compliance*** To produce an expiratory $\Delta P$–$V$ curve, the subject is instructed to inspire to TLC and then to exhale to successively smaller volumes, holding each volume while the pressure in an esophageal balloon is measured relative to pressure at the airway opening. This pressure difference is used as an estimate of transpulmonary pressure (Section 9.2). The lung volume corresponding to each measurement is obtained by spirometer in terms of a change from a reference volume (for example, FRC) determined independently either by gas washout (Section 9.4) or plethysmograph (Section 9.5).

Figure 9.9 shows a facsimile of statically determined expiratory $\Delta P$–$V$ curves for a normal subject, for a subject who has restricted, or stiff, lungs

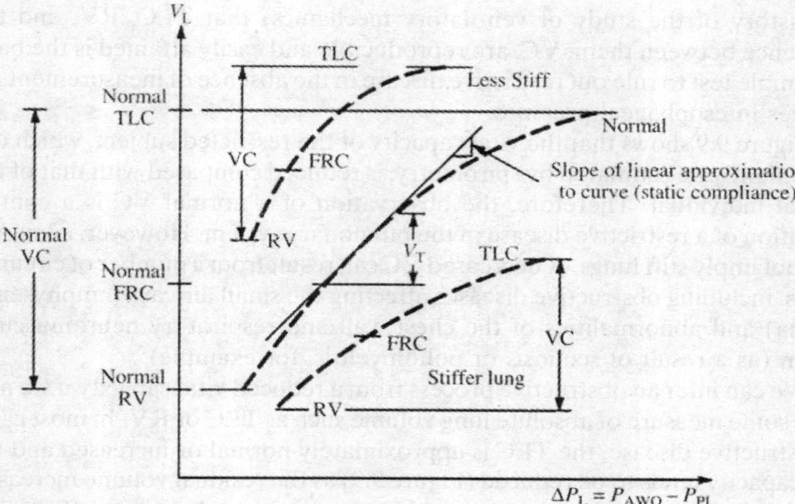


**Figure 9.9** Idealized statically determined expiratory pressure–volume relations for the lung. The positions and slopes for lungs with different elastic properties are shown relative to scales of absolute volume and pressure difference.

(from diseases such as pulmonary fibrosis or pneumonia), and for a subject who has very distensible lungs (from pulmonary emphysema, for example). The curves extend from TLC to RV for the corresponding individual and are seen to be nonlinear. Such relations are not routinely described for the entire vital capacity. Instead, for small changes in volume, on the order of a tidal volume, straight-line approximations about a volume operating point are used. The slope of the linear approximation to the statically determined $\Delta P$–$V$ curve is the static compliance, $C$st, as defined by (9.7).

Assuming that the compliance of each of the curves in Figure 9.9 is computed at the respective FRCs, we find, as would be expected, that the stiffer lung has a lower compliance and the less stiff lung a higher compliance than normal. Therefore, we can identify a restricted, or stiff, lung by computing lung compliance at a standardized lung volume. However, even though an increased compliance can be associated in certain cases with obstructive pulmonary diseases, such as emphysema, lungs affected by other obstructive diseases, such as those involving partial blockage of the lumen of large airways, frequently exhibit a normal compliance. Consequently, even when compliance is normal, the dynamic behavior of the system must also be studied to rule out obstruction.

***Static Lung Volumes*** Although pulmonary compliance is a desirable parameter to obtain when the physician suspects restrictive lung disease, it is not routinely measured because it requires the use of an esophageal balloon, which is very unpleasant for the subject. Instead, the observation (made very early in the history of the study of ventilatory mechanics) that TLC, RV, and the difference between them, VC, are reproducible and easily attained is the basis of a simple test to rule out restrictive disease in the absence of measurements of changes in esophageal pressure.

Figure 9.9 shows that the vital capacity of the restricted subject, which can conveniently be estimated by spirometry, is reduced compared with that of the normal individual. Therefore, the observation of a normal VC is a contra-indication of a restrictive disease in the pulmonary system. However, a low VC does not imply stiff lungs. A decreased VC can result from a number of circumstances, including obstructive diseases affecting the small airways (emphysema, asthma) and abnormalities of the chest wall and respiratory neuromuscular system (as a result of scoliosis or poliomyelitis, for example).

We can infer an obstructive process from a reduced vital capacity if we also know some measure of absolute lung volume such as TLC or RV. In most cases of obstructive disease, the TLC is approximately normal or increased and the vital capacity tends to be reduced (Figure 9.9) as the residual volume increases, because the obstructed patient is unable to empty his or her lungs effectively. However, some obstructive processes, such as those in the larger airways or the initial phases of small airways disease, may not lead to a reduced vital capacity. Consequently, the dynamic behavior of the system should also be studied.

***Maximal Inspiratory and Expiratory Static Pressures*** When the vital capacity is reduced and a restrictive process is suspected, the clinician can investigate extrapulmonary abnormality by measuring the maximal static inspiratory and expiratory pressures that can be produced at the airway opening at a given lung volume by forceful efforts against a blocked airway opening. By combining (9.3a) to (9.3c), we note that for no flows in the system,

$$p_{\text{AWO}} - p_{\text{BS}} = \left(\frac{1}{Cst_{\text{L}}} + \frac{1}{Cst_{\text{W}}}\right) v_{\text{L}} - \Delta p_{\text{MUS}} \tag{9.34}$$

in which the pressure on the body surface is usually taken to be atmospheric. If a patient is instructed to try to exhale or inhale maximally against a closed nose and mouthpiece while the pressure changes in the mouth are measured, changes in lung volume $v_{\text{L}}$ should be negligible, and the measured changes in mouth pressure will reflect the forces produced by the respiratory muscles during these efforts. If the respiratory muscles, the nerve cells controlling them, and the kinematics of the chest wall are not impaired, then $p_{\text{AWO}} - p_{\text{BS}}$ should approximate that attained by a normal person at the corresponding point in his or her vital capacity (usually FRC) at which the test is performed.

## DYNAMIC MECHANICS DURING SMALL VOLUME CHANGES AND FLOWS

Equations (9.3a) and (9.3b) indicate that, during resting breathing, changes in transpulmonary pressure can be expressed as a function of the changes in lung volume and gas volume flow rate that would occur if the alveoli were purely elastic structures. However, the alveoli are not purely elastic, in that they are able to exhibit a viscoelastic type of behavior. Inclusion of this in (9.3a) and (9.3b) yields

$$p_{\mathrm{AWO}} - p_{\mathrm{PL}} = \frac{1}{C\mathrm{st}_{\mathrm{L}}} v_{\mathrm{L}} + R_{\mathrm{LT}} \dot{v}_{\mathrm{L}} + R_{\mathrm{AW}} q_{\mathrm{AWO}} \tag{9.35}$$

in which $R_{\mathrm{LT}}$ is the resistance of the lung tissue and $R_{\mathrm{AW}}$ is the airway resistance defined by (9.6). $R_{\mathrm{AW}}$ represents a direct measure of obstruction in the airways. Because of the viscoelastic behavior of the alveolar tissue, the computation of $R_{\mathrm{AW}}$ from (9.35) is not convenient. Instead, we compute $R_{\mathrm{AW}}$ directly from (9.6). The pressure and flow at the airway opening required by (9.6) are easily measured. However, estimating changes in a representative alveolar pressure while there is flow in the airways requires the total-body plethysmograph, as discussed in Section 9.5.

***Airway Resistance*** As an example of a TBP procedure for estimating $R_{\mathrm{AW}}$, consider a subject situated inside a pressure plethysmograph (Figure 9.8). The individual (with nose blocked) breathes within the box through a mouthpiece and flowmeter with an associated shutter that can be closed to block flow at the mouth. While the shutter is open, the pressure at the airway opening (external to the mouthpiece and flowmeter) is the pressure within the plethysmograph $P_{\mathrm{B}}$. That portion of the pressure drop between the alveoli and box that results from the mouthpiece assembly is taken into account by expressing the total alveolar-to-box resistance [given by (9.6) for this arrangement] as the sum of $R_{\mathrm{AW}}$ and the mouthpiece assembly resistance $R_{\mathrm{MP}}$. For a panting maneuver, (9.33) indicates that changes in the representative alveolar pressure are proportional to changes in $P_{\mathrm{B}}$. Consequently, (9.6) can be rewritten

$$R_{\mathrm{AW}} + R_{\mathrm{MP}} = \left(1 + \frac{(P_{\mathrm{atm}} - P_{\mathrm{AH_2O}})\, V_{\mathrm{B}}}{V_{\mathrm{L}} \alpha_{\mathrm{B}} P_{\mathrm{B}}}\right) \frac{\partial P_{\mathrm{B}}}{\partial Q_{\mathrm{AWO}}} \tag{9.36}$$

The fraction within the large parentheses in (9.36) is much greater than unity because $V_{\mathrm{B}}$, the volume of the gas space in the box, is much larger ($> 100:1$) than $V_{\mathrm{L}}$, the volume within the lungs [$(P_{\mathrm{atm}} - P_{\mathrm{AH_2O}})/\alpha_{\mathrm{B}} P_{\mathrm{B}}$ being of order 1]. Consequently, as shown by (9.31), a closed-shutter panting maneuver, in which mouth pressure (behind the shutter) and box pressure are measured simultaneously, can be used to evaluate the term in the large parentheses in (9.36). We can obtain an approximation to the partial derivative of box pressure $P_{\mathrm{B}}$ with respect to gas flow rate at the airway opening $Q_{\mathrm{AWO}}$ by displaying these two variables, measured simultaneously with the shutter open, on orthogonal axes of an oscilloscope (Figure 9.8). For very small changes in volume (a condition of the panting maneuver) and the accelerations associated with panting, normal lungs exhibit a relatively straight $P_{\mathrm{B}}$–$Q_{\mathrm{AWO}}$ relationship with very slight looping. Changes in box pressure are then essentially a function of flow in the airways alone. Thus $\partial P_B/\partial Q_{AWO}$ can be evaluated as the inverse of the slope of the oscilloscope figure, $dP_B/dQ_{AWO}$, and $R_{AW}$ can be computed as

$$R_{AW} = \left(-\frac{(dP_M)_0}{(dP_B)_0}\right)\frac{dP_B}{dQ_{AWO}} - R_{MP} \tag{9.37}$$

for which $R_{MP}$ can be evaluated independently.

In some instances, however, the $P_B$–$Q_{AWO}$ plot produced on the oscilloscope screen is highly nonlinear and can display exaggerated looping (dynamic hysteresis). Because of this, it is difficult to determine a representative slope for the plot. A convention has therefore been adopted for the evaluation of $R_{AW}$. The representative slope is that which corresponds to a straight line drawn between the points on the plot at which flow is +0.5 liter/s and −0.5 liter/s in the region corresponding to the end of inspiration and the beginning of expiration. This straddles the point $Q_{AWO} = 0$; it is usually fairly straight and involves small changes in volume. The representative slope and the parameter $R_{AW}$ computed from it are the only pieces of information from this procedure that are routinely used for the clinical evaluation of airway mechanics.

At least three phenomena associated with the respiratory system can cause exaggerated looping and/or nonlinearity of the $P_B$–$Q_{AWO}$ relationship in this experiment. (1) Equation (9.33) may not be a good approximation to (9.30) for the conditions of the experiment. (2) The pulmonary system being tested may not act as a single mechanical unit. Hence the concept of a single representative alveolar pressure in phase with flow may be inappropriate. (3) The mechanical properties of the lungs and airways may be so abnormal that even during a panting maneuver, significant changes in dimension (primarily in diameter) of the airways occur, so that the $P_B$–$Q_{AWO}$ relationship becomes quite bizarre (nonlinear). The latter two situations can be evaluated by additional independent pulmonary function tests.

The aggregate resistance of the smaller airways that play a major role in the final distribution of gas to the alveoli is small compared with that of the larger, upper airways. Consequently, $R_{AW}$ easily reflects obstruction in the larger airways. However, only when the smaller airways are so affected by pulmonary disease that their aggregate resistance is drastically increased do they significantly affect $R_{AW}$. Thus the parameter $R_{AW}$ is not a sensitive indicator of the initial phases of diseases of the small airways.

***Pulmonary Mechanics Evaluated during Breathing*** For a normal pulmonary system that can be represented by a first-order linear differential equation such as (9.11), mechanical properties (the coefficients $C$ and $R$) can be estimated by direct substitution of pressure difference, flow, and volume. Measuring the pressure difference across the pulmonary system, i.e., between the airway opening and the thoracic esophagus, and the flow at the airway opening, and integrating this flow (as a measure of volume change) for breathing at voluntarily achieved frequencies permits calculation of the total pulmonary (lung) properties. For example, total lung resistance can be calculated from

$$R_{\mathrm{L}} = \frac{\Delta p_{\mathrm{L}}(t_2) - \Delta p_{\mathrm{L}}(t_1)}{q_{\mathrm{AWO}}(t_2) - q_{\mathrm{AWO}}(t_1)} \tag{9.38}$$

if $t_2$ and $t_1$ are successive instants at which $V_{\mathrm{L}}(t_2) = V_{\mathrm{L}}(t_1)$. ($R_{\mathrm{L}}$ generally would be expected to be greater than $R_{\mathrm{AW}}$ because of the resistive component of the viscoelastic lung tissue.) Similarly,

$$C_{\mathrm{L}} = \frac{v_{\mathrm{L}}(t_4) - v_{\mathrm{L}}(t_3)}{\Delta p_{\mathrm{L}}(t_4) - \Delta p_{\mathrm{L}}(t_3)} \tag{9.39}$$

for which $t_4$ and $t_3$ are successive instants at which flow at the airway opening, $Q_{\mathrm{AWO}}$ is zero. (In general, when flow at the airway opening is instantaneously zero, there still can be motions and flows at other places within the pulmonary system so that the system may not be truly "static.")

If the lungs have a uniform distribution of mechanical properties so that all parts act in unison (exhibit a single degree of freedom), then $R_{\mathrm{L}}$ and $C_{\mathrm{L}}$ will be constants, independent of the breathing pattern the patient produces and frequency at which he or she breathes. In this case, $C_{\mathrm{L}}$ will equal the static compliance, $C\mathrm{st}_{\mathrm{L}}$, (see Figure 9.9) at all frequencies and the combination of both lungs can be characterized by a single viscoelastic unit and a single time constant, $\tau_{\mathrm{L}} = R_{\mathrm{L}} C\mathrm{st}_{\mathrm{L}}$.

However, if the lungs have a nonuniform distribution of mechanical properties, the values computed for $R_{\mathrm{L}}$ and $C_{\mathrm{L}}$ from (9.38) and (9.39), respectively, will decrease from their static (zero frequency) values as breathing frequency increases. In this case, a single degree-of-freedom pulmonary system can be ruled out, and the lungs can be represented by a combination of viscoelastic units, each with its own time constant. Because $C_{\mathrm{L}}$ is calculated from data obtained while the subject is breathing and does not necessarily have the same value as $C\mathrm{st}_{\mathrm{L}}$, it is given the name *dynamic compliance* and the symbol $C\mathrm{dyn}_{\mathrm{L}}$.

A test that is sensitive to the nonuniform mechanical changes caused by the onset of small airways disease is based on the values of $C\mathrm{dyn}_{\mathrm{L}}$ obtained at several breathing frequencies. If $C\mathrm{st}_{\mathrm{L}}$ and $R_{\mathrm{AW}}$ or $R_{\mathrm{L}}$ are normal, and $C\mathrm{dyn}_{\mathrm{L}}$ obtained for breathing frequencies between 2 and 4 breath/s is less than 80% of $C\mathrm{st}_{\mathrm{L}}$, then small airways disease is indicated.

## HIGH-FREQUENCY BEHAVIOR OF THE RESPIRATORY SYSTEM

Mechanical properties of the respiratory system have been inferred from its response to high frequency perturbations. Two procedures have been developed: the "forced oscillation" and the "interrupter" techniques.

***Forced Oscillation Technique*** As with any system whose behavior can be approximated over a given operating range by a linear model, for example, (9.3a) to (9.3b), the respiratory system can be characterized over very small volume changes by its (complex) mechanical impedance. For a pneumatic system, such as the respiratory system, the total respiratory impedance, $Z_{TR}(j\omega)$, can be expressed in terms of the sinusoidal components of the imposed changes in pressure difference across the system $(p_{AWO} - p_{BS})$ and the resulting rate of change in volume, $\dot{v}_L$ (measured, in practice, as change in flow, $q_{AWO}$).

At frequencies higher than those that can be achieved by voluntary movements of the chest wall, the forces to accelerate the masses of the respiratory tissues and the air in the airways become measurable. The simplest model for the respiratory system, then, must include a second order term that accounts for the inertance $I$ (pneumatic analog of mass) of the system. In complex form this can be written:

$$(p_{AWO} - p_{BS})(j\omega) = \left[R_{TR} + j\left(I_{TR}\omega - \frac{1}{\omega C_{TR}}\right)\right]\dot{v}_L(j\omega)$$
$$= Z_{TR}(j\omega)\dot{v}_L(j\omega) \quad (9.40)$$

The real part of the impedance is interpreted as the total respiratory resistance and the imaginary part as the total respiratory reactance. The use of this equation requires either that measurements be made when the respiratory muscles are completely relaxed so that the forces produced by the chest wall muscles, $\Delta p_{MUS}$, which should appear on the left hand side, are zero, or that, at the frequencies of interest, active participation of the muscles is negligible.

The simplest method of imposing high-frequency forcing on the respiratory system uses a speaker system. Small sinusoidal pressure waves at individual frequencies are superimposed on tidal flow at the airway opening while the subject is breathing normally. An apparatus such as that shown in Figure 9.10 has been used to do this (Hyatt *et al.*, 1970). This approach is especially useful in subjects, such as comatose patients and young children, who are unable to provide the cooperation required by most pulmonary function tests. More complicated wave shapes with broad frequency content, from repeated short duration square waves [called *impulse oscillometry* (Frei *et al.*, 2005)] to random noise (Michaelson *et al.*, 1975), have been superimposed on breathing using variations of the same type system. The resulting measurements have been analyzed using Fourier transforms to evaluate the real and imaginary parts of the impedance spectrum at discrete frequencies. Analyses of these data with more complicated models than (9.40) have produced inferences about the mechanical properties and disease status of various parts of the lungs, airways and chest wall. Standardization of the technique for clinical practice has begun (Oostveen *et al.*, 2003).

***Interrupter Technique*** Instead of superimposing a controlled pressure variation on breathing, interrupter techniques produce momentary complete or partial blockage of flow into and out of the airway, thereby causing pressure fluctuations at the airway opening. The device used to produce this flow interruption is a form of high-speed shutter or "chopper," usually a spinning

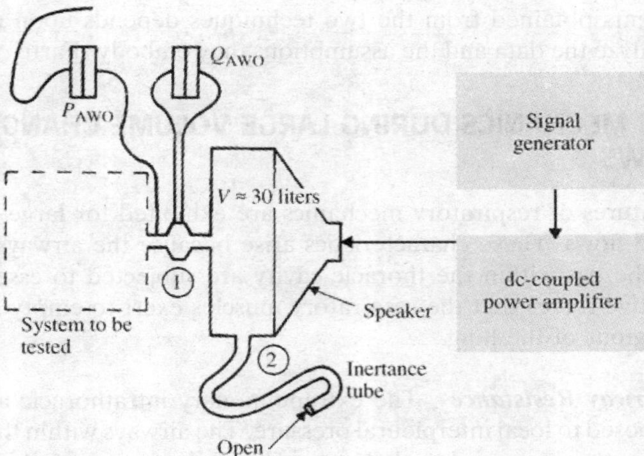


**Figure 9.10** A speaker-driven forced oscillation system can be used to obtain the mechanical impedance of the total respiratory system during spontaneous breathing and to measure the acoustic impedance and/or frequency responses of laboratory apparatus. The high inertance of the long (8.5 m) tube at port 2 acts as a low-pass filter for flow. As the subject breathes normally, the low-frequency flow produced passes through port 1 and port 2. However, the small, high-frequency pressure variations generated by the speaker are blocked by the inertance at port 2 and are preferentially transmitted to the subject through port 1.

disk that intersects the outlet of the mouthpiece through which the subject is breathing. Carefully shaped and spaced apertures and a variable speed drive allow the disk to produce specific variations in flow and pressure during inspiration and/or expiration, at selected repetition rates. The resulting patterns of flow through the mouthpiece and pressure on the subject side of the shutter are continuously recorded simultaneously.

The original approach to the analysis was to assume that the pressure change that resulted from the momentary complete occlusion of the flow is related to the resistance of the total respiratory system. Then the ratio of the pressure perturbation, to the flow before the occlusion, was identified as a characteristic resistance of the system. As the technique has been modified and adapted, the interpretation of the parameters computed from the measured variables have evolved (Bates *et al.,* 1988). To produce clinically useful procedures based on the technique, various procedures and data analyses have been developed (Lausted and Johnson, 1999).

Even though forced oscillation and interrupter techniques are similar in that they impose high frequency pressure and/or flow disturbances at the airway opening during breathing, they appear sensitive to the effects of different combinations of mechanical properties of the various respiratory structural components (Delacourt *et al.*, 2001). The interpretation of the measurements obtained from the two techniques depends upon the models used to analyze the data and the assumptions they embody (Farre *et al.*, 1998).

## DYNAMIC MECHANICS DURING LARGE VOLUME CHANGES AND FLOWS

Several features of respiratory mechanics are exhibited for large changes in volume and flows. These characteristics arise because the airways that must distribute the gas within the thoracic cavity are subjected to essentially the same effective forces that the respiratory muscles exert to empty and fill the alveolar regions of the lung.

***Specific Airway Resistance*** The extrapulmonary intrathoracic airways are directly exposed to local interpleural pressure. The airways within the lungs are subjected to the increased and decreased tensile forces produced by the stretching of their parenchymal attachments as the lung regions in which they are embedded inflate and deflate. Consequently, as the alveolar regions are expanded and compressed, the length and cross-sectional area of each airway generation undergo corresponding changes. One manifestation of this is an approximately inverse relationship between plethysmographically determined airway resistance and the lung volume at which it is measured. The larger the volume of the lung, the more expanded the airways and the lower the resistance to flows produced during a panting maneuver, and vice versa. Hence

$$R_{\mathrm{AW}} \cong \frac{(SR_{\mathrm{AW}})}{V_{\mathrm{TG}}} \tag{9.41}$$

where $SR_{\mathrm{AW}}$ is a constant of proportionality referred to as *specific airway resistance* and $V_{\mathrm{TG}}$ is volume of thoracic gas. $SR_{\mathrm{AW}}$ represents a property of a subject's airways normalized for his or her lung volume.

***Flow Limitation*** Another manifestation of the effects of changes in airway dimensions during ventilatory maneuvers is the *flow limitation* exhibited during forced expirations. If it were possible to keep the volume of the lung constant and vary the pressure drop and flow through the airways, characteristic *isovolume pressure–flow curves* would result, depending on the volume of the lung for which the curve was obtained. Figure 9.11 gives idealized examples of such curves for normal lungs. In practice these curves are obtained by cycling the lungs through a succession of increasing volume amplitudes and flows. The pressure–flow curve for each cycle is plotted, and points on each curve corresponding to the same volume are connected.

Three features generally appear: (1) Inspiratory flow continually increases as the difference in pressure is increased at any lung volume. (2) For high lung volumes (near TLC), expiratory flow increases as the difference in pressure becomes more negative. (3) For lung volumes below about 80% of the TLC, the expiratory flow reaches a value that is never exceeded, even though the

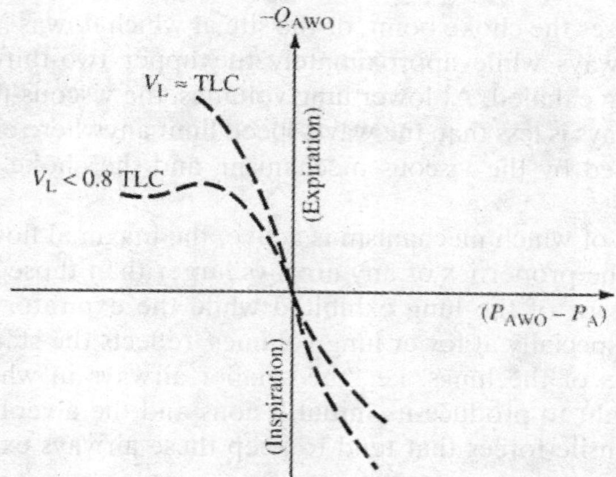


**Figure 9.11** Idealized isovolume pressure-flow curves for two lung volumes for a normal respiratory system. Each curve represents a composite from numerous inspiratory–expiratory cycles, each with successively increased efforts. The pressure and flow values measured as the lungs passed through the respective volumes of interest are plotted and connected to yield the corresponding curves.

difference in pressure becomes more negative. This condition is referred to as *flow limitation* in which the flow is *effort independent.* That is, expiratory flow cannot be increased, no matter how much expiratory efforts are increased.

The flow limit that can be achieved at any given lung volume is dependent on the characteristics of the intrathoracic pulmonary system and the physical properties (viscosity, density) of the gas it contains. Two basic flow-limiting mechanisms appear to be operating (Hyatt, 1986). Central to both is the viscoelastic behavior of the pulmonary airways by which the cross-sectional area of the airways changes in response to changes in transmural pressure.

The first flow-limiting mechanism, accounted for by what is referred to as the *wave-speed theory,* involves the coupling of airway compliance to the pressure drop due to the inertial properties of the gas and convective acceleration of flow in the airways. This coupling determines the wave speed in the compliant airways—that is, the speed at which a small pressure disturbance, or wave, can propagate along the airway. Flow in a compliant tube cannot exceed that at which the local fluid velocity equals the local wave speed at any point in the tube. The second mechanism, termed *viscous-flow limitation,* involves the coupling between airway compliance and viscous-flow losses; that is, under appropriate conditions, laminar and turbulent dissipation dominate the pressure distribution that causes airway compression.

At larger lung volumes, for which the driving pressure and local flows are high and airways are held open by the stretched parenchyma, the viscous limit for the peripheral, smaller airways is greater than the wave speed for the central, larger airways. Consequently, in normal lungs, the wave-speed mechanism causes the choke point, or the site at which flow is limited, to be in the central airways while approximately the upper two-thirds of the vital capacity is being exhaled. At lower lung volumes, the viscous-flow limit in the peripheral airways is less than the wave-speed limit anywhere else in the lungs, so flow is limited by the viscous mechanism, and the choke point is in the smaller airways.

Regardless of which mechanism is active, the maximal flow is not greatly influenced by the properties of any airways larger than those that limit flow. Thus the behavior of the lung exhibited while the expiratory flow is effort independent, especially at lower lung volumes, reflects the status of the more peripheral parts of the lungs, i.e., the smaller airways in which obstructive disease is thought to produce its initial lesions and the alveolar parenchyma that provide tensile forces that tend to keep these airways expanded.

***The Forced Expiratory Vital Capacity Maneuver: the Maximal Expiratory Flow Volume Curve and Timed Vital Capacity Spirogram*** Flow limitation phenomena can be displayed in two clinically useful ways, both based on measures of only volume flow of gas at the airway opening during a forced expiration from TLC to RV (referred to as a forced expiratory vital capacity maneuver). The equivalent volume of gas expired during this maneuver is the *forced vital capacity* (FVC). Two alternative (and equivalent) methods of displaying the events within a forced expiration involve either (1) plotting volume flow of gas at the airway opening against its integral (or volume change in a spirometer) subtracted from FVC, or (2) plotting the integral of expired-gas volume flow (or spirometer volume change) subtracted from FVC against time (Figure 9.12). The first method produces the *maximal expiratory flow volume* (MEFV) curve, and the second corresponds to the spirogram of the *timed vital capacity* (TVC) routinely performed as part of standard spirometry tests.

The normal MEFV curve reaches a maximal flow at a volume slightly below TLC, and as the forced expiration continues below about 25% of FVC (below TLC), the expired flow rate decreases nearly linearly with decreasing volume. This linear region corresponds to effort-independent flow; it is reproducible and characteristic of the state of the lungs. The MEFV curve represents the relationship between a variable ($\mathrm{FVC} - \int Q_{\mathrm{AWO}}\,dt$) and its derivative ($-Q_{\mathrm{AWO}}$). When this relationship is a straight line through the origin, it represents a homogeneous, linear, first-order differential equation:

$$Q_{\mathrm{AWO}} = -K\left(\mathrm{FVC} - \int Q_{\mathrm{AWO}}\,dt\right) \tag{9.42}$$

Because the coefficient (slope of the linear part of the MEFV curve, $-K$) is negative, it corresponds to an exponential decay from the initial value of ($\mathrm{FVC} - \int Q_{\mathrm{AWO}}\,dt$) at which the relationship became linear. Thus the latter part of the TVC spirogram from 25% FVC below TLC to RV is approximately exponential, corresponding to the effort-independent region of the MEFV

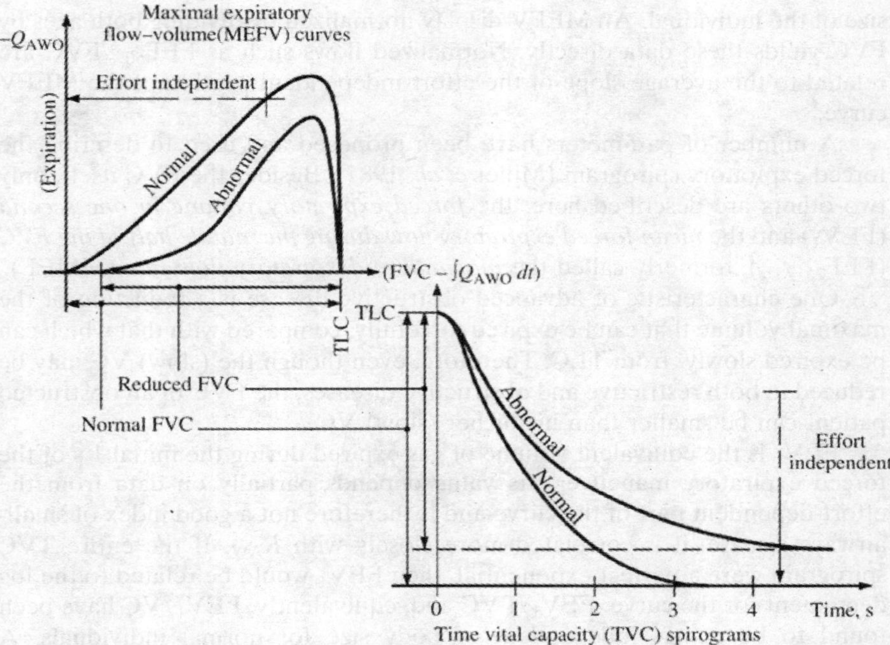


**Figure 9.12** Alternative methods of displaying data produced during FVC expiration. Equivalent information can be obtained from each type of curve; however, reductions in expiratory flow are subjectively more apparent on the MEFV curve than on the timed spirogram.

curve, and is reproducible and unique for a given subject. The region of each curve between TLC and approximately 25% of the FVC below TLC is effort-*dependent*. It provides information about the larger, upper airways and the extrapulmonary parts of the ventilatory system (chest wall, respiratory muscles, and so on). The effort-independent region reflects mechanics of the smaller airways and parenchyma of the lungs. We can make comparable inferences about the state of these various parts of the respiratory system from either the MEFV curve or the TVC spirogram.

***Forced Expiratory Flows and Forced Expiratory Volume*** The MEFV curve has gained popularity because it provides a dramatic visual display compatible with subjective evaluation of lung impairment. We can easily recognize decreases in maximal flows or the concave effort-independent region characteristic of even minimal small airways (obstructive) disease. These are harder to detect visually in a spirogram (Figure 9.12). The parameters used to describe the MEFV curve are basically the maximal flow at a given lung volume—for example, *forced expiratory flow* after 50 or 75% of the FVC has been expired, $FEF_{50\%}$ and $FEF_{75\%}$, respectively. It is especially useful when studying children to normalize these flows to a measure of lung volume to compensate for the size of the individual. An MEFV display normalized by dividing both axes by FVC yields these data directly. Normalized flows such as $FEF_{50\%}/FVC$ are related to the average slope of the effort-independent portion of the MEFV curve.

A number of parameters have been proposed and used to describe the forced expiratory spirogram (Miller *et al.*, 1987). Besides the FVC itself, only two others are described here: the *forced expiratory volume in one second* ($FEV_1$) and the *mean forced expiratory flow during the middle half of the FVC* ($FEF_{25-75\%}$), formerly called the *maximal midexpiratory flow rate* (MMEF).

One characteristic of advanced obstructive disease is a reduction of the maximal volume that can be expired forcefully, compared with that which can be expired slowly, from TLC. Therefore, even though the (slow) VC may be reduced in both restrictive and obstructive diseases, the FVC of an obstructed patient can be smaller than his or her (slow) VC.

$FEV_1$ is the equivalent volume of gas expired during the initial 1 s of the forced expiratory maneuver. Its value depends partially on data from the effort-dependent part of the curve and is therefore not a good index of small-airways disease; it is correlated more closely with $R_{AW}$. If the entire TVC spirogram were a perfect exponential, then $FEV_1$ would be related to the log decrement for the curve. $FEV_1/FVC$ and, equivalently, $FEV_1/VC$ have been found to be nearly independent of body size for normal individuals. A decreased $FEV_1/FVC$ can suggest obstruction, and $FEV_1/VC$ can be reduced even more than $FEV_1/FVC$ in obstructive disease.

The $FEF_{25-75\%}$ represents an average flow produced during the middle half of the FVC. It is computed as follows:

$$FEF_{25-75\%} = \frac{0.5\,FVC}{t_{25\%FVC} - t_{75\%FVC}} \tag{9.43}$$

where $t_{25\%FVC}$ and $t_{75\%FVC}$ are the times at which 25% and 75% of the FVC, respectively, have been exhaled. It is an estimate of the maximal flow at 50% of the FVC, that is, $FEF_{50\%}$—which is obtained from the MEFV curve. It is therefore no less valuable as an indicator of small-airways disease. Dividing $FEF_{25-75\%}$ by FVC is a useful normalization for differences in size among individuals.

***Peak Expiratory Flow and Maximal Voluntary Ventilation*** Two other parameters that yield information about obstruction in the larger airways are *the peak expiratory flow* (PEF) and the *maximal voluntary ventilation* (MVV). The PEF is the highest instantaneous flow at the airway opening that a subject can produce during a maximally forced expiration from TLC. The MVV is the average expiratory flow produced by a subject who is instructed to continually inhale and exhale as deeply and rapidly as possible. Usually this maneuver is performed for only 12 to 15 s to prevent a large reduction in arterial $PCO_2$. The gas expired during this time period is collected, and its volume is measured by spirometer. Using (9.21), the clinician converts this volume to the volume that the gas would occupy at the temperature and pressure existing within the lungs and routinely expresses the result on a per-minute basis. Like $R_{AW}$, the PEF and MVV reflect small airway obstruction only when it is major. However, unlike $R_{AW}$, these parameters can also be affected by neuromuscular impairment.

## 9.7 MEASUREMENT OF GAS CONCENTRATION

Analysis of the composition of gas mixtures is one of the primary methods of obtaining information about lung function. In respiratory studies, the concentration of a component in a gas mixture is not routinely expressed as mass per volume. It is most frequently given in terms of partial pressure or molar fraction [which can be expressed as an equivalent volume fraction, as shown by (9.23)].

Discrete samples of gas are all that is required in certain circumstances. However, as analytical devices with fast response times have been developed, continuous measurement of intrabreath events has become possible and desirable.

Input systems for continuous sampling usually consist of a thin (capillary) tube or catheter and an input connector (which may include a valve or a mixing chamber). Depending on the particular instrument and the application, the transport pathway can vary from centimeters to meters. This introduces transit delays and mixing within the sample and requires that the characteristics of the catheter and connector be matched to those of the instrument. Adjustment of the delay time, which depends on the mean velocity of the sample through the catheter, requires consideration of the following: the pressure drop along the catheter, the pressure within the instrument, the length and diameter of the catheter, the geometry of the input connector, the composition of the sampled gas, and the volume flow of sample required by the instrument for accurate results. Some minimal time delay is always produced by catheter sampling systems, so electrical or numerical signal processing is required if a gas analyzer's output is to be synchronized with the output from another, independent instrument, such as a flowmeter.

Water vapor presents a major problem in sampling respiratory gas by catheter. Investigators have used thin, flexible, stainless steel inlet tubing, carrying sufficient current through its length to heat its wall above body temperature, to prevent changes of gas composition and plugging of its lumen by water condensation. However, heating of the sample within the catheter increases axial diffusion, which can effectively filter out high-frequency components of fast-changing concentration waveshapes. An additional difficulty in measurement is introduced by the tendency of water vapor to be adsorbed and desorbed from surfaces within the system. The establishment of equilibrium between the water molecules on these surfaces and in the moving sample lags behind changes in partial pressures in the sample. Therefore, the gas delivered to the sensor does not represent the gas entering the inlet tube until after that equilibrium is reached. For precision measurements in some applications, the sampled gas is passed through a tube filled with a drying agent. This effectively eliminates water vapor but prolongs the overall response time of the measurement system.

The pH and partial pressures of $O_2$ and $CO_2$ dissolved in blood are routinely measured clinically *in vitro* in discrete samples withdrawn from the circulatory system. The instruments used are specifically adapted electrode systems such as those discussed in Section 10.2. Indwelling, intravascular monitoring systems designed to provide continuous measurements of blood gases and pH using electro-optical techniques, as described in Section 10.3, have been introduced. Their commercial and clinical viability has yet to be demonstrated, at least in part, due to the cost of the disposable sensor-tipped catheters.

Devices for measurements in the gas phase vary in complexity and capabilities from those that can continuously detect and analyze several gas species simultaneously (such as the mass spectrometer) to those that can be modified to test for a few gases individually (such as the infrared analyzer) to those sensitive to a particular property possessed by only one gas that is important to the respiratory system (such as the paramagnetic $O_2$ sensor). Increasing versatility usually entails increasing cost.

## MASS SPECTROSCOPY

A *mass spectrometer* is an apparatus that produces a stream of charged particles (ions) from a substance being analyzed, separates the ions into a spectrum according to their mass-to-charge ratios, and determines the relative abundance of each type of ion present. Medical mass-spectrometer systems include the following elements (Figure 9.13): a sample-inlet assembly, an ionization chamber, a dispersion chamber, and an ion-detection (collector) system (Sodal *et al.*, 1988).

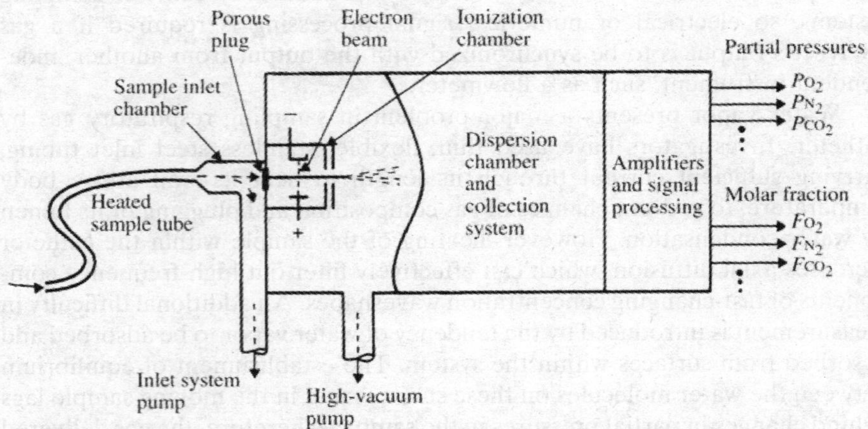


**Figure 9.13 Essential elements of a medical mass spectrometer**

The sample-inlet assembly consists of a heated or unheated capillary tube [approximately 0.25 mm inside diameter (ID)] and sample-inlet chamber. Gas is drawn through this system by a rotary pump that reduces the pressure in the inlet chamber to about 10 to 20 mm Hg (1.3 to 1.7 kPa) absolute. A small amount of gas in the inlet chamber leaks by diffusion through a porous plug into the ionization chamber, which, along with the dispersion chamber, is evacuated to approximately $10^{-7}$ mm Hg ($10^{-5}$ Pa) by a high-vacuum, high-capacity pump. A stream of electrons traveling between a heated filament and an anode bombards the gas entering the ionization chamber and causes the molecules to lose electrons, thereby producing positive ions. These ions are focused into a beam and accelerated by an electric field into the dispersion chamber, where the ion beam is sorted into its components on a molecular mass basis.

Dispersion techniques incorporated into commercially available systems include a magnetic field, a quadrupole electric field, or measurement of time of flight. The separated ion beams fall on the collector system that produces the output signal of the instrument. A mass spectrometer is of real value in respiratory applications only if it simultaneously produces separate continuous outputs for the several chemical species of interest. This has been achieved in two ways. One method uses a single collector that is swept sequentially by the component beams at a high repetition rate. Individual sample-and-hold circuits, each corresponding to a particular species, register the ion current as the beam for their respective species falls on the collector. The second approach employs multiple collectors, the positions of which can be adjusted so that each continuously receives the ions of only one of the components of interest.

The ion current measured by the collector is proportional to the partial pressure of the corresponding component in the gas mixture. Online signal processing, in conjunction with an appropriate calibration procedure, makes it possible for the output to be expressed in terms of molar fractions.

The range of molecular weight that is adequate for most respiratory measurements extends from 4 (He) to 44 ($CO_2$) atomic mass units. Expanded ranges make possible the monitoring of gases such as sulfur hexafluoride (146) and halothane (196). Several important gases produce outputs for the same atomic mass units. In particular, $O_2$ and $CO_2$ cannot be measured in the presence of $N_2O$. Also, CO interferes with $N_2$. CO and $N_2O$ can be quickly and easily measured with infrared instruments, as described in the following paragraphs.

The sensitivity, linearity, and SNR quoted by manufacturers are appropriate for precision measurements. The response time (2% to 90%) for a step change in input is typically less than 100 ms (except for water vapor, which is longer). Transport delays associated with 1.3 m to 1.6 m inlet catheters are on the order of 200 ms (with sample flow rates of 10 to 30 ml/min). Systems that can measure numerous component gases are available.

## THERMAL-CONDUCTIVITY DETECTORS

One of the properties of a gas mixture that changes with composition is its *thermal conductivity*. In general, the thermal conductivity of a gas is inversely related to its molecular weight. For example, $H_2$ and He have thermal conductivities approximately 6.5 times greater than those of $N_2$ and $O_2$. As we noted in Section 9.3, heat transfer between a stationary heated body and a fluid moving past it is related to the velocity, the thermal conductivity, and the temperature of the fluid, among other factors.

*Thermal-conductivity detectors* (TCD) have been developed for use in gas chromatography and in instruments designed to analyze gas mixtures for He or $H_2$. In both applications, heated sensing elements operated in the constant-current mode (Section 8.5) are connected in a Wheatstone bridge. The heated elements can be either thermistors or coiled wires made of a metal with a high temperature coefficient of resistance (such as platinum, tungsten, or nickel). Thermal-conductivity detectors incorporating heated wires are called *katharometers.*

## INFRARED SPECTROSCOPY

Various chemical species, whether in the gas phase or in liquid solution, absorb energy from specific ranges of the electromagnetic radiation spectrum. The infrared region, spanning wavelengths from 3 to 30 μm, is very useful in the study of gases. This is because most gases absorb infrared "light" and do so only at distinct, highly characteristic wavelengths, thus yielding what has been called a molecular fingerprint (Lord, 1987). The energy absorbed is transformed into heat and increases the temperature of the absorbing gas. However, infrared light is absorbed only by molecules made up of dissimilar atoms, because only such molecules possess an electric dipole moment with which the electromagnetic wave can interact. $CO_2$, CO, $N_2O$, $H_2O$, and volatile anesthetic agents are examples of such molecules. Symmetric molecules (such as $O_2$, $N_2$, and $H_2$) and the noble gases (such as He and Ne) do not have an electric dipole moment and do not absorb infrared radiation.

In general, when light of wavelengths characteristic of a particular gas falls on a sample of that gas, only some is absorbed. The remainder is transmitted through the gas. For light of a specific wavelength, the power per unit area transmitted, $P_t$, by the sample relative to that entering the sample, $P_0$, is given by Beer's law (we use $P$ here for power per unit area to be consistent with Section 11.1):

$$P_t = P_0 e^{-aLC} \tag{9.44}$$

where $a$ is the absorption coefficient, $L$ is the length of the light path through the gas, and $C$ is the concentration of the absorbing gas. Consequently, we can measure the concentration of the components of a gas mixture by determining the power that is either *absorbed* or *transmitted* by the mixture. Instruments based on each of these approaches have been developed to measure gases important in respiration—most notably $CO_2$, but also CO, water vapor, and anesthetic agents.

**EXAMPLE 9.4** Using Beer's law (9.44), show that the power absorbed by a component of a gas mixture is approximately proportional to the concentration of that component in the mixture.

**ANSWER** $P_t$ = power transmitted; $P_0$ = power entering; $P_a$ = power absorbed.

$$P_a = P_0 - P_t = P_0(1 - e^{-aLC}) \approx P_0 aLC \text{ for low absorption, e.g., } P_a/P_0 < 0.1$$

The conventional technique that we will refer to here as *transmission analysis* measures the power *transmitted* at wavelengths corresponding to the substances under study. In contrast, photoacoustic principles have been utilized to measure directly the power *absorbed* by a sample. Both types of instruments have employed wide-band (black-body) sources to irradiate the sample. However, neither produces an entire spectrum of absorption or transmission by which to identify the components of the sample, as "dispersive" spectroscopy does (Lord, 1987). Instead, they measure the behavior at only a well-defined set of wavelengths chosen to maximize the response for the substance of interest and to minimize interference with other substances. Such instruments fall into the category of nondispersive infrared (NDIR) analyzers.

Both transmission systems and photoacoustic systems have a minimum of five essential components, as shown in Figure 9.14: (1) a source of radiation of the required wavelengths; (2) a means, usually a mechanical "chopper," of periodically varying the power and/or wavelength of the source radiation; (3) a sample cell; (4) a detector; and (5) signal processing and display equipment. The relative positions of the components vary from one instrument to another.

***Transmission Analysis*** An NDIR system used to analyze a gas mixture for the presence of a single species of test gas has two identical intermittently interrupted (10 to 90 times per second, depending on the particular instrument) infrared (IR) beams. The IR power pulses produced travel two parallel paths, one of which includes a test cell. A sample of the gas mixture to be analyzed is continuously drawn through the test cell from a sampling catheter. The second path includes an interference filter, either a thin film filter that transmits selected wavelengths or, in older systems, a reference cell that has windows exactly the same as those of the test cell but containing a gas mixture free of the test gas.

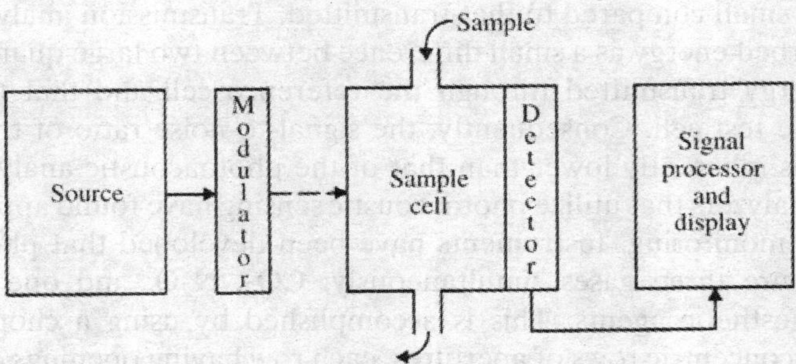


**Figure 9.14** General arrangement of the components of an infrared spectroscopy system.

A detector measures the difference between the powers transmitted through the reference pathway and through the test pathway for each pulse of the IR beams. The rms power difference between the two pathways is *approximately* proportional to the concentration of the absorbing gas in the test cell. The output of the detector circuit is demodulated and processed to produce a signal proportional to the concentration (molar density) of the test gas. At flow rates through the sampling catheter on the order of 0.5 to 1 liter/min, a 90% full-scale step-response time of approximately 100 ms can be achieved. However, newer devices are sufficiently small to be used in-line with the gas stream during breathing (Coombes and Halsall, 1988). IR transmission instruments have been developed to measure gases with the following full-scale molar fractions: 10% $CO_2$, 0.3% CO, 100% $N_2O$, 7.5% halothane, enflurane, isoflurane, and sevoflurane, and 20% desflurane.

***Photoacoustic Analysis*** West *et al.* (1983) define the photoacoustic effect as the process of sound generation in a gas that results from the absorption of photons. They point out that Alexander Graham Bell, among others, described this phenomenon in 1880. Bell was able to produce sound by repeatedly interrupting a beam of sunlight that was focused on a test tube filled with tobacco smoke. The sound pressure waves were caused by the expansion of gas resulting from the absorption of the incident infrared radiation and by the interspersed contraction of the gas when the light source was blocked. This observation has formed the basis for gas analysis, because the radiant energy absorbed by a gas is approximately proportional to the concentration of that gas. Consequently, the higher the gas concentration is, the louder is the sound for the same input of light.

Figure 9.14 shows the general scheme for a photoacoustic gas analyzer. Broadband infrared light is modulated by a mechanical chopper and filtered to permit pulses of light of selected wavelengths to be focused on the gas mixture in the test cell. The resulting pressure fluctuations recur at the mechanical chopper's repetition rate, which is in the audio-frequency range. An extremely sensitive, stable capacitance microphone detects the sound generated.

The photoacoustic analyzer measures the IR energy absorbed by a test gas by sensing the sound pressure waves produced. The IR energy absorbed by a gas is very small compared to that transmitted. Transmission analyzers determine absorbed energy as a small difference between two large quantities, such as the energy transmitted through the reference cell and that transmitted through the test cell. Consequently, the signal-to-noise ratio of transmission analyzers is inherently lower than that of the photoacoustic analyzer.

Gas analyzers that utilize photoacoustic sensing have found applications in anesthesia monitoring. Instruments have been developed that photoacoustically measure three gases simultaneously: $CO_2$, $N_2O$, and one of several volatile anesthetic agents. This is accomplished by using a chopper wheel with three concentric rows of apertures, each row having openings of different spacing and size. Thus, for the same rotational velocity of the wheel, three beams are created, each interrupted at its own frequency. Each beam is filtered so that it contains only wavelengths that will be absorbed by a particular gas of interest. The beams are focused into the cell and simultaneously excite specific constituents of the mixture. Three sounds are produced, each with a characteristic pitch corresponding to one chopping frequency and with amplitude approximately proportional to the concentration of the gas producing it. The concentration of each gas component of interest can be continuously determined by filtering the sensing microphone's output for its Fourier components at the chopper frequencies and demodulating the resulting amplitude-modulated signals.

Such instruments claim remarkable stability (calibration at 1 to 3 month intervals), 1 min warm-up, high accuracy (less than 1% full scale error), and 10% to 90% response time of 250 to 300 ms at a 90 ml/min sample flow rate (Møllgaard, 1989).

## EMISSION SPECTROSCOPY

Figure 9.15 depicts a device used to detect the concentration of a single gas species in a mixture by measuring the intensity of the light in a given wavelength range produced when the gas mixture is ionized at very low pressures. The respiratory gas routinely measured by such a device is $N_2$ (East and East, 1988). The system is evacuated by a high-capacity vacuum pump, and the pressure [1 to 4 mm Hg (150 to 550 Pa)] is regulated by a needle valve that allows a small flow of gas to be drawn through the ionization chamber.

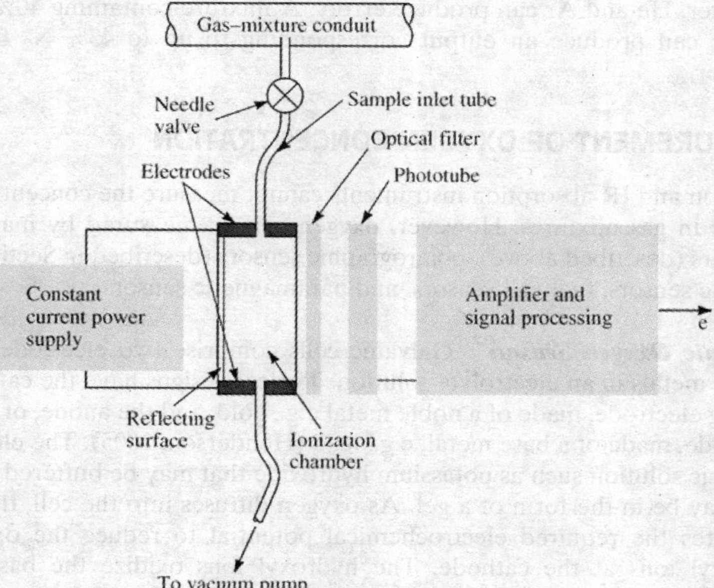


**Figure 9.15** $N_2$ analyzer employing emission spectroscopy

Respiratory gases ionized by the voltage difference (600 to 1500 V dc) between the electrodes in the ionization chamber emit light in the range of 310 to 480 nm. Reflecting surfaces direct the light through a selective optical filter that absorbs unwanted wavelengths. A photoelectric tube produces a current proportional to the intensity of the light passed by the filter. For a fixed ionization-chamber geometry, vacuum, gas flow, and current, the amplified output of the phototube is a nonlinear function of the molar fraction of the gas species of interest. The output is processed to produce a signal, $e$, proportional to this molar fraction.

Spectroscopic $N_2$ analyzers yield the $N_2$ molar fraction in a gas mixture on a wet basis. Calibration procedures must take into account the humidity of the sample. The needle valve and conduit from which the sample is withdrawn may have to be heated to prevent plugging or loss of water vapor by condensation. The high vacuum within the system prevents condensation of water vapor in the transport tubing that leads from the needle value to the ionization chamber, but it may not prevent adsorption and desorption during changes in the partial pressure of the water vapor.

Commercially available $N_2$ analyzers can produce a steady-state output that has as little as 0.5% rms error over the range of 0% to 80% $N_2$. In response to a step change in $N_2$ molar fraction, the transport delay and rise time (between 10% and 90% of the steady-state output) can each be on the order of 40 ms. Variation in output to a constant input can be less than 1.5% over 24 h. Deposition of electrode material on the glass walls of the ionization chamber over a long period of time eventually degrades the instrument's performance. $O_2$ and $CO_2$ do not interfere with the accuracy of $N_2$ determinations. However, He and Ar can produce errors. A mixture containing 40% $N_2$ and 5% He can produce an output corresponding to up to 43% $N_2$ from the analyzer.

## MEASUREMENT OF OXYGEN CONCENTRATION

Emission and IR absorption instruments cannot measure the concentration of oxygen in gas mixtures. However, oxygen can be measured by mass spectrometers (described above), polarographic sensors (described in Section 10.2), galvanic sensors, fuel-cell sensors, and paramagnetic sensors.

***Galvanic Oxygen Sensors*** Galvanic cells comprise two electrodes of dissimilar metals in an electrolyte solution. Typical designs have the cathode, or sensing electrode, made of a noble metal e.g., gold, and the anode, or working electrode, made of a base metal, e.g., lead (Henderson, 2005). The electrolyte is a basic solution such as potassium hydroxide that may be buffered and that also may be in the form of a gel. As oxygen diffuses into the cell, the anode generates the required electrochemical potential to reduce the oxygen to hydroxyl ions at the cathode. The hydroxyl ions oxidize the base anode producing electrons that, if the electrodes are connected by an external conductor, travel to the cathode and can be measured as a current. Two oxygen permeable membranes cover the oxygen inlet to the cell. One, usually made of Teflon, is porous but hydrophobic and prevents the formation of a water film on its surface when used in a humid environment. The second membrane is a diffusion barrier that causes the current produced by the cathode to be diffusion limited. In this configuration, the current flowing from the cell is approximately proportional to the partial pressure of the oxygen at the inlet to the cell. If the ambient pressure changes, e.g., with altitude, the output will change for the same $O_2$ concentration.

A galvanic sensor is relatively low in cost, light in weight, has minimal power requirements and can be used in any orientation. Its life is limited by the depletion of the electrodes or electrolyte. It can measure from the parts per million to pure $O_2$, and depending on its design, can have a step response time from less than a second to seconds.

***Fuel-Cell Oxygen Sensors*** A fuel cell that has found respiratory applications uses a heated zirconia membrane to separate a reference gas (can be ambient air) from the oxygen-containing test gas (Anonymous, 2003). Platinum electrodes are deposited on each side of the membrane and are connected to each other through an external circuit. Zirconia (zirconium oxide, $ZrO_2$) is a ceramic. When it is doped with trace amounts of yttrium oxide and heated above 575 °C it becomes a solid electrolyte, permitting ions to pass from one side to the other. Ions are generated on the high concentration side and pass through the membrane to the opposite electrode while electrons pass through the external circuit. The potential difference between the two sides of the membrane is given by the Nernst equation (4.1) and is related to the logarithm of the ratio of the *concentration* of $O_2$ on each side of the membrane. Therefore, if the total (ambient) pressure (and temperature) of the gases are the same on both sides of the membrane, the output voltage (concentration reading) will be unaffected by changes in ambient pressure. The oxygen readings for the test gas can be linearized computationally in the output circuitry.

Since the zirconia membrane is very brittle, care must be taken in the design of the device to protect it from vibration, and thermal and mechanical shock. A zirconia fuel-cell sensor can measure $O_2$ concentrations ranging from the ppb to 100%, with millisecond response times fast enough for intrabreath measurements. Unlike the galvanic sensor, neither electrode nor the electrolyte membrane is depleted during operation. However, these components can be poisoned by contaminants in the test gas and can deteriorate eventually because of the high operating temperature.

***Paramagnetic Oxygen Sensors*** Oxygen is unusual among gases in that it is attracted by a magnetic field. This property, referred to as paramagnetism, is characterized by a positive magnetic susceptibility. The high magnetic susceptibility of iron, ferromagnetism, is a special case of paramagnetism (McGrath and Wendelken, 2006). Most gases are diamagnetic, being repulsed by a magnetic field, and thus exhibit negative susceptibilities.

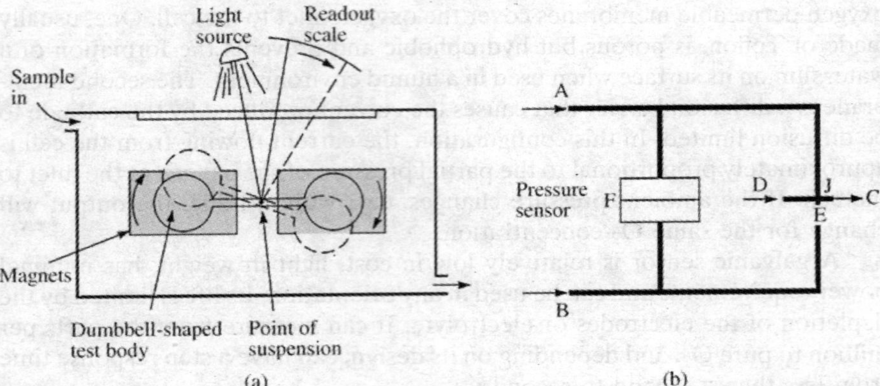


**Figure 9.16 Oxygen analyzers** (a) Diagram of the top view of a balance-type paramagnetic oxygen analyzer. The magnetic field is perpendicular to the plane of the diagram. The test body either is allowed to rotate (as shown) or is held in place by countertorque, which is measured to determine the oxygen concentration in the gas mixture. (b) Diagram of a differential pressure and a magnetoacoustic oxygen analyzer (see text for descriptions).

Several instruments exploit the paramagnetic property of oxygen. The first to have been developed is a *balance-type* device that has a diamagnetic, nitrogen-filled, hollow, thin-walled, glass test body situated in a nonuniform magnetic field within a gas-sample chamber. The test body is shaped like a dumbbell [Figure 9.16(a)] and is suspended by a taut fiber attached to the midpoint of the bar connecting its two globes. The fiber acts as a torsional spring and permits the dumbbell to rotate in a plane perpendicular to the magnetic field. When at undisturbed equilibrium, the globes of the test body are positioned in the region of highest magnetic-field concentration—that is, between the poles of the magnet producing the field. When a gas mixture with no paramagnetic components is introduced into the sample chamber, the density of the mixture remains uniform within the chamber, and the dumbbell maintains its equilibrium position. When a paramagnetic gas such as oxygen is in the mixture, however, it is attracted by the field, causing the local gas density between the poles of the magnet to increase. This causes the test body to be displaced in much the same way as a fishing bobber is forced to the surface of the much denser water into which it is cast. The more oxygen, the larger the region of increased density, the higher the density gradient, and the more the force on the test body tending to displace it.

The concentration of oxygen can thus be determined either by measuring the deflection of the test body about its suspension axis (via the reflection of a light beam by a mirror placed on the test body at its center of rotation [Figure 9.16(a)] or by measuring the torque required to maintain the dumbbell in its oxygen-free equilibrium position. This type of system is very accurate (repeatability and linearity are both to within 0.1%), but it has a long (on the order of 10 s) response time (Kocache, 1988).

Another paramagnetic approach involves measuring the pressure required to maintain the flow of an oxygen-containing gas mixture through a magnetic field. In one instrument [Figure 9.16(b)], two reference gas streams meet and mix at a junction point J and exit through a common pathway C. A pulsating magnetic field is focused on one of the reference gas streams at its point of entry E into the junction. The sample to be analyzed is introduced through D into the junction, where it mixes with the reference gases and flows through the exit C. Any oxygen in the gas sample is attracted by the magnetic field at E and increases the local density in the outlet of that reference pathway, retarding flow by effectively increasing flow resistance and causing an increased back-pressure in that branch. This produces a pressure difference between the two reference pathways, and that difference is sensed by a differential pressure sensor at F. The output of the sensor is proportional to the difference in $PO_2$ between the reference gas and the sample gas (East, 1990). Their performance is slightly inferior to that of paramagnetic balance-type analyzers, but the *differential pressure-type analyzers* display a response time of less than 200 ms, which is adequate for breath-by-breath measurements (Kocache, 1988).

A variation of the differential pressure analyzer is used in a commercial instrument in conjunction with the photoacoustic spectrometer we have described (Møllgaard, 1989). Termed *magnetoacoustic spectroscopy,* this technique employs the same general configuration shown in Figure 9.16(b), with a few modifications. The sample is introduced directly into one of the pathways, such as at A, that leads to the mixing junction J. (D is not used.) An alternating magnetic field with a frequency in the audio range is imposed across the junction J, not just across the end of one of the pathways. Consequently, the gas from both pathways is exposed to the same magnetic field. If the sample introduced at A contains some oxygen, then when it reaches J, the oxygen portion of the mixture is alternately expanded and compressed, causing acoustic waves to propagate through the two gas pathways. The amplitude of these sound pressure waves is proportional to the concentration of oxygen in the mixture. Finally, instead of using a single differential pressure sensor to measure the pressure difference between the two pathways, this system has two capacitance microphones to measure the sound in the sample gas and that in the reference gas separately. The sample-gas microphone is the same one used to measure the photoacoustic disturbances caused by the absorption of IR energy by other components in the sample gas. The alternating magnetic-field frequency is different from the frequencies of the modulated IR beams exciting these other gas components. Thus the magnetically generated sound pressure waves can be digitally bandpass-filtered from the output of the sample-gas microphone and compared to the signal emanating from the reference gas to determine the absolute concentration of oxygen in the sample gas. The resulting instrument is stable (gain drift: $<2\%$ full scale/30 days, temperature drift $<0.1\%$ of reading/°C), is accurate (better than 1% full scale or 2% of reading), and has a 10% to 90% rise time of less than 250 ms at a sample flow rate of 90 ml/min.

**EXAMPLE 9.5** You are to specify the requirements for an inhalation anesthesia monitor. Besides analyzers for the various volatile anesthetics and nitrous oxide, analyzers for which other two gases should the monitor include and why? Where should the gas concentrations be measured?

**ANSWER** Surgical patients are typically ventilated through an endotracheal tube (ET). Assuming that the response times of the analyzers are sufficiently fast to detect intrabreath variations in concentrations, inspired gas composition should be monitored at the connection of the ET and the patient circuit coming from the anesthesia machine. The monitor should include an oxygen sensor to give a continuous readout of inspired oxygen concentration. A carbon dioxide sensor is used to verify that the patient's lungs are being ventilated properly during the procedure. It is also used to verify placement of the ET during insertion. If the ET were inserted into the patient's esophagus instead of the airway, the stomach would be ventilated rather than the lungs, and no $CO_2$ would be detected.

## 9.8 SOME TESTS OF GAS TRANSPORT

The pulmonary function tests to be discussed in this section are concerned primarily with gas-phase transport between the airway opening and the alveoli and with interphase (or membrane) transport between alveolar gas and pulmonary capillary blood. Gas-transport tests are designed to achieve one or more of the following objectives:

1. Determine the homogeneity of the distribution of inspired gas (ventilation).
2. Determine the matching of ventilation to perfusion.
3. Evaluate the ability of the alveolar membrane to allow gas transfer.

Because of the architecture of the respiratory system, it is usually impossible to isolate the processes involved or to make direct measurements at sites of interest. Access is available only at the boundaries of the system—that is, at the airway opening and the systemic circulation.

An overall evaluation of gas transport by the lungs can be obtained from a measurement of the partial pressures of $O_2$ and $CO_2$ in a sample of systemic arterial blood drawn while the subject is breathing air. If the gas-exchange ratio $\dot{V}_{CO_2}/\dot{V}_{O_2}$ is approximately 0.8, then the sum of the arterial partial pressures, $P_{aO_2}$ and $P_{aCO_2}$, should be approximately 140 mm Hg (18.7 kPa). If this sum is below 120 mm Hg (16 kPa), it is considered abnormal. Because the acquisition of these data requires puncturing an artery, it is not used routinely as a pulmonary-function test, especially for children.

Further discussion of arterial blood gases is limited here to the observation that they can be used in a procedure to distinguish between two possible causes of abnormally low partial pressures: (1) the shunting of blood past the gas-exchange regions in the lung and (2) a mismatch between local alveolar ventilation and blood perfusion. Besides a sample of arterial blood gas, the procedure requires an estimate of the mean $P_{O_2}$ in the alveoli. This is obtained from an end-expired gas sample collected as the subject exhales to RV. If the steady-state alveolar-arterial (A–a) difference in $O_2$ partial pressure does not appreciably change when the subject breathes 100% $O_2$ instead of air, then a shunt is assumed to be present. If the A–a difference decreases, then a ventilation–perfusion mismatch is implied.

## GAS-PHASE TRANSPORT

Tests of gas-phase transport are concerned with questions arising from two of the objectives mentioned above: (1) How is the inspired gas (ventilation) distributed in the lungs? (2) What is the equivalent volume of inspired gas that is not taking part in the exchange of gas with the blood? In other words, what is the effective dead space of the lung?

We can assess the distribution of gas in the lungs from multibreath and single-breath maneuvers by using a tracer gas that is insoluble in the pulmonary tissues and blood. The assumption can then be made that the tracer gas can enter or leave the lung only through the airway opening. Gases that fulfill this requirement are He, $N_2$, Ar, Ne, and Xe.

***Multibreath $N_2$ Washout*** The multibreath He-dilution and $N_2$-washout procedures used to estimate lung volume (FRC) as described in Section 9.4 can also provide information about the efficiency of gas mixing in the lungs: whether the gas in all ventilated alveoli is diluted at the same rate by gas inspired during resting breathing. As an example, consider the washout of $N_2$ from the lungs during resting breathing of 100% $O_2$. A set of one-way valves, as shown in Figure 9.7, is used to prevent mixing of the inspired $O_2$ with the expirate. If a pulmonary system were to act as a single, well-mixed compartment ventilated at a constant breathing rate and tidal volume, a time plot of the end-tidal expired-nitrogen molar fraction $F_{N_2}$ would exhibit an exponential decay. Normal lungs exhibit a washout curve that can be approximated rather closely by a single exponential. The shape of the washout curve is not routinely used as a test of abnormal ventilation because it is difficult to compensate for the effects of variations in tidal volume and breathing frequency on the shape of the curve. However, abnormality is indicated if the $F_{N_2}$ of a sample of gas obtained at the end of an expiration to RV after 7 min of $O_2$ breathing has not been reduced to 0.02. This procedure is obviously highly dependent on cooperation, because it is sensitive to changes in the tidal volume and frequency of breathing of the subject.

***Single-Breath $N_2$ Washout*** The single-breath $N_2$ washout can yield as many as three useful pieces of information: (1) an estimate of the anatomical dead space (approximately the volume of the conducting airways); (2) a measure of the distribution of ventilation—that is, the relative local rates of filling and emptying of the regions of the lungs; and (3) an index of small-airway mechanical function, the closing volume CV.

The procedure requires that, after having reached a steady state while breathing air, the subject inspires 100% $O_2$ from RV to TLC. A setup similar to Figure 9.7 can be used for this experiment. After a momentary pause at TLC, the individual is instructed to exhale very slowly to residual volume. The $F_{N_2}$ in the expired gas, $F_{EN_2}$, and the volume of the expired gas are continuously measured and displayed against each other on an $x$–$y$ plot. The interpretation of these plots requires a discussion of the events that occur in the lungs during both a vital-capacity inspiration and a slow vital-capacity expiration.

Consider the idealized normal upright lung (subject sitting or standing erect) (Figure 9.17). At residual volume, the *dependent* parts of the lungs

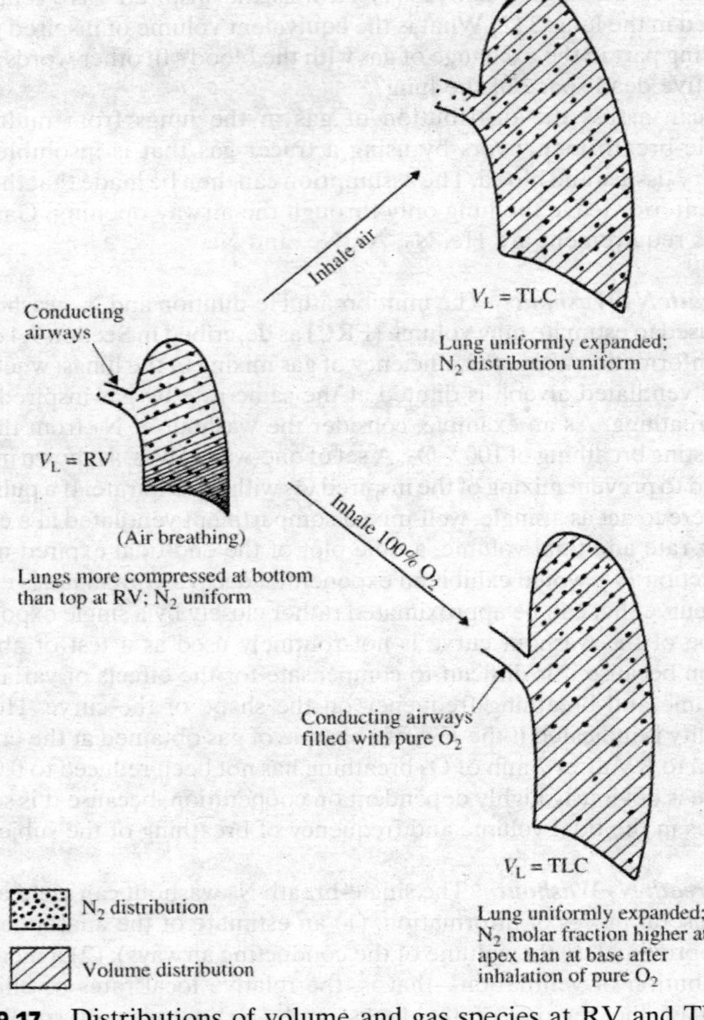


**Figure 9.17** Distributions of volume and gas species at RV and TLC for a vital-capacity inspiration of air or pure oxygen.

(those lowest with respect to gravity) are less expanded than the upper regions. Thus there is a distribution of local alveolar volumes corresponding roughly to the distribution of the pressure on the interpleural surface of the lungs. That is, there is lower pressure at the top of the lungs (larger alveoli) and higher pressure at the base (smaller alveoli).

After the lung has been expanded to and held at TLC, the lung is more uniformly inflated, with all regions having the same relative local volume. This means that the top parts of the lungs must have changed their volumes less during a vital-capacity inspiration of 100% $O_2$ than did the lower, dependent parts in order for the two regions to reach approximately the same final volume at TLC. Consequently, less inspired $O_2$ was added to the upper regions than to the lower. If the subject had achieved steady state while breathing air prior to performing this test, then it can be assumed that the $F\mathrm{N}_2$ in the gas within the lungs was the same throughout. Thus, because less diluting inspired $O_2$ is added to the upper regions than to the lower during a VC inspiration of pure $O_2$, the $F\mathrm{N}_2$ in the upper regions is higher than in the lower regions at the end of the inspiration. In addition, at TLC, the conducting airways (anatomical dead space) are filled with pure $O_2$.

For a slow vital-capacity expiration, following the inspiration of pure $O_2$, normal lungs exhibit four identifiable regions or phases on the $F_{\mathrm{E}}\mathrm{N}_2$-versus-volume plot [Figure 9.18(b)]. During phase I, lung volume changes but $F_{\mathrm{E}}\mathrm{N}_2$ is zero as pure $O_2$ is emptied from the conducting airways past the $N_2$ sensor. Phase III is a (sloping) plateau corresponding to the emptying of the mixed alveolar gas from all parts of the lungs. Oscillations of $F_{\mathrm{E}}\mathrm{N}_2$ during phase III have been attributed to local emptying of areas of different $F\mathrm{N}_2$ caused by the changes in volume associated with the heartbeat. Phase II is the transition between the emptying of the anatomical dead space and the arrival of mixed alveolar gas at the $N_2$ sensor. Phase IV signifies a drastic change in the rates of emptying of the dependent parts of the lungs. It is dramatically evident if the lung is normal or has only minimal small-airways disease.

A system consisting of a single, perfectly mixed compartment and a transport dead space [Figure 9.18 (a)] would exhibit a washout curve like that in Figure 9.18(b) (dashed line). By analogy, the anatomical dead space, $V'_{\mathrm{D}}$, is taken as the volume emptied to the point at which the $F_{\mathrm{E}}\mathrm{N}_2$ reaches one-half of a representative mixed alveolar value. For conditions in the spirometer in Figure 9.7, we can compute

$$V'_{\mathrm{D}} = \mathrm{VC} - \frac{\int_0^{\mathrm{VC}} F_{\mathrm{E}}\mathrm{N}_2 dv_{\mathrm{S}}}{\hat{F}_{\mathrm{E}}\mathrm{N}_2(\mathrm{III})} \tag{9.45}$$

Where

VC = expired vital capacity

$v_{\mathrm{S}}$ = volume change of spirometer used to estimate the integral of expired flow

$\hat{F}_{\mathrm{E}}\mathrm{N}_2(\mathrm{III})$ = mean value for $F_{\mathrm{E}}\mathrm{N}_2$ during phase III

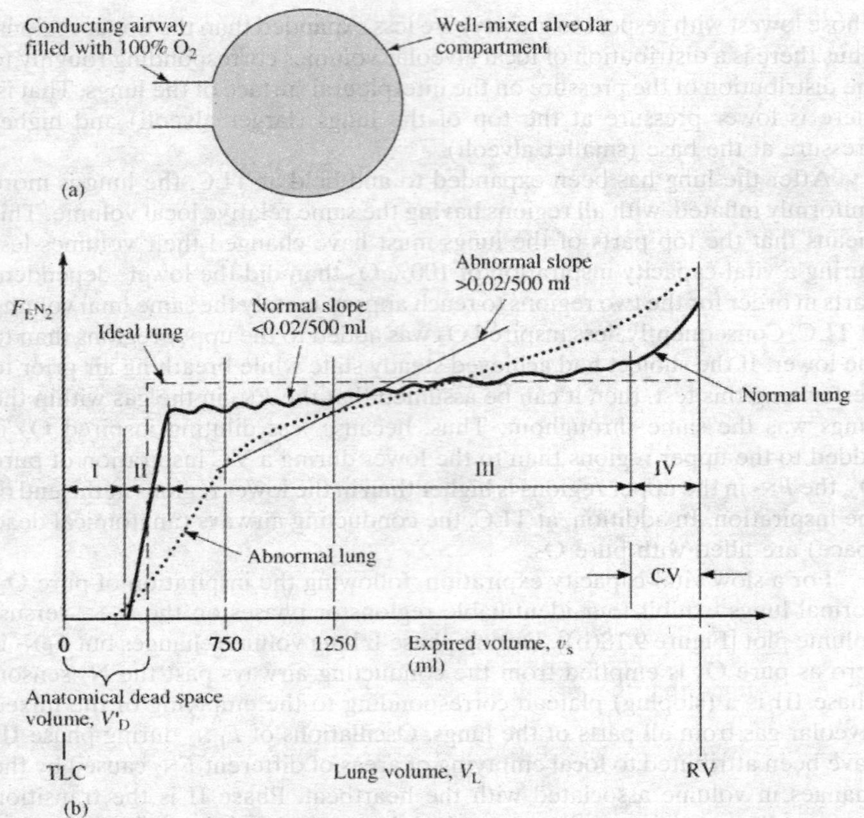


**Figure 9.18 Single-breath nitrogen-washout maneuver** (a) An idealized model of a lung at the end of a vital-capacity inspiration of pure $O_2$, preceded by breathing of normal air. (b) Single-breath $N_2$-washout curves for idealized lung, normal lung, and abnormal lung. Parameters of these curves include anatomical dead space, slope of phase III, and closing volume.

Normal lungs exhibit an average slope during phase III that does not exceed a 0.02 increase in $F_{E}N_2$ per 500 ml of expired volume for an interval of expired volume between 750 and 1250 ml below TLC. A greater increase than this is taken to indicate a nonuniformity of local alveolar emptying rates.

The volume above RV at which phase IV begins is designated the *closing volume,* CV. The absolute volume at which phase IV begins is the *closing capacity,* CC = RV + CV. As the lung volume approaches RV, the dependent gas spaces in the lung begin to cease emptying at the same rate at which they emptied during phase III. Therefore, the expirate at the airway opening contains a higher proportion of gas from the superior parts of the lungs and less from the dependent portions. Because the upper parts of the lung had the higher $F_{N_2}$ after the vital-capacity inspiration of pure $O_2$, the expirate passing the $N_2$ sensor at the airway opening has an increasing $F_{E}N_2$ as an increasing number of dependent lung units decrease their emptying rate as the lung approaches RV.

Inferences about the mechanical state of the small airways in the dependent parts of the lungs have been made from the size of the CV relative to the VC and of the CC relative to TLC. Closing volume varies with body position, age, and disease. In the initial phases of small-airways disease, CV increases. However, as the disease progresses, the slope of phase III increases, and the transition between phases III and IV becomes less distinct [Figure 9.18(b)]. The resulting ambiguity in determining the onset of phase IV limits the use of the CV, except as an indicator of the beginnings of abnormalities of the small airways.

## EFFECTIVE (PHYSIOLOGIC) DEAD SPACE DURING ALVEOLAR-CAPILLARY GAS EXCHANGE

When inspired gas cannot reach alveoli with well-perfused capillaries, and when blood cannot perfuse capillaries of alveoli that are ventilated with inspired gas, gas exchange is impaired. A tracer gas that is not diffusion-limited by the alveolar membrane can be used to evaluate the matching of ventilation and perfusion. The $CO_2$ added to the gas in the lungs from the pulmonary capillary blood satisfies this requirement. It diffuses so freely that it can be assumed that the alveoli and capillaries are in equilibrium during the entire expiration: that their respective $CO_2$ partial pressures are equal.

In the absence of significant right-to-left heart shunt, systemic arterial $CO_2$ partial pressure provides an excellent estimate of an average pulmonary capillary $P_{CO_2}$. Consequently, a conceptual *alveolar volume,* $V_A$, can be defined as the equivalent volume of gas in the lung that communicates with the airway opening and satisfies two conditions: (1) It contains all the $CO_2$ in the lungs at the end of inspiration. (2) This $CO_2$ exists at a partial pressure equal to that of systemic arterial blood. The *effective dead space,* $V_D$, sometimes called the *physiologic dead space,* is the remainder of the gas space in the lungs that is in excess of the alveolar volume. If we consider that none of the $CO_2$ expired during a breath is contributed by the dead space—that all of it is coming from the alveolar volume—then we can obtain an estimate of the volume of the effective dead space as a fraction of the expired tidal volume, $V_T$, from a mass balance of expired $CO_2$. Thus

$$\frac{V_D}{V_T} = 1 - \frac{\hat{P}_{E}CO_2}{\hat{P}_{a}CO_2} \tag{9.46}$$

where $\hat{P}_{E}CO_2$ is the mean $CO_2$ partial pressure in the expirate, and $\hat{P}_{a}CO_2$ is the mean partial pressure of systemic arterial $CO_2$, each determined over several breaths.

The $V_D/V_T$ is important in inferring the etiology of diseases involving poor gas exchange.

## DIFFUSION PROCESSES

To complete the description of gas exchange in the lungs, we need to characterize the transport processes that occur between the alveolar gas space and the pulmonary capillary blood. Gas moves between these regions by diffusion. A parameter used to describe the diffusion processes in the vicinity of the alveolar membrane is the *diffusing capacity of the lung, $D_L$*. This is the constant of proportionality between the rate of uptake of tracer gas by the blood (obtained from measurements at the airway opening) and the difference in partial pressure of the tracer gas between the alveolar gas space and the capillary blood. Because it is impossible to measure alveolar partial pressures directly, and because they are affected by convective transport between the airway opening and the alveoli, diffusing capacity is not independent of the pattern of ventilation distribution in the lungs.

***Carbon Monoxide Diffusing Capacity*** $CO_2$ diffuses across the alveolar membrane much more easily than $O_2$, so a diffusion defect would affect $O_2$ transfer first. Because of this and the prime role $O_2$ plays in sustaining life, it is important to evaluate a diffusing capacity for $O_2$. However, obtaining the required $P_aO_2$ requires a sample of arterial blood. To avoid this, clinicians use CO as the tracer gas because its properties are sufficiently close to those of $O_2$ for its diffusing capacity, $D_LCO$, to provide a meaningful estimate of $D_LO_2$. In addition, because of its affinity for hemoglobin (at low concentrations essentially all CO that enters the blood chemically combines with the hemoglobin in the red blood cells), $P$CO exhibited by the blood is negligibly small and need not be measured.

One of the various methods that have been used to estimate $D_LCO$ involves a single-breath maneuver. The subject inspires a mixture of air, 0.3% CO (or less), and He (approximately 10%) from RV to TLC. The subject holds his or her breath at TLC for about 10 s and then forcefully exhales down to RV. Even though it necessitates subject cooperation, this procedure can be performed quickly and can be repeated easily. In addition, it does not require samples of arterial blood or an estimate of dead space before the clinician can obtain a value of alveolar $P_ACO$. The computation of $D_LCO$ from measurements made during this single-breath maneuver is based on a one-compartment model of the lung. If a well-mixed alveolar compartment is filled with a mixture of gases containing some initial $F_ACO$, then during breath holding with the airway open, the CO diffuses into the blood in the pulmonary capillaries, and the alveolar $F_ACO$ decreases exponentially with time:

$$F_ACO(t_2) = F_ACO(t_1) \times \exp\left(-\frac{D_LCO(P_{atm} - P_AH_2O)(t_2 - t_1)}{V_A}\right) \quad (9.47)$$

where $V_A$ is the equivalent volume of the alveolar gas space throughout which the inspired CO is assumed to be distributed; and $t_1$ and $t_2$ are the times corresponding to the end of the inspiration to TLC and the beginning of expiration to RV, respectively. That is, $t_2 - t_1$ is the duration of the breath holding.

The fraction of alveolar CO at the end of the breath holding, $F_{A}\text{CO}(t_2)$, is taken as that of the gas expired at the end of the expiration to RV. The $F\text{HE}$ of this end-expiratory gas is also measured. Because the inspired He is insoluble in the lung tissues and blood, none of it should have left the lung during the breath holding. It can be assumed that, during inspiration, both the He and the CO were similarly distributed throughout the lungs and that the dilution of the He in the alveoli at the end of inspiration is the same as that for the CO. The end-inspiratory $F\text{He}$ should not change during breath holding, so it can be estimated from the measured end-expiratory value, $F_{EE}\text{He}$. The end-inspiratory alveolar $F_{A}\text{CO}$ can be estimated from

$$\frac{F_{A}\text{CO}(t_1)}{F_{I}\text{CO}(t_0)} = \frac{F_{A}\text{He}(t_1)}{F_{I}\text{He}(t_0)} = \frac{F_{EE}\text{He}}{F_{I}\text{He}(t_0)} \tag{9.48}$$

where $F_{I}\text{CO}(t_0)$ and $F_{I}\text{He}(t_0)$ are the fractions of CO and He, respectively, in the inspired gas. In addition, the equivalent alveolar volume to which the gas is distributed can be estimated using a mass balance on the He:

$$V_{A} \cdot F_{EE}\text{He} = \text{VC} \cdot F_{I}\text{He}(t_0) \tag{9.49}$$

Diffusing capacity depends on many factors besides the distribution of ventilation to the alveoli and the properties of the alveolar membrane. The distribution of pulmonary perfusion, cardiac output (flow rate), and volume of blood in the pulmonary capillaries also affect it. These, in turn, are related not only to disease processes but also to exertion during exercise or excitement and to the patient's body position when the measurements are made. $D_{L}\text{CO}$ also varies with hematocrit and type of hemoglobin in the blood. The American Thoracic Society has recommended a standard technique for the single breath $D_{L}\text{CO}$ and has extensively discussed practical considerations for obtaining reproducible, consistent values (Anonymous, 1995b).

## PROBLEMS

**9.1** State three reasons why abstract models are important in respiratory physiology, pulmonary function testing, and patient monitoring.

**9.2** For a single mechanical unit lung, assume that the relationship among pressure, volume, and number of moles of ideal gas in the lung is given by

$$P_{A}\left(\frac{V_{L}}{N_{L}}\right)^{\alpha} = K$$

where $\alpha = 1$ and $K$ is a constant. Derive the lowest-order (linear) approximation to the relationship among changes in pressure, changes in volume, and changes in moles of gas within the lung.

**9.3** Define the acoustic compliance of a gas mixture as

$$C_g = -\frac{\partial V}{\partial P}$$

Using the relationship given in Problem 9.2, evaluate the acoustic compliance, in liter/cm $H_2O$, for a lung with volume 2 liters and with an ideal-dry-gas alveolar pressure of 713 mm Hg (95 kPa).

**9.4** Assuming zero net gas exchange with the blood and using (9.2), (9.3a) to (9.3c), and the results of Problem 9.2 and Problem 9.3, draw an analogous equivalent circuit model for the lung represented by Figure 9.2(a) with gas compression included.

**9.5** Gas concentration is interchangeably expressed in units of mass density $\gamma$ (such as mg/m$^3$) and molar fraction $F$ [such as parts per million (ppm)]. For a given gas at 1 atm and 25 °C, mass density in mg/m$^3$ can be converted to molar fraction in ppm as follows:

$$\gamma(\text{mg/m}^3) \times \frac{24.44}{\text{MW}} = F(\text{ppm})$$

where MW is the gram molecular weight of the gas in question. Derive this equation from the ideal gas law, using the fact that 1 mole of gas occupies 24.44 dm$^3$ at 1 atm and 25 °C.

**9.6** Show that the output of an instrument that is related to test-gas molar density is related in the same way to test-gas molar fraction (on a wet-gas basis) only if the ratio of the pressure of the total gas mixture to its absolute temperature remains constant.

**9.7** Assume that the chest-wall static compliance is 0.31 liter/cm $H_2O$ and that the pulmonary static compliance is 0.19 liter/cm $H_2O$ when the ventilatory system described by Figure 9.2 is at its resting volume (FRC). Evaluate the static compliance for the total respiratory system.

**9.8** Discuss the (qualitative) effects of the placement of a container filled with 6 mm-diameter beads of soda lime in (a) the inlet side of a spirometer and (b) the outlet side of a spirometer on the dynamics of the spirometer response and the accuracy of continuous measurements of changes in lung volume: (1) during very slow maneuvers (in the limit) from one static volume to another and (2) during very fast maneuvers, such as a forced-vital-capacity expiration—that is, a maximal-effort exhalation from TLC down to RV.

**9.9** Evaluate the effect on an estimate of FRC from (9.23) when the experiment is terminated at a lung volume other than FRC. Evaluate the effect on an estimate of FRC from (9.24) when the final volume of the spirometer does not equal its original volume.

**9.10** Discuss the subject of accuracy of measurement, especially of flow rate, by a single instrument over the wide range required for the FVC and $N_2$-washout experiments.

**9.11** Derive an expression for TLC, using static mass balances on the lungs between the beginning and end of a slow inspiration of $O_2$ from RV to TLC and between the subsequent TLC and the end of the slow expiration to RV at the finish of the $N_2$-washout test. Discuss the accuracy of this estimate.

(*Answer*):

$$\mathrm{TLC} = \frac{\mathrm{VC_I} F_{\mathrm{A}}\mathrm{N_2}(t_0) - V'_{\mathrm{D}} F_{\mathrm{A}}\mathrm{N_2}(t_1)}{F_{\mathrm{A}}\mathrm{N_2}(t_0) - F_{\mathrm{A}}\mathrm{N_2}(t_1)}$$

in which

$$F_{\mathrm{A}}\mathrm{N_2}(t_1) = \frac{\int_{t_1}^{t_2} F_{\mathrm{E}}\mathrm{N_2} Q_{\mathrm{AWO}}\, dt}{\mathrm{VC_E} - V'_{\mathrm{D}}}$$

where $\mathrm{VC_I}$ is the volume inspired from RV at $t_0$ to TLC at $t_1$ and $\mathrm{VC_E}$ is the volume expired from TLC at $t_1$ to RV at $t_2$. $F_{\mathrm{E}}\mathrm{N_2}$ is the instantaneous expired $N_2$ molar fraction measured at the AWO between $t_1$ and $t_2$. $F_{\mathrm{A}}\mathrm{N_2}(t_0)$ is the $N_2$ molar fraction in the alveolar gas before the test began ($t_0$), and $V'_D$ is the anatomical dead space.] Which terms must be estimated, and which terms are accessible for measurement?

**9.12** In an He-dilution experiment, a spirometer is preloaded with 10 liters of 5% He at room temperature, 25 °C. After the patient has rebreathed, the He concentration in the spirometer is 4%. What is the FRC? [Assume $T_{\mathrm{S}}(t_2) = 305\,\mathrm{K}$.]

**9.13** In a 1000 liter-body plethysmograph, a 100 liter person blows into a pressure sensor, raising mouth pressure 30 cm $H_2O$ (3 kPa). The pressure in the box drops 0.1 cm $H_2O$ (10 Pa). Calculate the person's lung volume assuming that $a_{\mathrm{B}} = 1.4$ and that atmospheric pressure is 760 mm Hg (101 kPa).

**9.14** Derive the governing equation for the TBP for breathing within the box, including nonnegligible exchange of gases between the alveoli and pulmonary capillary blood.

**9.15** Derive the governing equation for the TBP for breathing within the box for a lung characterized by two alveolar compartments (Figure P9.1). Assume that the net exchange of gases through the alveolar-capillary membrane is zero.

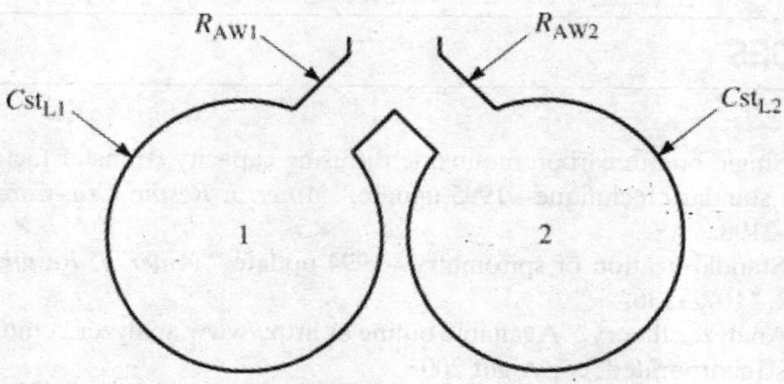


**Figure P9.1**

**9.16** We want to measure the tissue density of a human being, from which we can estimate the volume of body fat as required in metabolic studies. Describe a dry method, using three steps: (a) Measure the total volume of the body. (b) Measure the volume of the lungs. (c) Make an additional measurement, then calculate tissue density.

**9.17** Name three instruments for monitoring changes in thoracic volume, and cite the physical dimension from which each infers volume change.

**9.18** Describe the experimental tests that yield a measure of the obstruction of the large airways.

**9.19** Describe three tests that yield measures of obstruction in small airways.

**9.20** Design an experiment that requires no surgery and measures *in vivo* the mechanical time constant ($\tau = RC$) of the lungs of an anesthetized, paralyzed animal (assume normal lungs).

**9.21** Describe an experiment that could be used to estimate $R_L$ from (9.38). Why would the estimate of $R_L$ be expected to differ from that obtained from (9.37)?

**9.22** Assume that an abnormal pulmonary system can be represented as two airway-alveolar-compartment units (negligible gas compression) connected in parallel (Figure P9.1). Derive expressions for the effective compliance $Ceff_L$ and effective resistance $Reff_L$ for voluntary breathing frequencies.

**9.23** Which gases can be measured by IR absorption spectroscopy?

**9.24** An instrument requires 10 ml/min of flow to analyze a gas properly. Assuming a blunt flow profile, and given that the transit delay time of a sample is to be 200 ms, what is the relationship between length and diameter for an inlet tube?

**9.25** Name three instruments that can be used to measure oxygen in gas mixtures in respiratory experiments and that do not involve chemical reactions. On which physical phenomenon or property is each based?

**9.26** Sketch a normal single-breath $N_2$-washout curve, and explain why it has this shape.

**9.27** Derive and discuss (9.45) and (9.46).

**9.28** Derive (9.47 and describe how you could evaluate diffusing capacity of the lung.

## REFERENCES

Anonymous, "Single-breath carbon monoxide diffusing capacity (transfer factor), recommendations for a standard technique—1995 update." *Amer. J. Respir. Crit. Care Med. Dis.*,1995b, 152, 2185–2198.

Anonymous, "Standardization of spirometry—1994 update." *Amer. J. Respir. Crit. Care Med.*, 1995a, 152, 1107–1136.

Anonymous, "Analyzer theory." Available online at http://www.analyzer.com/theory/. Analytical Specialties Incorporated, copyright 2003.

Bates, J. H., P. Baconnier, and J. Milic-Emili, "A theoretical analysis of interrupter technique for measuring respiratory mechanics." *J. Appl. Physiol.*, 1988, 64, 2204–2214.

Broughton, R. J., "Polysomnography: Principles and applications in sleep and arousal disorders." In E. Niedermeyer and F. L. da Silva (eds.), *Electroencephalography: Basic Principles, Clinical Applications, and Related Fields*, 3rd ed. Baltimore: Williams & Wilkins, 1993.

Chatburn, R. L., and F. P. Primiano, Jr., "Mathematical models of respiratory mechanics." In R. L. Chatburn and K. C. Craig (eds.), *Fundamentals of Respiratory Care Research*. Norwalk, CT: Appleton & Lange, 1988, pp. 59–100.

Coombes, R. G., and D. Halsall, "Carbon dioxide analyzers." In J. G. Webster (ed.), *Encyclopedia of Medical Devices and Instrumentation*. New York: Wiley, 1988, pp. 556–564.

Delacourt, C., H. Lorino, C. Fuhrman, M. Herve-Guillot, P. Reinert, A. Harf, and B. Housset, "Comparison of the forced oscillation technique and the interrupter technique for assessing airway obstruction and its reversibility in children." *Am. J. Respir. Crit. Care Med.*, 2001, 164, 965–972.

DuBois, A. B., S. Y. Botelho, and J. H. Comroe, Jr., "A new method for measuring airway resistance in man using a body plethysmograph: Values in normal subjects and in patients with respiratory disease." *J. Clin. Inv.*, 1956b, 35, 327–336.

DuBois, A. B., S. Y. Botelho, G. N. Bedell, R. Marshall, and J. H. Comroe, Jr., "A rapid plethysmographic method for measuring thoracic gas volume. A comparison with a nitrogen-washout method for measuring functional residual capacity in normal subjects." *J. Clin. Inv.*, 1956a, 35, 322–326.

East, T. D., "What makes noninvasive monitoring tick? A review of basic engineering principles." *Respiratory Care*, 1990, 35, 500–519.

East, T. D., and K. A. East, "Nitrogen analyzers." In J. G. Webster (ed.), *Encyclopedia of Medical Devices and Instrumentation*. New York: Wiley, 1988, pp. 2052–2058.

Farre, R., M. Ferrer, M. Rotger, A. Torres, and D. Navajas, "Respiratory mechanics in ventilated COPD patients: Forced oscillation versus occlusion techniques." *Eur. Respir. J.*, 1998, 12, 170–176.

Finucane, K. E., B. A. Egan, and S. V. Dawson, "Linearity and frequency response of pneumotachographs." *J. Appl. Physiol.*, 1972, 10(2), 210–214.

Fleisch, A., "Der Pneumotachograph: ein Apparat zur Beischwindigkeitregstrierung der Atemluft." *Arch. Ges. Physiol.*, 1925, 209, 713–722.

Frei, J., J. Jutla, G. Kramer, G. E. Hatzakis, F. M. Ducharme, and G. M. Davis, "Impulse oscillometry: Reference values in children 100 to 150 cm in height and 3 to 10 years of age." *Chest*, 2005, 128, 1266–1273.

Hänninen, H., "Continuous patient spirometry during anesthesia." Presented at the 1st European Conference on Biomedical Engineering, Nice, France. February 17–20, 1991.

Henderson, R., "Understanding oxygen sensor performance." *Occupational Health & Safety*, May, 2005. Available online at http://www.ohsonline.com/articles/44859. 1105 Media Inc., copyright 2008.

Hyatt, R. E., "Forced expiration," Chapter 19. In P. T. Macklem and J. Mead (eds.), *Handbook of Physiology*, Section 3: The Respiratory System. Vol. III: *Mechanics of Breathing*, Part 1. Bethesda, MD: American Physiological Society, 1986, pp. 295–314.

Hyatt, R. E., I. R. Zimmerman, G. M. Peters, and W. J. Sullivan, "Direct write-out of total respiratory resistance." *J. Appl. Physiol.*, 1970, 28(5), 675–678.

Jones, W., "Characteristics of the disposable transducer/mouthpiece for the new Jones Satellite spirometer." *Product Literature*, 1990, Jones Medical Instrument Co., Oakbrook, IL.

Kreit, J. W., and F. C. Sciurba, "The accuracy of pneumotachograph measurements during mechanical ventilation." *Am. J. Respir. Crit. Care Med.*, 1996, 154, 913–917.

Kryger, M. H., "Monitoring respiratory and cardiac function." In M. H. Kryger, T. Roth, and W. C. Dement (eds.), *Principles and Practice of Sleep Medicine*, 4th ed., Philadelphia: W. B. Saunders, 2005.

Lausted, C. G., and A. T. Johnson, "Respiratory resistance measured by an airflow perturbation device." *Physiol. Meas.*, 1999, 20, 21–35.

Ligas, J. R., "Respiratory mechanics and gas exchange." In J. G. Webster (ed.), *Encyclopedia of Medical Devices and Instrumentation*, 2nd ed., New York: Wiley, 2006, Vol. 6, pp. 99–108.

Lord, R. C., "Infrared spectroscopy." In *McGraw-Hill Encyclopedia of Science and Technology*, 6th ed. New York: McGraw-Hill, 1987, Vol. 9, pp. 162–167.

Macia, N. F., "Pneumotachometers." In J. G. Webster (ed.), *Encyclopedia of Medical Devices and Instrumentation*, 2nd ed. New York: Wiley, 2006, Vol. 5, pp. 367–379.

Macklem, P. T., "Symbols and abbreviations." In P. T. Macklem and J. Mead (eds.), *Handbook of Physiology*, Section 3: The Respiratory System, Vol. III: *Mechanics of Breathing,* Part 1. Bethesda, MD: American Physiological Society, 1986, p. ix.

Macklem, P. T., *Procedures for Standardized Measurements of Lung Mechanics*. Bethesda, MD: NHLI, Division of Lung Diseases, 1974.

McGrath, S., and S. Wendelken, "Oxygen analyzers." In J. G. Webster (ed.), *Encyclopedia of Medical Devices and Instrumentation*. 2nd ed., New York: Wiley, 2006, Vol. 5, pp. 198–209.

Michaelson, E. D., E. D. Grassman, and W. R. Peters, "Pulmonary mechanics by spectral analyses of forced random noise." *J. Clin. Invest.*, 1975, 56, 1210–1230.

Miller, W. F., R. Scacci, and L. R. Gast, *Laboratory Evaluation of Pulmonary Function*. Philadelphia: J. B. Lippincott, 1987.

Møllgaard, K., "Acoustic gas measurement." *Biomed. Instrum. Technol.*, 1989, 23, 495–497.

Oostveen, E., D. MacLeod, H. Lorino, R. Farré, Z. Hantos, K. Desager, and R. Marchal, "The forced oscillation technique in clinical practice: methodology, recommendations and future developments." *Eur. Respir. J.*, 2003, 22, 1026–1041.

Peslin, R., J. Morinet-Lambert, and C. Duvivier, "Frequency response of pneumotachographs." *Bull. Physio-path. Resp.*, 1972, 8, 1363–1376.

Petrini, M. F., "Pulmonary function testing." In J. G. Webster (ed.), *Encyclopedia of Medical Devices and Instrumentation*. New York: Wiley, 1988, pp. 2379–2395.

Primiano, F. P., Jr., "A conceptual framework for pulmonary function testing." *Ann. Biomed. Eng.*, 1981, 9, 621–632.

Primiano, F. P., Jr., and I. Greber, "Analysis of plethysmographic estimation of alveolar pressure." *IEEE Trans. Biomed. Eng.*, 1975, 22(5), 393–399.

Primiano, F. P., Jr., and R. L. Chatburn, "The use of models in pulmonary physiology." In R. L. Chatburn and K. C. Craig (eds.), *Fundamentals of Respiratory Care Research*, Norwalk, CT: Appleton and Lange, 1988, pp. 39–57.

Primiano, F. P., Jr., and R. L. Chatburn, "Zen and the art of nomenclature maintenance: A revised approach to respiratory symbols and terminology." *Respiratory Care*, 2006, 51, 1458–1470.

Sackner, M. A., "Monitoring of ventilation without a physical connection to the airway." In M. A. Sackner (ed.), *Diagnostic Techniques in Pulmonary Disease*, Part I. New York: Marcel Dekker, 1980, pp. 503–537.

Silverman, L., and J. L. Whittenberger, "Clinical pneumotachograph." In J. H. Comroe, Jr. (ed.), in *Methods in Medical Research*, Vol. 2. Chicago: Year Book, 1950, pp. 104–112.

Sodal, I. E., J. S. Clark, and G. D. Swanson, "Mass spectrometers in medical monitoring." In J. G. Webster (ed.), *Encyclopedia of Medical Devices and Instrumentation*. New York: Wiley, 1988, pp. 1848–1859.

Sullivan, W. J., G. M. Peters, and P. L. Enright, "Pneumotachographs: Theory and clinical application." *Respiratory Care*, 1984, 29, 736–749.

Turney, S. Z., and W. Blumenfeld, "Heated Fleisch pneumotachometer: A calibration procedure." *J. Appl. Physiol.*, 1973, 34, 117–121.

Verschakelen, J. A., K. Deschepper, I. Clarysse, and M. Demedts, "The effect of breath size and posture on calibration of the respiratory inductive plethysmograph by multiple linear regression." *Eur. Respir. J.*, 1989, 2, 71–77.

West, G. A., J. J. Barrett, D. R. Siebert, and K. V. Reddy, "Photoacoustic spectroscopy." *Rev. Sci. Instrum.*, 1983, 54, 797–817.

# 10

# CHEMICAL BIOSENSORS

Robert A. Peura

A chemical biosensor is a sensor that produces an electric signal proportional to the concentration of biochemical analytes. These biosensors use chemical as well as physical principles in their operation.

The body is composed of living cells. These cells, which are essentially chemical factories, the input to which is metabolic food and the output waste products, are the building blocks for the organ systems in the body. The functional status of an organ system is determined by measuring the chemical input and output analytes of the cells. As a consequence, the majority of tests made in the hospital or the physician's office deal with analyzing the chemistry of the body.

The important critical-care analytes are the blood levels of pH; $Po_2$; $Pco_2$; hematocrit; total hemoglobin; $O_2$ saturation; electrolytes including sodium, potassium, calcium, and chloride; and various metabolites including glucose, lactate, creatinine, and urea. Table 10.1 gives the normal ranges in blood for these critical-care analytes.

These variables are normally analyzed in a central clinical-chemistry laboratory remote from the patient's bedside. This conventional approach provides only historical values of the patient's blood chemistry, because there is a delay between when the sample is obtained and when the result is reported. (The sample must be transported to the main clinical-chemistry laboratory, and the appropriate analyses must be performed.) This inherent delay is approximately 30 min or more. Other significant drawbacks plague central-laboratory analyses of patient chemistry, including potential errors in the origin of the sample and in sample-handling techniques, and (because of the delay) the timeliness of the therapeutic intervention.

For these reasons, there has been a movement to decentralize clinical testing of the patient's chemistry (Collison and Meyerhoff, 1990). This is particularly important in the critical-care and surgical settings. The decentralized approach has resulted from a number of improvements in biosensor technology, including the development of blood-gas and electrolyte monitoring systems equipped with self-calibration for measuring the patient's blood chemistry at the bedside.

Economic pressures have also encouraged movement of sophisticated chemical-analysis and diagnostic equipment from the central laboratory to

**Table 10.1 Critical-Care Analytes and Their Normal Ranges in Blood**

| Blood Gases and Related Parameters | | Electrolytes | | Metabolites | |
|---|---|---|---|---|---|
| $P_{O_2}$ | 80–104 mm Hg | $Na^+$ | 135–155 mmol/l | Glucose | 70–110 mg/100 ml |
| $P_{CO_2}$ | 33–48 mm Hg | $K^+$ | 3.6–5.5 mmol/l | Lactate | 3–7 mg/100 ml |
| pH | 7.31–7.45 | $Ca^{2+}$ | 1.14–1.31 mmol/l | Creatinine | 0.9–1.4 mg/100 ml |
| Hematocrit | 40–54% | $Cl^-$ | 98–109 mmol/l | Urea | 8–26 mg/100 ml |
| Total hemoglobin | 13–18 g/100 ml | | | | |
| $O_2$-saturation | 95–100% | | | | |

SOURCE: M. E. Collison and M. E. Meyerhoff, "Chemical sensors for bedside monitoring of critically ill patients," *Anal. Chem.*, 1990, 62, 425A–437A.

specific clinical areas. Such sites include the operating room, where patient blood gases and electrolytes must be monitored continuously, and dialysis centers, where patients are treated on an outpatient basis and measurements of uric acid and other blood analytes must be made in a timely manner. In addition, self-contained, small, economical blood-chemistry units have been developed for use in the physician's office and the patient's home.

In the future, integrated-circuit and optoelectronic technology will be used to develop miniaturized biosensors, which are sensitive to body analytes for real-time, *in vivo* measurements of body chemistry (Turner *et al.*, 1987). Self-contained biosensor units for closed-loop drug-delivery systems will also become available. Examples of future applications of closed-loop systems with chemical biosensors include (1) control of implantable pacemakers and defibrillators, (2) regulation of anesthesia during operations, and (3) control of insulin secretion from an artificial pancreas. Note that moving laboratory devices from a central location to a decentralized location in the hospital, physician's office, or patient's home poses significant challenges. These involve stability, calibration, quality control of the measurements, and ease of instrument use.

Noninvasive measurement of the biochemistry of the body will increase tremendously in the future. The advances in and burgeoning applications of pulse oximetry offer just one example of the impact that noninvasive measurement can have on patient monitoring. Pulse oximetry has become the standard of care in a number of clinical situations, which include monitoring during administration of anesthesia (to assess functioning of the cardiopulmonary system) and during the administration of oxygen to neonates (to avoid high arterial oxygen levels, which can lead to serious damage to retinal and pulmonary tissue). The future will see applications for noninvasive monitoring of the blood biochemistry in the standard blood-chemistry tests for glucose, cholesterol, urea, electrolytes, and so on.

## 10.1 BLOOD-GAS AND ACID–BASE PHYSIOLOGY

The fast and accurate measurements of the blood levels of the partial pressure of oxygen ($P_{O_2}$), the partial pressure of $CO_2$ ($P_{CO_2}$), and the concentration of hydrogen ions (pH) are vital in the diagnosis and treatment of many pathological conditions. Significant abnormalities of these quantities can rapidly be fatal if not treated appropriately. These measurements are usually made on specimens of arterial blood, though "arterialized" venous samples are often obtained from infants.

Oxygen is carried in the blood in two separate states. Normally, approximately 98% of the $O_2$ in the blood is combined with hemoglobin (Hb) in the red blood cells. The remaining 2% is physically dissolved in the plasma. The amount (saturation, $S$) of $O_2$ bound to Hb in arterial blood is defined as the ratio of the concentration of oxyhemoglobin ($HbO_2$) to the total concentration of Hb. That is,

$$S_{O_2}(\%) = \frac{[HbO_2]}{[\text{total Hb}]} \times 100 \qquad (10.1)$$

The sigmoid-shaped oxyhemoglobin dissociation curve (ODC), shown in Figure 10.1, graphically illustrates the relationship between the percent oxygen saturation of hemoglobin and the partial pressure of oxygen in the plasma. The total content of $O_2$ in blood is directly related to $S_{O_2}$ for any given Hb concentration, because the amount of $O_2$ that is physically dissolved in the blood is relatively small.

Arterial $P_{O_2}$ and $S_{O_2}$ have different physiological meanings. Arterial $P_{O_2}$ determines the efficiency of alveolar ventilation; $S_{O_2}$ indicates the amount of $O_2$ per unit of blood. It is possible to derive $S_{O_2}$ from $P_{O_2}$ measurements by using an ODC, but significant errors result for abnormal physiological situations unless the temperature and pH of the blood, the type of Hb derivative, and 2,3-diphosphoglycerate (DPG) are known. Direct measurement of $S_{O_2}$ is more accurate than an indirect calculation, because the affinity of Hb for $O_2$ is affected by these several variables.

For young adults, the normal range of $P_{O_2}$ in arterial blood is from 90 to 100 mm Hg (12 to 13.3 kPa). As a result of the sigmoid nature of the $O_2$ disassociation curve, a $P_{O_2}$ of 60 mm Hg (8 kPa) still provides an $O_2$ saturation of 85%. Decreases in $P_{O_2}$ are seen in a variety of settings. These can be divided into two groups: (1) decreased delivery of $O_2$ to the site of $O_2$ exchange between the inspired air and the blood (the lung alveoli) and (2) decreased delivery of blood to the alveoli to which $O_2$ is being supplied. Examples of the first group include decreased overall ventilation (such as caused by narcotic overdose or paralysis of the ventilatory muscles), obstruction of major airways

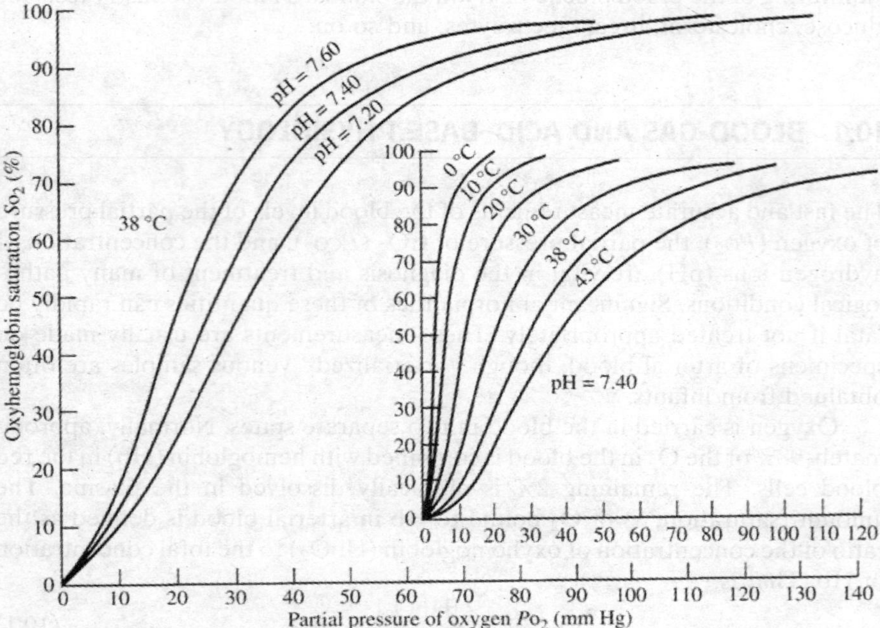


**Figure 10.1** The oxyhemoglobin dissociation curve shows the effect of pH and temperature on the relationship between $S_{O_2}$ and $P_{O_2}$.

(such as by aspirated foreign objects such as food; by spasm of the airway muscles, such as that which occurs in an acute attack of asthma); or by filling of the alveoli and small airways with fluid (such as in pneumonia or pulmonary edema). Examples of the second group include congenital cardiac abnormalities, in which blood is shunted past the lungs (the Tetralogy of Fallot, for example), and obstruction of flow through the pulmonary blood vessels (such as caused by pulmonary emboli). The important lung diseases of emphysema and chronic bronchitis usually display characteristics of both these types of abnormalities.

The $P_{CO_2}$ level is an indicator of the adequacy of ventilation and is therefore increased in the first group of disorders discussed above, but it is generally normal in the second group unless the defect is massive in nature. In young adults, the normal range of $P_{CO_2}$ in arterial blood is 35 to 40 mm Hg (4.7 to 5.3 kPa).

The acid–base status of the blood is assessed by measuring the hydrogen ion concentration $[H^+]$. It is conventional to use the negative logarithm to the base 10 (pH) to report this quantity; that is,

$$pH = -\log_{10}[H^+] \tag{10.2}$$

The normal range of pH in arterial blood is 7.38 to 7.44. Decreases in pH (increased quantity of hydrogen ions) occur with a decreased rate of excretion of $CO_2$ (respiratory acidosis) and/or with increased production of fixed acid (such as occurs in diabetic ketoacidosis) or abnormal losses of bicarbonate (the principal hydrogen ion buffer in the blood). Acidosis resulting from the last two processes is called *metabolic acidosis*. Increases in pH (decreased quantity of hydrogen ions) occur with an increased rate of excretion of $CO_2$ (respiratory alkalosis) and/or abnormal losses of acid (such as result from prolonged vomiting), which is called *metabolic alkalosis*. Table 10.2 gives examples of arterial-blood gases in different clinical situations. Note that a measurement of $P_{CO_2}$, or the level of bicarbonate in the blood, along with a measurement of pH, must be done in order to classify the type of acid–base abnormality (Davenport, 1975).

**EXAMPLE 10.1** A blood specimen has a hydrogen ion concentration of 40 nmol/liter and a $P_{CO_2}$ of 60 mm Hg. What is the pH? What type of acid–base abnormality does the patient exhibit?

**ANSWER**

$$\text{pH} = -\log_{10}[\text{H}^+] = -\log_{10}\left[40 \times 10^{-9}\right] \text{ mol/liter} = -[1.6 - 9.0] = 7.4.$$

So pH is in the normal range 7.38 to 7.44. However, the $P_{CO_2}$ is 60 mm Hg, which is high compared to the normal value of 40 mm Hg. Table 10.2 shows that the patient has decreased overall ventilation.

The basic concepts of ions, electrochemical cells, and reference cells are discussed in Chapter 5. This section shows how these concepts are used to design electrodes for the measurement of pH, $P_{CO_2}$ and $P_{O_2}$.

## 10.2 ELECTROCHEMICAL SENSORS

### MEASUREMENT OF pH

The measurement of pH is accomplished by utilizing a glass electrode that generates an electric potential when solutions of differing pH are placed on the two sides of its membrane (Von Cremer, 1906). Figure 10.2 is a schematic diagram of a pH electrode.

The glass electrode is a member of the class of ion-specific electrodes that react to any extent only with a specific ion.

The approach of a hydrogen ion to the outside of the membrane causes the silicate structure of the glass to conduct a positive charge (hole) into the ionic solution inside the electrode. The Nernst equation, (4.1), applies, so the voltage across the membrane changes by 60 mV/pH unit. Because the range of physiological pH is only 0.06 pH units, the pH meter must be capable of accurately measuring changes of 0.1 mV.

**Table 10.2 Examples of Arterial Blood Gases in Different Clinical Situations**

| Example | $PCO_2$, mm Hg | pH | $PO_2$, mm Hg | Interpretation | Likely Causes |
|---|---|---|---|---|---|
| 1 | $40 \pm 3$ | $7.40 \pm 0.03$ | $90 \pm 5$ | Normal blood gas | |
| 2 | $44 \pm 3$ | $7.37 \pm 0.03$ | $88 \pm 5$ | Normal blood gas while asleep | |
| 3 | 22 | 7.57 | 106 | Hyperventilation | Anxiety |
| 4 | 68 | 7.10 | 58 | Hypoventilation | Central nervous system depression; blockage of upper airway |
| 5 | 58 | 7.21 | 39 | Hypoventilation and hypoxemia | Pneumonia; small-airway obstruction; severe asthma |
| 6 | 61 | 6.99 | 29 | Combined respiratory and metabolic acidosis and hypoxemia | Birth asphyxia; near-drowning |
| 7 | 60 | 7.37 | 106 | Chronic respiratory acidosis with metabolic compensation; patient is receiving supplemental oxygen | Patient has chronic lung disease and is on oxygen |
| 8 | 29 | 7.31 | 106 | Metabolic acidosis with respiratory compensation | Diabetic; ketoacidosis; dehydration |

SOURCE: B. G. Nickerson and F. Monaco, "Carbon dioxide electrodes, arterial and transcutaneous," in J. G. Webster (ed.), Encyclo
Instrumentation. New York: Wiley, 1988, pp. 564–569.

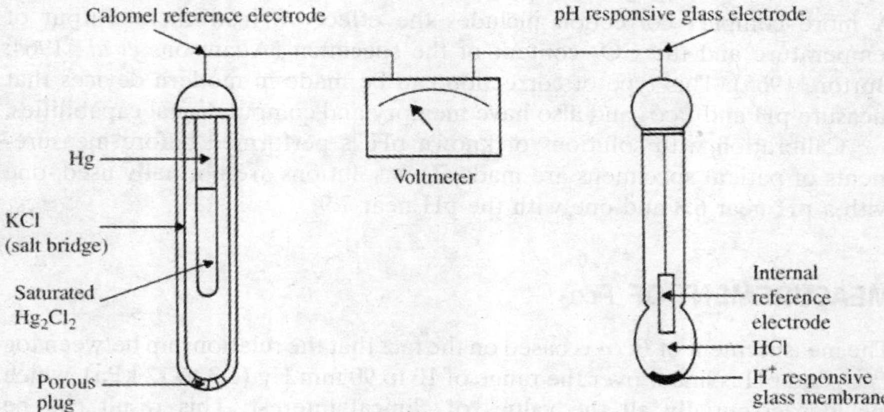


**Figure 10.2 pH electrode** (From R. Hicks, J. R. Schenken, and M. A. Steinrauf, Laboratory Instrumentation. Hagerstown, MD: Harper & Row, 1974. Used with permission of C. A. McWhorter.)

The basic approach is to place a solution of known pH on the inside of the membrane and the unknown solution on the outside. Hydrochloric acid is generally used as the solution of known pH. A reference electrode, usually an Ag/AgCl or a saturated calomel electrode, is placed in this solution. A second reference electrode is placed in the specimen chamber. A salt bridge is included within the reference to prevent the chemical constituents of the specimen from affecting the voltage of the reference electrode. The potential developed across the membrane of the glass electrode is read by a pH meter. This pH meter must have extremely high input impedance, because the internal impedance of the pH electrode is in the 10 to 100 MΩ range.

**EXAMPLE 10.2** Design an amplifier for use with the pH electrode. An output in the range of 1 to 2 mV is desired for the normal pH variation of blood.

**ANSWER** Because the internal impedance of the pH electrode is in the 10 to 100 MΩ range, we need an amplifier with extremely high input impedance and extremely small bias current. Thus, select a field-effect transistor (FET) op amp that has specifications for extremely low bias current and extremely low offset voltage drift. To achieve high input impedance, connect it as a noninverting amplifier with a gain of 101.

The Nernst equation shows that the voltage produced by a pH electrode varies with the temperature of the specimen and the reference solution. Some pH electrodes include a water bath that allows the pH determination to be made at 37 °C; others require a temperature correction. This temperature correction can be made by changing the constant used to convert from the electrode voltage to the meter scale reading in pH units by setting a temperature-control knob to the temperature at which the pH measurement is being made.

A more complex correction includes the effect on instrument output of temperature and the $CO_2$ content of the specimen (Adamsons *et al.*, 1964; Burton, 1965). This type of correction can be made in modern devices that measure pH and $P_{CO_2}$ and also have memory and computational capabilities.

Calibration with solutions of known pH is performed before measurements of patient specimens are made. Two solutions are normally used: one with a pH near 6.8 and one with the pH near 7.9.

## MEASUREMENT OF $P_{CO_2}$

The measurement of $P_{CO_2}$ is based on the fact that the relationship between log $P_{CO_2}$ and pH is linear over the range of 10 to 90 mm Hg (1.3 to 12 kPa), which includes essentially all the values of clinical interest. This result can be established by examining some fundamental chemical relationships among $H^+$, $H_2CO_3$, $HCO_3^-$, and $P_{CO_2}$. The first three quantities are related by the equilibrium equation

$$H_2O + CO_2 \rightleftharpoons H_2CO_3 \rightleftharpoons H^+ + HCO_3^- \tag{10.3}$$

In addition, the relationship between $P_{CO_2}$ and the concentration of $CO_2$ dissolved in the blood, $[co_2]$, is given by

$$[CO_2] = a(P_{CO_2}) \tag{10.4}$$

where $a = 0.0301$ mmol/liter per mm Hg $P_{CO_2}$. The mass relationship corresponding to (10.3) can then be written as

$$k' = \frac{[H^+][HCO_3^-]}{[H_2CO_3]} \tag{10.5}$$

Next we use the fact that $[H_2CO_3]$ is proportional to $[CO_2]$ to obtain the result

$$k = \frac{[H^+][HCO_3^-]}{[CO_2]} \tag{10.6}$$

where $k$ represents the combined values of $k'$ and the proportionality constant between $[H_2CO_3]$ and $[CO_2]$. Now, using (10.4), we obtain the following result:

$$k = \frac{[H^+][HCO_3^-]}{aP_{CO_2}} \tag{10.7}$$

Next, taking the base-10 logarithm of (10.7) and rearranging, we obtain

$$\log[H^+] + \log[HCO_3^-] - \log k - \log a - \log P_{CO_2} = 0 \tag{10.8}$$

Using the definition of pH yields

$$\text{pH} = \log[HCO_3^-] - \log k - \log a - \log P_{CO_2} \tag{10.9}$$

This shows that pH has a linear dependence on the negative of log $P_{CO_2}$.

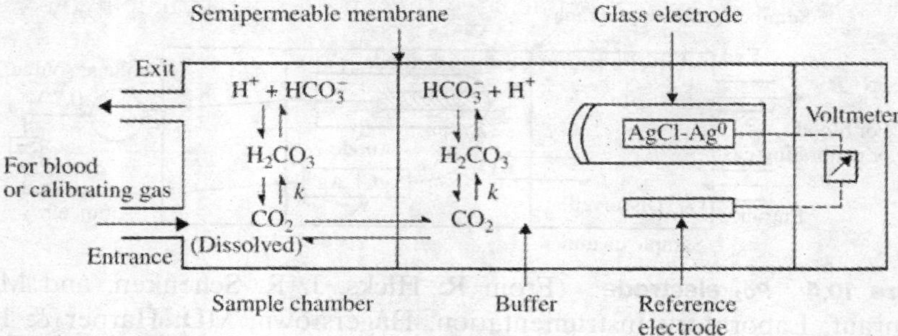


**Figure 10.3** ***P*$_{CO_2}$ electrode** (From R. Hicks, J. R. Schenken, and M. A. Steinrauf, Laboratory Instrumentation. Hagerstown, MD: Harper & Row, 1974. Used with permission of C. A. McWhorter.)

This result is used in the construction of the $P_{CO_2}$ electrode shown in Figure 10.3 (Severinghaus, 1965). The assembly includes two chambers, one for the specimen and a second containing a pH electrode of the type discussed. In contrast to the basic pH-measurement device in which the pH electrode is placed in the specimen, in this case the pH electrode is bathed by a buffer solution of bicarbonate and NaCl.

The two chambers are separated by a semipermeable membrane, usually made of Teflon or silicone rubber. This membrane allows dissolved $CO_2$ to pass through but blocks the passage of charged particles, in particular $H^+$ and $HCO_3^-$. When the specimen is placed in its chamber, $CO_2$ diffuses across the membrane to establish the same concentration in both chambers. If there is a net movement of $CO_2$ into (or out of) the chamber containing the buffer, $[H^+]$ increases (or decreases), and the pH meter detects this change. Because the relationship between pH and the negative log $P_{CO_2}$ is only a proportional one, it is necessary to calibrate the instrument before each use with two gases of known $P_{CO_2}$.

Using the values of pH obtained by processing these two standards, we obtain a calibration curve of $P_{CO_2}$ versus pH. We then use the measured pH value to obtain the specimen's $P_{CO_2}$ from this curve. With some instruments, the capability of calibrating the $P_{CO_2}$ electrode is built into the instrument so that the calibration curve is set up in the electronics of the instrument by setting the values of two potentiometers.

## THE $P_{O_2}$ ELECTRODE

Figure 10.4 shows the basic components of the Clark-type polarographic electrode. The measurement of $P_{O_2}$ is based on the following reactions. At the cathode, reduction occurs:

$$O_2 + 2H_2O + 4e^- \rightarrow 2H_2O_2 + 4e^- \rightarrow 4OH^-$$

$$4OH^- + 4KCl \rightarrow 4KOH + 4Cl^- \qquad (10.10)$$

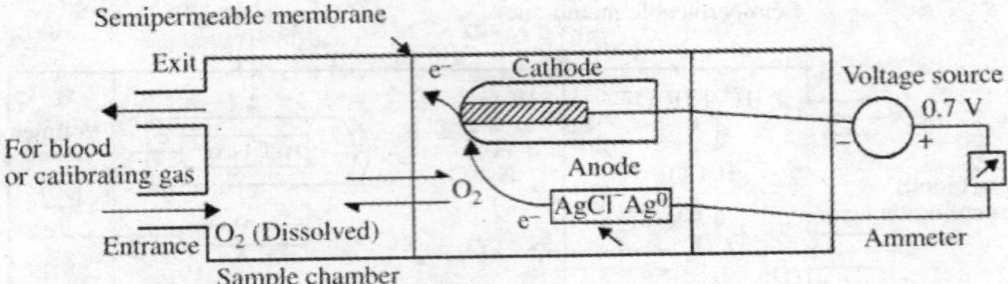


**Figure 10.4** ***$P_{O_2}$* electrode** (From R. Hicks, J. R. Schenken, and M. A. Steinrauf, Laboratory Instrumentation. Hagerstown, MD: Harper & Row, 1974. Used with permission of C. A. McWhorter.)

The hydroxyl ions created in this reaction are buffered by the electrolyte. At the anode, which in this $P_{O_2}$ electrode is the reference electrode, oxidation occurs.

$$4Ag + 4Cl^- \rightarrow 4AgCl + 4e^- \tag{10.11}$$

This produces the four electrons required for the reaction in (10.10).

The cathode is constructed of glass-coated Pt, and the reference electrode is made of Ag/AgCl.

The plot of current versus polarizing voltage of a typical $P_{O_2}$ electrode (polarogram) is shown in Figure 10.5(a). The polarizing voltage is selected in the "plateau" region to provide a sufficient potential to drive the reaction, without permitting other electrochemical reactions that would be driven by greater voltages to take place. Thus the resulting current is linearly proportional to the number of $O_2$ molecules in solution [see Figure 10.5(b)]. The $O_2$ membrane is permeable to $O_2$ and other gases and separates the electrode from its surroundings.

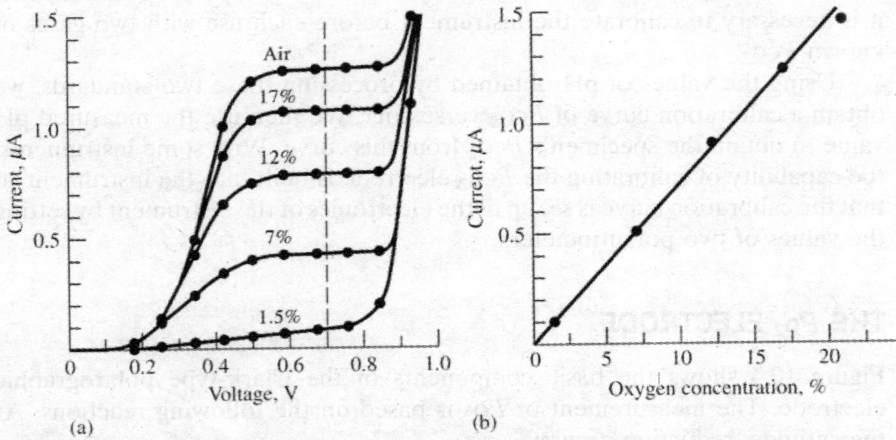


**Figure 10.5** (a) Current plotted against polarizing voltage for a typical $P_{O_2}$ electrode for the percents $O_2$ shown. (b) Electrode operation with a polarizing voltage of 0.68 V gives a linear relationship between current output and percent $O_2$.

A polarizing voltage of 600 to 800 mV is required for these reactions to occur. This voltage is usually supplied by a mercury cell.

We determine the value of $Po_2$ by using the fact that the flow of current through the external circuit connecting the electrodes is proportional to $Po_2$. The presence of $O_2$ and the resulting chemical reaction can be thought of as producing in the circuit a variable source of current the value of which is directly proportional to the $Po_2$ level. When the $Po_2$ level is zero, the current flowing through the circuit is called the background current. Part of the calibration sequence involves setting the $Po_2$ meter to zero when a $CO_2/N_2$ gas is bubbled through the specimen chamber. Slow bubbling is used to ensure proper temperature equilibration.

**EXAMPLE 10.3** Design an amplifier and a power source for an $O_2$ electrode. The output of your device should range from 0 to 10 V for an oxygen range from 0% to 100%. At a 20% $O_2$ level, the electrode current is 50 nA.

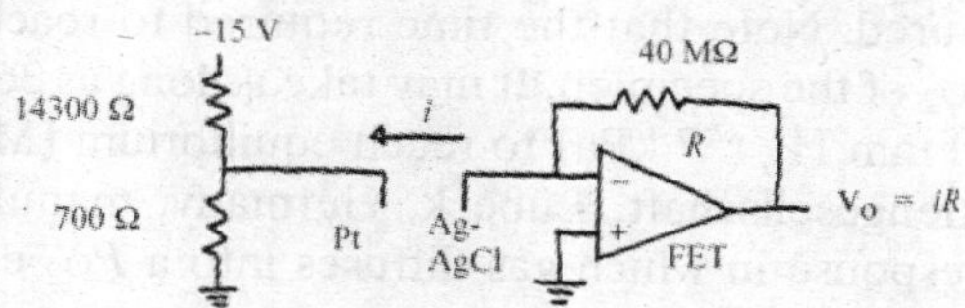


**ANSWER** From a –15 V power supply use a 14,300 Ω and 700 Ω resistor voltage divider to yield –0.7 V to bias the Pt electrode. Feed the Ag/AgCl electrode output into an FET current-to-voltage converter with a feedback resistor $= V/I = 10\,\text{V}/250\,\text{nA} = 40\,\text{M}\Omega$.

Equation (10.10) shows that the reaction consumes $O_2$. This loss is a direct function of the area of the Pt electrode that is exposed to the reaction solution and the permeability of the semipermeable membrane to $O_2$. The exposed area of the Pt electrode usually has a diameter of 20 μm.

The choice of the semipermeable membrane is based on a trade-off between consumption of $O_2$ and the time required for the $Po_2$ values in the specimen and measurement chambers to equilibrate. The more permeable the membrane is to $O_2$, the higher the consumption of $O_2$ and the faster the response. Polypropylene is less permeable than Teflon and is preferable in most applications. Polypropylene is also quite durable, and it maintains its position over the electrode more reliably than other membrane materials.

The membrane thickness and composition determine the $O_2$ diffusion rate; thicker membranes extend the sensor time response by significantly increasing the diffusion time and produce smaller currents.

Because the electrode consumes $O_2$, it partially depletes the oxygen in the immediate vicinity of the membrane. If movement of the sample takes place, undepleted solution brought to the membrane causes a higher instrument reading—the "stirring" artifact. This is avoided by waiting for a stagnant equilibrium to occur.

The reaction is very sensitive to temperature. To maintain a linear relationship between $P_{O_2}$ and current, the temperature of the electrode must be controlled to $\pm 0.1$ °C. This has been traditionally accomplished by using a water jacket. However, new blood-gas analyzers are now available that use precision electronic heat sources. The current through the meter is approximately 10 nA/mm Hg (75 nA/kPa) $O_2$ at 37 °C, so the instruments must be designed to be accurate at very low current levels.

The system is calibrated by using two gases of known $O_2$ concentration. One gas with no $O_2$ (typically a $CO_2$–$N_2$ mixture) and a second with a known $O_2$ content (usually an $O_2$–$CO_2$–$N_2$ mixture) are used. The specimen chamber is filled with water, and the calibrating gas containing no $O_2$ is bubbled through it. The $P_{O_2}$ meter output is set to zero after equilibrium of $O_2$ content is achieved—usually in about 90 s. Next the second calibrating gas is used to determine the second point on the $P_{O_2}$-versus-electrode-current calibration scale, which is electrically set in the machine. Then the value of the specimen $P_{O_2}$ can be measured. Note that the time required to reach equilibrium is a function of the $P_{O_2}$ of the specimen. It may take as long as 360 s for a specimen with a $P_{O_2}$ of 430 mm Hg (57 kPa) to reach equilibrium (Moran *et al.*, 1966). Drägerwerk Aktiengesellschaft, Lübeck, Germany, manufactures a gas $O_2$ sensor with 2 s response in which gas diffuses into a $P_{O_2}$ electrode.

**EXAMPLE 10.4** Because the average venous-arterial oxygen tension is about 70 mm Hg and that of air is about 155 mm Hg, there exists an inward flux of oxygen from the air to all surfaces of the mammalian body. Normally insignificant compared to that of the lungs, this oxygen uptake is, however, significant for the cornea, which obtains its metabolic oxygen not from blood but rather from the inward flux of oxygen from the air. Design a system to measure the inward flux of oxygen across the cornea. Specify what parameters you would monitor, and indicate how you would determine the oxygen influx across the cornea in liters of $O_2$ per square centimeter of cornea surface per hour.

**ANSWER** Place a cup-shaped contact lens, which is filled with a known concentration of oxygen (volume of $O_2$/volume in contact lens) in physiologic saline, on the eye. The inner surface of the contact lens that is in contact with the eye should be permeable to $O_2$. The $O_2$ flux into the eye is determined by the following:

1. Flux $= Q/(At)$, where $Q =$ volume of $O_2$, $A =$ contact area, $t =$ time.
2. $Q = VC$, where $V =$ volume in contact lens, $C =$difference in concentration of $O_2$ between initial value and value after 1 h.

Thus, measure $O_2$ concentration in solution initially and after 1 h using $P_{O_2}$ electrode. Note that the $P_{O_2}$ electrode measures the partial pressure of $O_2$, which is directly proportional to the $O_2$ concentration in physiologic saline.

## 10.3 CHEMICAL FIBROSENSORS

Rapid advances in the communications industry have provided appropriate small optical fibers, high-energy sources such as lasers, and wavelength detectors. The fiber-optic sensors that were developed were called *optodes*, a term coined by Lübbers and Opitz (1975), which implies that optical sensors are very similar to electrodes. As we shall see, however, the properties and operating principles for optical fibrosensors are quite different from those for electrodes. The term *optrode*, with an *r*, is currently used.

Chemical fibrosensors offer several desirable features.

1. They can be made small in size.
2. Multiple sensors can be introduced together, through a catheter, for intracranial or intravascular measurements.
3. Because optical measurements are being made, there are no electric hazards to the patient.
4. The measurements are immune to external electric interference, provided that the electronic instrumentation is properly shielded.
5. No reference electrode is necessary.

In addition, fibrosensors have a high degree of flexibility and good thermal stability, and low-cost manufacturing and disposable usage are possible. In reversible sensors, the reagent phase is not consumed by its reaction with the analyte. In nonreversible sensors, the reagent phase is consumed. The consumption of the reagent phase for nonreversible sensors must be small, or there must be a way to replenish the reagent.

Optical-fiber sensors have several limitations when compared with electrode sensors. Optical sensors are sensitive to ambient light, so they must be used in a dark environment or must be optically shielded via opaque materials. The optical signal may also have to be modulated in order to code it and make it distinguishable from the ambient light. The dynamic response of optical sensors is normally limited compared with that of electrodes. Reversible indicator sensors are based on an equilibrium measurement rather than a diffusion-dependent one, so they are less susceptible to changes in flow concentration at the sensor (Seitz, 1988).

Long-term stability for optical sensors may be a problem for reagent-based systems. However, this can be compensated for by the use of multiple-wavelength detection and by the ease of changing reagent phases. In addition, because the reagent and the analyte are in different phases, a mass-transfer step is necessary before constant response is achieved (Seitz, 1988). This limits the temporal response of an optical sensor. Another consideration with optical sensors is that for several types of optical sensors, the response is proportional to the amount of reagent phase. For small amounts of reagent, an increased response can be achieved by increasing the intensity of the source. An increased response, however, results in an increase in the photodegradation process of the reagent. Designers of optical sensors, then, must consider amount of the reagent phase, intensity of the light source, and system stability (Seitz, 1984).

These limitations can be alleviated by an appropriate design of the optical sensor and instrumentation system (Wise, 1990). The systems described in the following paragraphs incorporate many features specifically for this purpose.

## INTRAVASCULAR MEASUREMENTS OF OXYGEN SATURATION

Blood oxygen can be monitored by means of an intravascular fiber-optic catheter. These catheters are used to monitor mixed venous oxygen saturation during cardiac surgery and in the intensive-care unit. A Swan–Ganz catheter is used (see Section 7.11), in which a flow-directed fiber-optic catheter is placed into the right jugular vein. The catheter is advanced until its distal tip is in the right atrium, at which time the balloon is inflated. The rapid flow of blood carries the catheter into the pulmonary artery.

Measurements of mixed venous oxygen saturation give an indication of the effectiveness of a cardiopulmonary system. Measurements of high oxygen saturation in the right side of the heart may indicate congenital abnormalities of the heart and major vessels or the inability of tissue to metabolize oxygen. Low saturation readings on the left side of the heart may indicate a reduced ability of the lungs to oxygenate the blood or of the cardiopulmonary system to deliver oxygen from the lungs. Low saturation readings in the arterial system indicate a compromised cardiac output or reduced oxygen-carrying capacity of the blood.

Figure 10.6 shows the optical-absorption spectra for oxyhemoglobin, carboxyhemoglobin, hemoglobin, and methemoglobin. Measurements in the red region are possible because the absorption coefficient of blood at these wavelengths is sufficiently low that light can be transmitted through whole blood over distances such that feasible measurements can be made with fiber-optic catheters. Note that the 805 nm wavelength provides a measurement independent of the degree of oxygenation. This isosbestic wavelength is used to compensate for the scattering properties of the whole blood and to normalize the measurement signal with any changes in hemoglobin from patient to patient.

Oxygen saturation is measured by taking the ratio of the diffusely backscattered light intensities at two wavelengths. The first wavelength is in the red region (660 nm); the second is in the infrared region (805 nm), which is known as the isosbestic point for Hb and $HbO_2$. Oxygen saturation is given by (10.1), which considers the optical density of the blood—the light

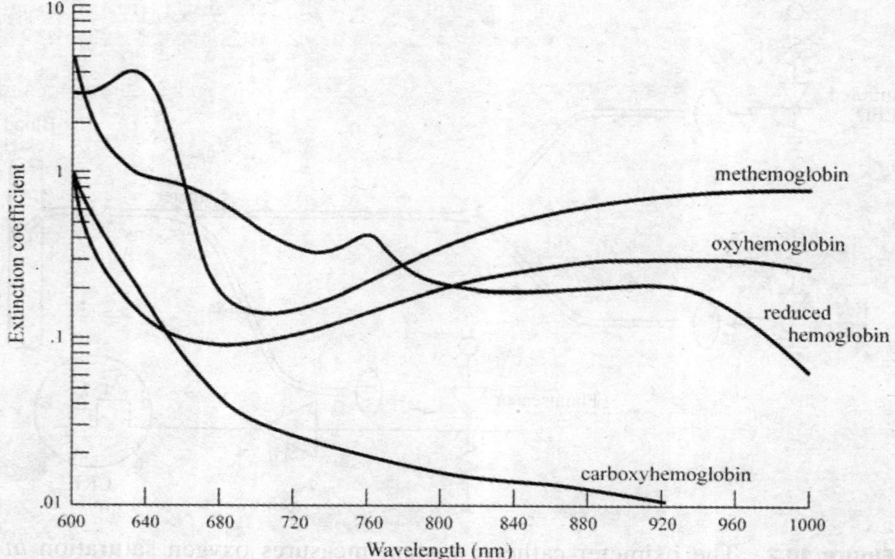


**Figure 10.6** Absorptivities (extinction coefficients) in liter/(mmol·cm) of the four most common hemoglobin species at the wavelengths of interest in pulse oximetry. (Courtesy of Susan Manson, Biox/Ohmeda, Boulder, CO.)

transmitted through the blood—according to Beer's law. For hemolyzed blood (blood with red cells ruptured), Beer's law (Section 11.1) holds, and the absorbance (optical density) at any wavelength is (Allan, 1973)

$$A(\lambda) = WL[a_o(\lambda)C_o + a_r(\lambda)C_r] \tag{10.12}$$

where

$W$ = weight of homoglobin per unit volume
$L$ = optical path length
$a_o$ and $a_r$ = absorptivities of $HbO_2$ and Hb
$C_o = C_r$ = relative concentrations of $HbO_2$ and Hb ($C_o + C_r = 1.0$)

Figure 10.6 shows that $a_o$ and $a_r$ are equal at 805 nm, called the *isosbestic* wavelength. If this wavelength is $\lambda_2$, then

$$WL = \frac{A(\lambda_2)}{a(\lambda_2)} \tag{10.13}$$

where

$$a(\lambda_2) = a_o(\lambda_2) = a_r(\lambda_2) \tag{10.14}$$

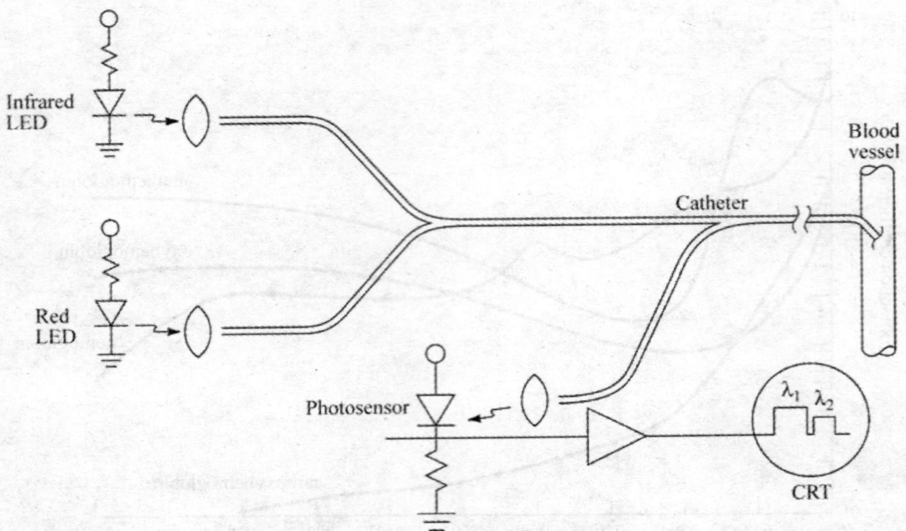


**Figure 10.7** The oximeter catheter system measures oxygen saturation *in vivo*, using red and infrared light-emitting diodes (LEDs) and a photosensor. The red and infrared LEDs are alternately pulsed in order to use a single photosensor.

Therefore,

$$A(\lambda) = \frac{A(\lambda_2)}{a(\lambda_2)}[a_o(\lambda)C_o + a_r(\lambda)C_r] \tag{10.15}$$

When absorbance is measured at a second wavelength $\lambda_1$, the oxygen saturation is given by

$$C_o = x + \frac{yA(\lambda_1)}{A(\lambda_2)} \tag{10.16}$$

where $x$ and $y$ are constants that depend only on the optical characteristics of blood. In practice, $\lambda_1$ is chosen to be that wavelength at which the difference between $a_o$ and $a_r$ is a maximum, which occurs at 660 nm [see Figure 10.6].

Figure 10.7 shows a fiber-optic instrument devised to measure oxygen saturation in the blood. This device, which could also be used for measuring cardiac output with a dye injected, is described here. The instrument consists of red and infrared light-emitting diodes (LEDs) and a photosensor. Plastic optical fibers are well adapted to these wavelengths. Figure 10.8 shows a fiber-optic oximeter catheter that is flow directed. After insertion, the balloon is inflated, and blood flow drags the tip through the chambers of the heart.

In addition to measuring blood-oxygen saturation through reflectance, the same dual-wavelength optics can be used to measure blood flow by dye dilution. Indo/cyanine/green, which absorbs light at 805 nm (the isosbestic wavelength of oxyhemoglobin), is used as the indicator. This is a dual-fiber system. Light at 805 nm is emitted from one fiber, scattered by the blood cells,

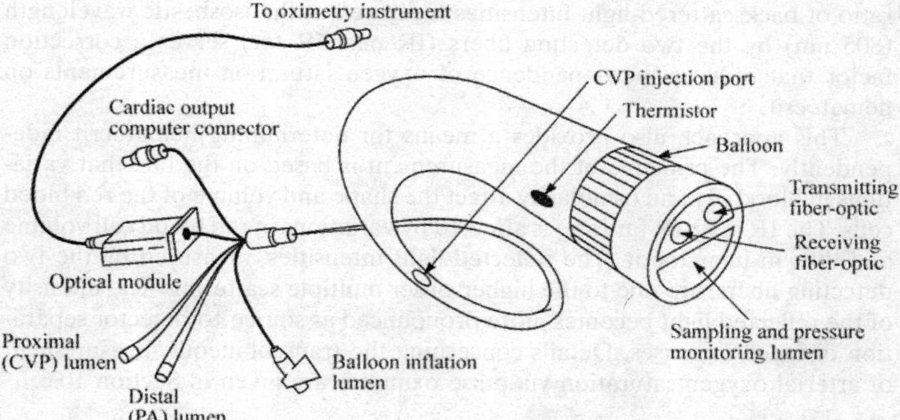


**Figure 10.8** The catheter used with the Abbott Opticath Oximetry System transmits light to the blood through a transmitting optical fiber and returns the reflected light through a receiving optical fiber. The catheter is optically connected to the oximetry processor through the optical module. (From Abbott Critical Care Systems. Used by permission.)

attenuated by the dye in the blood, and partially collected by the other fiber for measurement. The second wavelength, above 900 nm, is used as a reference; this is the region where the light is absorbed by the dye. It is used to compare the effect of flow-rate light scattering. In effect, a dual-beam ratiometric system is developed for dye-dilution measurements of blood flow. Cardiac output is determined via the dye-dilution method described in Section 8.2.

A significant difference exists between two-wavelength oximetry systems and the Abbott three-wavelength Oximetry Opticath System. In two-wavelength systems an important limitation, in the *in vivo* measurement of oxygen saturation below 80%, is the dependence of the reflected light's intensity on the patient's hematocrit. Hematocrit varies from subject to subject, and within one subject it varies for different physiological conditions. Catheter tip oximeters require frequent updates of a patient's hematocrit. Various correction techniques have been devised to correct the oxygen-saturation measurements for errors due to hematocrit variations. (This limitation is eliminated in the three-wavelength Abbott Opticath Oximetry System.) False readings occur in situations in which hemoglobin combines with another substance besides oxygen, such as carbon monoxide. Hemoglobin has a strong affinity for carbon monoxide, so oxygen is displaced. The optical spectra for $HbO_2$ and HbCO overlap at 660 nm (Figure 10.6), causing an error in $So_2$ if CO is present in the blood.

A three-fiber intravascular fiber-optic catheter that measures mixed venous oxygen saturation and hematocrit simultaneously has been developed and tested (Mendelson *et al.*, 1990). The system consists of a catheter with a single light source in two equally spaced, near and far detecting fibers. The ratio of backscattered-light intensities measured at the isosbestic wavelength (805 nm) by the two detecting fibers (IR near/IR far) serves a correction factor that reduces the dependence of oxygen-saturation measurements on hematocrit.

This approach also provides a means for determining hematocrit independently. The principle of the measurement is based on the fact that variations in blood pH and osmolarity affect the shape and volume of the red blood cells. The IR near/IR far ratio is affected by variations in red blood cell volume and thus in hematocrit. The reflected-light intensities, measured by the two detecting fibers, are due to the higher-order multiple scattering. The intensity of the reflected light becomes more pronounced as source-to-detector separation distance increases. Details concerning the transcutaneous measurement of arterial oxygen saturation via pulse oximetry are given in Section 10.6.

## REVERSIBLE-DYE OPTICAL MEASUREMENT OF pH

The continuous monitoring of blood pH is essential for the proper treatment of patients who have metabolic and respiratory problems. Small pH probes have been developed for intravascular measurement of the pH of the blood (Peterson *et al.*, 1980). These instruments require a range of 7.0 to 7.6 pH units and a resolution of 0.01 pH unit.

Figure 10.9 shows an early version of a pH sensor, in which a reversible colorimetric indicator system is fixed inside an ion-permeable envelope at the distal tip of the two plastic optical fibers. Light-scattering microspheres are mixed with the indicator dye inside the ion-permeable envelope in order to optimize the backscattering of light to the collection fiber that leads to the detector.

The reversible indicator dye, phenol red, is a typical pH-sensitive dye. The dye exists in two tautomeric (having different isomers) forms, depending on whether it is in an acidic or a basic solution. The two forms have different optical spectra. In Figure 10.10, the absorbance is plotted against wavelength for phenol red for the base form of the dye, indicating that the optical-

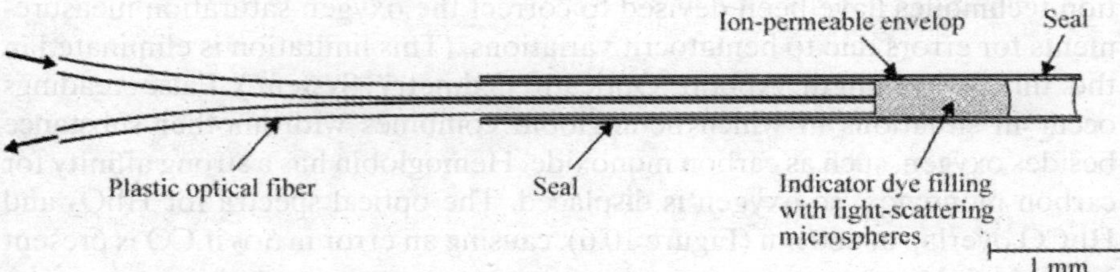


**Figure 10.9** A reversible fiber-optic chemical sensor measures light scattered from phenol red indicator dye to yield pH. [From J. I. Peterson, "Optical sensors," in J. G. Webster (ed.), Encyclopedia of Medical Devices and Instrumentation. New York: Wiley, 1988, pp. 2121–2133. Used by permission.]

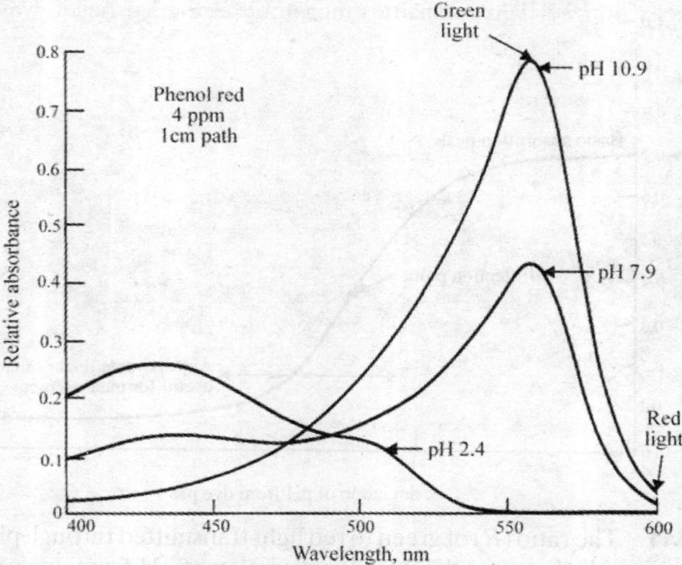


**Figure 10.10** The plot of absorbance against wavelength of phenol red (base form) increases with pH for green light but is constant for red light.

absorbance peak increases with increasing pH. The ratio of green to red light transmitted through the dye is (Peterson, 1988)

$$R = k \times 10^{\left[-C/\left(10^{-\Delta}+1\right)\right]} \tag{10.17}$$

where

$\Delta =$ difference between pH and pK of the dye

$R = I(\text{green})/I(\text{red})$ =measured ratio of light intensities

$k = I_0(\text{green})/I_0(\text{red})$ = a constant ($I_0$ = initial light intensity)

$C =$ a constant determined by (1) the probe geometry, (2) the total dye concentration, and (3) the absorption coefficient of the dye's basic tautomer

Equation (10.17) shows that the ratio of green to red light transmitted through the dye can be expressed as a function of (1) the ionization constant of the dye—that is, the $pK_a$ where "a" indicates the dye is a weak acid; (2) Beer's law for optical absorption; and (3) the use of the definition of pH. The constants are $k$, the optical constant; $A$, the absorbance of the probe when the dye is completely in the base form; and pK, the inverse log of the ionization constant of the dye. The ratio of green to red light is used because the green light transmitted varies with pH, whereas the red light is an isosbestic wavelength and does not vary with pH. In effect, this system is a dual-beam spectrometer.

Figure 10.11 shows a plot of $R$, the ratio of green to red light, against $\Delta$, the deviation of the pH from the pK of the dye. The curve shows that over a range

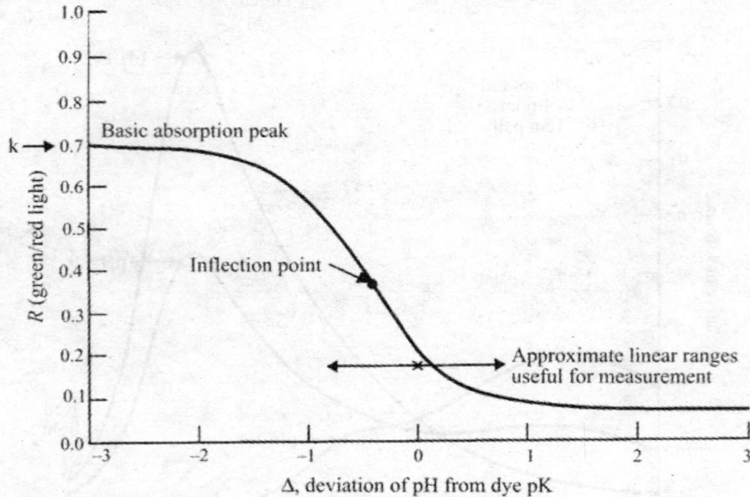


**Figure 10.11** The ratio ($R$) of green to red light transmitted through phenol red for basic and acidic forms of the dye. $\Delta$ =deviation of pH from dye pK. (From J. I. Peterson, S. R. Goldstein, and R. V. Fitzgerald, "Fiber-optic pH probe for physiological use." *Anal. Chem.*, 1980, 52, 864–869. Used by permission.)

of about 1 pH unit, a nearly linear region for the S-shaped curve results. The instrument for pH measurement via the fiber-optic sensor uses a 100 W quartz halogen light as the source, and a rotating filter wheel selects between green and red light to illuminate the sample under study. Light passes down the fiber-optic input fiber and is scattered from the polystyrene light-scattering microspheres so that adequate light is collected and sent back to the receiving fiber (Peterson and Vurek, 1984).

The green light returning to the sensor varies as a function of the pH, whereas the red light does not vary with pH. Because the red light is generated by the same source as the green light and travels the same optical path to the detector, any changes in the optical system are reflected in changes in the red light received by the detector. Thus, when the intensity of the green light received by the detector is divided by the intensity of the red light received, any changes in the optical system are compensated for by this ratiometric method.

## FLUORESCENCE OPTICAL pH SENSOR (IRREVERSIBLE)

Many colorimetric or fluorometric approaches are irreversible because of the tight binding between reagent and analyte or the formation of an irreversible product of the reaction. The pH sensor described below is based on irreversible chemistry, so either a long-lasting reagent or a continuous reagent-delivery system is necessary for long periods of operation. A fluorescence pH sensor based on the pH-sensitive dye hydroxypyrene trisulfonic acid (HPTS), which is a water-soluble fluorescent dye with a $pK_a$ of 7.0, has been used as an

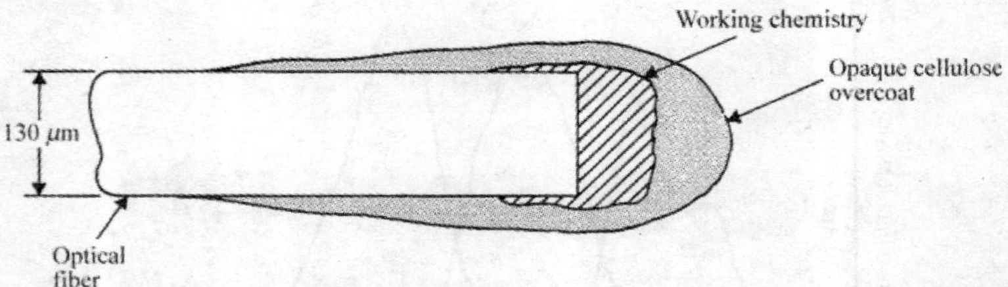


**Figure 10.12** A single-fiber intravascular blood-gas sensor excites fluorescent dye at one wavelength and detects emission at a different wavelength. The following modifications are made to the sensor tip: pH: Chemistry—pH-sensitive dye bound to hydrophilic matrix. $P\text{CO}_2$: Chemistry—Bicarbonate buffer containing pH-sensitive dye with silicone. $P\text{O}_2$: Chemistry—Oxygen-sensitive dye in silicone. (From J. L. Gehrich, D. W. Lübbers, N. Optiz, D. R. Hansmann, W. E. Miller, J. K. Tusa, and M. Yafuso, "Optical fluorescence and its application to an intravascular blood gas monitoring system," *IEEE Trans. Biomed. Eng.*, 1986, BME-33, 117–132. Used by permission.)

intravascular blood-gas probe for pH (Gehrich *et al.*, 1986). The pH-sensitivity range is approximately equal to $\text{pK}_a \pm 1$.

Figure 10.12 is a diagram of the intravascular blood-gas sensor, in which chemistries are covalently bonded through a cellulose matrix attached to the fiber tip. An opaque cellulose overcoat formed over the matrix provides mechanical integrity and optical isolation from the environment.

The underlying principle of fluorescent measurement is that fluorescent dyes emit light energy at a wavelength different from that of the excitation wavelength, which they absorb. This can be seen in Figure 10.13, which gives the fluorescence spectra of a pH-sensitive dye. The excitation peak wavelength for the acidic form of the dye is 410 nm, whereas the excitation peak wavelength for the basic form of the dye is 460 nm. It is also apparent that the emission spectra for both the acidic and the basic forms of the dye have a peak at 520 nm. Because of the separation between the excitation and emission wavelengths, it is possible to use a single optical fiber both for the delivery of light energy to the sensor and for its reception from that sensor.

Intravascular dye fluorescence sensors must be stable enough to maintain accuracy for up to three days of use within the patient. Cost and shelf life of this disposable product must also be considered. In addition, the dye must be able to follow physiological changes in the blood-gas parameters and thus must have sufficient dynamic range and time response (Gehrich *et al.*, 1986).

The ratiometric principle, or two-wavelength approach, is used to design an optical measurement system that is independent of system and other parameters, which include (1) loss of the optical signal as a result of fiber bending, (2) optical misalignment, and (3) other changes in the optical path that could be incorrectly interpreted as changes in the concentration of the analyte being measured. The ratiometric approach is undertaken by selecting fluorescent dyes with two absorption or emission peaks or by providing a

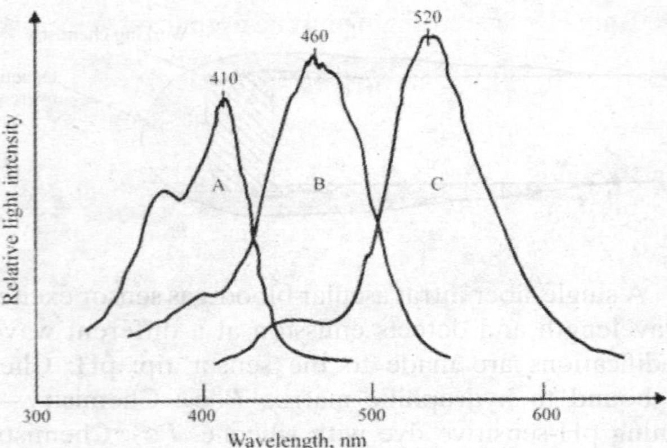


**Figure 10.13** This pH-sensitive dye is excited at 410 and 460 nm and fluoresces at 520 nm: (A) the excitation spectrum of the acidic form of the dye, (B) the excitation spectrum of the basic form of the dye, and (C) the emission spectrum of the acidic and basic forms of the dye. (From J. L. Gehrich, D. W. Lübbers, N. Optiz, D. R. Hansmann, W. E. Miller, J. K. Tusa, and M. Yafuso, "Optical fluorescence and its application to an intravascular blood gas monitoring system,"- *IEEE Trans. Biomed. Eng.*, 1986, BME-33, 117–132. Used by permission.)

mixture of dyes at the sensor tip, one that is sensitive to the measured parameter and one that is not (reference wavelength, which is affected only by the optical system parameters). In the foregoing example, the emission due to excitation at 410 nm represents the relative amount of the basic phase, and the emission due to excitation at 460 nm represents the relative amount of the acidic phase. The ratio of these phases represents the pH.

## FLUORESCENCE OPTICAL $P_{CO_2}$ SENSOR

The $P_{CO_2}$ sensor uses the same pH-sensitive fluorescent dye as the pH sensor described before. The operation of this sensor is similar to that of the electrochemical Severinghaus $P_{CO_2}$ electrode described in the previous section in that a pH-type sensor is used as the basic sensing element to detect $P_{CO_2}$. Carbon dioxide comes to equilibrium with a mixture of a pH indicator in bicarbonate buffer. There is a direct relationship, based on the Henderson–Hasselbach equation, between the pH change in a bicarbonate solution and the $CO_2$ concentration in that solution. Thus a change in pH in an isolated bicarbonate buffer with a changing $P_{CO_2}$ is measured. This buffer is encapsulated by a hydrophobic gas-permeable silicone matrix that provides ionic isolation and mechanical stability for the measurement system.

As before, an optical cellulose overcoat ensures optical isolation of the sensor chemistry from the environment. $CO_2$ equilibrates rapidly across the silicone membrane and causes a change in the pH. The concentration of the bicarbonate buffer is selected such that a sufficient pH change is detectable with appropriate accuracy and sensitivity over the physiological range for $CO_2$, which is 10 to 100 mm Hg. Dye strength must be optimized to increase the signal-to-noise ratio, and there is a trade-off between ionic strength and pK.

## FLUORESCENCE OPTICAL $P_{O_2}$ SENSOR

One approach for a fiber-optic $P_{O_2}$, or oxygen partial pressure, sensor makes use of the principle of fluorescence or luminescence quenching of oxygen. In this quenching process, energy is absorbed and lost by various processes, such as vibration of the molecule (heat) and emission of the light as fluorescence or phosphofluorescence. With oxygen present, these molecules provide collision paths and transfer of energy to the oxygen molecule, which competes with the energy decay modes, and luminescence is decreased by the increasing loss of energy to oxygen.

Figure 10.14 shows the fluorescent spectra of oxygen-sensitive dye for both the excitation and the emission.

The $P_{O_2}$ probe is similar in design to the pH sensor. The principle of its operation is that when these fluorescent quenching dyes are irradiated by light at an appropriate wavelength, they fluoresce in a nonoxygen atmosphere for a given period of time. However, when oxygen is present the fluorescence is quenched—that is, the dye fluoresces for a shorter period of time. The period of dye fluorescence is inversely proportional to the partial pressure of oxygen in the environment. This leads to a poor signal-to-noise ratio at high $P_{O_2}$ values, because the high $O_2$ levels quench the luminescence, which results in a small signal at the detector. In Figure 10.15, fibers and inert beads are enclosed in an oxygen-permeable hydrophobic sheet such as porous polypropylene.

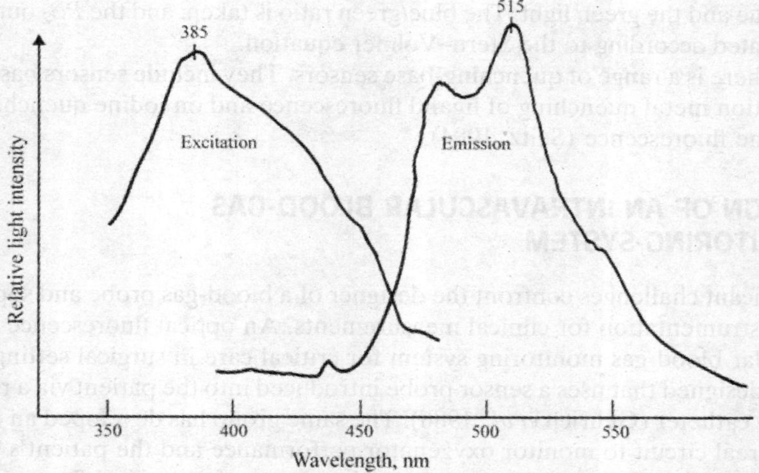


**Figure 10.14** The emission spectrum of oxygen-sensitive dye can be separated from the excitation spectrum by a filter. (From J. L. Gehrich, D. W. Lübbers, N. Opitz, D. R. Hansmann, W. W. Miller, J. K. Tusa, and M. Yafuso, "Optical fluorescence and its application to an intravascular blood gas monitoring system," *IEEE Trans. Biomed. Eng.*, 1986, BME-33. 117–132. Used by permission.)

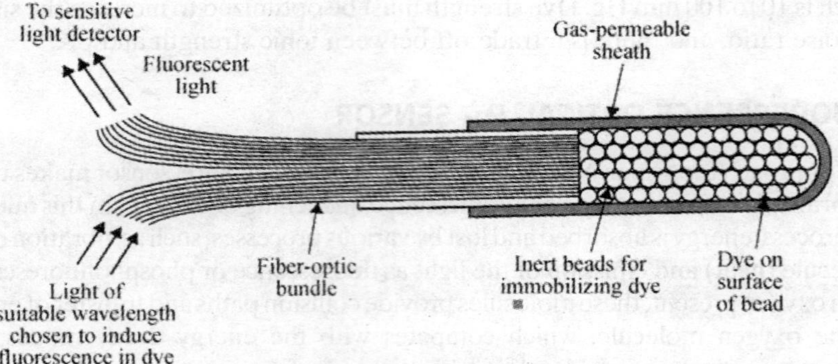


**Figure 10.15** In a fiber-optic oxygen sensor, irradiation of dyes causes fluorescence that decreases with $P_{O_2}$. [From R. Kocache "Oxygen analyzers." in J. G. Webster (ed.), Encyclopedia of Medical Devices and Instrumentation. New York: Wiley, 1988, pp. 2154–2161. Used by permission.]

The $P_{O_2}$-measurement instrument includes both optical and electronic systems. The instrumentation system as designed uses plastic optical fibers because of their mechanical strength and flexibility; they allow for a sharp bending radius. The light returning from the sensor passes through a dichroic filter, which separates the green fluorescent light from the blue excitation light, and the latter is scattered by the probe back into the return fiber. Photomultiplier tubes are used in this application to convert the light signal into a current, and then a current-to-voltage converter is used to provide the voltage proportional to the blue and the green light. The blue/green ratio is taken, and the $P_{O_2}$ output is calculated according to the Stern–Volmer equation.

There is a range of quenching-base sensors. They include sensors based on transition metal quenching of ligand fluorescence and on iodine quenching of rubrene fluorescence (Seitz, 1984).

## DESIGN OF AN INTRAVASCULAR BLOOD-GAS MONITORING SYSTEM

Significant challenges confront the designer of a blood-gas probe and supporting instrumentation for clinical measurements. An optical fluorescence intravascular blood-gas monitoring system for critical care in surgical settings has been designed that uses a sensor probe introduced into the patient via a radial-artery catheter (Gehrich *et al.*, 1986). The same group has developed an extracorporeal circuit to monitor oxygenator performance and the patient's status during cardiopulmonary bypass surgery by means of an optical fluorescence-based blood-gas monitoring system. The following discussion deals with the development of an intravascular blood-gas monitoring system intended for continuous monitoring of arterial pH, $P_{CO_2}$, and $P_{O_2}$ in critical-care and surgical settings. The fluorescence-based blood-gas probe is introduced into the patient's vasculature by means of the radial-artery catheter. This approach is normally used for drawing blood-gas samples and for arterial pressure measurements (see Section 7.1).

## SYSTEM DESIGN CONSIDERATIONS

The system design considerations are given for the intravascular blood-gas monitoring system, which comprises a blood-gas probe, an optoelectronic instrument, and a probe calibration (Gehrich *et al.*, 1986).

***Blood-Gas Probe Design*** The design requirements for an ideal blood-gas probe include the following: (1) operating temperature range of 15 °C to 42 °C, (2) pH from 6.8 to 7.8, (3) $P\text{CO}_2$ from 10 to 100 mm Hg, and (4) $P\text{O}_2$ from 20 to 300 mm Hg. The $P\text{O}_2$ value may reach 500 mm Hg for procedures that require high levels of supplemental oxygen, such as open-heart surgery. The probe must be fabricated from materials that are sterilizable and biocompatible. Carcinogenicity and toxicity must be avoided, and the blood-contact surfaces must exhibit nonthrombogenic and nonhemolytic properties.

One of the most significant requirements in designing an intravascular probe is that it not be affected by such naturally occurring substances as proteins in the blood and those introduced during the surgical or therapeutic procedures (Regnault and Picciolo, 1987). In addition, the probe must be immune to absorption of the components in the blood and to their deposition on the sensor surfaces. The probe must have a small diameter so that it can be introduced into the radial artery. At the same time, blood pressure must be measured through the lumen of the blood-gas probe.

***Mechanical Design Considerations*** Figure 10.16 shows the design of the intravascular blood-gas probe. It consists of three single fiber-optic sensors and a thermocouple integral to a polymer structure that achieves the required strength. Fused silicon fibers are used for the three fiber-optic sensors, which measure pH, $P\text{CO}_2$, and $P\text{O}_2$, respectively. The thermocouple gives a direct

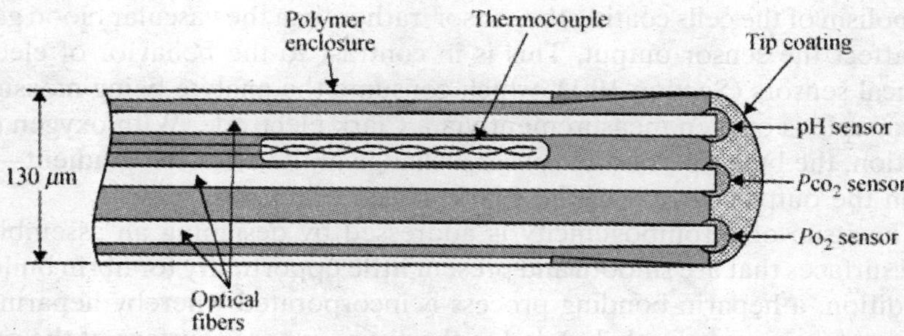


**Figure 10.16** An intravascular blood-gas probe measure pH, $P\text{CO}_2$, and $P\text{O}_2$ by means of single fiber-optic fluorescent sensors. (From J. L. Gehrich, D. W. Lübbers, N. Optiz, D. R. Hansmann, W. W. Miller, J. K. Tusa, and M. Yafuso, "Optical fluorescence and its application to an intravascular blood gas monitoring system," *IEEE Trans. Biomed. Eng.*, 1986, BME-33, 117–132. Used by permission.)

readout of the probe and of blood temperature at the probe tip. Temperature measurements are important in that the blood solubility of $O_2$ and $CO_2$ are temperature dependent. In addition, the fluorescence chemistry varies slightly with temperature and requires temperature compensation. *In vitro* blood-gas measurements in a laboratory are standardized to the normal body temperature of 37 °C. In the case of the intravascular blood-gas measurement system, the patient's core temperature during surgery may vary from hypothermia (say, 15 °C) to hyperthermia (say, 42 °C). The operator of the instrument must know the patient's temperature in order to make adjustments and report blood-gas values at the standardized temperature of 37 °C.

It is essential that the catheter be small, because the intravascular blood-gas probe will be inserted into a radial-artery catheter of a size consistent with clinical practice. That is, it must be possible to determine blood pressure, as well as to withdraw blood-gas samples, with the catheter in place. A viable blood pressure signal can be maintained by using a 20-gage radial-artery catheter if the diameter of the blood-gas probe is limited to 600 μm. With the probe described in Figure 10.16, this restricts the fiber diameter to 130 μm when three optical fibers and a thermocouple are included.

A major challenge is the selection of nontoxic materials the physical configuration and composition of which minimize the formation of blood clots on the blood-contact surfaces. This is important in order to prevent blockage of the residual lumen between the probe and catheter wall, which would compromise blood pressure measurements, and to reduce the risk that an embolus might form, slough off the probe/catheter, and cause trauma "downstream" in a cerebral or pulmonary capillary bed. In addition, formation of a thrombus at the site of the fluorescence sensors would affect the blood-gas measurement itself (Gehrich *et al.*, 1986).

This last issue is of least concern, because the fluorescence sensors are characterized as equilibrium sensors; that is, the parameter being measured is in equilibrium with the dye but is not being consumed. Thus thrombosis buildup on the probe would increase the time response of the sensors but would not affect the equilibrium accuracy. It has been proposed that the local metabolism of the cells coating the sensor, rather than the vascular blood gases, may affect the sensor output. This is in contrast to the behavior of electrochemical sensors (Section 10.1), which consume the analyte being measured. An example is oxygen measurement via a Clark electrode. With oxygen consumption, the buildup of fibrin causes a change in the diffusion gradient—and thus in the output current of the Clark oxygen electrode.

The issue of thrombogenicity is addressed by designing an assembly of blood surfaces that are smooth and present little opportunity for fibrin buildup. In addition, a heparin-bonding process is incorporated whereby heparin (an anticoagulant) is covalently bonded to the entire exposed surface of the probe (Gehrich *et al.*, 1986).

***Fluorescence Sensor Design*** The system design requires a single optical fiber for both the delivery of light energy to the sensor dye and its reception from that dye. Two fibers are not necessary, because the sensor input and output signals are of different wavelengths. The design challenge is to select dyes that offer the appropriate absorption and emission wavelength characteristics, are nontoxic, can be attached to an optical fiber, have sufficient sensitivity to the physiological parameters being measured, and exhibit high fluorescent intensity for signal strength over the physiological measurement range of interest. In addition, fluorescent dyes must not be affected by drugs or other blood constituents and must be stable enough to maintain accuracy for up to 3 days. Because this dye is a disposable product, consideration must also be given to its cost and shelf life. Finally, the dye must have a dynamic time response such that physiological changes in the blood-gas parameters can be followed (Gehrich *et al.*, 1986).

***Instrument Design*** The intravascular blood-gas system instrument design has three sections (Gehrich *et al.*, 1986). The first section is an analyzer module; the second is a patient interface module (PIM); and the third is the display. The illuminator consists of a broadband xenon-arc source lamp (350 to 750 nm), a collimating lens system, a filter wheel, and a condensing lens to direct the xenon emission onto the interface fibers. The xenon arc and filter wheel are synchronized at a flash rate of 20 Hz. The pulsating light source provides a more stable energy source than can be achieved with a constant, steady-state input signal. Light energy at specific wavelengths travels along the fiber optics to the PIM and is coupled by the graded index (GRIN) lens to the interface optics.

In order to maximize the energy delivered to and from each fiber-optic sensor, the following design approach was taken: (1) The number of optical connections was kept to a minimum. (2) The length of the fibers, especially those returning the fluorescent energy from the sensors, was kept to a minimum. (3) Transduction of the optical signal to an electric signal was made to occur at the distal end of the subsystem as near as possible to the patient. (4) The analog front-end circuitry in the PIM was located such that the analog signal is converted into a digital signal and multiplexed and then sent along approximately 4 m of cable to the analyzer section. All signals are normalized against the intensity, and ratiometric techniques are used to compare the active fluorescence wavelength to the reference wavelength before the blood-gas concentration is calculated.

***Calibration Device*** For all blood-gas detection systems, it is essential that an independent calibration of the probe be made prior to its use in the patient. This is done by utilizing tonometric techniques and a fluid-filled calibration cuvette that is an integral part of the packaging of the probe, in that the sensors must remain hydrated. The calibration device uses two gas cylinders, each with appropriate, precisely controlled values of oxygen and carbon dioxide (Gehrich *et al.*, 1986).

## 10.4 ION-SENSITIVE FIELD-EFFECT TRANSISTOR

The potential for low-cost, reliable microminiature sensors that utilizes ion-sensitive field-effect transistors (ISFETs) was first recognized over 30 years ago (Bergveld, 1970). Ion-sensitive field-effect transistors employ the same electrochemical principles in their measurement as ion-sensitive electrodes (ISE). The ISFET is produced by removal of the metal gate region that is normally present on a FET (Rolfe, 1988).

A metal oxide–semiconductor field-effect transistor (MOSFET) is composed of two diodes separated by a gate region. The gate is a thin insulator—usually silicon dioxide—upon which a metallic material is deposited. This gate material can be any conducting material that is compatible with IC processing. Voltage applied to the gate controls the electric field in the dielectric and thus the charge on the silicon surface. This field effect is the basis of operation of the MOSFET and ISFET. The high-input impedance results from the gate insulator, which is essential for operation of the ISFET device (Janata, 1989).

Figure 10.17(a) is a schematic diagram of an ISFET with the sample under measurement in contact with an ion-selective membrane and a reference electrode. To improve the pH-sensitivity and stability of the silicon dioxide layer, a silicon nitride layer is placed over the silicon dioxide.

The potential developed across the insulator depends on the electrolyte concentration of the solution in contact with the ion-selective membrane. The ISFET measures the potential at the gate; this potential is derived through an ion-selective process, in which ions passing through the ion-selective membrane modulate the current between the source and the drain. The voltage across the gate region changes, and thus the field-effect transistor current flows (Arnold and Meyerhoff, 1988).

The ISFET is of considerable interest because it offers the potential for low-cost microminiature sensors. These devices can be produced by microfabrication of silicon integrated circuits (ICs). Figure 10.17(b) shows a plan view, with dimensions, for a microfabricated ISFET. The IC manufacturing technology makes use of photolithographic techniques for producing unique properties of IC silicon substrates. ISFETs are particularly attractive, because they can be made in very small sizes and because multiple analytes can be measured on a single chip. Note that ISFET sensors are in the development stage.

In one device for measuring $CO_2$, an Ag/AgCl reference is incorporated on the ISFET chip, and polyvinyl alcohol gel (which contains NaCl and $NaHCO_3$) is deposited over the ISFET and reference (Rolfe, 1990). These regions are then coated with a thin silicone resin. Measurements have been made for a 24 h period for intravascular experiments with animals and humans. However, encapsulation problems arose. Other ISFET sensors have been developed for potassium ion measurements; here the gate region is covered with a glass potassium-selective membrane or with a balinomycin–PVC polymer membrane. Figure 10.18 is a plot of drain current versus potassium ion activity for an ISFET. Calcium ISFET sensors have been developed to monitor $Ca^{2+}$ activity in venous blood of dogs.

The initial use of ISFETs will involve small volumes of analytes and measurement times of only a few seconds (Hammond and Cumming, 2006). This measurement speed is fast compared to the several minutes required in a typical laboratory analysis. ISFETs are suited for monitoring blood

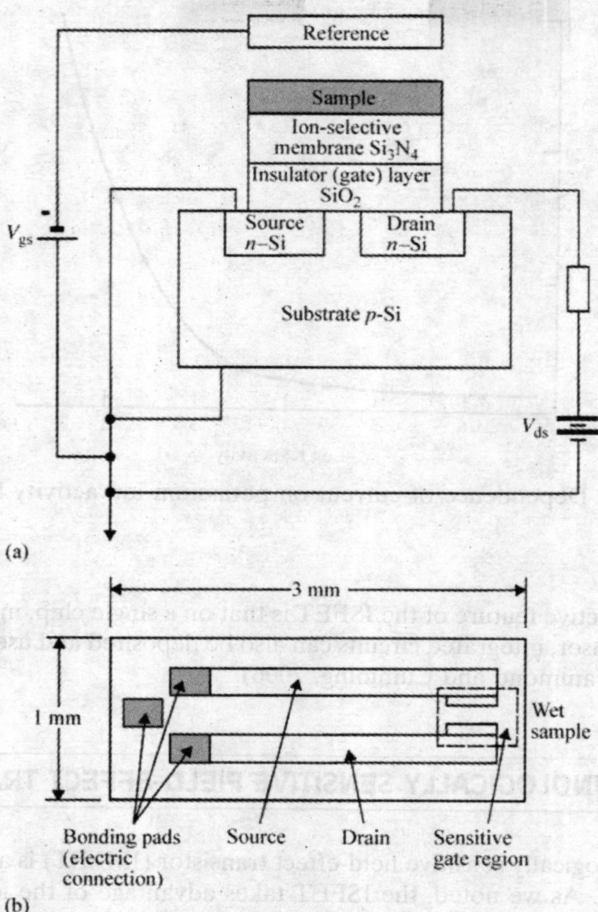


**Figure 10.17** (a) In a chemically sensitive field-effect transistor, the ion-selective membrane modulates the current between the source and the drain. (b) A stretched ISFET maximizes the spacing between the "wet" sample region and the electric connections. (Part (b) from P. Rolfe, "In vivo chemical sensors for intensive-care monitoring," *Med. Biol. Eng. Comput.*, 1990, 28. Used by permission.)

electrolytes and could perhaps be used for measurements inside a cell, provided that workable fabrication techniques are developed.

The main challenge of designing ISFET devices is satisfactory encapsulation of the ISFETs in order to protect the electric characteristics of the ISFET, which deteriorate as a result of water vapor entering from the environment.

Multiple-species ISFETs for up to eight different sensors have been fabricated on silicon chips a few square millimeters in size. In addition, probes 50 μm in diameter have been fabricated for on-chip circuitry that can measure pH, glucose, oxygen saturation, and pressure for biomedical applications.

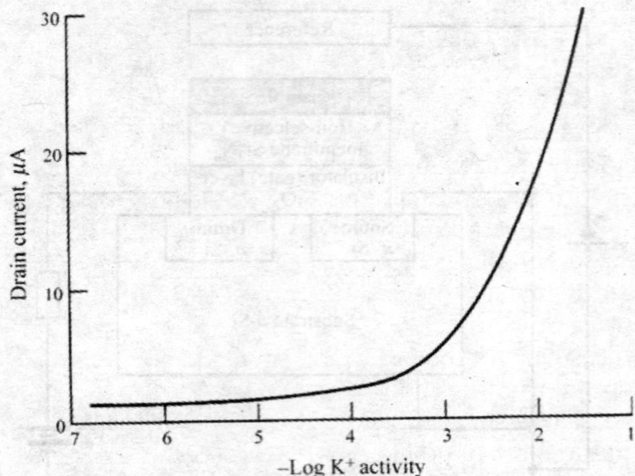


**Figure 10.18** Dependence of current on potassium ion activity for a potassium ISFET.

Another attractive feature of the ISFET is that on a single chip, in addition to the ISFET sensor, integrated circuits can also be deposited and used for signal processing (Hammond and Cumming, 2006).

## 10.5 IMMUNOLOGICALLY SENSITIVE FIELD-EFFECT TRANSISTOR

The immunologically sensitive field-effect transistor (IMFET) is an extension of the ISFET. As we noted, the ISFET takes advantage of the ion-sensitive or chemical sensitive properties of the field-effect transistor. As described above, the ISFET design makes use of the properties of the metal-insulator-semiconductor structure, in which the gate metal layer and the semiconductor layer form a capacitive sandwich by framing an insulating layer—normally $SiO_2$. Essentially, the system is a capacitor with a totally impermeable dielectric through which no charge passes.

The IMFET is similar in structure to the ISFET except that the solution-membrane interface is polarized rather than unpolarized; that is, charged species cannot cross the membrane (Zachariah *et al.*, 2006). The ISFET interacts through an ion-exchange mechanism with the chemical analyte that is being measured, whereas the IMFET operation is based on an antigen–antibody reaction. An antibody is immobilized on the membrane that is attached to the insulator of a FET. In this way the device is used as an antigen sensor. An antibody could be detected in a similar way: by immobilizing an antigen on the membrane. The IMFET measures charge, so in order to be sensed, the absorbing species on the membrane must possess a net electric charge.

## 10.6 NONINVASIVE BLOOD-GAS MONITORING

Blood-gas determination can provide valuable information about the efficiency of pulmonary gas exchange, the adequacy of alveolar ventilation, blood-gas transport, and tissue oxygenation. Although invasive techniques to determine arterial blood gases are still widely practiced in many clinical situations, it is becoming apparent that simple, real-time, continuous, and noninvasive techniques offer many advantages. Most important, intermittent blood sampling provides historical data valid only at the time the sample was drawn. Delays between when the blood sample is drawn and when the blood-gas values are reported average about 30 min. Furthermore, invasive techniques are painful and have associated risks.

These limitations are particularly serious in critically ill patients for whom close monitoring of arterial blood gases is essential. Continuous noninvasive monitoring of blood gases, on the other hand, makes it possible to recognize changes in tissue oxygenation immediately and to take corrective action before irreversible cell damage occurs.

Various noninvasive techniques for monitoring arterial $O_2$ and $CO_2$ have been developed. This section describes the basic sensor principles, instrumentation, and clinical applications of the noninvasive monitoring of arterial oxygen saturation ($SO_2$), oxygen tension ($PO_2$), and carbon dioxide tension ($PCO_2$).

### SKIN CHARACTERISTICS

In order to appreciate the challenges of noninvasive measurement of the blood chemistry, it is important to understand the structure of the human skin. The human skin has three principal layers: the stratum corneum, epidermis, and dermis (Mendelson and Peura, 1984). These layers form a cohesive structure that typically varies in thickness from 0.2 to 2 mm, depending on the position on the body. Figure 5.7 is a schematic diagram that represents a cross section of the human skin.

The stratum corneum is the nonliving, outer layer of the skin. It is composed of a supple, protective layer of dehydrated cells. The nonvascular epidermis layer is a living tissue underneath the stratum corneum. It consists of proteins, lipids, and the melanin-forming cells (melanocytes) that give skin its color. The average thickness of the epidermis is 0.1 to 0.2 mm.

Dense connective tissue, hair follicles, sweat glands, nerve endings, fat cells, and a profuse system of capillaries make up the dermis. Here vertical capillary loops approximately 200 to 400 μm in length provide nutrients for the upper layers of the skin. Blood is supplied to these capillaries by arterioles that form a flat network parallel to the surface of the skin below the dermis. Larger arteries located in the subcutaneous tissue supply these arterioles. Venous blood in the skin is drained by venules in the upper and middle dermis and by larger veins in the subcutaneous tissue.

Arteriovenous anastomoses are innervated by nerve fibers. These shunts are found largely in the dermis of the palms, ears, and face. They regulate blood flow through the skin in response to heat; blood flow through these channels can increase to nearly 30 times the basal rate. Normal gas diffusion through the skin is low, but with increased heat—at 40 °C and above—the skin becomes more permeable to gases.

## TRANSCUTANEOUS ARTERIAL OXYGEN SATURATION MONITORING (PULSE OXIMETRY)

Attempts to apply the nonpulsed two-wavelengths approach that we have discussed, which was successful for intravascular oximetry applications, to the transilluminated ear or fingertip resulted in unacceptable errors due to light attenuation by tissue and blood absorption, refraction, and multiple scattering. In addition, because of differences in the properties of skin and tissue, variation from individual to individual in attenuation of light caused large calibration problems. Oximeters can be used to measure $So_2$ noninvasively by passing light through the pinna of the ear (Merrick and Hayes, 1976). Because of the complications caused by the light-absorbing characteristics of skin pigment and other absorbers, measurements are made at eight wavelengths and are computer-processed. The ear is warmed to 41 °C to stimulate arterial blood flow.

A two-wavelength transmission noninvasive pulse oximeter was introduced (Yoshiya *et al.*, 1980). This instrument determines $So_2$ by analyzing the time-varying, or ac, component of the light transmitted through the skin during the systolic phase of the blood flow in the tissue (Figure 10.19). This approach achieves measurement of the arterial oxygen content with only two

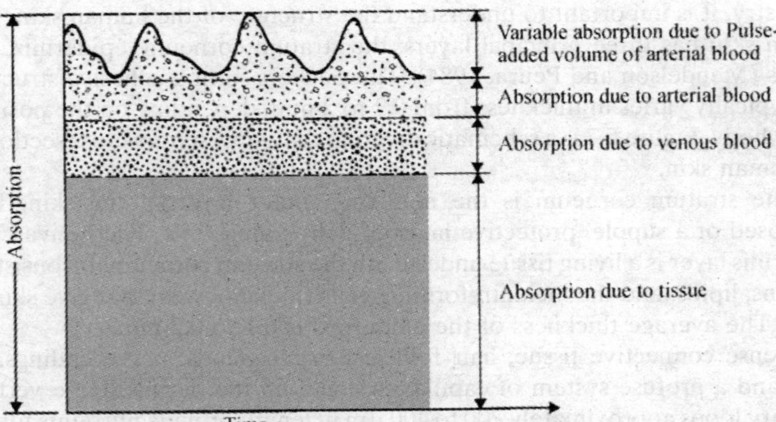


**Figure 10.19** The pulse oximeter analyzes the light absorption at two wavelengths of only the pulse-added volume of oxygenated arterial blood. [From Y. M. Mendelson, "Blood gas measurement, transcutaneous,"in J. G. Webster (ed.), *Encyclopedia of Medical Devices and Instrumentation.* New York: Wiley, 1988, pp. 448–459. Used by permission.]

wavelengths (660 and 940 nm, for instance). The dc component of the transmitted light, which represents light absorption by the skin pigments and other tissues, is used to normalize the ac signals.

A transcutaneous reflectance oximeter based on a similar photoplethysmographic technique has been developed (Mendelson *et al.*, 1983). The advantage of the reflectance oximeter is that it can monitor $So_2$ transcutaneously at various locations on the body surface, including more central locations (such as the chest, forehead, and limbs) that are not accessible via conventional transmission oximetry.

Because of these and other significant improvements in the instruments, measurements of ear, toe, and fingertip oximetry are widely used. Noninvasive measurements of $So_2$ can be made with 2.5% accuracy for saturation values from 50% to 100%.

***Transcutaneous So₂ Sensor*** The basic transcutaneous $So_2$ sensor, for both the transmission and the reflective mode, makes use of a light source and a photodiode. In the transmission mode, the two face each other and a segment of the body is interposed; in the reflection mode, the light source and photodiode are mounted adjacent to each other on the surface of the body (Webster, 1997).

Figure 10.20 shows an example of a transcutaneous transmission $So_2$ sensor and monitor. These transmission sensors are placed on the fingertips, toes, ear lobes, or nose. A pair of red and infrared light-emitting diodes are used for the light source, with peak emission wavelengths of 660 nm (red) and 940 nm (infrared). These detected signals are processed, in the form of transmission photoplethysmograms, by the oximeter, which determines the $So_2$.

***Applications of So₂ Monitoring*** As we have noted, the applications of noninvasive $So_2$ monitoring have blossomed rapidly to the point where it has become the standard of clinical care in a number of areas. Direct assessment and trending of the adequacy of tissue oxygenation can be made by determining the $So_2$ value. Oximetry is applied during the administration of anesthesia, pulmonary function tests, bronchoscopy, intensive care, and oral surgery and in neonatal monitoring, sleep apnea studies, and aviation medicine.

Noninvasive oximetry is also used in the home for monitoring self-administered oxygen therapy. Noninvasive oximetry provides time-averaged blood oxygenation values and can be used to determine when immediate therapeutic intervention is necessary. A lightweight (less than 3 g) and small (20 mm diameter) optical sensor makes this transcutaneous reflectance sensor appropriate for monitoring newborns, ambulatory patients, and patients in whom a digit or earlobe is not accessible. Problems with both transmission and reflectance oximetry include poor signal with shock, interference from lights in the environment and from the presence of carboxyhemoglobin, and poor trending of transients (Payne and Severinghaus, 1986, Moyle, 1994).

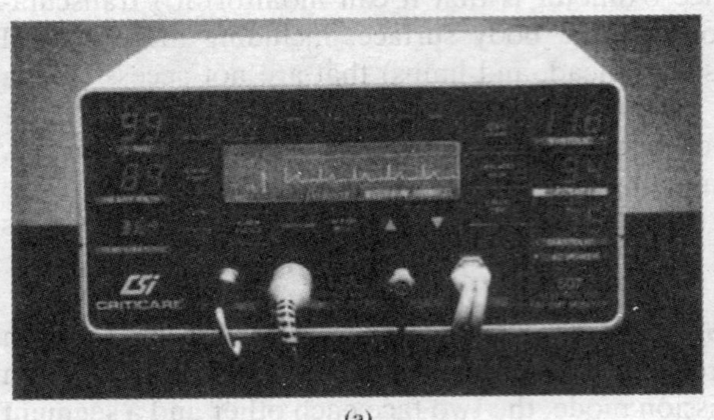

(a)

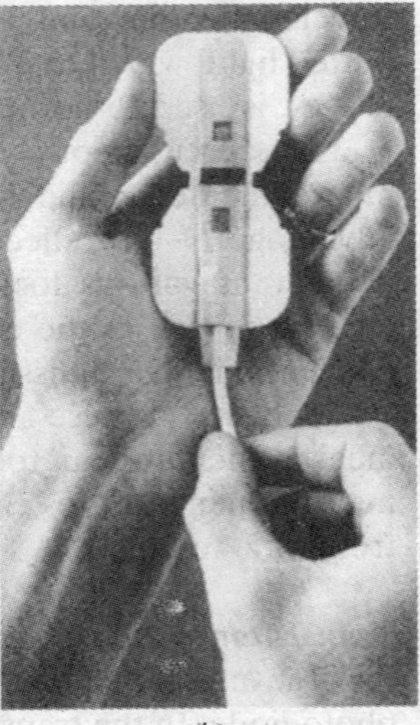

(b)

**Figure 10.20** (a) Noninvasive patient monitor capable of measuring ECG, noninvasive blood pressure (using automatic oscillometry), respiration (using impedance pneumography), transmission pulse oximetry, and temperature. (From Criticare Systems, Inc. Used by permission.) (b) Disposable transmission $SO_2$ sensor in open position. Note the light sources and detector, which can be placed on each side of the finger. (From Datascope Corporation. Used by permission.)

## TRANSCUTANEOUS ARTERIAL OXYGEN TENSION (tc$PO_2$) Monitoring

Measurement of tc$PO_2$ is similar in principle to the conventional in vitro $PO_2$ determination we have described. A Clark electrode is used in a sensor unit that is placed in contact with the skin. The oxygen electrode principle of operation has already been discussed.

Only two known gas mixtures are required to calibrate the sensor, because the relationship between $O_2$-dependent current and $PO_2$ is linear. Two calibration procedures are commonly used. One employs two precision medical gas mixtures, such as nitrogen and oxygen. The other employs sodium sulfite, which is a "zero-$O_2$ solution," and ambient air. Good stability of the sensor is usually maintained; a drift of 1 to 2 mm Hg/h for the tc$PO_2$ sensor is typical.

***Transcutaneous $PO_2$ Sensor*** Figure 10.21 shows a cross-sectional view of a typical Clark-type tc$PO_2$ sensor in which three glass-sealed Pt cathodes are separately connected via current amplifiers to an Ag/AgCl anode ring (Huch and Huch, 1976). A buffered KC1 electrolyte, which has a low water content to reduce drying of the sensor during storage, is used to provide a medium in which the chemical reactions can occur. Under normal physiological

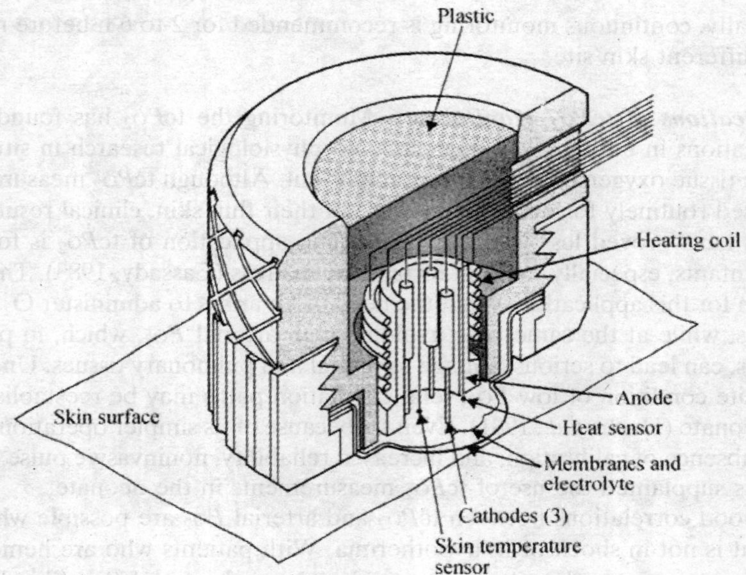


**Figure 10.21** Cross-sectional view of a transcutaneous oxygen sensor. Heating promotes arterialization. (From A. Huch and R. Huch, "Transcutaneous, noninvasive monitoring of $P\text{O}_2$," *Hospital Practice*, 1976, 6, 43–52. Used by permission.)

conditions, the $P\text{O}_2$ at the skin surface is essentially atmospheric regardless of the $P\text{O}_2$ in the underlying tissue.

Hyperemia of the skin causes the skin $P\text{O}_2$ to approach the arterial $P\text{O}_2$. Hyperemia can be induced by the administration of certain drugs, by the heating or abrasion of the skin, or by the application of nicotinic acid cream. Because heating gives the most readily controllable and consistent effect, a heating element and a thermistor sensor are used to control the skin temperature beneath the tc$P\text{O}_2$ sensor. Sufficient arterialization results when the skin is heated to temperatures between 43 °C and 44 °C. These temperatures cause minimal skin damage, but with neonates it is still necessary to reposition the sensor frequently to avoid burns.

Heating the skin has two beneficial effects: $O_2$ diffusion through the stratum corneum increases, and vasodilation of the dermal capillaries increases blood flow to skin at the sensor site where the heat is applied. Increased blood flow delivers more $O_2$ to the heated skin region, making the excess $O_2$ diffuse through the skin more easily. As Figure 10.1 suggests, heating the blood also causes the ODC to shift to the right, resulting in a decreased binding of Hb with $O_2$. Accordingly, the amount of $O_2$ released to the cells for a given $P\text{O}_2$ is increased. Note that heat also increases local tissue $O_2$ consumption, which tends to decrease oxygen levels in the skin tissue. Opportunely, these two opposing factors approximately cancel each other. Duration of monitoring is a function of the skin's sensitivity to possible burns, as well as to electrode drift.

Typically, continuous monitoring is recommended for 2 to 6 h before moving to a different skin site.

***Applications of tc$P$o$_2$ Monitoring*** Monitoring the tc$P$o$_2$ has found many applications in both clinical medicine and physiological research in situations where tissue oxygenation values are important. Although tc$P$o$_2$ measurements are used routinely for neonates because of their thin skin, clinical results with adults have proved less valuable. The prime application of tc$P$o$_2$ is for newborn infants, especially those in respiratory distress (Cassady, 1983). The main reason for this application is that the need often arises to administer $O_2$ to sick infants, while at the same time avoiding high arterial $P$o$_2$, which, in preterm infants, can lead to serious damage to retinal and pulmonary tissues. Under the opposite condition of low $P$o$_2$, fetal circulation paths may be reestablished in the neonate (Huch *et al.*, 1981). Even so, because of its simpler operation, lower cost, absence of calibration, and increased reliability, noninvasive pulse oximetry has supplanted the use of tc$P$o$_2$ measurements in the neonate.

Good correlations between tc$P$o$_2$ and arterial $P$o$_2$ are possible when the patient is not in shock or in hypothermia. With patients who are hemodynamically compromised, tc$P$o$_2$ does not always equal arterial $P$o$_2$. Skin heating in situations where there are significant decreases in skin blood perfusion cannot compensate for the low blood flow and the attendant low delivery of oxygen to the tissue. The result is low transcutaneous $P$o$_2$ readings. Examples of conditions in which skin perfusion is compromised—and tc$P$o$_2$ readings therefore do not represent tissue $P$o$_2$ values—include severe hypothermia, acidemia, anemia, and shock. Adult tc$P$o$_2$ values have not been found to equal arterial $P$o$_2$, even when the skin is heated to 45 °C. This is due to the greater skin thickness of the adult; heating of the skin to intolerably high temperatures would be necessary to compensate for the increased metabolism. Studies have, however, demonstrated the clinical usefulness of this technique for evaluating the adequacy of cutaneous circulation in patients with peripheral resuscitation (Huch *et al.*, 1981).

Maintaining the seal between the tc$P$o$_2$ probe and the skin surface can be a problem with long-term monitoring. If the seal is compromised, the sensor is exposed to the atmosphere and will yield a $P$o$_2$ of approximately 155 mm Hg, instead of lower physiological values.

## TRANSCUTANEOUS CARBON DIOXIDE TENSION (tc$P$co$_2$) MONITORING

Monitoring tc$P$co$_2$ gives more accurate results than tc$P$o$_2$ measurements in adult patients, because tc$P$co$_2$ measurements are much less dependent on skin blood flow.

***Transcutaneous $P$co$_2$ Sensor*** Figure 10.22 shows a typical tc$P$co$_2$ sensor, which is similar to a tc$P$o$_2$ sensor except for the sensing element. Its operation

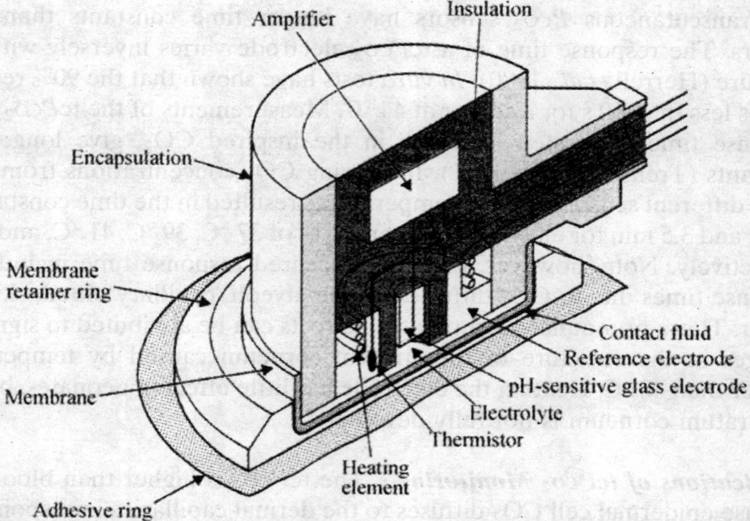


**Figure 10.22** Cross-sectional view of a transcutaneous carbon dioxide sensor. Heating the skin promotes arterialization. (From A. Huch, D. W. Lübbers, and R. Huch, "Patientenuberwachung durch transcutane $P\text{CO}_2$ Messung bei gleiechzeiliger koutrolle der relatiuen Iokalen perfusion," *Anaesthetist*, 1973, 22, 379. Used by permission.)

is similar to that of the electrochemical $P\text{CO}_2$ sensor described earlier. The $CO_2$ sensor is a glass pH electrode with a concentric Ag/AgCl reference electrode that is used as a heating element. The electrolyte, a bicarbonate buffer, is placed on the electrode surface. A $CO_2$-permeable Teflon membrane separates the sensor from its environment.

As we noted before, the tc$P\text{CO}_2$ sensor operates according to the Stow–Severinghaus principle; that is, a pH electrode senses a change in the $CO_2$ concentration. The system is calibrated with a known $CO_2$ concentration solution. Because a $CO_2$ electrode has a negative temperature coefficient, calibration must be performed at the temperature at which the device will be used. The effects of heating the skin beneath the tc$P\text{CO}_2$ sensor must be determined before the measurements can be properly interpreted.

Heating the skin beneath the sensor causes an increase in (1) $P\text{CO}_2$, because the solubility of $CO_2$ decreases with an increase in temperature; (2) local tissue metabolism, because cell metabolism is directly correlated with temperature; and (3) the rate of $CO_2$ diffusion through the stratum corneum, which increases with temperature. As a consequence of these three effects, which all work in the same direction to increase tc$P\text{CO}_2$ values, heating the skin yields tc$P\text{CO}_2$ values larger than the corresponding arterial $P\text{CO}_2$. Nevertheless, the correlation between tc$P\text{CO}_2$ and arterial $P\text{CO}_2$ is usually satisfactory. Because the slope of the $CO_2$ electrode calibration line is essentially that of the Nernst equation, a two-point calibration (as for the $P\text{O}_2$ electrode) is not needed.

Transcutaneous $P\text{CO}_2$ sensors have longer time constants than tc$P\text{O}_2$ sensors. The response time of a tc$P\text{CO}_2$ electrode varies inversely with temperature (Herrell *et al.*, 1980). *In vitro* tests have shown that the 90% response time is less than 60 s for a sensor at 44 °C. Measurements of the tc$P\text{CO}_2$ sensor response time, with step increases in the inspired $CO_2$, give longer time constants (Tremper *et al.*, 1981). Increasing $CO_2$ concentrations from 0% to 7% at different sensor and skin temperatures resulted in the time constants 15, 7.5, 5, and 3.5 min for electrode temperatures of 37 °C, 39 °C, 41 °C, and 44 °C, respectively. Note, however, that the measured response time included the response times due to $CO_2$ diffusion in the alveoli, capillary blood, skin, and sensor. These pronounced temperature effects can be attributed to significant changes in the structure of the stratum corneum caused by temperatures greater than 40 °C. Heating the electrode has little effect in neonates, because the stratum corneum is not fully developed.

***Applications of tc$P\text{CO}_2$ Monitoring*** The tc$P\text{CO}_2$ is higher than blood $P\text{CO}_2$ because epidermal cell $CO_2$ diffuses to the dermal capillaries in response to a diffusion gradient. A countercurrent-exchange mechanism in the dermal capillaries causes $CO_2$ diffusion between the parallel arterial and venous sides of the capillary bed. Arterial blood entering the rising segment of the capillary loop picks up $CO_2$ from the exiting venous side. As a consequence, the venous $P\text{CO}_2$ is lowered, and a maximal $P\text{CO}_2$ gradient is established at the top of the countercurrent capillary loops. Because of this phenomenon, $P\text{CO}_2$ at the skin surface is higher than venous $P\text{CO}_2$, even when the electrode is not heated (Tremper *et al.*, 1981).

Generally, it is accepted that tc$P\text{CO}_2$ is a valuable trend monitor in neonates and adults who are not in shock. Since arterial $P\text{CO}_2$ varies linearly with alveolar ventilation, tc$P\text{CO}_2$ provides information concerning the effectiveness of spontaneous or mechanical ventilation for individuals. The extent of impaired tissue perfusion, i.e. circulation to a limb, or response to therapy may be monitored by observing the change in tc$P\text{CO}_2$.

## 10.7 BLOOD-GLUCOSE SENSORS

Accurate measurement of blood glucose is essential in the diagnosis and long-term management of diabetes. This section reviews the use of biosensors for continuous measurement of glucose levels in blood and other body fluids.

Glucose is the main circulating carbohydrate in the body. In normal, fasting individuals, the concentration of glucose in blood is very tightly regulated—usually between 80 and 90 mg/100 ml, during the first hour or so following a meal. The hormone insulin, which is normally produced by beta cells in the pancreas, promotes glucose transport into skeletal muscle and adipose tissue. In those suffering from diabetes mellitus, insulin-regulated uptake is compromised, and blood glucose can reach concentrations ranging from 300 to 700 mg/100 ml (hyperglycemia).

Accurate determination of glucose levels in body fluids, such as blood, urine, and cerebrospinal fluid, is a major aid in diagnosing diabetes and improving the treatment of this disease. Blood glucose levels rise and fall several times a day, so it is difficult to maintain normoglycemia by means of an "open-loop" insulin delivery approach. One solution to this problem would be to "close the loop" by using a self-adapting insulin infusion device with a glucose-controlled biosensor that could continuously sense the need for insulin and dispense it at the correct rate and time. Unfortunately, present-day glucose sensors cannot meet this stringent requirement (Peura and Mendelson, 1984).

***Glucose Oxidase Method*** The glucose oxidase method used in a large number of commercially available simple test strip meters allows quick and easy blood glucose measurements. A test strip product, One Touch UltraMini (www.LifeScan.com), depends on the glucose oxidase–peroxidase chromogenic reaction. After a drop of blood is combined with reagents on the test strip, the reaction shown in (10.18) occurs.

$$\text{Glucose} + 2\text{H}_2\text{O} + \text{O}_2 \xrightarrow{\text{glucose oxidase}} \text{Gluconic Acid} + 2\text{H}_2\text{O}_2 \tag{10.18}$$

Adding the enzymes peroxidase and o-dianiside, a chromogenic oxygen, results in the formation of a colored compound that can be evaluated visually.

$$\text{o-dianisine} + \text{H}_2\text{O}_2 \xrightarrow{\text{peroxidase}} \text{oxidized o-dianisine} + \text{H}_2\text{O} \tag{10.19}$$

Glucose oxidase chemistry in conjunction with reflectance photometry produces a system for monitoring blood glucose levels (Burtis and Ashwood, 1994). In the One Touch system (Figure 10.23), a test strip is inserted into the meter, a drop of blood is applied to end of the test strip, and a digital screen displays the results 5 s later.

***Electroenzymatic Approach*** Electroenzymatic sensors based on polarographic principles utilize the phenomenon of glucose oxidation with a glucose oxidase enzyme (Clark and Lyons, 1962). The chemical reaction of glucose with oxygen is catalyzed in the presence of glucose oxidase. This causes a decrease in the partial pressure of oxygen ($Po_2$), an increase in pH, and the production of hydrogen peroxide by the oxidation of glucose to gluconic acid according to equation (10.18).

Investigators measure changes in all of these chemical components in order to determine the concentration of glucose. The basic glucose enzyme electrode utilizes a glucose oxidase enzyme immobilized on a membrane or a gel matrix, and an oxygen-sensitive polarographic electrode. Changes in oxygen concentration at the electrode, which are due to the catalytic reaction of glucose and oxygen, can be measured either amperometrically or potentiometrically.

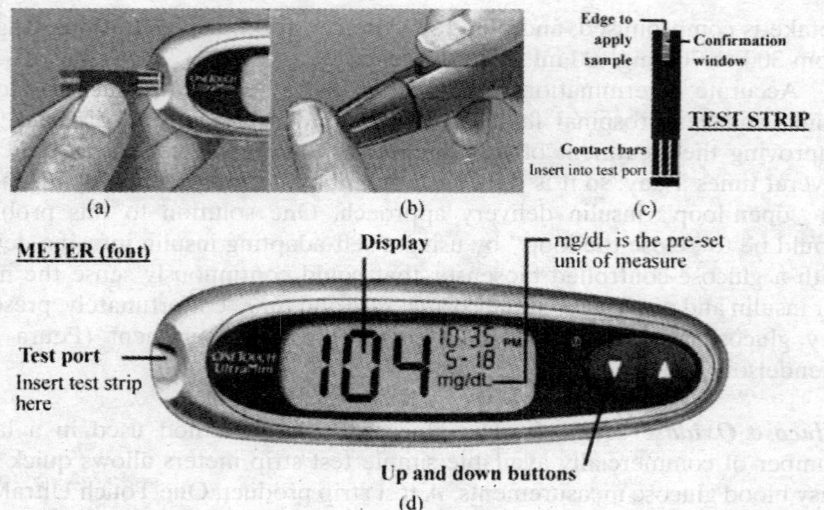


**Figure 10.23** (a) A test strip is inserted into the meter. (b) A lance is released to lance the skin less than 1 mm. (c) The 1 μL blood sample is applied to the end of the test strip and drawn into it by capillary action. (d) Then 5 s later, the meter displays the blood glucose in mg/dL.

Because a single-electrode technique is sensitive both to glucose and to the amount of oxygen present in the solution, a modification to remove the oxygen response by using two polarographic oxygen electrodes has been suggested (Updike and Hicks, 1967). Figure 10.24 illustrates both the principle of the enzyme electrode and the dual-cathode enzyme electrode. An active enzyme is placed over the glucose electrode, which senses glucose and oxygen. The other electrode senses only oxygen. The amount of glucose is determined as a function of the difference between the readings of these two electrodes. More recently, development of hydrophobic membranes that are more permeable to oxygen than to glucose has been described (Gilligan *et al.*, 2004). Placing these membranes over a glucose enzyme electrode solves the problem associated with oxygen limitation and increases the linear response of the sensor to glucose.

The major problem with enzymatic glucose sensors is the instability of the immobilized enzyme and the fouling of the membrane surface under physiological conditions. Most glucose sensors operate effectively only for short periods of time. In order to improve the present sensor technologies, more highly selective membranes must be developed. The features that must be taken into account in designing and fabricating these membranes include the diffusion rate of both oxygen and glucose from the external medium to the surface of the membrane, diffusion and concentration gradients within the membrane, immobilization of the enzyme, and the stability of the enzymatic reaction (Jaffari and Turner, 1995).

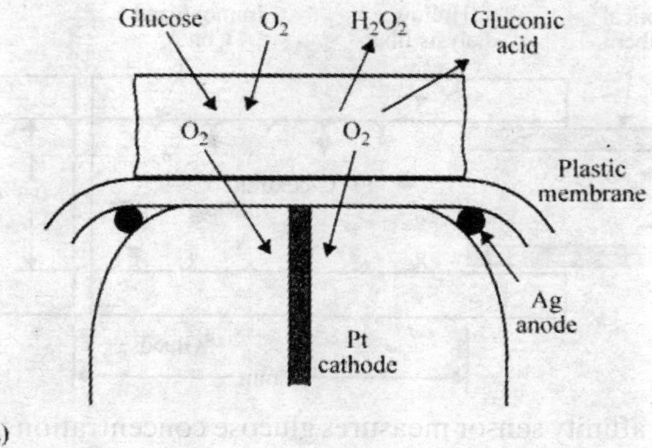


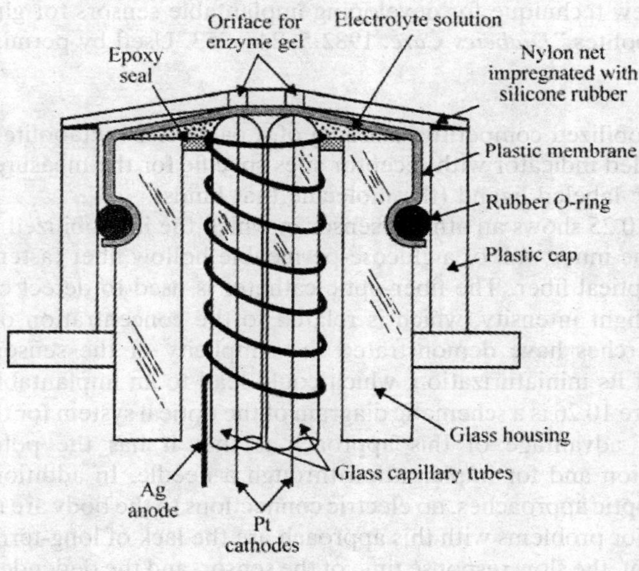


**Figure 10.24** (a) In the enzyme electrode, when glucose is present it combines with $O_2$, so less $O_2$ arrives at the cathode. (b) In the dual-cathode enzyme electrode, one electrode senses only $O_2$ and the difference signal measures glucose independent of $O_2$ fluctuations. (From S. J. Updike and G. P. Hicks, "The enzyme electrode, a miniature chemical transducer using immobilized enzyme activity," *Nature*, 1967, 214, 986–988. Used by permission.)

***Optical Approach*** A number of innovative glucose sensors, based on different optical techniques, has been developed in recent years. A new fluorescence-based affinity sensor has been designed for monitoring various metabolites, especially glucose in the blood plasma (Schultz *et al.*, 1982). The method is similar in principle to that used in radioimmunoassays. It is based

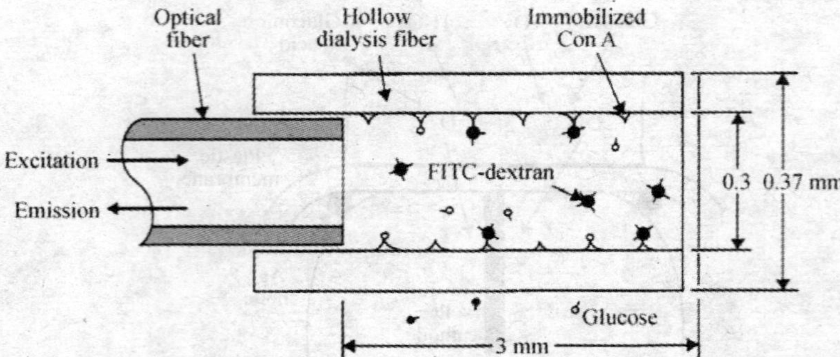


**Figure 10.25** The affinity sensor measures glucose concentration by detecting changes in fluorescent light intensity caused by competitive binding of a fluorescein-labeled indicator. (From J. S. Schultz, S. Manouri, *et al.*, "Affinity sensor: A new technique for developing implantable sensors for glucose and other metabolites," *Diabetes Care*, 1982 5, 245–253. Used by permission.)

on the immobilized competitive binding of a particular metabolite and fluorescein-labeled indicator with receptor sites specific for the measured metabolite and the labeled ligand (the molecule that binds).

Figure 10.25 shows an affinity sensor in which the immobilized reagent is coated on the inner wall of a glucose-permeable hollow fiber fastened to the end of an optical fiber. The fiber-optic catheter is used to detect changes in fluorescent light intensity, which is related to the concentration of glucose. These researches have demonstrated the simplicity of the sensor and the feasibility of its miniaturization, which could lead to an implantable glucose sensor. Figure 10.26 is a schematic diagram of the optical system for the affinity sensor. The advantage of this approach is that it has the potential for miniaturization and for implantation through a needle. In addition, as with other fiber-optic approaches, no electric connections to the body are necessary.

The major problems with this approach are the lack of long-term stability of the reagent, the slow response time of the sensor, and the dependence of the measured light intensity on the amount of reagent, which is usually very small and may change over time.

***Attenuated Total Reflection (ATR) and Infrared Absorption Spectroscopy***
The application of multiple infrared ATR spectroscopy to biological media is another potentially attractive noninvasive technique. By this means, the infrared spectra of blood can be recorded from tissue independently of the sample thickness, whereas other optical-transmission techniques are strongly dependent on the optical-transmission properties of the medium. Furthermore, employing a laser light source makes possible considerable improvement of the measuring sensitivity. This is of particular interest when one is measuring the transmission of light in aqueous solutions, because it counteracts the intrinsic attenuation of water, which is high in most wavelength ranges.

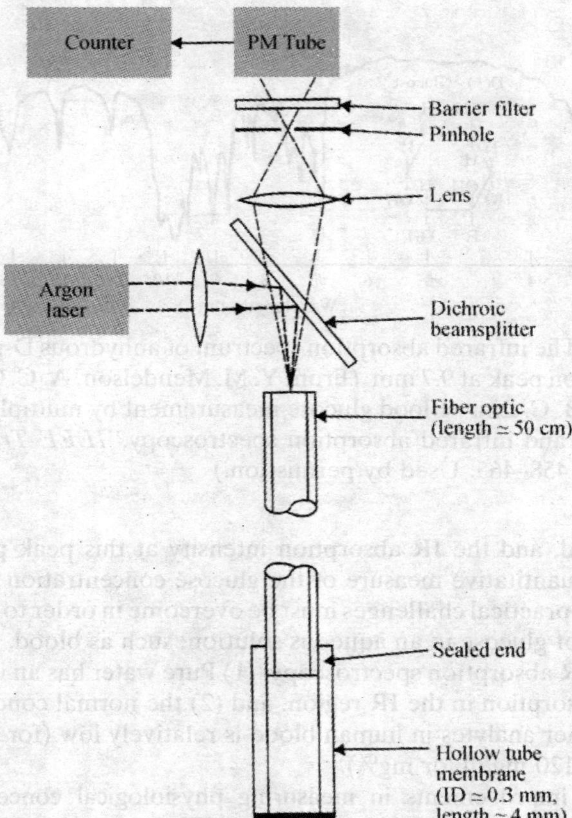


**Figure 10.26** The optical system for a glucose affinity sensor uses an argon leaser and a fiber-optic catheter. (From J. S. Schulz, S. Manouri, *et al.*, "Affinity sensor: A new technique for developing implantable sensors for glucose and other metabolites," *Diabetes Care*, 1982, 5, 245–253. Used by permission.)

Absorption spectroscopy in the infrared (IR) region is an important technique for the identification of unknown biological substances in aqueous solutions. Because of vibrational and rotational oscillations of the molecule, each molecule has specific resonance absorption peaks, which are known as *fingerprints*. These spectra are not uniquely identified; rather, the IR absorption peaks of biological molecules often overlap. An example of such a spectrum is shown in Figure 10.27, which is the characteristic IR spectrum of anhydrous D-glucose in the wavelength region 2.5 to 10 μm. The strongest absorption peak, around 9.7 μm, is due to the carbon–oxygen–carbon bond in the molecule's pyran ring.

The absorption-peak magnitude is directly related to the glucose concentration in the sample, and its spectral position is within the wavelength range emitted by a $CO_2$ laser. Thus a $CO_2$ laser can be used as a source of energy to

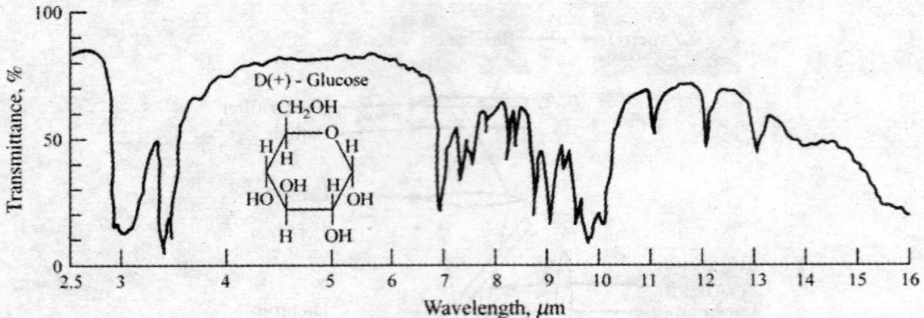


**Figure 10.27** The infrared absorption spectrum of anhydrous D-glucose has a strong absorption peak at 9.7 mm. (From Y. M. Mendelson, A. C. Clermont, R. A. Peura, and B. C. Lin, "Blood glucose measurement by multiple attenuated total reflection and infrared absorption spectroscopy,"*IEEE Trans. Biomed Eng.*, 1990, 37, 458–465. Used by permission.)

excite this bond, and the IR absorption intensity at this peak provides, via Beer's law, a quantitative measure of the glucose concentration in a sample.

Two major practical challenges must be overcome in order to measure the concentration of glucose in an aqueous solution, such as blood, by means of conventional IR absorption spectroscopy. (1) Pure water has an intrinsic high background absorption in the IR region, and (2) the normal concentration of glucose and other analytes in human blood is relatively low (for glucose, it is typically 90 to 120 mg/dl, or mg%).

Significant improvements in measuring physiological concentrations of glucose and other blood analytes by conventional IR spectrometers have resulted from the use of high-power sources of light energy at specific active wavelengths. In the case of glucose, the $CO_2$ laser serves as an appropriate IR source.

## 10.8 ELECTRONIC NOSES

Physicians can diagnose diabetes by the sweet smell of a patient's breath. A handheld breathalyzer senses only a single compound and sells for $50 and up. Electronic noses (e-noses) have been developed that use an array of 10 to 50 sensors and pattern recognition algorithms to distinguish many odors, and are use in the pharmaceutical, food, and cosmetics industry, but they cost about $10,000. Figure 10.28 shows a printed organic thin-film transistor (OTFT) that may lower the cost and bring e-noses into more widespread use. Vapor molecules in the odor change a conducting polymer active material conductance of a thin-film transistor. Soluble polymers can be printed to yield many sensors on a single substrate using ink-jet techniques. Carbon black or polypyrrole is placed in the soluble polymer to change the conductance (Chang *et al.*, 2006; Chang and Subramanian, 2008).

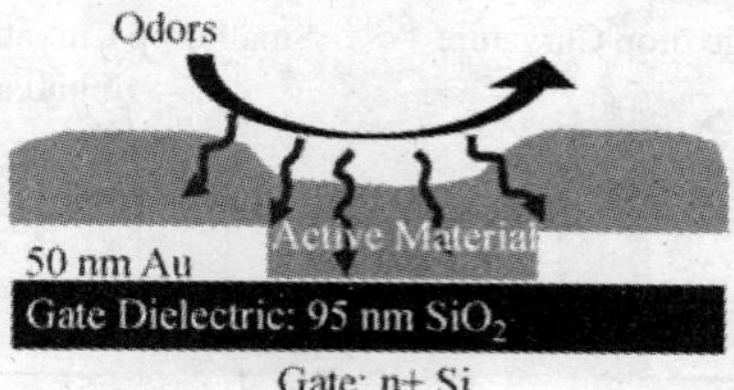


**Figure 10.28** A printed organic thin-film transistor senses volatile organic compounds to yield an affordable electronic nose. A 2.5 nm chrome adhesion layer and 50 nm thick gold source and drain pads are thermally evaporated onto 95 nm of thermally grown wet oxide. The active material is spun cast or drop cast. From J. B. Chang, V. Liu, V. Subramanian, K. Sivula, C. Luscombe, A. Murphy, J. Liu, and J. M. J. Fréchet, Printable polythiophene gas sensor array for low-cost electronic noses, *J. Appl, Phys.*, 2006, 100, 014506.

## 10.9 LAB-ON-A-CHIP

Lab-on-a-chip (LOC) describes devices that integrate (multiple) laboratory functions on a single chip of only millimeters to a few square centimeters in size and that are capable of handling extremely small fluid volumes down to less than picoliters. They are fabricated using MEMS techniqes and use microfluidics.

The basis for most LOC fabrication processes is photolithography. Initially most processes were in silicon, as these well-developed technologies were directly derived from semiconductor fabrication. Because of demands for e.g. specific optical characteristics, bio- or chemical compatibility, lower production costs and faster prototyping, new processes have been developed such as glass, ceramics and metal etching, deposition and bonding, PDMS processing (e.g., soft lithography), thick-film and stereolithography as well as fast replication methods via electroplating, injection molding, and embossing. Furthermore the LOC field more and more exceeds the borders between lithography-based microsystem technology, nanotechnology and precision engineering.

LOCs may provide advantages, very specifically for their applications. Typical advantages are: low fluid volumes consumption, faster analysis and response times due to short diffusion distances, compactness of the systems, massive parallelization due to compactness, which allows high-throughput analysis, lower fabrication costs, and safer platform for chemical, radioactive or biological studies.

LOCs use novel technology and therefore are not fully developed. Some examples that have been demonstrated include real-time PCR, detect bacteria, viruses and cancers, immunoassay, detect bacteria, viruses and cancers based on antigen–antibody reactions, dielectrophoresis detecting cancer cells and bacteria, blood sample preparation, crack cells to extract DNA, cellular lab-on-a-chip for single-cell analysis, and ion channel screening (Wikipedia, 2008).

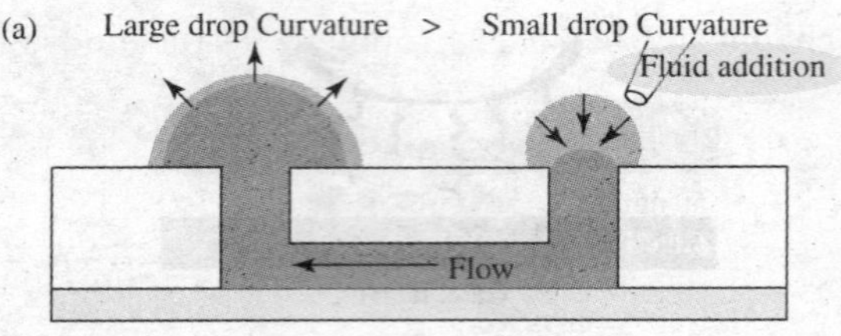


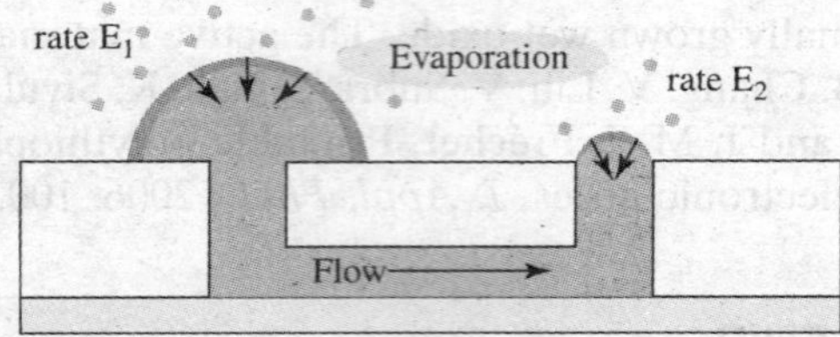


**Figure 10.29** Schematic of a passive pumping device. A. Flowing fluid in the channel is effectuated by adding a drop to the port opposing the large drop. The subsequent increase of pressure due to the small curvature of the added drop provokes its flow towards the large drop until curvatures match. This happens in seconds to minutes. B. During the storage of the channel, as evaporation occurs both at the large and small drop, a decrease in volume will provoke more decrease in curvature in the small drop, and thus an unbalance of pressure in its favor. A flow will be generated from the large to the small drop, thus ensuring constant wetting of the port. From Berthier, E., J. Warrick, H. Yu and D. J. Beebe, Managing evaporation for more robust microscale assays. Part 2. Characterization of convection and diffusion for cell biology, *Lab Chip*, 2008, 8, 860–864. Reproduced by permission of The Royal Society of Chemistry.

Proposed LOCs include HIV tests, methicillin-resistant staph bacteria test, a screening test that can detect the chromosome mutations of various cancers (Choi, 2007). One of the problems is providing flow through LOCs. Figure 10.29 shows that instead of using external pumps, passive flow occurs when different sized drops are used and larger surface tension of the small drop provides the pressure to cause the flow.

## 10.10 SUMMARY

Many biosensors produce signals that are correlated with the concentration of glucose in body fluids. It may be possible to miniaturize some small sensors for implantation. Nevertheless, further progress must be made before these sensors can be used reliably for long-term monitoring of glucose in the body. The problems that have yet to be solved involve operating implanted sensors in the chemically harsh environment of the body, where they are subject to continuous degradation by blood and tissue components. The device must be biocompatible, properly encapsulated, and well protected against elevated temperatures and saline conditions. Furthermore, it should be possible to calibrate the sensor *in situ*.

## PROBLEMS

**10.1** Sketch the arrangement of a $P\text{CO}_2$ electrode. Explain briefly how it works.

**10.2** What affects the response time of the $CO_2$ electrode?

**10.3** What affects the response time of the $O_2$ electrode?

**10.4** As described in the text, glucose concentration can be determined enzymatically by a glucose oxidase procedure. An oxygen electrode can be used if the plastic electrode membrane is coated with a layer of glucose oxidase immobilized in acrylamide gel. When the electrode is placed in a solution containing glucose and oxygen, the glucose and oxygen diffuse into the gel layer of immobilized enzyme. The diffusion flow of oxygen through the plastic membrane to the oxygen electrode is decreased in the presence of the glucose. One difficulty with this electrode design is that it responds to changes in oxygen concentration as well as to changes in glucose concentration. Design an instrumentation system for *in vivo* measurement that responds only to the change in glucose concentration and not to changes in oxygen concentration. Your design should include circuit diagrams, the equations for all reactions occurring at the electrodes, and explanations of how your system would work.

**10.5** Explain what a double-beam optical instrument is. Give an example of a medical instrument that operates on this principle, and explain how it improves the instrument's performance.

## REFERENCES


Adamsons, K., S. D. Salha, G. Gillian, and A. Games, "Influence of temperature on blood pH of the human adult and newborn." *J. Appl. Physiol.*, 1964, 19, 894.

Allan, W. B., *Fibre Optics Theory and Practice*. New York: Plenum, 1973.

Arnold, M. A., and M. E. Meyerhoff, "Recent advances in the development and analytical applications of biosensing probes." *CRC Crit. Rev. Anal. Chem.*, 1988, 20, 149–196.

Bergveld, P., "Development of an ion-sensitive solid-state device for neurophysiological measurement." *IEEE Trans. Biomed. Eng.*, 1970, BME-17, 70–71.

Berthier, E., J. Warrick, H. Yu, and D. J. Beebe, "Managing evaporation for more robust microscale assays. Part 2. Characterization of convection and diffusion for cell biology." *Lab Chip*, 2008, DOI: 10.1039/b717423c.

Burtis, C. A., and E. R. Ashwood, (eds.) 1994. *Tietz Textbook of Clinical Chemistry*. 2nd ed. Philadelphia: W. B. Saunders.

Burton, G. W., "Effects of the acid-base state upon the temperature coefficient of pH of blood." *Brit. J. Anesth.*, 1965, 37, 89.

Cassady, G., "Transcutaneous monitoring in the newborn infant." *J. Pediatr.*, 1983, 103, 837–848.

Chang, J. B., and V. Subramanian, "Electronic noses sniff success." *IEEE Spectrum*, 2008, 45(3), 51–56.

Chang, J. B., V. Liu, V. Subramanian, K. Sivula, C. Luscombe, A. Murphy, J. Liu, and J. M. J. Fréchet, "Printable polythiophene gas sensor array for low-cost electronic noses." *J. Appl. Phys.*, 2006, 100, 014506.

Choi, C. Q., "Big lab on a tiny chip." *Sci. Amer.*, 2007, 297(4), 100–103.

Clark, L. D., Jr., and C. Lyons, "Electrode systems for continuous monitoring in cardiovascular surgery." *Ann. N. Y. Acad. Sci.*, 1962, 102, 29–45.

Collison, M. E., and M. E. Meyerhoff, "Chemical sensors for bedside monitoring of critically ill patients." *Anal. Chem.*, 1990, 62, 7, 425A–437A.

Davenport, H. W., *The ABC of Acid-Base Chemistry*. 6th ed. Chicago: University of Chicago Press, 1975.

Gehrich, J. L., D. W. Lübbers, N. Opitz, D. R. Hansmann, W. W. Miller, J. K. Tusa, and M. Yafuso, "Optical fluorescence and its application to an intravascular blood-gas monitoring system." *IEEE Trans. Biomed. Eng.*, 1986, BME-33, 117–132.

Hammond, P. A., and D. R. S. Cumming, "Ion-sensitive field-effect devices." In J. G. Webster (ed.), *Encyclopedia of Medical Devices and Instrumentation*. 2nd ed. New York: Wiley, 2006, Vol. 4, pp. 185–198.

Herrell, N., R. J. Martin, M. Pultusker, M. Lough, and A. Fanaroff, "Optimal temperature for the measurement of transcutaneous carbon dioxide tension in the neonate." *J. Pediatr.*, 1980, 97, 114–117.

Hicks, R., J. R. Schenken, and M. A. Steinrauf, *Laboratory Instrumentation*. New York: Harper & Row, 1974.

Huch, A., and R. Huch, "Transcutaneous, noninvasive monitoring of $Po_2$." *Hospital Practice*, 1976, 6, 43–52.

Huch, R., A. Huch, and D. W. Lübbers, *Transcutaneous $Po_2$*. New York: Thieme-Stratton, 1981.

Huch, A., D. W. Lübbers, and R. Huch, "Patientenuberwachung durch transcutane $Pco_2$ Messung bei gleiechzeiliger koutrolle der relatiuen Iokalen perfusion." *Anaesthetist*, 1973, 22, 379.

Jaffari, S. A., and A. P. F. Turner, "Recent advances in amperometric glucose biosensor for in vivo monitoring." *Physiol. Meas.*, 1995, 16, 1–15.

Janata, J., *Principles of Chemical Sensors*. New York: Plenum, 1989.

Kocache, R., "Oxygen analyzers." In J. G. Webster (ed.), *Encyclopedia of Medical Devices and Instrumentation*. New York: Wiley, 1988, pp. 2154–2161.

Lübbers, D. W., and N. Opitz, "Die $pCO_2/pO_2$ Optode: Eine Neue $pCO_2$—bzw. $pO_2$—Messonde zur Messung des $pCO_2$ oder $pO_2$ von Gasen und Flüssigkeiten." *Z. Naturfors*, 1975, 30c, 532–533.

Mendelson, Y. M., "Blood gas measurement, transcutaneous." In J. G. Webster (ed.), *Encyclopedia of Medical Devices and Instrumentation*. New York: Wiley, 1988, pp. 448–459.

Mendelson, Y. M., A. C. Clermont, R. A. Peura, and B. C. Lin, "Blood glucose measurement by multiple attenuated total reflection and infrared absorption spectroscopy." *IEEE Trans. Biomed Eng.*, 1990, 37, 458–465.

Mendelson, Y. M., and R. A. Peura, "Noninvasive transcutaneous monitoring of arterial blood gases." *IEEE Trans. Biomed. Eng.*, 1984, BME-31, 792–800.

Mendelson, Y. M., J. J. Galvin, and Y. Wang, "In-vitro evaluation of a dual oxygen saturation/hematocrit intravascular fiberoptic catheter." *Biomed. Instrum. & Technol.*, 1990, 24, 199–206.

Mendelson, Y. M., P. Cheung, M. R. Neuman, D. G. Fleming, and S. D. Cahn, "Spectrophotometric investigation of pulsatile blood flow for transcutaneous reflectance oximetry." *Adv. Exp. Med. Biol.*, 1983, 159, 93–102.

Mendelson, Y., "Optical sensors." In J. G. Webster (ed.), *Encyclopedia of Medical Devices and Instrumentation*. 2nd ed. New York: Wiley, 2006, Vol. 5, pp. 160–175.

Merrick, E. B., and T. J. Hayes, "Continuous, noninvasive measurements of arterial blood oxygen levels." *Hewlett-Packard J.*, 1976, 28(2), 2–9.

Moran, F., L. J. Kettel, and D. W. Dugell, "Measurement of blood $P_{O_2}$ with the microcathode electrode." *J. Appl. Physiol.*, 1966, 21, 725–728.

Moyle, J. T. B., *Pulse Oximetry*. London: BMJ Publishing, 1994.

Nickerson, B. G., and F. Monaco, "Carbon dioxide electrodes, arterial and transcutaneous." In J. G. Webster (ed.), *Encyclopedia of Medical Devices and Instrumentation*. New York: Wiley, 1988, pp. 564–569.

Payne, J. P., and J. W. Severinghaus, *Pulse Oximetry*. Berlin: Springer, 1986.

Peterson, J. I., "Optical sensors." In J. G. Webster (ed.), *Encyclopedia of Medical Devices and Instrumentation*. New York: Wiley, 1988, pp. 2121–2133.

Peterson, J. I., and Vurek, G. G., "Fiber-optic sensors for biomedical applications." *Science*, 1984, 224, 123–127.

Peterson, J. I., S. R. Goldstein, and R. V. Fitzgerald, "Fiber-optic pH probe for physiological use." *Anal. Chem.*, 1980, 52, 864–869.

Peura, R. A., and Y. Mendelson, "Blood glucose sensors: An overview." *In Proceedings of the Symposium on Biosensors*. Piscataway, N.J.: IEEE, 1984, pp. 63–68.

Regnault, W. R., and G. L. Picciolo, "Review of medical biosensors and associated materials problems." *J. Biomed. Mater. Res.: Applied Biomaterials*, 1987, 21, 163–180.

Rolfe, P., "In vivo chemical sensors for intensive-care monitoring." *Med. Biol. Eng. Comput.*, 1990, 28, B34–B47.

Rolfe, R., "Review of chemical sensors for physiological measurement." *J. Biomed. Eng.*, 1988, 10, 138–145.

Schultz, J. S., S. Mansouri and I. J. Goldstein, "Affinity sensor: A new technique for developing implantable sensors for glucose and other metabolites." *Diabetes Care*, 1982, 5, 245–253.

Seitz, W. R., "Chemical sensors based on fiber optics." *Anal. Chem.*, 1984, 56, 16A–34A.

Seitz, W. R., "Chemical sensors based on immobilized indicators and fiber optics." *CRC Crit. Rev. Anal. Chem.*, 1988, 19, 135–173.

Severinghaus, J. W., "Blood gas concentrations." In W. O. Fenn and H. Rahn (eds.), *Handbook of Physiology*, Vol. II, Sec. 3. Washington, D.C.: American Physiological Society, 1965, pp. 1475–1482.

Tremper, K. K., R. A. Mentelos, and W. C. Shoemaker, "Clinical and experimental transcutaneous $P_{CO_2}$ monitoring." *J. Clin. Eng.*, 1981, 6, 143–147.

Turner, A. P. F., I. Karube, and G. Wilson, *"Biosensors: Fundamentals and Applications."* New York: Oxford University Press, 1987.

Updike, S. J., and G. P. Hicks, "The enzyme electrode, a miniature chemical transducer using immobilized enzyme activity." *Nature*, 1967, 214, 986–988.

Gilligan, B. C., M. Shults, R. K. Rhodes, P. G. Jacobs, J. H. Brauker, T. J. Pintar, and S. J. Updike, "Feasibility of continuous long-term glucose monitoring from a subcutaneous glucose sensor in humans." *Diabetes Technol Ther.*, 2004, 6, 378–386.

VonCremer, M., "Uber die Ursache der elektromotorischen Eigenschaften der Gewbe, zuglelchein Beitrag zur Lehre von den polyphasischen Elektrolytketten." *Zeitschrift fuer Biologie*, 1906, 47, 564–608.

Webster, J. G. (ed.), *Design of Pulse Oximeters*. Bristol, UK: IOP Publishing, 1997.

Wikipedia, *"Lab-on-a-chip."* 2008. http://en.wikipedia.org/wiki/Lab-on-a-chip.

Wise, D. L. (ed.), *Bioinstrumentation: Research, Developments and Applications*. Stoneham, MA: Butterworth, 1990.

Yoshiya, I., Y. Shimada, and K. Tanaka, "Spectrophotometric monitoring of arterial oxygen saturation in the fingertip." *Med. Biol. Eng. Comput.*, 1980, 18, 27–32.

Zachariah, E. S., P. Gopalakrishakone, and P. Neuzil, "Immunologically sensitive field-effect transistors." In J. G. Webster (ed.), *Encyclopedia of Medical Devices and Instrumentation*. 2nd ed. New York: Wiley, 2006, Vol. 4, pp. 98–110.

# 11

# CLINICAL LABORATORY INSTRUMENTATION

Lawrence A. Wheeler

The clinical laboratory is responsible for analyzing patient specimens in order to provide information to aid in the diagnosis of disease and evaluate the effectiveness of therapy. The hospital department that performs these functions may also be called the department of clinical pathology or the department of laboratory medicine. The major sections of the clinical laboratory are the chemistry, hematology, and microbiology sections and the blood bank.

The chemistry section performs analyses on blood, urine, cerebrospinal fluid (CSF), and other fluids to determine how much of various clinically important substances they contain. Most applications of electronic instrumentation in the clinical laboratory take place in the chemistry section. The hematology section performs determinations of the numbers and characteristics of the formed elements in the blood (red blood cells, white blood cells, and platelets) as well as tests of the function of physiological systems in the blood (clotting studies are an example). Many of the most frequently ordered of these tests have been automated on the Coulter Counter (see Section 11.5). The microbiology section performs studies on various body tissues and fluids to determine whether pathological microorganisms are present. Until quite recently, there were essentially no applications of electronic instrumentation in microbiology. However, devices that automatically monitor the status of blood cultures (tests for the presence of microorganisms) and tests that semiautomatically measure the sensitivity of microorganisms to antibiotics (susceptibility tests) are now being used in many microbiology laboratories. The application of electronic instrumentation for the blood bank is in its infancy. A few systems that automate the basic classification of the type of the blood product (ABO grouping) are currently being developed.

Because many critical patient-care decisions are based on test results supplied by the clinical laboratory, the accuracy and precision of these results are of great importance. Excellent equipment design and effective quality-control programs are essential. Everyone involved in the design or use of clinical laboratory instruments must be constantly aware that erroneous test results can lead to a tragic outcome.

A second important characteristic of many test procedures is fast response, because in many critical clinical situations, the therapy selected by the physician depends on the test results. The application of electronics in the clinical laboratory has greatly reduced the time required to perform a wide variety of crucial tests.

A major application of electronics in the clinical laboratory is the use of computer systems for information management. Mainframes, minicomputers, and microcomputers are used in commercial systems. Laboratory information systems keep track of patient specimens, organize the flow of work, automatically acquire test results from some types of instruments, maintain test-result databases, report results to on-line devices in patient-care areas, prepare printed reports, assist in quality control, and support a variety of management functions. We shall not discuss laboratory information management systems in detail. The current design trend in laboratory instrumentation, however, is to include data-processing capability in essentially every instrument. Therefore, our discussions of specific laboratory instruments will cover some aspects of laboratory information management.

## 11.1 SPECTROPHOTOMETRY

Spectrophotometry is the basis for many of the instruments used in clinical chemistry. The primary reasons for this are ease of measurement, satisfactory accuracy and precision, and the suitability of spectrophotometric techniques to use in automated instruments. In this section, *spectrophotometer* is used as a general term for a class of instruments. Photometers and colorimeters are members of this class (Shen *et al.*, 2006).

Spectrophotometry is based on the fact that substances of clinical interest selectively absorb or emit electromagnetic energy at different wavelengths. For most laboratory applications, wavelengths in the range of the ultraviolet (200 to 400 nm), the visible (400 to 700 nm), or the near infrared (700 to 800 nm) are used; the majority of the instruments operate in the visible range.

Figure 11.1 is a general block diagram for a spectrophotometer-type instrument. The source supplies the radiant energy used to analyze the sample. The wavelength selector allows energy in a limited wavelength band to pass through. The cuvette holds the sample to be analyzed in the path of the energy. The detector produces an electric output that is proportional to the amount of energy it receives, and the readout device indicates the received energy or some function of it (such as the concentration, in the sample, of a substance of interest).

The basic principle of a spectrophotometer is that if we examine an appropriately chosen, sufficiently small portion of the electromagnetic spectrum, we can use the energy-absorption properties of a substance of interest to measure the concentration of that substance. In the vast majority of cases, these substances, as they are normally found in a patient's samples (of serum,

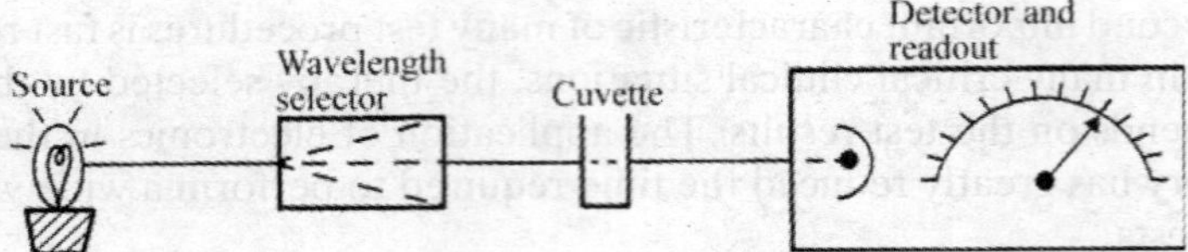


**Figure 11.1 Block diagrams of a spectrophotometer** (Based on R. J. Henry, D. C. Cannon, and J. W. Winkelman, eds., *Clinical Chemistry,* 2nd ed. Hagerstown, MD: Harper & Row, 1974.)

urine, or CSF, for instance), do *not* exhibit the desired energy-absorption characteristics. In such cases, reagents are added to the sample, causing a reaction to occur. This reaction yields a product that *does* have the desired characteristics. The reaction products are then placed in the cuvette for analysis. The instrument-calibration procedures take into account the possible difference in concentration between the reaction product and the original quantity of interest.

Let us discuss in detail the characteristics of each of the subsystems shown in Figure 11.1.

***Power Sources*** Hydrogen or deuterium discharge lamps are used to provide power in the 200-to-360 nm range, and tungsten filament lamps are used for the 360-to-800 nm range. Hydrogen and deuterium lamps both produce a continuous spectrum; but a problem with these power sources is that they produce about 90% of their power in the infrared range. The output in the ultraviolet and visible ranges can be increased by operating the lamp at voltages above the rated value, but this stratagem significantly reduces the expected life of the lamp. Another problem with tungsten lamps is that, during operation, the tungsten progressively vaporizes from the filaments and condenses on the glass envelope. This coating, which is generally uneven, alters the spectral characteristics of the lamp and can cause errors in determinations.

***Wavelength Selectors*** A variety of devices are used to select those portions of the power spectrum produced by the power source that are to be used to analyze the sample. These devices can be divided into two classes: filters and monochromators. There are two basic types of filters: glass filters and interference filters.

Glass filters function by absorbing power. For example, a blue-colored filter absorbs in the higher-wavelength visible range (red region) and transmits in the lower-wavelength visible range (blue-green region). These filters (consisting of one or more layers of glass plates) are designed to be low-pass, high-pass, or bandpass (a combination of low- and high -pass) filters.

Interference filters are made by spacing reflecting surfaces such that the incident light is reflected back and forth a short distance. The distance is selected such that light in the wavelength band of interest tends to be in phase and to be reinforced; light outside this band is out of phase and is canceled (the interference effect). Harmonics of the frequencies in this band are also passed and must be eliminated by glass cutoff filters.

Glass filters are used in applications in which only modest accuracy is required. Interference filters are used in many spectrophotometers, including those used in the SMAC (Technicon Instrument Corporation) and the CentrifiChem (Union Carbide). Devices that use filters as their wavelength selectors are called colorimeters or photometers.

*Monochromators* are devices that utilize prisms and diffraction gratings. They provide very narrow bandwidths and have adjustable nominal wavelengths. The basic principle of operation of these devices is that they disperse the input beam spatially as a function of wavelength. A mechanical device is then used to allow wavelengths in the band of interest to pass through a slit.

Prisms are constructed from glass and quartz. Quartz is required for wavelengths below 350 nm. A convergent lens system is used to direct the light from the source through an entrance slit. The prism bends the light as a function of wavelength. The smaller wavelengths (ultraviolet) are bent the most. This produces an output beam in which the wavelength band of interest can be selectively passed by placing in the light path an opaque substance with a slit in it. The wavelength spectrum of the power passing through the slit is nominally triangle shaped. In prisms, as in filters, the wavelength at which maximal transmittance occurs is the nominal central wavelength. Bandwidths of 0.5 nm can be obtained with this type of device. Prisms have been used over the wavelength range of 220 to 950 nm. The nonlinear spatial distribution of the power emerging from a prism requires relatively complex mechanical devices for control of the slit position to select different nominal wavelengths.

Diffraction gratings are constructed by inscribing a large number of closely spaced parallel lines on glass or metal. A grating exploits the fact that rays of light bend around sharp corners. The degree of bending is a function of wavelength. This results in separation of the light into a spectrum at each line. As these wave fronts move and interact, reinforcement and cancellation occur. The light emerging from a grating is resolved spatially in a linear fashion, unlike the light from a prism, in which the separation of wavelengths is less at longer wavelengths. As in the case of the prism, a slit is used to select the desired bandwidth. The mechanics of the slit-positioning mechanism of a grating are less complicated than those of a prism because of the linearity of the spatial separation of the wavelengths. Gratings can achieve bandwidths down to 0.5 nm and can operate over the range of 200 to 800 nm.

***Cuvette*** The cuvette (Figure 11.1) holds the substance being analyzed. Its optical characteristics must be such that it does not significantly alter the spectral characteristics of the light as that light enters or leaves the cuvette. The degree of care and expense involved in cuvette design is a function of the overall accuracy required of the spectrophotometer.

***Sample*** The sample (actually, in most cases, the substances resulting from the interaction of the patient specimen and appropriate reagents) absorbs light selectively according to the laws of Lambert, Bouguer, Bunsen, Roscoe, and Beer. The principles stated in these laws are usually grouped together and called Beer's law. The essence of the law was stated by Bouguer: "Equal thickness of an absorbing material will absorb a constant fraction of the energy incident upon it." This relationship can be stated formally as follows:

$$P = P_0 10^{-aLC} \tag{11.1}$$

where

$P_0$ = radiant power arriving at the cuvette
$P$ = radiant power leaving the cuvette
$a$ = absorptivity of the sample (extinction coefficient)
$L$ = length of the path through the sample
$C$ = concentration of the absorbing substance

Absorptivity is a function of the characteristics of the sample and the wavelength content of the incident light. This relationship is often rewritten in the form

$$\%T = 100P/P_0 = (100)10^{-aLC} \tag{11.2}$$

where $\%T$ is the percent transmittance. The value of $a$ is constant for a particular unknown, and the cuvette and cuvette holder are designed to keep $L$ as nearly constant as possible. Therefore, changes in $P$ should reflect changes in the concentration of the absorbing substance in the sample.

Percent transmittance is often reported as the result of the determination. However, because the relationship between concentration and percent transmittance is logarithmic, it has been found convenient to report absorbance. Absorbance $A$ is defined as $\log(P_0/P)$, so

$$A = \log\left(\frac{P_0}{P}\right) = \log\left(\frac{100}{\%T}\right) = 2 - \log(\%T) \tag{11.3}$$

Note that the relationship

$$A = aLC \tag{11.4}$$

follows from (11.1) and (11.3). As previously stated, the spectrophotometer is designed to keep $a$ and $L$ as nearly constant as possible so that a particular determination $A$ ideally varies only with $C$. Therefore, the concentration of an unknown can be determined as follows. The absorbance $A_s$ of a standard with known concentration of the substance of interest, $C_s$, is determined. Next the absorbance of the unknown, $A_u$, is determined. Finally, the concentration of the unknown, $C_u$, is computed via the relationship

$$C_u = C_s\left(\frac{A_u}{A_s}\right) \tag{11.5}$$

If this relationship holds over the possible range of concentration of the unknown substance in patient samples, then the determination is said to obey Beer's law. This relationship may not hold, however, because of absorption by the solvent or reflections at the cuvette. Then a relatively large number of standards with concentration values spanning the range of interest must be used to compute a calibration curve of concentration versus absorbance. This curve is then employed to obtain a concentration value for the absorbance value of the unknown.

**EXAMPLE 11.1** A filter photometer is being used to determine total concentration of serum protein (grams per deciliter). A technologist runs one standard with a known total protein concentration of 8 g/dl and obtains a $\%T$ reading of 20%, processes a patient sample and gets a $\%T$ reading of 30%, assumes the instrument's operation satisfies Beer's law, and calculates the patient value. What value should be obtained? Do you agree with the methodology? If not, what would you do differently and why?

**ANSWER** From (11.3), $A_s = 2 - \log \%T = 2 - \log 20 = 2 - 1.30 = 0.70$. $A_u = 2 - \log 30 = 2 - 1.48 = 0.52$. From (11.5)

$$C_u = C_s \frac{A_s}{A_u} = 8 \frac{0.52}{0.70} = 5.9 \text{ g/dl}$$

Do not agree with the methodology. Because of absorption by the solvent or reflections at the cuvette, Beer's law may not hold. Run more than one standard of known concentration to ensure that Beer's law holds.

**EXAMPLE 11.2** A spectrophotometer is being calibrated before being used to determine concentration of serum calcium. Four standards (samples of known calcium concentration) are analyzed, and the following values emerge.

| Standards | % Transmittance | Calcium Concentration, mg/dl |
|---|---|---|
| 1 | 79.4 | 2 |
| 2 | 39.8 | 8 |
| 3 | 31.6 | 10 |
| 4 | 20.0 | 14 |

Does this determination follow Beer's law? If a patient sample was processed and a percentage of 35 were obtained, what would the calcium concentration be?

**ANSWER**

$$A_1 = 2 - \log 79.4 = 2 - 1.90 = 0.10$$
$$A_2 = 2 - \log 39.8 = 2 - 1.60 = 0.40$$
$$A_3 = 2 - \log 31.6 = 2 - 1.50 = 0.50$$
$$A_4 = 2 - \log 20 = 2 - 1.30 = 0.70$$

For all four samples ratio of concentration to Absorbance is given as:

$$\frac{2}{0.1} = \frac{8}{0.4} = \frac{10}{0.5} = \frac{14}{0.7} = 20$$

Therefore, the samples follow Beer's law. For $\%T = 35$,

1. Absorbance $= 2 - \log(\%T) = 2 - \log 35 = 0.46$.
2. Concentration is given as $C_u = C_s(A_u/A_s) = 2(0.46/0.1) = 9.1$ mg/dl.

The amount of light absorbed by a compound is generally a function of wavelength. The chemical reaction used in preparing the sample for spectrophotometry is designed to produce a compound (1) the concentration of which is proportional to that of the compound of interest and (2) the peak of the absorption spectrum of which is separated from the absorption peaks of the other compounds in the sample.

The wavelength band of light allowed to pass through the wavelength selector is generally chosen to cover the peak of the absorption curve symmetrically. There are a number of other factors to consider, however, including the absolute level of absorbance at the peak and its wavelength value. If the absorbance is too great ($A > 1.0$) or too small ($A < 0.11$), the errors of the photometric system become unacceptably large (Henry, 1984). In the case in which the absorbance is very large, the sample can be diluted, but this procedure is time-consuming and can result in errors. The wavelength of the peak must be within the range of the spectrophotometer's capabilities.

***Photometric System*** A spectrophotometer's photometric system includes detectors to measure the amount of power leaving the cuvette (Radiation Sensors, Section 2.16), circuits for amplification of the low currents developed by detectors (Amplifiers and Signal Processing, Chapter 3), and devices to present the results of the determination to the technologist operating the instrument (meters or recorders). Commonly used detectors include barrier layer cells, phototubes, and photoconductive cells.

The design of meters for this application has been somewhat of a problem in the past as a result of the need for precision and the nonlinear relationship between the detected quantity (power) and the quantity of interest (absorption). Now, thanks to the development of low-cost digital electronics, the problems of computation and data presentation have been largely eliminated.

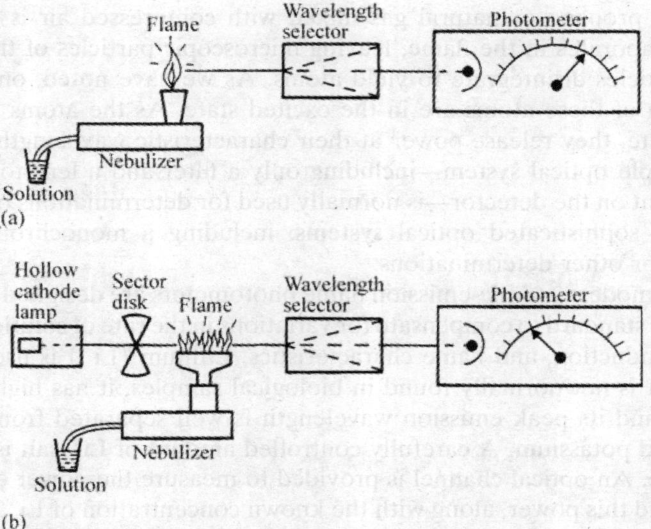


**Figure 11.2** Block diagrams of instruments for (a) flame emission and (b) flame absorption. (Based on R. J. Henry, D. C. Cannon, and J. W. Winkelman, eds., *Clinical Chemistry,* 2nd ed. Hagerstown, MD: Harper & Row, 1974.)

## FLAME PHOTOMETERS

Flame photometers differ in three important ways from the instruments we have already discussed. First, the power source and the sample-holder function are combined in the flame. Second, in most applications of flame photometry, the objective is measurement of the sample's emission of light rather than its absorption of light, although we shall also discuss atomic absorption-type flame photometers. (Schematic representations of these two types of instruments are shown in Figure 11.2.) Third, flame photometers can determine only the concentrations of pure metals (Lyon and Lyon, 2006).

## ATOMIC EMISSION

At the normal levels of power used in flame photometers, only about 1% of the atoms are raised to an excited state. In addition, only a few elements produce enough power at a single wavelength as they move from higher-energy to lower-energy orbits. These two factors have limited the use of atomic-emission flame photometry largely to determinations of $Na^+$, $K^+$, and $Li^+$. Instruments have been developed that can make determinations of other elements, such as $Ca^{2+}$, but relatively complicated optical systems are required.

As shown in Figure 11.2(a), the sample, combined with a solvent, is drawn into a nebulizer that converts the liquid into a fine aerosol that is injected into the flame. Several types of fuels have been used in flame photometers.

Currently, propane or natural gas mixed with compressed air is used. The solvent evaporates in the flame, leaving microscopic particles of the sample. These particles disintegrate to yield atoms. As we have noted, only a small proportion of these atoms are in the excited state. As the atoms fall to the ground state, they release power at their characteristic wavelength.

A simple optical system—including only a filter and a lens to focus the filtered light on the detector—is normally used for determinations of $Na^+$ and $K^+$. More sophisticated optical systems, including a monochromator, are required for other determinations.

Many modern atomic-emission flame photometers are designed to include an internal standard to compensate for variations in the rate of solution uptake, aerosol production, and flame characteristics. Lithium ($Li^+$) is used for this purpose. It is not normally found in biological samples, it has high emission intensity, and its peak emission wavelength is well separated from those of sodium and potassium. A carefully controlled amount of $Li^+$ salt is added to the sample. An optical channel is provided to measure the power emitted by the $Li^+$, and this power, along with the known concentration of $Li^+$, is used to correct the determination of $Na^+$ or $K^+$ for variations in the instrument. Actually, in most applications, the determinations of $Na^+$, $K^+$, and $Li^+$ are done in parallel.

A few problems arise in the use of $Li^+$ as the internal standard. First, although correction for small variations in the characteristics of the instrument is possible, there is no way to correct for large variations. Second, $Li^+$ is being used increasingly for treatment of an important psychotic disorder, manic-depressive psychosis. If patients who are receiving $Li^+$ are not identified to the clinical laboratory, significant errors in determinations of $Na^+$ and $K^+$ can occur. It is an unfortunate fact that the clinical laboratory is rarely given any clinical information to use in assessing the accuracy of determinations.

## ATOMIC ABSORPTION

This technique has shown great promise for the very accurate determination of the concentration of a variety of elements, including calcium, lead, copper, zinc, iron, and magnesium. It is based on the fact that the vast majority of atoms in a flame absorb energy at a characteristic wavelength. A special power source is used that emits power at the characteristic wavelength of the atom the concentration of which is being determined. This source is a hollow cathode lamp. Such lamps are constructed from the metal to be determined or are lined with a coating of it. In most cases, a separate lamp is needed for each metal determination, but the special characteristics of a few metals make it possible to use one lamp for combinations of two or three of them. The cathode is placed in an atmosphere of an inert gas. When the cathode is heated, the atoms of the cathode leave the surface of the cathode and fill the cathode cavity with an atomic vapor. These atoms become excited as a result of collisions with electrons and ions, and when they return to the ground state, each releases power at its characteristic wavelength, as previously discussed. This power is directed through the flame [see Figure 11.2(b)], and the amount of absorption is proportional to the amount of the atom present.

Atomic-absorption flame photometers normally require a monochromator and use a photomultiplier as the detector. One additional feature of these devices is that, because the atoms in the flame emit as well as absorb power at the characteristic wavelength, it is necessary to be able to differentiate between the two sources of power reaching the detector. This is accomplished by designing the source to produce pulses of power rather than a steady output. A rotating-sector disk between the source and the flame is generally used for this purpose. The detection electronics incorporate the phase-sensitive demodulator described in Section 3.15 to eliminate the dc component and analyze only the ac signal.

## FLUOROMETRY

Fluorometry is based on the fact that a number of molecules emit light in a characteristic spectrum—the emission spectrum—immediately after absorbing radiant energy and being raised to an excited state. The degree to which the molecules are excited depends on the amplitude and wavelength of the radiant power in the excitation spectrum. Small amounts of power are lost in this process, which results in the emission spectrum's being generally higher in wavelength content than the excitation spectrum (Klebe, 2006).

Various power sources, wavelength selectors, and detection circuits are used in fluorometers of varying sensitivity. Mercury arc lamps are commonly used power sources. They produce major line spectra at 365, 405, 436, and 546 nm. Photomultipliers are normally used as detectors. A unique feature of these devices is the need to select operational bandwidths for two spectra—excitation and emission. Figure 11.3 shows a fluorometer block diagram. The

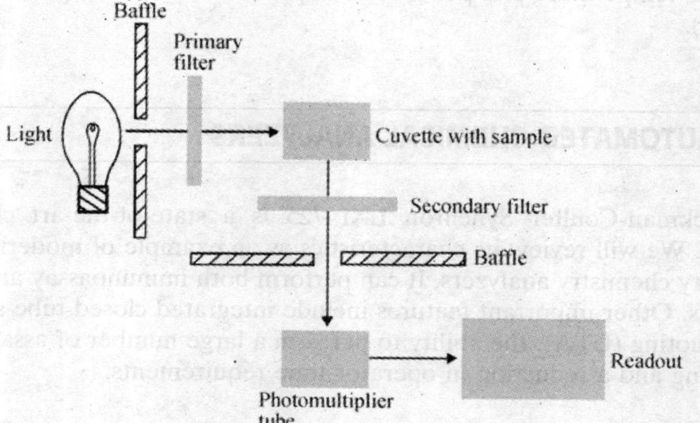


**Figure 11.3 Block diagram of a fluorometer** (From R. Hicks, J. R. Schenken, and M. A. Steinrauf, *Laboratory Instrumentation.* Hagerstown, MD: Harper & Row, 1974. Used with permission of C. A. McWhorter.)

detector is placed at a right angle to the power source to minimize the chance of direct transmission of light from source to detector. The wavelength characteristics of the wavelength selectors are also chosen such that there is little or no overlap in the wavelengths they pass.

One advantage fluorometry offers is its much greater sensitivity, which may exceed that of spectrophotometric methods by as much as four orders of magnitude. This is because in spectrophotometric methods, the difference between the absorption of a solution assumed to have a zero concentration ($\%T = 100$) of the unknown substance and the absorption of the sample is used as a measure of the concentration of the unknown substance. With highly dilute samples (such as one wherein $\%T = 98$), small errors in the process can cause large percent errors in the determination. In fluorometry, by contrast, a direct measurement of the fluorescence of the sample is used to determine the concentration of the unknown substance.

A special advantage of fluorometry is its great specificity. In spectrophotometric methods, the light absorbed in the wavelength band may be from substances other than the unknown. Only a relatively small number of substances, however, have the property of fluorescence. Thus many substances that might interfere with a spectrophotmetric measurement cannot interfere with a determination of fluorescence. Also, substances that have similar excitation spectra may have different emission spectra, and vice versa. Therefore, appropriate selection of the bandwidths of the two wavelengths selectors can provide additional rejection of noise.

The combination of these characteristics makes fluorometry capable of detecting picogram amounts of unknown substances. Highly dilute samples are used to prevent the light produced by fluorescence from being absorbed by other molecules as it passes through the sample solution.

The principal disadvantage of fluorometry is the sensitivity of its determinations to temperature and pH of the sample (fluorescence in general is pH-sensitive).

## 11.2 AUTOMATED CHEMICAL ANALYZERS

The Beckman-Coulter Synchron LXi 725 is a state-of-the-art chemistry analyzer. We will review its characteristics as an example of modern clinical laboratory chemistry analyzers. It can perform both immunoassay and chemistry tests. Other important features include integrated closed tube sampling and aliquoting (CTA), the ability to perform a large number of assays, rapid stat testing and a reduction in operator time requirements.

### SPECIMEN HANDLING

The LXi 725 utilizes Beckman–Coulter's rack technology to improve workflow by reducing manual processes. Sample tubes are placed in racks and put directly into a Spinchron DLX centrifuge. The rack is then loaded onto the analyzer. The racks can accommodate multiple tube sizes, sample cups, open or closed tubes. This provides increased efficiency.

Integrated parallel processing of general chemistry and immunoassay testing maximizes the productivity of the system. Both the immunoassay and chemistry analytical units on the LXi 725 can accommodate plasma samples to help improve turnaround time. Specimens that require both the immunoassay and chemistry testing are initially processed in the immunoassay unit. The sample is routed to the chemistry analyzer after an aliquot is obtained for immunoassay testing.

The immunoassay CTA system has the capacity for 100 aliquots per hour. Built-in data management capability tracks the aliquot vessel throughout the testing process. Aliquoting and routing of tests is done automatically without operator intervention. This translates into less labor and lower operating costs with increased output and increased efficiency. Laboratory operating safety is improved by reducing exposure to biohazards and minimizing repetitive motions.

The rack and sample barcodes are read as the rack is queued on the sample-handling carousel. In the CTA system, tubes are positioned for the cap piercing mechanism. The system adapts to a mixed batch of tubes in a single rack.

The CTA includes a piercing probe and a sampling probe. Once a tube is pierced, the sample probe aspirates the proper amount of sample based on the volume required for requested tests and dispenses it into an aliquot vessel.

The CTA reduces the potential for sample carry over by washing both the piercing and sample probe after each pierce and sample aspiration. By reducing the potential for carry over accurate results are obtained even the most sensitive assays such as beta HCG.

A radio sensor in the sample probe automatically determines sample levels within tubes. It detects when there is insufficient sample for the requested tests and the operator is notified when this situation exists.

The LXi 725 also features clot detection at both the immunoassay and the general chemistry sections. When the LXi 725 aspirates a sample the probe is extended into the sample tube. A sample is withdrawn. A pressure transducer detects blockage. If the probe is blocked, a wash solution is flushed through the probe forcing out any obstructions. The probe is now ready to re-aspirate the sample. If the clot is still detected, the operator is alerted, the sample is bypassed, and the system will continue to the next sample.

As soon as the immunoassay aliquots are dispensed, the LXi 725 releases the rack for general chemistry testing. Aliquots for general chemistry tests are prepared using the open tube aliquoting.

After the aliquots have been prepared for the chemistry tests, the rack is sent to the rack output area unless a test result triggers rerun or reflex rules (see below), then the rack is held until all results are delivered.

## TEST PERFORMANCE

The LXi 725 has a menu (i.e., list of types of tests) of 145 assays. The system allows 65 test types (24 immunoassays and 41 general chemistries) to be onboard simultaneously. In addition, the general chemistry section accepts programming for over 100 user-defined chemistries. This wide menu enables the laboratory to consolidate workstations. General chemistry, STAT, cardiac, thyroid and other test panels can be performed on the LXi 725.

The immunoassay analysis throughput is up to 100 tests per hour, while general chemistry testing runs at speeds up to 1440 tests per hour. Dual processing enables the LXi 725 to perform a basic metabolic panel in less than 2 min from standby. Troponin results are delivered in less than 14 min. Troponin levels are used in the evaluation of a possible myocardial infarct (MI) so a fast response time is very important. When the troponin value supports the diagnosis of an MI, therapy can be immediately initiated.

Conventional instruments require visual inspection by the technologist to determine the presence of sample interferences from icterus, hemolysis, or lipemia. This determination is highly subjective. The LXi 725 performs an automatic polychromatic analysis on a diluted reagent-free sample using near infrared particle immunoassay (NIPIA) methodology. The system calculates a set of equations that are related to a standard concentration graph. Each index reading can be related to a semiquantitative concentration expressed as a number. This system alerts the operator to a potentially compromised test result.

Paramagnetic particle separation and chemiluminescent detection provide precision, broad dynamic range and excellent sensitivity. Paramagnetic particle separation helps maximize small sample volumes and allows for multiple assay formats for improved performance

Chemiluminescent detector uses alluminometry to take 10 readings of the reaction. The system uses the median response to help eliminate reaction noise and deliver a more accurate result. Chemiluminescence is the generation of light by a chemical reaction, a light source is not used. This eliminates the need to filter out the source light and allows very low concentrations of substances to be detected.

When a stat test is ordered the operator loads the sample into a rack and pushes the priority button. The system will interrupt routine programming to load the new rack, improving the laboratory's delivery of critical test results. It takes approximately 60 s for the CTA to process a sample. Tests results for 11 critical care chemistries are available in less than 2 min from sample introduction. This eliminates the need for a separate instrument to perform stat testing.

## SYSTEM CONTROL

The primary system console performs two functions, operation of the analyzer and management of data. The system software offers simple touch screen operation and single point control of the entire LXi 725 workstation. The DL200 data manager helps improve workflow and results management. It offers a dynamic pending list, add-on tests, review by exception, and automatic reflex testing.

The *dynamic pending list* identifies tests that have not been completed. If an additional test is ordered after the initial specimen submission, this test is called an *add-on test*. The system operator can order the test for a specimen currently in the instrument.

*Review by exception* is a process that identifies test results that satisfy specified rules (for example a test result that is outside of the reference range for the test) for review by the operator. Often the test is repeated, if the repeat test result agrees with the initial result, the test results may be reviewed by a pathologist. The pathologist may prepare an interpretive report for the patient's clinician.

The review by exception feature is based on user-defined criteria and delta checking, only tests with abnormal results are flagged for operator review. This helps to prevent workflow bottlenecks and improves efficiency. Delta checking is a process in which the current test result is compared with the most recent test result of the same type from the patient (e.g. a potassium level). If the two values differ by a specified amount (the delta value), the test result will be repeated even though the current result is within the reference range. This technique can help identify situations such as specimen identification errors (e.g. the specimen as obtained from the wrong patient).

*Automatic reflex testing* is a method of computer-based algorithmic test performance. The use of the clinical laboratory to diagnose disease states is often based on an algorithmic approach. An initial set of tests is performed to identify the presence of abnormality in organ function. For example the diagnosis of thyroid disorders. When an initial abnormal value is obtained, the next test(s) in the algorithm is performed. Some algorithms have more than two stages. This approach is more cost effective than if the clinician initially orders all of the tests in the algorithm (so-called shotgun approach) since when the initial test is normal, the performance of the other tests in the algorithm is unnecessary. The advantage of the shotgun approach is that it eliminates the delay resulting from the clinician receiving an initial abnormal result and then ordering the next test in the algorithm.

Automatic reflex testing is implemented by automatically performing the next test(s) in the algorithm when the initial (or subsequent) test in the algorithm yields an abnormal value. This process can decrease the time needed to diagnose a disease condition and eliminate the need for shotgun test ordering. If a result meets the laboratory's criteria for reflex testing, the additional test(s) is ordered automatically.

The LXi 725 holds the primary tube until all testing is final. Controlled through the DL2000 data manager, this feature allows for automatic reflex testing with no operator intervention. If an immunoassay test order contains reflex rules, the CTA system will automatically aliquot the extra volume required for the potential reflux test.

With dynamic download from the LIS to the DL2000, LXi 725 test requests are continuously updated. From this information and the sample barcode, the LXi 725 workstation determines the type of tests required and schedules the system accordingly. After the tests are run, the DL2000 validates the results. Normal results are automatically forwarded to the LIS.

### REAGENT AND CALIBRATION

Bar-coded liquid reagents can be loaded at any time during a run maximizing efficiency. Manual tracking of onboard reagent inventory is eliminated. The system tracks identification, lot number expiration date, calibration frequency and precise number of tests remaining in the cartridge or pack.

For around the clock accessibility, the immunoassays stores 24 assays packs at a constant 4 °C to 10 °C. Self resealing immunoassays packs contain enough reagent volume for up to 50 tests. General chemistries cartridges can supply reagents for anywhere from 40 to 400 tests. Easy to use liquid calibrators, for both immunoassay and general chemistry testing, improve productivity by reducing manual processes. Calibration can be performed as needed.

## 11.3 CHROMATOLOGY

Chromatology is basically a group of methods for separating a mixture of substances into component parts. (Although the use of the term *chromatography* is firmly established, it is really a misnomer: In modern techniques, the colors of the mixture's components are not really used to identify substances.) One phase is fixed—liquid or solid—and the other is mobile—gas or liquid. When a liquid stationary phase is used, the process is called partition. When a solid stationary phase is used, the process is called adsorption.

In all chromatology, differences in the rate of movement of components of the mixture in the mobile phase, caused by interaction of these components with the stationary phase, are used to separate the components. The four possible combinations of stationary and mobile phases have been used in chromatographic methods.

From the viewpoint of the clinical laboratory, these methods are used primarily for the detection of complex substances such as drugs and hormones. For example, gas–liquid chromatographs (GLC) and thin-layer chromatographs (TLC) have been useful in determining what drug or drugs have been taken in overdose cases. The availability of this information is vitally important to the clinician who must select appropriate therapy. The characteristics of the GLC are presented here as an important example of the use of chromatographic methods in the clinical laboratory.

## GAS–LIQUID CHROMATOGRAPHS

The basic components of a GLC are shown in Figure 11.4. Prior to being injected into the GLC, the patient sample usually must undergo some initial purification, the extent of which depends on the determination that is being performed. The functions of the major subsystems are as follows:

***Injector*** The injector is used to introduce into the GLC 1 to 5 ml of the patient sample including the solvent in which it is contained (usually a volatile organic solvent). The temperature of the injector is set to flash-evaporate the sample and solvent.

***Carrier Gas*** The inert carrier gas (usually $N_2$ or He) is the mobile phase of the chromatograph. It sweeps the evaporated sample and solvent gas down the column.

***Column*** The column typically is 1 m long and less than 7 mm in diameter. It is packed with the solid support material (such as diatomaceous earth). The solid support is coated with the liquid phase. The small size of the solid beads produces the separation of the components. The column is enclosed in an oven the temperature of which is carefully controlled. A temperature programmer gradually increases the temperature of the column in a sequence designed for maximal efficiency of separation for the type of substance being analyzed.

***Detector*** The detector is located at the end of the column. Its function is to provide an electric output proportional to the quantity of the compound in the effluent gas. A number of types of detectors are available for use with different types of samples. They include ionization detectors, thermal-conductivity detectors, and electron-capture detectors. Ionization detectors are most commonly used in clinical laboratory applications (Littlewood, 1970).

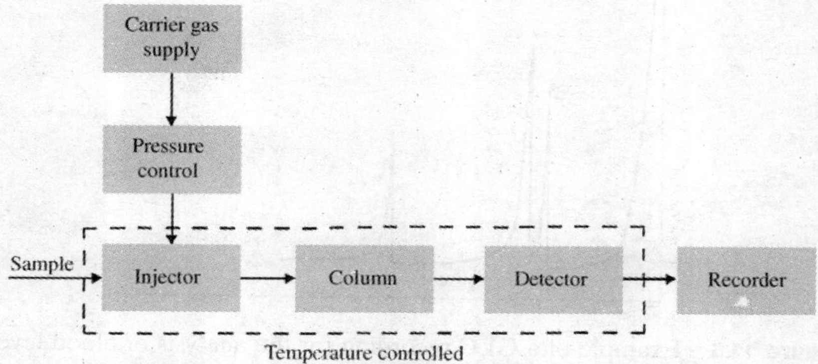


**Figure 11.4** **Block diagram of a gas–liquid chromatograph (GLC)**

All the detectors are sensitive to classes of compounds, not only to some particular component of interest. Therefore, both the concentrations of the detected compounds and the times during the operation of the column when those concentrations occurred (that is, a plot of concentration versus time) are used in determining the types and quantities of components present in the sample. The output of the detector is connected to a recorder.

***Recorder*** In the recorder, the $x$ axis represents time, and the $y$ axis the output of the detector. The recording thus provides a display of both the quantity of a component that was present (the area under the peak) and the time at which it was eluted off the column. From this information, the components present can be identified by the time they took to leave the column or, preferably, by comparison with recordings obtained by analyzing compounds of known composition with the GLC.

Figure 11.5 shows a recording obtained from the analysis of a blood specimen for the levels of the important anticonvulsant drugs phenobarbital and phenytoin. A measured amount of heptabarbital was added to the specimen to serve as an internal standard. The area under the phenobarbital and phenytoin peaks is compared with the area under the heptabarbital peak to compute the blood levels of these drugs.

Gas–liquid chromatography offers a number of important advantages in the analysis of complex compounds. They include speed, ability to operate with small amounts of sample, and great sensitivity. Most instruments can complete analyses of clinically important substances in less than 1 h, and often in 15 min or less. Only milliliter amounts of the sample are needed. The sensitivity of the device depends on the detector used, but high-quality instruments can detect 1 ng quantities of a compound.

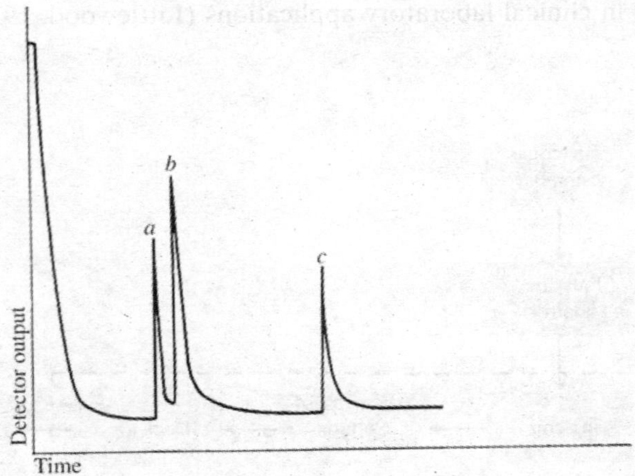


**Figure 11.5** Example of a GLC recording for the analysis of blood levels of phenobarbital (peak $a$) and phenytoin (peak $c$). Peak $b$ corresponds to the level of heptabarbital (the internal standard).

## 11.4 ELECTROPHORESIS

Devices based on electrophoretic principles are used in the clinical laboratory to measure quantities of the various types of proteins in plasma, urine, and CSF; to separate enzymes into their component isoenzymes; to identify antibodies; and to serve in a variety of other applications.

### BASIC PRINCIPLES

Electrophoresis may in general be defined as the movement of a solid phase with respect to a liquid (the buffer solution). The main functions of the buffer solution are to carry the current and to keep the pH of the solution constant during the migration. The buffer solution is supported by a solid substance called the medium.

Our discussion in this section is limited to zone electrophoresis. In this technique, the sample is applied to the medium; and under the effect of the electric field, groups of particles that are similar in charge, size, and shape migrate at similar rates. This results in separation of the particles into zones. The factors that affect the speed of migration of the particles in the field are discussed in the following paragraphs.

***Magnitude of Charge*** The mobility of a given particle is directly related to the net magnitude of the particle's charge. Mobility is defined as "the distance in centimeters a particle moves in unit time per unit field strength, expressed as voltage drop per centimeter" [mobility = $cm^2/(V{\cdot}s)$] (Henry *et al.*,1974).

***Ionic Strength of Buffer*** The more concentrated the buffer, the slower the rate of migration of the particles. This is because the greater the proportion of buffer ions present, the greater the proportion of the current they carry. It is also due to interaction between the buffer ions and the particles.

***Temperature*** Mobility is directly related to temperature. The flow of current through the resistance of the medium produces heat. This heat has two important effects on the electrophoresis. First, it causes the temperature of the medium to increase, which decreases its resistance and thereby causes the rate of migration to increase. Second, the heat causes water to evaporate from the surface of the medium. This increases the concentration of the particles and further boosts the rate of migration. Because of these effects, either the applied voltage or the current must be held constant in order to maintain acceptable reproducibility of the procedures. For short runs at relatively low voltage levels, either can be held constant. However, when a gel is used as the medium, heating is a significant problem. With this type of medium, constant-current sources are normally used to minimize the production of heat.

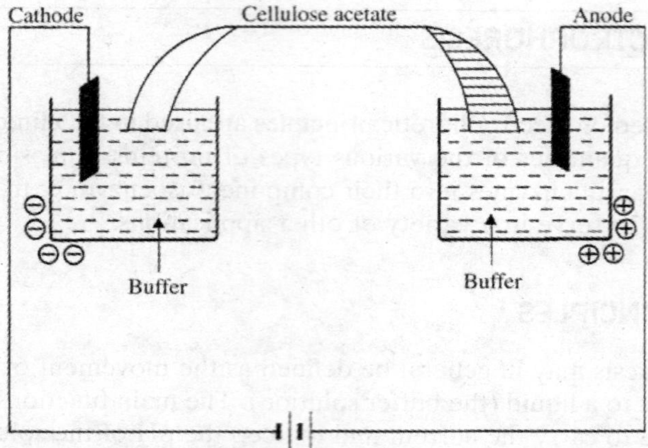


**Figure 11.6 Cellulose acetate electrophoresis** (From R. Hicks, J. R. Schenken, and M. A. Steinrauf, *Laboratory Instrumentation.* Hagerstown, MD: Harper & Row, 1974. Used with permission of C. A. McWhorter.)

***Time*** The distance of migration is directly related to the time the electrophoresis takes. Other factors that influence migration include electroendosmosis, chromatography, particle shape, "barrier" effect, "wick flow," and streaming potential (Henry *et al.,* 1974; Hicks *et al.,*1974).

***Types of Support Media*** A large variety of support media have been used in various electrophoretic applications. They include paper, cellulose acetate, starch gel, agar gel, acrylamide gel, and sucrose. We discuss cellulose acetate electrophoresis here, because it is used extensively in clinical laboratories and because the same general method is used with other media.

Cellulose acetate has a number of desirable properties compared with the paper that was the medium first used in electrophoresis.

Figure 11.6 illustrates the basic process of cellulose acetate electrophoresis. The cellulose acetate strip is saturated with the buffer solution and placed in the membrane holder (the "bridge"). The bridge is placed in the "cell" with both ends of the strip in the buffer wells.

A number of electrophoreses (typically eight) can be done on one strip. The sample for each test is placed on the strip at a marked location. Then the electric potential is applied across the strip. With this type of electrophoresis, constant-voltage-source power supplies are often used. A typical voltage is 250 V, which results in an initial current of 4 to 6 mA. As we have noted, this current increases slightly during the procedure. After 15 to 20 min, depending on the device used, the electric voltage is removed. The next step is to fix the migrated protein bands to the buffer and to stain them so that they can be seen as well as subsequently quantified. This may be done in separate or combined exposures to a fixative and a dye. The membrane is now "cleared" to make it transparent. The densities due to the dyed-specimen fractions are not affected. The membrane is dried in preparation for densitometry.

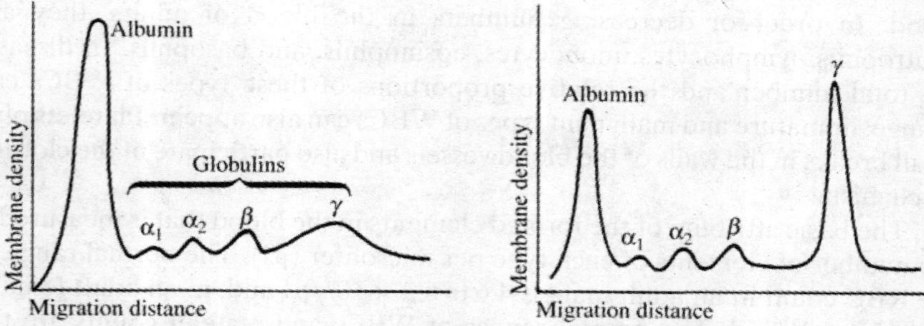


**Figure 11.7 Examples of patterns of serum protein electrophoresis** The left-hand pattern is normal; the right-hand pattern is seen when there is an overproduction of a single type of gamma globulin.

The densitometer is a device that consists of a light source, filter, and detector (typically a photodiode). The design and operation of this type of device are discussed in Section 11.1.

The membrane is placed in a holder in the densitometer. The path of migration of one of the specimens is then scanned. The low-voltage output of the detector is amplified by a very stable analog preamplifier. The output of the preamplifier is sent to an analog *x–y* recorder and to an analog integrator circuit. The *x–y* recorder produces a plot whereon the *x* coordinate represents migration distance and the *y* coordinate represents membrane density (which is directly proportional to the amount of specimen component that has moved the corresponding migration distance). The integrator has circuitry that detects the beginning and end of each significant peak and computes the area under the peak. These numbers are printed on the analog recording next to the corresponding peak. This process is repeated for each of the specimens on the membrane.

Figure 11.7 shows examples of the types of plots that are obtained via electrophoresis. These plots are for serum protein electrophoresis.

## 11.5 HEMATOLOGY

### BASIC CONCEPTS

The blood consists of formed elements, substances in solution, and water. This section covers only devices that measure characteristics of the formed elements: red blood cells (RBCs), white blood cells (WBCs), and platelets. The primary functions of the RBCs are to carry oxygen from the lungs to the various organs and to carry carbon dioxide back from these organs to the lungs for excretion. The primary function of the WBCs is to help defend the body against infections. Five types of WBCs are normally found in the peripheral blood. In order of decreasing numbers in the blood of adults, they are neutrophils, lymphocytes, monocytes, eosinophils, and basophils. In disease, the total number and the relative proportions of these types of WBCs can change; immature and malignant types of WBCs can also appear. Platelets plug small breaks in the walls of the blood vessels and also participate in the clotting mechanism.

The basic attribute of the formed elements in the blood that is measured is the number of elements of each type per microliter (μl). The normal range of the RBC count in an adult male is 4.6 to $6.2 \times 10^6/\mu l$ and, in an adult female, 4.2 to $5.4 \times 10^6/\mu l$. The normal ranges of WBCs and platelet counts are the same for men and women. The normal range of the WBC count is 4,500 to 11,000/μl; that for the platelet count is 150,000 to 400,000/μl. The hematocrit (HCT) is the ratio of the volume of all the formed elements in a sample of blood to the total volume of the blood sample. It is reported as a percentage, the normal range in adult men being 40 to 54% and, in adult women, 35 to 47%. Hemoglobin (Hb) is a conjugated protein within the RBCs that transports most of the $O_2$ and a portion of the $CO_2$ that is carried in the blood. It is reported in grams per deciliter. The normal range in adult men is 13.5 to 18 g/dl, and that in adult women is 12 to 16 g/dl.

A second group of measurements is made to characterize the RBC volume and Hb concentration. These measurements include the mean corpuscular volume (MCV) in cubic micrometers, the mean corpuscular hemoglobin (MCH) content in picograms, and the mean corpuscular hemoglobin concentration (MCHC) in percent. These values are called the RBC indices. Normal ranges for these parameters are as follows:

$$\begin{aligned} \text{MCV}: &\quad 82\text{–}98\ \mu\text{m}^3 \\ \text{MCH}: &\quad 27\text{–}31\ \text{pg} \\ \text{MCHC}: &\quad 32\text{–}36\% \end{aligned}$$

The RBC count (in millions per microliter), HCT (in percent), MCV (in cubic micrometers), Hb (in grams per deciliter), MCH (in picograms), and MCHC (in percent) are related as follows:

$$\text{MCV} = \frac{10\,\text{HCT}}{\text{RBC count}} \tag{11.6}$$

$$\text{MCH} = \frac{10\,\text{Hb}}{\text{RBC count}} \tag{11.7}$$

$$\text{MCHC} = \frac{100\text{Hb}}{\text{HCT}} \tag{11.8}$$

The units for RBC count, Hb, and HCT that are employed in these calculations are such that the units for MCV, MCH, and MCHC are those given above.

**EXAMPLE 11.3** Calculate the RBC indices from the following data.

$$\text{RBC} = 5\ \text{million}/\mu\text{l}$$
$$\text{Hb} = 15\ \text{g/dl}$$
$$\text{HCT} = 45\%$$

**ANSWER**

$$\text{MCV} = \frac{10\,\text{HCT}}{\text{RBC count}} = \frac{450}{5} = 90\ \mu\text{m}^3$$

$$\text{MCH} = \frac{10\,\text{Hb}}{\text{RBC count}} = \frac{150}{5} = 30\ \text{pg}$$

$$\text{MCHC} = \frac{100\,\text{Hb}}{\text{HCT}} = \frac{1500}{45} = 33.3\%$$

A new RBC characteristic that is assuming increasing importance in hematology is the volume distribution width [called the *red blood cell distribution width* (RDW)]. Somewhat similar to the standard deviation of a Gaussian distribution, it is a measure of the spread of the RBC volume distribution. In many RBC disorders, RBC production is disordered and a wider range than usual of RBC sizes is produced, leading to an increased RDW value.

Using the RDW with other RBC parameters can aid in the diagnosis of RBC disorders. For example, in iron deficiency anemia (an acquired disorder in which hemoglobin production is reduced due to a lack of iron) the RDW is high and the MCV is low or normal, while in heterozygous thalassemia (an inherited disorder in hemoglobin synthesis is abnormal) the RDW is normal and MCV is low.

## ELECTRONIC DEVICES FOR MEASURING BLOOD CHARACTERISTICS

There are two major classes of electronic devices for measuring blood characteristics. One type is based on changes in the electric resistance of a solution when a formed blood element passes through an aperture. Beckman Coulter, Abbott Diagnostics, and others manufacture hematology instruments based on this technique. The other type utilizes deflections of a light beam caused by the passage of formed blood elements to make its measurements. Bayer-Technicon Corporation is a leading manufacturer of hematology instruments that use this approach. Bayer Coulter Corporation has been a leader in blood analyzers for many years and it has developed a large series of instruments. Let us review two of these instruments: the very widely used Coulter STKS and the newest instrument in this series, the Coulter LH 755. The features of the STKS will be presented first, and then the added capabilities of the LH 755 will be discussed.

## COULTER STKS

The analyzed sample is blood that has been anticoagulated, with ethylenediaminetetraacetic acid (EDTA). Anticoagulants are substances that interfere with the normal clot-forming mechanism of the blood. They keep the formed elements from clumping together, which would prevent them from being counted accurately. Ethylenediaminetetraacetic acid does this by removing calcium from the blood. The initial step in the analysis procedure is the automatic aspiration of a carefully measured portion of the specimen. Next the specimen is diluted to 1:224 with a solution of approximately the same osmolality as the plasma in Diluter I, Figure 11.8. The diluted specimen is then split, part going to the mixing and lyzing chamber and part to Diluter II.

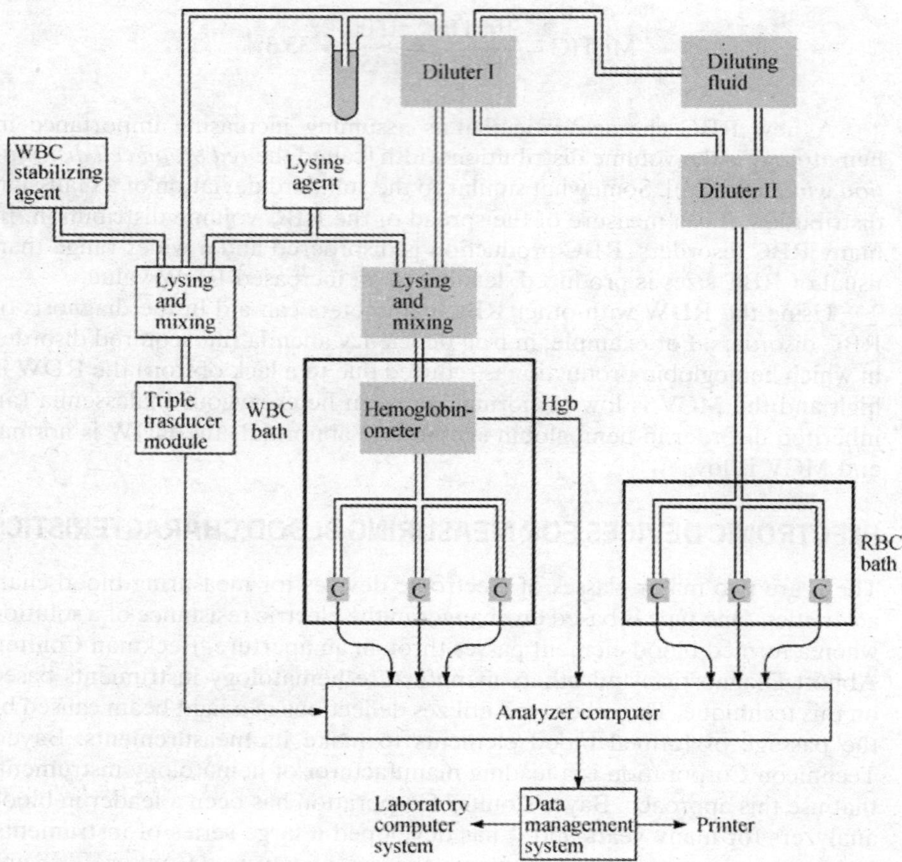


**Figure 11.8 A block diagram of a Coulter Model STKS** (Modified from J. Davidsohn and J. B. Henry, Todd Sanford Clinical Diagnosis by Laboratory Methods, 15 ed. Philadelphia: W. B. Saunders Co, 1974.)

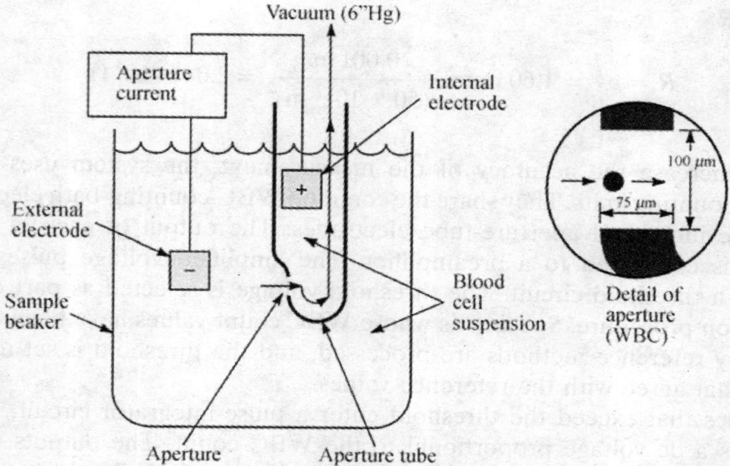


**Figure 11.9** Coulter STKS aperture bath.

The function of the diluting and lyzing chamber is to prepare the specimen for the measurement of its hemoglobin content and WBC count. The lyzing agent causes the cell membranes of the RBCs to rupture and release their hemoglobin into the solution. The WBCs are not lyzed by this agent. Adding the volume of lyzing agent increases the dilution to 1:250. A second substance, Drabkin's solution, is present; it converts hemoglobin to cyanmethemoglobin. This is done to conform to the accepted standard method for determining hemoglobin concentration. The advantage of this method is that it includes essentially all forms of hemoglobin found in the blood. The specimen is next passed through the WBC bath, which functions as a cuvette for the spectrophotometric determination (see Section 11.1) of the hemoglobin content. The final step in this process is measurement of the WBC count.

Figure 11.9 outlines the method that is used in making this determination. The same method is used for counting RBCs. A vacuum pump draws a carefully controlled volume of fluid from the WBC-counting bath through the aperture. A constant current passes from the electrode in the WBC-counting bath through the aperture to the second electrode in the aperture tube. As each WBC passes through the aperture, it displaces a volume of the solution equal to its own volume. The resistance of the WBC is much greater than that of the fluid, so a voltage pulse is created in the circuit connecting the two electrodes. The magnitude of that voltage pulse is related to the volume of the WBC (Zhanf, 2006).

**EXAMPLE 11.4** Diluted blood with a resistivity of 160 $\Omega\cdot$cm passes through a Coulter Counter cylindrical aperture 100 $\mu$m in diameter and 1 mm long. Calculate the resistance of the liquid-filled aperture.

**ANSWER**

$$R = \rho \frac{l}{a} = 1.60\,\Omega \cdot \text{m} \frac{0.001\text{ m}}{\pi(50 \times 10^{-6}\text{ m})^2} = 2.04 \times 10^5\,\Omega$$

To increase the accuracy of the measurement, the system uses three parallel counting units. They share the common WBC-counting-bath electrode and have individual aperture-tube electrodes. The output of each of these circuits is connected to a preamplifier. The amplified voltage pulses pass through a threshold circuit. The threshold voltage is selected as part of the calibration procedure. Specimens whose WBC count values have been determined by reference methods are processed, and the threshold is set to give counts that agree with the reference values.

Pulses that exceed the threshold enter a pulse-integrator circuit, which produces a dc voltage proportional to the WBC count. The outputs of the three pulse-integrator circuits are sent to a voting circuit. If the three outputs agree within a specified range, they are averaged. If one output disagrees with the other two by more than the specified range, it is not used in computing the average. If all three outputs disagree by more than the specified range, an error indicator is set, and a zero value is produced.

The next step in the signal processing is to correct the average-count signal for coincidence. Coincidence is the passage of two or more WBCs through the aperture at the same time. Statistical analysis is used to estimate the average level of coincidence for the aperture size and any uncorrected count level. An analog circuit makes this conversion. The digital WBC count value is displayed and also recorded on a printer.

We will now examine the right side of Figure 11.8. The first step is the further dilution of the specimen to 1:224 in Diluter II. This second dilution is required because of the much greater concentration of RBC than of WBC in the blood. A system identical to the one described for the WBC count is used to obtain the RBC count.

Cells with volumes greater than 35.9 fl are classified as RBCs. A 256-channel RBC size histogram is prepared. The MCV and RDW are computed from this histogram. The RDW is the coefficient of variation of the RBC volume distribution.

Cells whose volumes are in the 2 to 20 fl range are classified as platelets. The volumes of these cells from each aperture are transformed into a 64-channel histogram. These histograms are statistically processed to yield a platelet count along with a mean platelet volume (MPV) and platelet distribution width (PDW) from each channel. A voting process similar to that described for the WBC count is used to determine the final values for these parameters. The MPV and PDW values are primarily used for quality control functions at this time.

The RBC count, Hb and MCV are input to a special-purpose computer circuit that calculates the values of HCT, MCH, and MCHC by using the relationships given in (11.6) to (11.8).

The Coulter STKS performs a WBC differential count using a flow cytometry approach. At the same time portions of the specimen are being delivered to the WBC and RBC baths, another portion of the specimen is sent to the WBC differential mixing and lyzing chamber. Here the specimen is combined with (1) a lyzing agent to remove the RBCs and (2) a WBC stabilizing agent. The WBC stabilizing agent preserves the characteristics of the WBCs as they are processed in the triple transducer flow cell. Flow cytometry consists of evaluating cells moving in a fluid stream. The triple transducer module includes electronics to create a single line of cells that is passed through a measurement station. In the STKS measurements of low-frequency impedance, high-frequency conductivity and light scatter are made. The cell volume measurement is based on low-frequency impedance (the same approach used to measure RBC and WBC volume), and the internal conductivity is derived from the high-frequency conductivity. A laser illuminates the cells in the measurement station to create the light scatter. The light scatter measurement is made by a forward scatter detector. A measurement of cell internal structure and shape is based on the light scatter measurement. The cell volume, internal conductivity, and cell internal structure and shape measurements are sent to the analyzer computer for processing. The percent lymphocytes, monocytes, neutrophils, basophils, and eosinophils are calculated based on the cell position in a three-dimensional scatter plot. Figure 11.10 is one of the two-dimensional views of this three-dimensional scatter plot. These two-dimensional views can be displayed at the instrument to allow the operator to monitor the functioning of the instrument. The values for basophils and eosinophils are less reliable than those for the other cell types. If the percentage of these cell types exceeds laboratory specified limits (e.g., 10% for

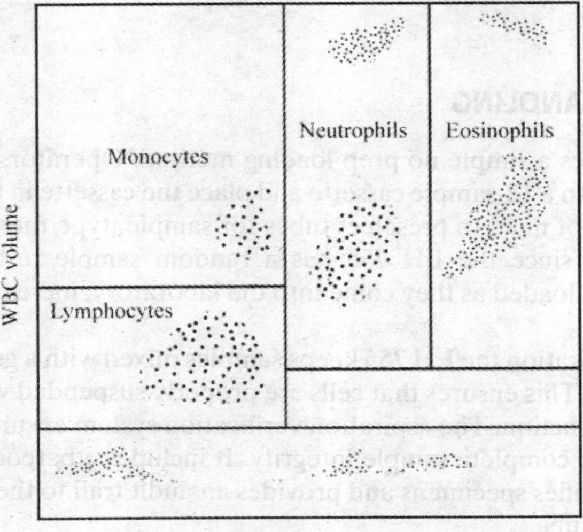


**Figure 11.10 Two-dimensional scatterplot**

eosinophils or 5% for basophils), a technologist will scan a peripheral blood smear slide to determine if the calculated value is correct. If it is not, a manual WBC differential will be performed. The STKS applies criteria to the scatter plot to determine if the computed WBC differential count appears to be accurate. In the majority of cases, the count is judged accurate and the need to perform a labor-intensive manual count is eliminated. Since the STKS cannot accurately identify immature WBCs (these cells are not normally found in the peripheral blood), the presence of these cells will trigger a message stating that a manual WBC count needs to be performed (Zelmanovic and Kunicka, 2006).

The STKS uses this same approach to measure the number of reticulocytes that are present. The RBCs are dyed before the specimen is placed in the STKS with New Methylene Blue to enhance the differences in characteristics measured in the flow cell between reticulocytes and mature RBCs. The reticulocyte count measurement is made as a separate run of the instrument. This is a very useful capability since a manual reticulocyte count is a time-consuming and relatively inaccurate process.

The blood parameters are printed on a result-report card. The printer includes a patient-identification number that is input to the STKS by the technologist. In computerized clinical laboratory systems, this identifying number, and the blood parameters are directly transmitted to the laboratory computer system.

## COULTER LH 755

The LH 755 is a workstation that blends sample handling, advanced testing accuracy and integrated postanalytical slide making and slide staining in real time.

## SPECIMEN HANDLING

The LH 755 uses a simple no prep loading method. Operators take a sample tube, place it into a 12-sample cassette and place the cassette in the instrument. Operators do not need to preselect tubes for sample, type them, or sort them before loading since the LH 755 has a random sample testing capability. Samples can be loaded as they come into the laboratory, increasing laboratory productivity.

Before aspiration the LH 755 keeps samples mixed with a gentle motion of the rocker bed. This ensures that cells are properly suspended without the risk of cellular destruction. The aspiration verification system ensures both sample verification and complete sample integrity. It includes a barcode scanner that positively identifies specimens and provides an audit trail to the exact location of the sample tube.

The LH 755 confirms sample integrity using dual optical blood detectors that check every sample for the presence of clots or microbubbles. The LH 755 also features a totally sealed aspiration and dilution system to protect laboratory staff from blood born pathogens. While the LH 755 enclosed needle simultaneously vents and aspirates the sample, it withdraws an aliquot of blood that is sufficient to analyze a sample and make a slide. This eliminates the need for redundant sample processing should a slide be needed.

The aliquot of blood is kept mixed by repetitive gentle inversion in a heated core to ensure proper cellular distribution without damaging the cells. These mechanisms and automated processes minimize operator procedures while improving productivity. Operator safety is increased by minimizing the chance of exposure to patient specimens.

## TEST PERFORMANCE

The LH 755 performs complete blood counts, WBC differential counts, and RBC morphology evaluation as well as nucleated RBC (NRBC), platelet and reticulocyte counts. The AccuCount technology delivers expanded linearity and high levels of accuracy, particularly at the clinical decision threshold, and virtually eliminates false-positive flagging. It is a set of mathematical algorithms that is used to process the individual cell volume, high-frequency conductivity, and laser-light scatter measurements made by the instrument.

The AccuCount WBC count has linearity from 0 to 400,000/μl and eliminates most interference from RBCs, NRBCs, giant platelets, and platelet clumps, which decrease the need for manual intervention. The AccuCount platelet count expands linearity from 0 to 3,000,000/μl. The accuracy of AccuCount has been validated against reference flow cytometry methods.

The LH 755 WBC differential allows laboratories to minimize manual slide reviews. It includes a six-part differential plus the enumeration of NRBCs. The determination of which cells are NRBCs is based on the location of the cell in the NRBC area of the differential plot (cell volume versus rotated light scatter) as well as the presence of cells in the far left (low cell volume) end of the WBC histogram. If cells are present in both locations, the NRBC count is derived from the WBC histogram.

AccuGate technology provides accurate enumeration of populations, blasts identification, and accurate flagging. It is based on using adaptive contouring methods to achieve optimal separation of overlapping clusters of data.

## SLIDE PREPARATION

When cells are present that can't be identified by the LH 755 differential method or when user defined decision rules specify that a manual review of the blood specimen is required, a blood smear is automatically prepared. This process is begun by the integrated slide labeling station attaching a label to the slide. The label can contain up to 7 lines of information, or three lines of text and a barcode. It is not affected by fixatives or stains. Once at the smearing station a second slide is released and is used as the spreader blade.

As a drop of blood is applied to the slide, an algorithm makes an intelligent viscosity calculation based on parameters of the CBC data. This calculation determines the amount of time the spreader blade waits for the blood to properly spread out across the slide, as well as the acceleration rate and the final velocity of the spreader blade, creating a slide with a consistent feathered edge. The feathered edge is the portion of the smear where the RBCs are just touching and is the best area in which to make cytologic evaluations.

The prepared smear is dried and stained. The LH 755 gently warms the slide from underneath accelerating the natural evaporation process without introducing drying artifacts. When a slide exits the drying lane it is automatically lowered into a basket. Completed baskets containing 6 to 12 slides are routed to the integrated slide-staining module. The slide stainer's robotic arm then retrieves the basket and moves it into the staining module for automatic fixing, staining and drying.

## SYSTEM CONTROL

Age, gender and location specific reference ranges, action and critical limits can be specified. These postanalytical sample review criteria are used so that every sample is assessed the same way every time by every person running the analyzer. Decision rules can be easily defined for parameter values, flags, system messages, location, specific physicians or a combination of these factors. The LH 755 provides fully automated testing that reduces technologist time requirements.

Normal results are auto validated without further technologist intervention. Abnormal results are held for review and follow-up as indicated by the message generator. Samples that require review are sorted and placed in various folders for quick retrieval. A pathologist will review the abnormal slides. He/she will prepare an interpretive report including possible etiologies of the abnormal smear results for the patient's clinician.

## PROBLEMS

**11.1** Discuss the differences between photometers or colorimeters and monochromators. What are the factors to consider in selecting one or the other for a particular determination?

**11.2** Sketch a double-beam spectrophotometer, and explain its operation.

**11.3** Explain why fluorometers can be used to detect much smaller quantities of substances than absorption spectrophotometers.

**11.4** Assume that you are the biomedical engineer at a 300-bed hospital. The director of the clinical laboratory plans to buy an automated chemical analyzer and wants your advice on which type to buy. What factors would you consider in preparing your response? (This is a broad question, but try to be as specific as possible.)

**11.5** The following values are obtained for a specimen of venous blood: MCV = 90 $\mu m^3$, HCT = 40%, and MCH = 30 pg. Compute the RBC count, the MCHC, and the Hb concentration.

**11.6** Design a circuit to perform the RBC-counting function in a Coulter Counter. Include the voting logic.

## REFERENCES

Brittin, G. M., and G. Brecher, "Instrumentation and automation in clinical hematology." *Prog. Hematol.*, 1971, 7, 299–341.

Davidsohn, J., and J. B. Henry, *Todd Sanford Clinical Diagnosis by Laboratory Methods*, 15th ed. Philadelphia: W. B. Saunders Co, 1974.

Dutcher, T. F., J. F. Benzel, J. J. Egan, D. F. Hart, and E. A. Christopher, "Evaluation of an automated differential leukocyte counting system." *Amer. J. Clin. Pathol.*, 1974, 62, 523–529.

Ellis, K. J., and J. F. Morrison, "Some sources of error and artifacts in spectrophotometric measurements." *Clin. Chem.*, 1975, 21, 776–779.

Henry, J. B., *Todd Sanford Clinical Diagnosis by Laboratory Methods*, 17th ed. Philadelphia: Saunders, 1984.

Henry, R. J., D. C. Cannon, and J. W. Winkelman, *Clinical Chemistry*. New York: Harper & Row, 1974.

Hicks, R., J. R. Schenken, and M. A. Steinrauf, *Laboratory Instrumentation*. New York: Harper & Row, 1974.

Klebe, R. J., G. Zardeneta, and P. M. Horowitz, "*Fluorescence measurements*" In J. G. Webster (ed.), *Encyclopedia of Medical Devices and Instrumentation*, 2nd ed. New York: Wiley, 2006, Vol. 3, pp. 342–347.

Littlewood, A. B., *Gas Chromatography*. New York: Academic, 1970.

Lyon, A. W., and M. E. Lyon, "Flame atomic emission spectrometry and atomic emission spectrometry." In J. G. Webster (ed.), *Encyclopedia of Medical Devices and Instrumentation*, 2nd ed. New York: Wiley, 2006, Vol. 3, pp. 315–322.

Shen, L.-J., R. Mandel, and W.-C. Shen, "Colorimetry." In J. G. Webster (ed.), *Encyclopedia of Medical Devices and Instrumentation*, 2nd ed. New York: Wiley, 2006, Vol. 2, pp. 187–197.

Zelmanovic, D., and J. Kunicka "Differential counts, automated." In J. G. Webster (ed.), *Encyclopedia of Medical Devices and Instrumentation*, 2nd ed. New York: Wiley, 2006, Vol. 2, pp. 410–421.

Zhanf, Y., "Cell counter, blood." In J. G. Webster (ed.), *Encyclopedia of Medical Devices and Instrumentation*, 2nd ed. New York: Wiley, 2006, Vol. 2, pp. 81–90.

# 12

# MEDICAL IMAGING SYSTEMS

Melvin P. Siedband

For many years, photographic film was the principal means for storing medical images. Computers have provided a new means for storing, processing, transferring, and displaying images. First used for computerized tomography, computers and digital image processing have engendered a revolution in the way medical images are produced and manipulated. Now it is possible to acquire data, perform mathematical operations to produce images, emphasize details or differences of images, and store and retrieve images from remote sites, all without film. Telephone lines and other communication means such as the Internet with common standards of image communication make possible the near instant display of the information needed for diagnosis.

Photographic, x-ray, ultrasonic, radionuclide, television, and other imaging systems can be thought of as cameras. All camera images are limited by resolution, amplitude scale, and noise content. The photographic image can be enlarged until it becomes quite grainy, and this graininess is the bound on both resolution and noise. The x-ray image is resolution limited by the dimensions of the x-ray source and noise limited by the beam intensity. The ultrasound image is limited by the angular resolution of the transducer and its ability to separate true signals from false signals and noise.

An image can be studied without regard to the camera that produced it. A camera can be considered a device that transfers an image from one surface to another. It can be defined as an aperture through which the signals related to all elements of the original image must pass to appear in the final image. A camera—whether a television, x-ray, or other image-forming device—can be described in terms of its spatial-transfer function.

## 12.1 INFORMATION CONTENT OF AN IMAGE

In most cases, the information content of an image is the product of the number of discrete picture elements (pixels) and the number of amplitude levels of each pixel. Because pixels may not be quantized into neat boxes, but overlap each other, some method of defining their dimensions is needed. Noise, whether originating from photographic grain, electric charge, or the statistical variations of the number of quanta (light, x ray, or gamma ray), limits the amplification permitted in a channel. For convenience, the number of amplitude steps within a channel is taken to be the same as the measured signal-to-noise ratio (SNR). The noise figure of a channel is the ratio of the theoretical or best possible SNR to the measured SNR.

## RESOLUTION

An image can be considered a surface of given dimension that has a spatial resolution expressed in terms of line pairs per millimeter (lp/mm). Resolution is defined this way so that objects and the spaces between them are counted equally. If we examine copper mesh having 10 holes/cm or 100 holes/cm$^2$, the system must resolve 1 lp/mm and must have at least 2 pixels/mm to show each mesh hole and each mesh wire. A single countable object requires at least one line pair (2 pixels) on each axis so that the space between objects as well as the object itself may be resolved.

Figure 12.1 shows the image of a set of round objects in a television frame. The first problem is to determine the number of television scanning lines

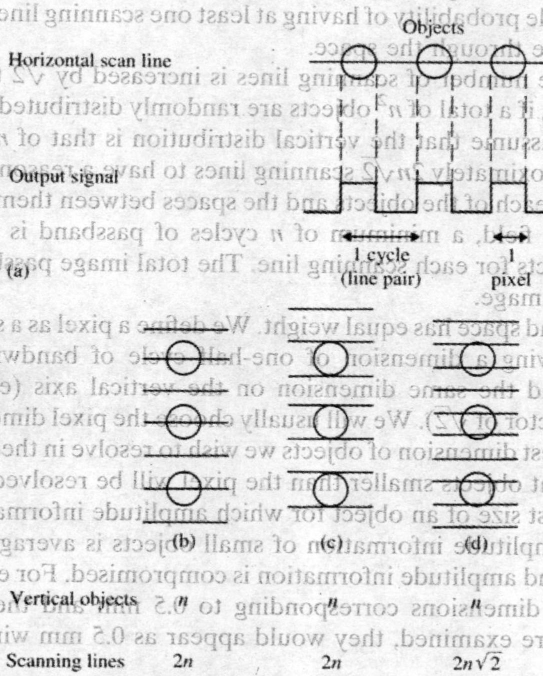

**Figure 12.1** **Scanning lines and round objects** (a) Each object represents 1 pixel, but each cycle of output signal represents 2 pixels, (b) For $n$ vertical objects, $2n$ scanning lines are required. (c) If objects are located between scanning lines, $2n$ lines are insufficient. (d) For adequate resolution, $2n\sqrt{2}$ lines are required.

needed to resolve these objects. We assume that the television scanner comprises a sensor that can be swept one line at a time across the image, stepped down to the next line, and so on, until the entire image is raster scanned. We assume that the output of the sensor will eventually feed a scanning light projector that paints a beam of light onto a photographic film to reproduce the original image as the light beam is modulated by the output of the sensor.

The first requirement of the scanner is to direct a line through each of the round objects. If the object is white, the output signal of the sensor is positive; if dark, then negative. For a succession of white objects with dark spaces between them, each object will be represented by a positive half cycle of the signal and each space by a negative half cycle. In general, a countable object requires one whole cycle of spatial frequency passband: the positive half cycle for the object and the negative half cycle for the space between objects.

In the vertical axis of columns of objects, a scanning line is needed for each row of objects and another scanning line is needed to detect the spaces. In any real system, we may not know the location of the object relative to the scanning lines. For a vertical column of $n$ objects, there must be at least $2n$ scanning lines. If the objects are disposed randomly, we must have more scanning lines to have a reasonable probability of having at least one scanning line through an object and one line through the space.

In general, the number of scanning lines is increased by $\sqrt{2}$ to allow for randomness. Thus, if a total of $n^2$ objects are randomly distributed in a square field of view, we assume that the vertical distribution is that of $n$ objects. A system needs approximately $2n\sqrt{2}$ scanning lines to have a reasonable probability of detecting each of the objects and the spaces between them. For the $n^2$ objects within the field, a minimum of $n$ cycles of passband is required to resolve these objects for each scanning line. The total image passband is thus $2n^2\sqrt{2}$ cycles per image.

Each object and space has equal weight. We define a pixel as a space on the image surface having a dimension of one-half cycle of bandwidth on the horizontal axis and the same dimension on the vertical axis (even though overscanned by factor of $\sqrt{2}$). We will usually choose the pixel dimension to be equal to the smallest dimension of objects we wish to resolve in the image. This does not mean that objects smaller than the pixel will be resolved. Rather, it defines the smallest size of an object for which amplitude information can be preserved. The amplitude information of small objects is averaged over the pixel dimension and amplitude information is compromised. For example, if a system had pixel dimensions corresponding to 0.5 mm and then 0.10 mm tungsten wires were examined, they would appear as 0.5 mm wires of lower contrast.

The bandwidth $\Delta f$ required for a television system is given by

$$\Delta f = \frac{n_h n_v 2\sqrt{2}}{F_h F_v T} \tag{12.1}$$

where

$n_h$ = maximal number of objects in a horizontal line
$n_v$ = maximal number of objects in a vertical line
$F_h$ = fraction of horizontal scan time spent on the picture (1.0 minus blanking fraction)
$F_v$ = fraction of vertical time spent on the picture
$T$ = total frame scanning time

**EXAMPLE 12.1** A standard United States closed-circuit television system has 240 objects in the horizontal direction, 180 in the vertical, $F_h = 0.82$, $F_v = 0.92$, and $T = 1/30$ s. Calculate the bandwidth.

**ANSWER**

$$\Delta f = \frac{(240)(180)(2)(2)^{1/2}}{(0.82)(0.92)(1/30)} = 4.85\,\text{MHz}$$

## IMAGE NOISE

All images are limited by both noise and spatial resolution. If we attempt to dissect an image into smaller and smaller areas, we soon find that the image is limited to some smallest element or that the lens or scanning aperture imposes a bound on how small an element we can resolve within the image. Further, within the smallest element, we can say that the image is either on or off. The on–off criterion certainly applies when we are considering silver grains of film. It also applies when we are considering a beam of electrons hitting a cathode-ray-tube phosphor: The beam is not continuous but rather consists of discrete electrons. The phosphor particles vary in size and in probability of being illuminated. For elements of larger size, we can say that the image has a gray, or amplitude, level, which can be defined by a digital number. This is another way of saying that the image is characterized by the number of on or off states of smaller elements.

If for each of a large number of trial measurements $q$, there is a small probability $p$ of a certain type of event; the average number of this type of event is simply $m = qp$. For example, if we wait $q$ seconds for randomly distributed raindrops to fall within a certain area, and for each second, the probability of observing a raindrop is $p$, then $m$ is the average number observed in several observations of $q$ seconds each. The relative probability of any *particular* number of drops $K$ in a measurement having an average $m$, $p(K;m)$, is given by the Poisson probability density distribution.

$$p(K;m) = \frac{e^{-m}m^k}{K!} \tag{12.2}$$

We can check that this distribution really has the average *m*.

$$\sum_{K=0}^{\infty} Kp(K;m) = m \tag{12.3}$$

The sum of $p(K;m)$ for all outcomes $K$ from zero to infinity is, of course, equal to 1. Finally, the variance of the distribution is also equal to $m$.

$$\sum_{K=0}^{\infty} Kp(K-m)^2 p(K;m) = m \tag{12.4}$$

Thus the rms fluctuation of outcomes around the average value $m$ is just $\sqrt{m}$. If we were to examine a succession of measurements that have an average outcome of 100 events, we would find very few with *exactly* 100 events, but they would be distributed about the average with a standard deviation of 10 events.

**EXAMPLE 12.2** For the Poisson probability density distribution, calculate $p(K;\ m)$ for $K = 0, 1, 2, 3, 4, 5$ and $m = 3$.

**ANSWER** Use the Poisson probability density distribution $P(K;m) = e^{-m}m^K/K!$ (12.2)

| K | m | P(k; m) |
|---|---|---|
| 0 | 3 | 0.049787 |
| 1 | 3 | 0.149361 |
| 2 | 3 | 0.224042 |
| 3 | 3 | 0.224042 |
| 4 | 3 | 0.168031 |
| 5 | 3 | 0.100819 |

When plotting, note that lines connecting points are not correct because $K$ takes on only integer values.

Independent raindrops falling on concrete squares and x-ray photons striking detector pixels have the same statistical properties. If the average number $r$ of raindrops per square is 100, the probability of finding exactly 100 is 0.040, even though the *average* is 100 per square. If we made a scanning voltmeter that read $N$ volts for $N$ events and used the scanning voltmeter to sample the output of the individual pixel, we would find a fluctuation of $\sqrt{N}$ rms volts.

Now we change from the steady signal $N$ to a modulated signal $N(1 \pm \overline{M})$, where $0 \le \overline{M} \le 1$ is the modulation and $N\overline{M}$ is the incremental increase representing the information-containing signal $S$. The maximal signal exists when $\overline{M} = 1$, so the maximal SNR equals $N/\sqrt{N} = \sqrt{N}$. Thus, for a time-average value of 100 events per pixel in 1 s, the maximal SNR equals 10. If the linear dimension of the cell is doubled, the area is multiplied by 4, and for the same time period, there are 400 events per larger pixel, for a maximal SNR of 20. Similarly, if only the integration time of the original cell is changed from 1 to 4 s, there is also the possibility of detecting 400 events per pixel and a maximal SNR of 20. For purely random signals having the same time average, time integration and spatial integration have the same effect. In other words, decreasing the resolution of an image (increasing the area of the pixel) either increases the SNR of the image or, for the same noise level, reduces the requirement for number of events. For those cases in which $\sqrt{M}$ is not equal to 1, the signal is $\overline{M}N$, but the noise level is still $\sqrt{N}$, so the SNR is $\overline{M}\sqrt{N}$.

The detection of low-contrast signals in a noisy field requires a fairly high SNR. See Figure 12.2, in which events correspond to gamma-ray photons, which register as counts on an image. We ask, "What is the probability that the number of photons per pixel randomly exceeds $N + J\sqrt{N}$ as a function of $J$ units of standard deviations?"

By referring to a table of integral values of the standard deviation, we find that where $J = 1$, 16% of the pixels exceed the bound; for $J = 2$, 2.3% of the pixels exceed the bound; for $J = 3$, 0.14% of the pixels exceed the bound; and for $J = 4$, 0.003% of the pixels exceed the bound. However, if we are looking at, say, the field of view of a typical television camera having $180 \times 240$ countable objects, or $360 \times 480 = 1.7 \times 10^5$ pixels, then even for $J = 4$, each television frame randomly has 5 pixels exceeding the bound. In other words, the modulation of TV must be greater than that required to produce the SNR $\overline{M}\sqrt{N}$ greater than 4 in order to simply detect the existence of a signal with fewer than five "false alarms," or random exceedances.

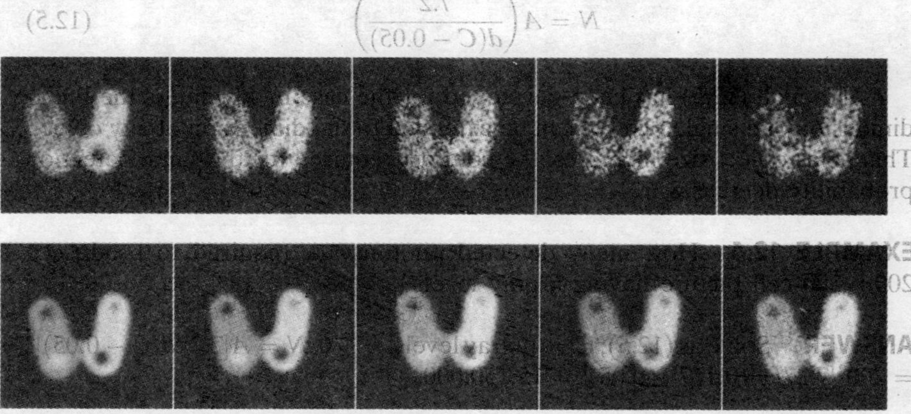

**Figure 12.2** In each successive gamma-camera picture of a thyroid phantom, the number of counts is increased by a factor of 2. The number of counts ranges from 1536 to 800,000. The Polaroid camera aperture was reduced to avoid overexposure as the number of counts was increased.

**EXAMPLE 12.3** A 100 × 100 pixel array has an average of 25 photons per pixel. How many picture elements will randomly exceed this average by more than 17 photons?

**ANSWER**

$$\overline{M} = 17/25 = 0.68,\ J = \overline{M}\sqrt{N} = 0.68(25)^{1/2} = 3.4.$$

From a table of single-ended probabilities of the normal (Gaussian) distribution http://www.math.unb.ca/~knight/utility/NormTble.htm or http://davidmlane.com/hyperstat/normal_distribution.html for $J = 3.4,\ p = 0.0003$.

$$\text{Exceedances} = 0.0003(10^4) = 3$$

If we define $C$ as the contrast of the $\overline{M}$ factor, the number of photons required must be at least equal to $bJ^2/C^2$, where $b$ is the total number of pixels. $J$ must be at least 4, for reasons cited earlier. If $d$ is the linear dimension of the pixel and $A$ is the area of the field, the total number of photons required equals $AJ^2/(d^2C^2)$. A good estimate for the number of photons of a grain-limited visual field would then be $N = 25A/(d^2C^2)$ under the assumption that $J = 5$. However, because of the presence of television scanning lines, phosphor granularity, and other factors, this number must actually be greater at low light levels and with low-contrast signals. The number approximately doubles to almost $50A/(d^2C^2)$. If we assume that, at the limit of resolution, an absolute-minimal contrast of approximately 5% is needed, then the number of photons required for detection is

$$N = A\left(\frac{7.2}{d(C - 0.05)}\right)^2 \tag{12.5}$$

Although (12.5) has been developed for the case in which $d$ is the linear dimension of a single pixel, $d$ can be extended to the dimension of any object. That is, as object size increases, the contrast required for the same detection probability decreases.

**EXAMPLE 12.4** How many detected photons are required to produce a 200 × 200 cell picture having 6 gray levels?

**ANSWER** Solve as (12.5); $C = 1/\text{gray levels} = 1/6$, $N = A[7.2/d(C - 0.05)]^2 = 200^2[7.2/(1)(0.167 - 0.05)]^2 = 15{,}150{,}000$.

Experiments have shown that (12.5) is true in most cases where the contrast is greater than 5%. However, when the number of scintillations or grains/pixel is very high, the observer can see objects of contrast below 5%. It is as if radiation requirements are increased greatly for objects below 5% contrast. For example, if the exposure is calculated for a small object at

10% contrast, the exposure may have to be increased by 50 or more times to clearly see an object at 2% contrast. Remember that contrast as used for radiation-produced or other noisy images is defined here as the number of scintillations or grains in the background reduced by a certain percentage (the contrast) by the presence of the object of interest. X-ray images are produced by subtracting quanta from the radiation field. Things would be far different if the objects produced quanta of their own against a dark field.

## 12.2 MODULATION TRANSFER FUNCTION

The *modulation transfer function* (MTF) is a modified form of the spatial-frequency response of an element or of the entire imaging system. The limiting resolution of a system, although it defines a system in terms of the smallest resolution element that can be seen, is not a sufficient indicator of system performance, because the system may resolve, say, a 2.0-mesh/mm copper screen at high contrast but perform poorly at showing the low-contrast image of a gall bladder. The MTF is plotted by measuring the amplitude response as a function of spatial frequency, assuming 100% response at zero frequency and ignoring phase shifts (see Figure 12.3). We assume that the amplitude is zero past the first phase rotation (crossover). The MTFs of each image transmission component may be combined as point-by-point products at each spatial frequency to obtain the MTF of the overall system.

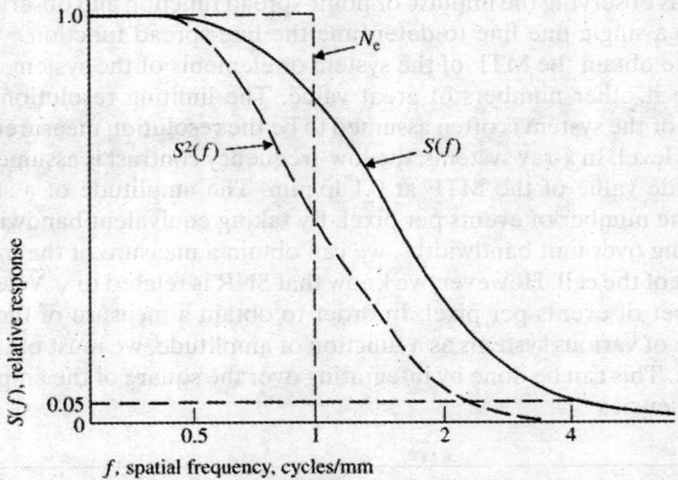


**Figure 12.3 Modulation transfer function $S(f)$ for a typical x-ray system** $S(f)$ is squared and integrated to yield $N_e$, the noise-equivalent bandwidth. The limiting resolution, 4 cycles/mm, is indicated at the 0.05 contrast level. The abscissa is plotted in cycles per millimeter, which is the same as line pairs per millimeter.

To measure MTF, we use a sinusoidal test object to modulate the input signal to cover the band of frequencies from zero to the maximal frequency. Sinusoidal test objects are hard to make, so a square-bar pattern is generally used. In the case of x-ray systems, the bar pattern is usually made of lead or tungsten alloys and consists of a series of bars and spaces starting at a low frequency and increasing in frequency (that is, decreasing in spacing). Such test objects are placed in front of the x-ray image detector, and the system is irradiated. Similar photographic bar patterns can be imaged by the various lenses of the system and tested independently by optical means. The detector consists of a microscope with a small slit in the local plane of the microscope lens, behind which is mounted a photomultiplier tube. The output of the tube is fed to a recorder, which may record the square-wave amplitude as a function of frequency.

A square-wave function can be analyzed in terms of its sine-wave components by means of a Fourier-series expansion. A matrix inversion of the Fourier-series expansion of square-wave terms yields an equation that defines sine-wave amplitudes in terms of square-wave amplitudes. In the following formula, $S(f)$ represents the amplitude of the sine wave at frequency $f$, obtained by substituting measured values $M(f)$ on the square-wave amplitudes at $f$, $3f$, $5f$, and so forth.

$$S(f) = \frac{\pi}{4}\left[M(f) + \frac{M(3f)}{3} - \frac{M(5f)}{5} + \frac{M(7f)}{7} - \cdots\right] \tag{12.6}$$

It is thus possible to convert the measured square-wave data to the sine-wave data required for obtaining the MTF. Other means exist for obtaining the MTF, such as observing the impulse or point-spread function and observing the response to a single fine line to determine the line-spread function.

Once we obtain the MTF of the system or elements of the system, we can derive from it other numbers of great value. The limiting resolution of the component or the system is often assumed to be the resolution measured at the 5% contrast level. In x-ray systems, the low-frequency contrast is assumed to be the amplitude value of the MTF at 0.1 lp/mm. The amplitude of a signal is related to the number of events per pixel. By taking equivalent bandwidths or by integrating over unit bandwidths, we can obtain a measure of the information content of the cell. However, we know that SNR is related to $\sqrt{N}$, where $N$ is the number of events per pixel. In order to obtain a measure of the visual equivalence of various systems as a function of amplitude, we must obtain rms equivalence. This can be done by integrating over the square of the amplitudes for all frequencies

## 12.3 NOISE-EQUIVALENT BANDWIDTH

Another way of looking at the information content of an image is to note that $N$ is related to area and that the square of the amplitude response is proportional to the number of events contained within an area defined by a given linear dimension. A noise-equivalent bandwidth $N_e$ is that of an equivalent system that has 100% amplitude response from zero frequency to $N_e$ and zero response above $N_e$ when compared with a system having an amplitude response as a function of spatial frequency, $S(f) = \text{MTF}$. The $N_e$ is obtained by integrating the square of the MTF amplitudes.

$$N_e = \int_0^\infty S^2(f)\,df \tag{12.7}$$

It is as though $N_e$ defines a mosaic of detectors of resolution $N_e$—say $N_e$ pixels/cm—that has the same SNR properties as a continuum of detectors having the MTF from which $N_e$ is derived. The value of $N_e$ is an excellent measure of the equivalent spatial resolution from the point of view of the noise performance of any system.

$$\frac{1}{N_e} = \left[\left(\frac{1}{N_{e1}}\right)^2 + \left(\frac{1}{N_{e2}}\right)^2 + \cdots\right]^{1/2} \tag{12.8}$$

The system $N_e$ can be estimated from elemental $N_e$'s. The $N_e$ concept becomes an extremely handy way to express the spatial-frequency response as a single number. As a useful and practical means for describing systems, $N_e$ ought to be preferred to limiting resolution.

## 12.4 TELEVISION SYSTEMS

A television system consists of a camera, optional image storage, signal processing means, and a display monitor. In a fluoroscopic system, the television camera is coupled through a lens or fiber optic to the output of the x-ray image intensifier. The camera detects the light signal, blanks it at the edges of the image frame, and adds synchronizing pulses so that storage and display devices will be synchronized to the camera scanning. Magnetic tape and disks, optical disks, and computer RAM are used to store image signals. Computer programs are used to process signals by emphasizing the edges of objects, by accumulating images to reduce noise, by showing differences within a group of images to enhance the outlines of blood vessels, or by showing the last image after x rays are turned off to reduce exposure. Computer processing makes possible rapid communication and diagnosis at a distance by way of the Internet or other data links. Data and image management systems combine the diagnostic images and their interpretation as well as other patient information in a complete hospital information system (HIS). During the diagnostic procedure, the display may show other vital information as well as the medical image. It is common to show the patient ECG, blood pressure, or other vital signs on the television screen during special or interventional fluoroscopic procedures.

## TELEVISION CAMERAS

The sensor of a television camera comprises a matrix or surface of photodetector and capacitors. The sensor accumulates information all of the time even though each element is interrogated to yield its information only once during each scanning frame. The characteristics and thickness of the photodetector determine the light sensitivity, and the capacitance determines the dynamic range and the noise properties of the sensor. The two most common geometries are of the form of an electron-beam-scanned camera tube or charge-coupled device. The sensor or target of a camera tube is a thin layer of a photoresistor such as antimony trisulphide where the sensitivity can be varied by adjustment of the target voltage $V_t$ or a photoconductor such as lead oxide where the sensitivity is constant. An analogy can be made with film where variable-gain film would have an ASA rating from 10 to 10,000 and fixed-gain film would be fixed at, say, 1000. Electron charges are stored in the capacity of the target determined by the thickness of the layer. The target material is deposited as a porous layer to increase its average resistance so that its dielectric constant is a minor factor in determining capacitance.

Figure 12.4 shows the construction of the vidicon and similar camera tubes. The tube has a hot cathode electron source, which operates at near ground potential. The control grid $G_1$ surrounds the cathode and modulates the electron beam. An accelerating electrode $G_2$ provides an electric field, which attracts the cathode electrons. The electrode has a very small hole: the beam-forming aperture. A metal cylinder $G_3$ may have a separate mesh at the end of the cylinder $G_4$ to provide a uniform electric field with room to magnetically deflect the beam by two orthogonal deflection coils and an axial magnetic field coil for focusing.

Digital still and motion picture cameras have almost made film obsolete. Solid-state sensors have achieved resolution and sensitivity approaching film and sensor sizes now permit an efficient optical match to the output screen of image intensifiers. The first of the successful solid-state cameras used an array of silicon photodiodes connected by CMOS switches so that individual photodiodes could be connected to an output signal amplifier. The usual

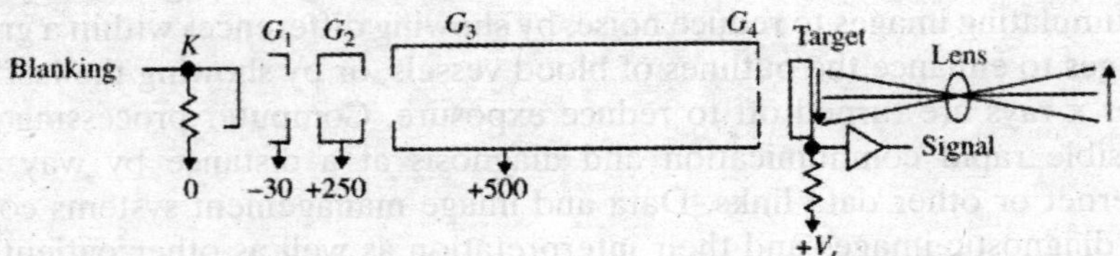


**Figure 12.4** The vidicon has a cathode and a series of grids to form, shape, and control an electron beam. Magnetic deflection (not shown) scans the beam over the target, which is mounted on the interior of the glass faceplate. From the target, light-modulated signal current flows through the load resistor and is amplified.

procedure is for a row of diodes to be connected in turn to the amplifier and then to scan the next row of diodes until the total sensor area has been scanned. Each diode has an associated capacitor so that signals could be stored long enough for the scanning process. These devices are called *charge-coupled devices* (CCDs).

While the CCD was made possible by progress in the technology associated with the development of complex integrated circuits containing many thousand transistors, further development of that technology led to devices incorporating transistor amplifiers for each of the thousands (later, millions) of photodiodes. The better of these more complex sensors used complimentary metal oxide semiconductor (CMOS) processes to achieve higher gain and higher signal levels. Both types of sensors are now used for medical imaging.

## IMAGE PROCESSING

Charge-coupled device images are already quantized as pixel-by-pixel information and analog camera tube information can be quantized by sampling and digitized for input to computers. A single frame can be stored in the computer and viewed continuously. Patient exposure can be reduced if the x-ray beam is pulsed on just long enough to acquire a picture and the images presented as a "slide show" rather than as a continuous image stream. During fluoroscopy, when the x-rays are turned off, the last image can be retained as a "last image hold" for close examination without irradiating the patient.

Pairs of images can be stored and compared. If one image is stored followed by an injection of a contrast medium (usually an iodine compound tolerated by the body) in a blood vessel, the differences between that first image and subsequent images will outline the blood vessels. Similar image subtraction methods may involve time differencing or differences of sharp and diffuse images (sharpens edges of objects). These differencing techniques together are called digital subtraction angiography (DSA). Images from different sources may be "fused". For example, an image from a nuclear camera may be superimposed on a radiographic image so that a view of functionality may be seen against a better image of the anatomy. If one image is stored and effectively defocused by "blending" neighboring stored pixels and compared to subsequent images, the resulting "harmonized" images will enhance the appearance of edges and small objects. Paired images can be used to show differences of energy absorption (images taken at different x-ray beam energies), useful for identifying tissue types. Images can be accumulated and averaged to reduce image noise.

Most importantly, the computer has become a regular component of hospital information systems so that the physician has ready access to patient information anywhere in the hospital or office. Medical images are treated as just another type of computer data, stored and accessed and available at once anywhere on request.

## 12.5 RADIOGRAPHY

Radiography produced the first medical images of the inside of the body. X-ray photons are electromagnetic radiation, as are light photons. However, light photons have an energy of 2 to 4 eV and x-ray photons have an energy of 20 to 150 keV, about $10^4$ times more energy than light photons. This higher energy makes x-ray photons more penetrating than light photons. Streams of x-ray photons can dissociate molecules by ionization and are thus called ionizing radiation. X rays damage the body in proportion to both the amount and rate of radiation as the body is normally in a constant state of damage and repair. Roentgen first observed x rays in 1895 as he experimented with a device that had a beam of electrons striking a metal target and he observed the fluorescence of some crystals several meters away.

### MEASUREMENT OF X RAYS

The Roentgen is defined as the incident radiation causing a conducted charge of $2.58 \times 10^{-4}$ C/kg in air, a definition which accounts for changes of temperature and pressure. The original unit of absorbed dose is the *rad*, defined as an absorbed energy of $10^{-2}$ J/kg. Because about 33.7 eV are needed to form one ion pair in dry air, one R is the equivalent of 0.87 r. Not all photon energies of ionizing radiation incident to a patient have the same effect: Beams of more energetic photons can produce greater tissue damage for the same measured radiation. To account for different biological effects, the absorbed dose in rad is multiplied by a "biological effect" factor of about 1.0 in the low energy range (up to 150 keV/photon) and about 4.0 (in the 4 MeV range) and the resulting absorbed dose is expressed in rem (radiation effect in man).

The modern unit of radiation replacing the rad is the *gray* (Gy), defined as 1 J/kg in dry air and the modern unit of exposure is the *sievert* (Sv), the number of grays times the biological effect factor. Both units are 100 times greater than their older equivalents, the rad and the rem.

### BACKGROUND RADIATION

We live in a world of background radiation, cosmic radiation, including that of the sun, and the natural radioactivity of the earth caused by disintegration of the heavier elements. A product of these disintegrations, *radon*, may seep through rock formations and invade the lower levels of our homes. Radon disintegration products may attach themselves to dust or smoke particles and find their way inside our bodies. The radiation of medical and dental x-ray machines, smoke detectors, package inspection machines, and other devices also affect the amount of background radiation. Like chlorine in water, very small amounts of radiation are not harmful, and may be beneficial. Large amounts can harm tissue, and this fact has been used to devise schemes to destroy cancerous tissue.

The natural background radiation ranges from $5 \times 10^{-3}$ to $2 \times 10^{-2}$ Sv/year. A few areas of the world have levels more than ten times higher. There is no statistically significant increase in deaths due to cancer for those living in areas of higher background. For people working with radiation, safe levels of occupational exposure are limited to $5 \times 10^{-2}$ Sv/year. Nonoccupational exposure is limited to $5 \times 10^{-3}$ Sv/year, a little above the background level. While ionizing radiation damages tissue, the slow rate of background exposure permits the body to repair the damage. A single whole body exposure of 6 Sv is the *mean lethal dose* (MLD); half of the people so exposed will die within a month. Yet, a lifetime exposure of 10 Sv appears harmless in that population exposures at this level will increase the incidence of cancer less than 1%. Not all tissue types are equally sensitive to the effects of exposure to ionizing radiation. A fetus is particularly sensitive as are the lens of the eye, bone marrow, the breast, and lung tissue. As a result, techniques have been developed to obtain radiographs with exposures as *low as* reasonably achievable, the ALARA principle.

## GENERATION OF X RAYS

A simple x-ray system consists of a high voltage generator, an x-ray tube, a collimator, the object or patient, an intensifying screen, and the film (see Figure 12.5). A simple x-ray generator has a line circuit breaker, a variable autotransformer, an exposure timer and contactor, a step-up transformer and rectifier, and a filament control for the tube. Medical exposures are of the order

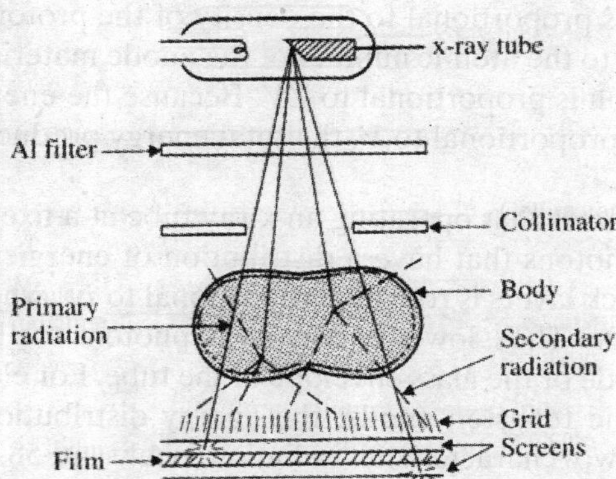


**Figure 12.5** The x-ray tube generates x rays that are restricted by the aperture in the collimator. The Al filter removes low-energy x rays that would not penetrate the body. Scattered secondary radiation is trapped by the grid, whereas primary radiation strikes the screen phosphor. The resulting light exposes the film.

of 80 kVp (peak kilovolts), 300 mA, 0.1 s. Power levels range up to more than 100 kW (Tornai, 2006).

The x-ray tube is a temperature-limited diode. Emission current is the smaller of the value defined by the Richardson–Dushman equation,

$$J_1 = AT^2 e^{-u/kT} \tag{12.9}$$

and that defined by the Langmuir equation

$$J_2 = BV^{3/2} \tag{12.10}$$

where $J$ is the current density, $T$ is the filament temperature, $u$ is the work function of the filament, $k$ is Boltzmann's constant, $A$ and $B$ are constants usually determined by experiment, and $V$ is the anode–cathode voltage. Because the filament cools primarily by radiation, filament power equals radiative heat dissipation

$$\sigma T^4 = I^2 R \tag{12.11}$$

where $\sigma$ is the Stefan–Boltzmann constant, and $I$ and $R$ are the current and resistance of the filament. Thus, electron beam current is controlled by adjusting the filament current, with compensation of filament current for variations of anode current. The fractional change of anode current is an order of magnitude greater than the change in filament current, so that circuits for filament control must be precisely regulated.

The beam electrons strike the anode and produce x rays through two mechanisms: *bremsstrahlung*, produced by the deceleration of the arriving electrons by the positively charged nuclei of the anode atoms, and *characteristic radiation*, produced when the anode's innermost electrons, knocked out of orbit by the arriving electrons, are replaced by outer shell electrons. Because the deceleration is proportional to the density of the protons of the nuclei, in turn proportional to the atomic number of the anode material $Z$, the efficiency of x-ray production is proportional to $ZV$. Because the energy of the photons produced will be proportional to $V$, the total energy produced will be proportional to $ZV^2$.

Figure 12.6 shows that operating an x-ray tube at a fixed anode voltage $V$ produces x-ray photons that have a distribution of energies. Transmission of x rays through thick layers is roughly proportional to $E^3$, where $E$ is the energy of the x-ray photon. Thus, lower energy x-ray photons are less readily able to penetrate the anode or the glass envelope of the tube. For electrons of 100 keV energy striking the tungsten anode, the energy distribution of exiting x-ray photons shows two characteristic radiation peaks at 58 and 68 keV, the *bremsstrahlung* and the absorption of the lower energies. (The 68 keV radiation is the energy given up by a distant electron from well outside the $l$-shell as it fills the hole left by an electron emitted from the $k$-shell, and the 58 keV radiation is the energy given up by an $l$-shell electron as it fills the hole in $k$-shell.)

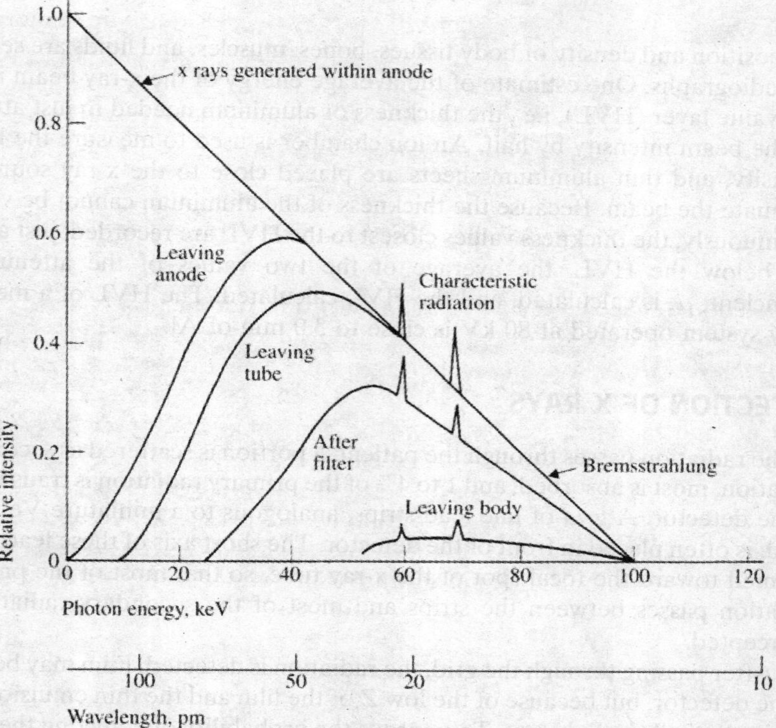


**Figure 12.6** The lowest-energy x rays are absorbed in the anode metal and the tube glass envelope. An Al filter further reduces the low-energy x rays that do not pass through the body and would just increase the patient dose. Only the highest-energy x rays are capable of penetrating the body and contributing to the film darkening required for a picture. Note that the average energy increases with the amount of filtration.

## ATTENUATION OF X RAYS

A beam of x rays covers a broad spectrum of energies similar to a beam of white light, which is the sum of beams of many colors. The attenuation of a beam of monochromatic x-ray photons, photons of the same energy, follows the same rules for, say, attenuation of light of one color in seawater:

$$I = I_0 e^{-\mu x} \tag{12.12}$$

where $I$ is the final beam intensity, $I_0$ is the initial beam intensity, $\mu$, is the attenuation coefficient, and $x$ is the thickness of the attenuator or layer of tissue. The attenuation coefficient depends on the photon energy, and the elemental composition and density of the layer of tissue. Differences in composition and density of body tissues, bones, muscles, and fluids are seen in the radiographs. One estimate of the average energy of the x-ray beam is the half-value layer (HVL), i.e., the thickness of aluminum needed to just attenuate the beam intensity by half. An ion chamber is used to measure the beam intensity, and thin aluminum sheets are placed close to the x-ray source to attenuate the beam. Because the thickness of the aluminum cannot be varied continuously, the thickness values closest to the HVL are recorded, just above and below the HVL, the average of the two values of the attenuation coefficient, $\mu$, is calculated, and the HVL calculated. The HVL of a medical x-ray system operated at 80 kV is close to 3.0 mm of Al.

## DETECTION OF X RAYS

As the radiation passes through the patient, a portion is scattered as secondary radiation, most is absorbed, and 1 to 4% of the primary radiation is transmitted to the detector. A *grid* of fine lead strips, analogous to a miniature Venetian blind, is often placed in front of the detector. The short axis of these lead strips is aimed toward the focal spot of the x-ray tube, so that most of the primary radiation passes between the strips and most of the secondary radiation is intercepted.

After passing through the grid, the radiation is detected. Film may be used as the detector, but because of the low $Z$ of the film and the thin emulsion, the film is relatively radiolucent. To improve the probability of detecting the x-ray photons, *intensifying screens* consisting of plastic sheets loaded or coated with high-$Z$ scintillation powders (for example, $CaWO_4$) are placed against each surface of a *double-emulsion film*. The use of screen-film techniques increases the sensitivity and reduces the exposure by a factor of 20 to 100, depending on the screens used. Two half-thick screens will have higher resolution than one thick screen.

From consideration of the radiation-noise limit, we know that there is a minimal value for the number of x-ray quanta required to produce an image at a given resolution. The object is to choose a detector that has the required resolution, determine an acceptable noise limit, and operate the detector in such a way as to meet those objectives.

The number of photons detected per square millimeter required to just see a fine object of dimension $d$ and contrast $C$ is found from (12.5). We assume that 1 R of typical radiation exposure is equivalent to about $3 \times 10^8$ $\phi_x > \text{mm}^2$, where $\phi_x > \text{mm}^2$ is the number of x-ray photons per square millimeter when the x-ray beam is not filtered by much material. Then the radiation exposure required to produce an image can be estimated by using

$$\text{cGy/image} = \frac{2 \times 10^{-7}}{(\text{QDE})(\text{RL})d^2(C - 0.05)^2} \tag{12.13}$$

where the *quantum detection efficiency* (QDE) is the fraction of x-ray photons detected and the *radiolucency* (RL) is the average fraction of incident x-ray photons that exit the object or patient and contribute to the image. Operation at values of x-ray exposure below that estimated by means of this formula results in noisy images. Operation above that value produces quieter images, but at the cost of unnecessary exposure of the patient to radiation.

In choosing an x-ray film-screen combination, we should choose a screen that will give the necessary resolution and a film that will provide adequate film density when sufficient radiation has been received to meet statistical requirements. If the film chosen is too sensitive, the film reaches maximal density before enough photons have been detected to meet the statistical requirements, and when the film is correctly exposed, it appears noisy. A better procedure is to use film of lower sensitivity, which permits an *increase* in the x radiation reaching the film. Then the statistical requirements are exceeded, and the film noise is acceptably low at correct exposure.

The more sensitive screens are thicker than the less sensitive ones. Screen thickness varies from 300 μm or more for high-sensitivity/low-resolution screens to less than 70 μm for detail screens of higher resolution. The value for $N_e$ of the screens is a function of screen thickness. The $N_e$ has values ranging from about 2.5 lp/mm for the most sensitive screens to about 7 lp/mm for detail screens. The film has a value of $N_e$ ranging from about 15 lp/mm for double-emulsion x-ray film to about 40 lp/mm for common photographic single-emulsion films. The screens obviously take precedence over the film when we are determining the MTF and $N_e$ of a radiographic system.

The use of detail screens and high-resolution film to view low-resolution objects results in unnecessary exposure of the patient. Certainly, high-resolution film-screen combinations are necessary for certain forms of arteriography, in which fine blood vessels must be seen, but they are not needed for discovering broad, soft-edge lesions of the lung. Measured in the plane to the film, there are very few body parts that have spatial resolutions in excess of 1 lp/mm. High resolution may not be the proper objective in the designing of a system. Trying to achieve high-contrast performance and the proper relationship between contrast and SNR may be a more worthwhile goal. Of course, there are exceptions. Mammography (radiography of the breast), for instance, requires resolution greater than 3 lp/mm.

The thicker, high sensitivity screens have a QDE of about 10%, and the thinner, detail screens have a QDE as low as 2%. Screens used for mammography are thin, but beam energies for that procedure are low, and the screens have a higher QDE, about 30%, at those energies.

The choice of screens for any application is a compromise: thinner screens/higher resolution/lower QDE and thicker screens/lower resolution/higher QDE. However, cesium iodide (sodium doped) screens have the unusual property of forming as a fiber optic and can be deposited as a thick layer, sufficient for QDE of 50% to 80%, with little lateral light scatter and high resolution. Unfortunately they absorb water and will deteriorate in air and cannot be used with film but function well in the vacuum of image intensifiers or as sealed coatings over large area solid-state flat panel detectors. Computed radiography (CR) screens store images for later scanning but have the same speed–thickness relations as conventional screens.

## AUTOMATIC EXPOSURE CONTROL

The diagnostic image requires a certain minimum exposure but overexposure may saturate the image receptor, i.e., exceed the receptor's dynamic range and underexposure may not yield images of diagnostic quality. Overexposure subjects the patient to unnecessary radiation with no benefit. While many CR screens have a very high dynamic range and their exposure may be measured with a low intensity pre-scan, reliance on this technique may be poor practice as the patient may be already be exposed more than necessary. Automatic exposure control (AEC) functions the same way as the automatic exposure option of a digital camera. For the camera, a light sensor sets the exposure time before the exposure. The AEC monitors the radiation to the image sensor during the exposure, usually by having three ion chambers in its sensor plate. Two chambers are positioned in front of the lung fields and the third or central chamber is in front of the spine. Current from the selected chambers is integrated and when enough charge has accumulated, the x-ray generator exposure is terminated. Because of charge stored in the x-ray tube cables, the AEC compensates by adding a rate correction based on the ion chamber current to the ion chamber charge to terminate the exposure earlier for fast exposures.

The ion chambers are usually made with thin plastic walls with painted graphite or vapor deposited metal electrodes. In some case, photoelectric emission from the electrodes augments the ionization current of the air in the chamber. in general, however, the ion current is most important as the electrodes are kept thin and to keep the AEC sensor indiscernible in the radiographic images. Typical chamber volumes are 100 to 200 ml/chamber. X-ray film-screen sensitivities are defined as 100 speed if exposure to 1 mR ($10^{-5}$ Sv) results in a film density of 1.0 (10% light transmission), 200 speed for density of 1.0 at 0.5 mR, etc. Because higher resolution images require higher exposures, lower sensitivity films and thinner screens are used. In the case of mammography, lower x-ray beam energy and thin screens are used. The AEC system must permit compensation for film and screen sensitivities as well as for variation of detector sensitivity vs. beam energy (the kVp setting of the x-ray generator).

## IMAGE INTENSIFIERS

X-ray image intensifiers are used in fluoroscopic systems and have replaced the old-fashioned fluoroscopic screens. One disadvantage of the fluoroscopic screen was that the radiologist's eyes had to be dark-adapted to see low-contrast objects. Other disadvantages include severe limitations of photographing the image. It can be shown that optical coupling (lens coupling) of a large area

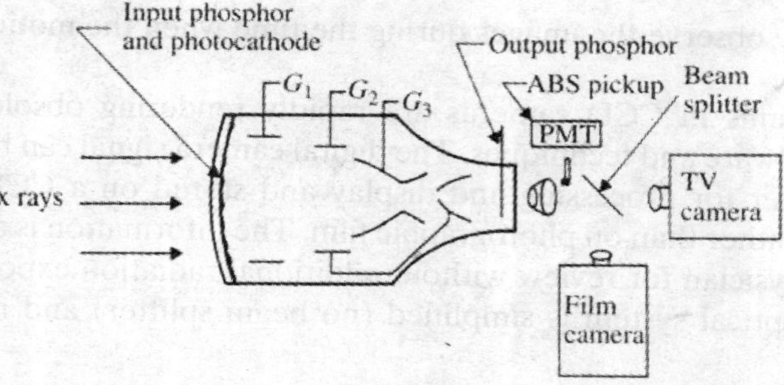


**Figure 12.7** In the image intensifier, x rays strike the input phosphor screen, thus generating light. Light stimulates the photocathode to emit electrons, which are accelerated through 25 kV to strike the output phosphor screen. Brightness gain is due to both geometric gain and electronic gain.

fluorescent screen to a small area detector is not possible without very large optical losses and order of magnitude increases of exposure to the patient.

The x-ray image intensifier combines the functions of x-ray detection and signal amplification in a single glass envelope. Figure 12.7 shows the construction of an x-ray image intensifier tube. X rays strike the input screen—usually a layer of cesium iodide, CsI,—which fluoresces in proportion to the x-ray intensity. The input phosphor is in close proximity to a photocathode, so the light stimulates the emission of electrons. These electrons are accelerated through the 25 kV electric field and focused by shaping the electric field. They strike the output phosphor, which produces an image that is smaller but brighter than that produced at the input phosphor. The ratio of image brightness of the two phosphors is called the *brightness gain* of the intensifier tube. The brightness gain is the product of the geometric gain (the ratio of the areas of the input and output phosphors) and the electronic gain (the product of input quantum efficiency, photocathode efficiency, potential difference between input and output phosphor, and output phosphor efficiency).

A lens mounted on the image intensifier serves to collimate or focus the output image to infinity. A lens used as a collimator has maximal light-gathering power when compared with the same lens used as a single re-imaging element. The objective lens for each camera collects the light of the collimating lens and refocuses it on the film plane. The advantage of the two-lens system, in addition to its optical speed, is that the distance between the two lenses does not influence the focusing of the systems and, furthermore, makes possible the use of a beam-splitting mirror so that light can be directed to more than one output port at a time and proportioned appropriately.

For example, in a two-port fluoroscopic system, all the light may be directed to the television camera during fluoroscopy. During cineradiography, the individual cine frames require a brighter image than that needed for the television camera, so the beam splitter is designed to direct 90% of the light to the cine camera and 10% of the light to the television camera. Thus the radiologist may observe the images during the time when the motion pictures are being made.

Improvements in CCD cameras are rapidly rendering obsolete cineradiography hardware and techniques. The digital camera signal can be acquired by the computer for processing and display and stored on a CCD or other digital means rather than on photographic film. The information is available at once to the physician for review without additional radiation exposure of the patient. The optical system is simplified (no beam splitter) and made more compact.

## SOLID-STATE IMAGERS

Large area amorphous silicon detectors coated with efficient scintillator crystals, such as CsI, all mounted on a ceramic substrate with $x$ and $y$ axis controls lines have been developed as alternatives to image intensifiers. A variation uses thin film transistors (TFT) arrays to amplify the diode signals before commutation. Another variation uses a layer of amorphous selenium over the TFT array and $x$–$y$ commutation lines. And still another solid-state imager comprises several tapered fiber optics coated with a scintillator on the large surface and optically cemented to CCD detectors. These assemblies are tiled and the computer splines, i.e., corrects the margins, the separate images into the full image. As the cost and yield of these methods improve, they will find more applications.

## IMAGE NOISE

If we use a film camera to photograph the output phosphor of an image intensifier with the objective-lens aperture wide open, the developed film may be too dark at the usual exposure levels. An operator might reduce the dose of x radiation to achieve proper darkening of the film. This would be a mistake, however, because the image would be statistically limited at the photocathode of the image intensifier, and would be noisy. The proper technique is to set the radiation dose or dose rate to achieve satisfactory image quality and then stop down the film objective lens to achieve proper darkening of the film. Similar arguments apply to all medical imaging: the statistical requirements of image quality determine the dose and adjustment of light or signal strength set the detector or sensor within its proper range.

## PATIENT EXPOSURE TO X-RAYS

As described earlier, background exposure is of the order of $10^{-2}$ Sv/yr. A typical chest x ray exposes the patient to $4 \times 10^{-4}$ Sv, about the equivalent of 25 days of background. Other diagnostic x-ray procedures involve single exposures ranging from $10^{-4}$ Sv (fingers) to $10^{-1}$ Sv (some heads) and are considered relatively safe. An excessive number of exposures or very long fluoroscopic times can subject the patient to high exposures, and the risk versus benefit of the procedure must be considered. Cineradiography or electronic serial radiography (where a video recorder or computer is used) records a succession of images, and each image is a separate radiograph. An extended study of the heart can subject the patient to very high incident radiation. We know that the MLD of a single exposure to the entire body is 6 Sv. Fractionated exposures or exposures to limited areas give the body time to recover but may increase the lifetime probability of cancer.

Interventional radiography permits the repair or modification of blood vessels or organs without conventional surgery. Guide wires and cannulae (small tubes) are threaded through blood vessels to reach the defect, and a small balloon is expanded to increase the effective diameter of a restricted blood vessel. Alternatively, a stent (an expanded metal retainer) can be threaded through a cannulus and positioned to keep a vessel from collapsing, all under the guidance of a fluoroscope. Unhappily, some interventional procedures take a long time and the exposure to the skin of the patient can exceed 1 Sv and cause skin reddening, *erythema*, and loss of hair, *epilation*. Higher exposures can cause ulceration, which can be severe enough to require skin grafts.

## 12.6 COMPUTED RADIOGRAPHY

Some early phosphors used in x-ray intensifier screens produced residual or afterimages. These appeared as faint shadows of previous images on new exposures. During the exposure to x rays, most of the excited phosphor electrons returned directly to the valence band. Some returned via an *f*-center with an energy gap in the visible light region so that the screen fluoresced. A few electrons were trapped and released thermally or by light excitation at a later time. Heating the screen removed electrons from the traps to erase the potential afterimage. Most modern phosphors are deficient in traps to reduce the effect.

However, the afterimage effect can be increased by making the screen rich in traps and then used in a practical way. After the screen has been exposed it can be scanned with a laser of energy close to the trap level. Then the trapped electrons will be released and will return to the valence band causing the screen to fluoresce in proportion to the initial exposure. When screens are used in this way without film they are called *storage phosphors* and make possible computed radiography.

Figure 12.8 shows that the storage phosphor screen can be mounted in a cassette of the same dimensions as a conventional x-ray cassette and exposed in the same way. The cassette is then placed in a laser scanner where the screen fluorescence is sensed by a phototube or photodiode, amplified, and converted to a digital signal for computer storage and processing. The screen can be scanned at a low level so that few electrons are removed from their traps in a single pass; but sufficient electrons are removed to estimate the

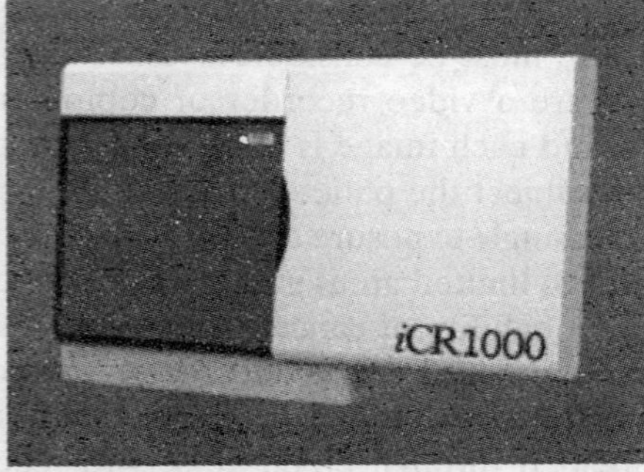


**Figure 12.8** Tabletop-computed radiography cassette scanner. The screen is removed from the cassette, scanned, erased, and returned to the cassette for the next exposure. The image information is sent to a computer for display and analysis. (Photo courtesy of iCRco.)

level of the stored signal, i.e., the exposure level to set the gain of the computer circuits that will process the signal. By scanning several times and accumulating the signals in the computer, it is possible to use an analog-to-digital converter (ADC) of lower bit capacity but faster response to generate clean signals of wide dynamic range which approach the quality of x-ray film. For example, a fast 10-bit ADC can be used over four scans to accumulate a 12-bit image in the computer.

Once high-quality x-ray images are stored within the computer, image processing is used to emphasize certain features of single images by unsharp masking (subtracting an out-of-focus image and amplifying the difference), line averaging, or interpolation to convert images from one scanning standard to another, or image fusion standardization where the dimensions and scan parameters are converted to standard values so that images from different sources can be superimposed. Other imaging systems, e.g., CT, ultrasound, magnetic resonance imaging (MRI), nuclear medicine cameras, digital fluoroscopy, store images in computer memory. However, the dynamic range and resolution requirements of these images vary with their source. It is simple to convert one image type to another. For example, a 512-line CT image can be converted to a 1024-line image by interpolation to produce the additional lines. While the new image will not contain any more information, it is compatible with high-resolution television images or those obtained from storage phosphor screens and then images from different sources may be compared, differenced, and displayed on the same bank of computer monitors.

The computer can be used for writing the diagnostic report and images and reports sorted and controlled in a database management system. The same methods used for transferring business information, technical drawings, or news photographs can be adapted for use in medical imaging for teleradiology or telemedicine. Using these methods, expert consultation is possible in the most remote areas of the world. However, image standards for communication and archiving engineering drawings or credit card information may not be adequate for the variety of medical images or the range of image compression schemes now in use.

Medical image diagnosis often requires examination of an entire high-resolution image followed by scrutiny of a portion of the image, the region of interest (ROI). A 1024-line display monitor may be used to display the entire image and the ROI magnified to fill a portion of the display. One system displays the ROI as if under a magnifying glass in its area of the original image. This means that the original image must have much higher resolution than the display monitor so that magnified portions will not be compromised. One system averages lines of a 4096-line image to 1024 lines for display and magnifies 1/4 field sections by a factor of 4 for ROI display.

Images can be transformed from real space to frequency space by means of the fast Fourier transformation, FFT. The coefficients of the FFT image are smaller than those of the real image and require less computer memory. Such "compressed" images can be converted back to the original form by an inverse transformation. Another compression scheme considers the original image in blocks of, say, $4 \times 4$ pixels of 1 byte/pixel. The mean and standard deviation of the 16-pixel block are calculated, and each pixel equal or greater than the mean is given a value of "1" or is otherwise valued as "0." The matrix of 1s and 0s requires two bytes to define the 16 pixels (the bit map) and the mean and standard deviation require 1.5 bytes (the standard deviation requires only 4 bits) to transmit. When reconstructed, the 1s are given the value of the mean plus the standard deviation and the 0s are given the value of the mean minus the standard deviation. Simple image filters are used to give the reconstructed image a more pleasing appearance. Thus, to store or transmit 16 pixels requires only 3.5 bytes where the original image requires 16 bytes, a compression ratio of about 4.7. This technique is called *filtered block compression*.

Computer techniques are also used to convert the dimensions of one image to conform to those of another. By mixing or comparing images from different medical imaging systems, a coarse image of the absorption of a metabolite taken by a nuclear camera can be seen against the high-resolution image of the brain taken by a CT machine. The technique of generating a composite image from more than one source is called *image fusion*. Figure 12.9 shows images from MRI and CT systems fused to show the details of the skull (CT) with enclosed brain tissue (MRI). Details, such as the distortion of the brain tissue flowing into an artifact of the skull are seen with clarity and certainty not possible in the separate images.

Computed radiography has been incorporated into *local area networks* (LANs) *as* part of a filmless medical imaging system. Systems that use a network of computers, optical disk archiving devices, and long line transmission have been assembled as *digital imaging network/picture archiving and communication systems* (DIN/PACS). In a DIN/PACS, an operator can call up any image and text file in the system for interactive display. *Teleradiology* enables a radiologist or other specialist at a distant site to view an image, make

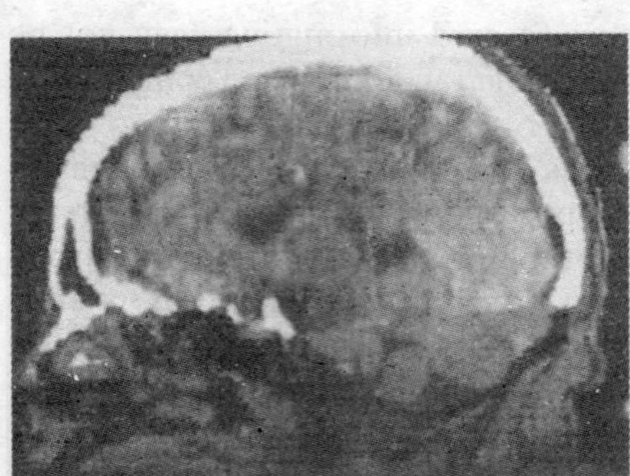
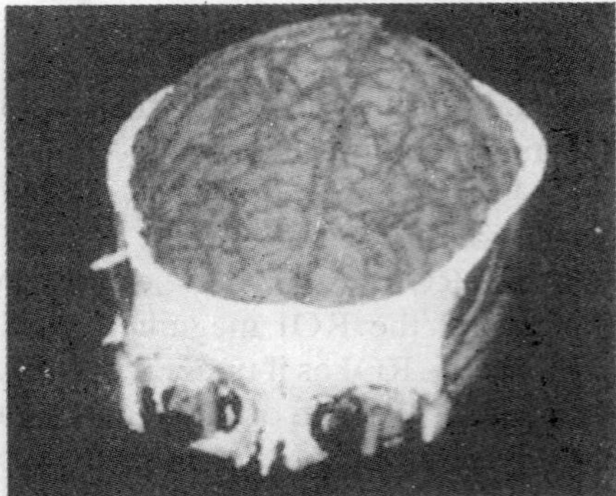

**Figure 12.9** Images of the skull taken using CT and images of the brain taken with MRI fused into composite images. (Courtesy of Rock Mackie, University of Wisconsin.)

a diagnosis, write a report, or obtain expert consultation. Figure 12.10 shows an example of computer presentation of an image that can be called up by anyone who has password access.

Standardization of DIN/PACS parameters is frequently done using the Digital Communications Standard, DICOM 3.0, to define the data header.

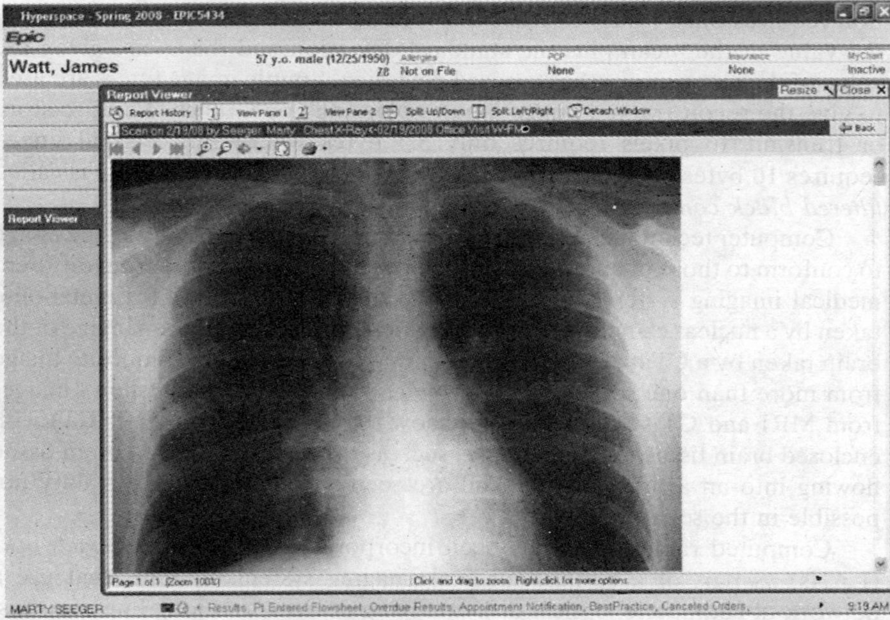


**Figure 12.10** Part of a patient report showing a chest x-ray image. Additional pages would give further diagnostic image and reference other images and reports. (Copyright 2008 Epic Systems Corporation.)

This describes the characteristics of the image and the compression method, and identifies the image. Manufacturers of imaging systems incorporate DICOM interfaces so that standard display consoles can show images from several sources for comparison. Optical scanners are used to scan and digitize film radiographs for entry into a DIN/PACS.

## 12.7 COMPUTED TOMOGRAPHY

A conventional x-ray image is limited because it is generated by projection from the x-ray source through the object onto the film. If there are regions of small and large variations in electron density along the same beam path, then small variations cannot be detected. An example of this is the conventional chest radiograph where dense bony structures make it difficult to derive information about the less-dense-tissue information in the lung fields.

One way to minimize this obstruction of one structure by another is to expose radiographs from several directions. This may not be practical because of the higher exposure received by the patient. In recent years, however, technology has yielded new ways of extracting more information from each transmitted photon so that better information on electron density of objects may be determined to reveal otherwise-hidden structures through multidirectional exposures.

*Computed tomography* is the name given to the diagnostic imaging procedure in which anatomical information is *digitally reconstructed* from x-ray transmission data obtained by scanning an area from many directions in the same plane to visualize information in that plane. The ideas involved were originally developed for imaging the brain. The dynamic range of densities in the brain is only a few percent, but the brain is encased in a bony structure so dense that most of the x rays are absorbed by the bony structure. Imaging of the brain by conventional radiography is difficult even when contrast is enhanced by injection of contrast materials or air. In concept, CT solves the set of simultaneous equations involving thousands of attenuation coefficients, $\mu_{ij}$, for each $ij$ element over the dozens of directions ("projections") used. Along a line of a given direction, the total attenuation is related to the sum of the individual attenuation coefficients:

For a single element, $I = I_0 e^{-\mu x}$ or $\ln I/I_0 = -\mu x$. For a series of elements of equal thickness,

$$\ln I/I_0 = -\Delta xe - Dx(\mu_1 + \mu_2 + \mu_3 + \mu_4 + \cdots)$$

where $I$ is the exit beam intensity, $I_0$ is the initial beam intensity, $x$ is the layer thickness, $\Delta x$ is the thickness of an element of constant size, $\mu$ is the attenuation coefficient, and $\mu_i$ is the absorption coefficient of a particular series element.

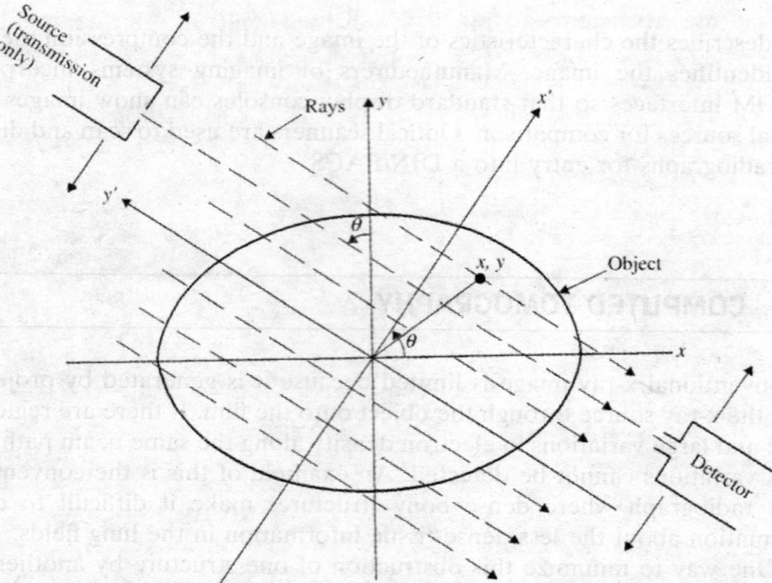


**Figure 12.11 Basic coordinates and geometry for computed tomography** The projection rays shown represent those measured at some angle $\theta$. The source and detector pair is rotated together through a small angle, and a new set of rays measured. The process is repeated through a total angle of 180°. [From Brooks and Di Chiro (1975).]

Figure 12.11 is a schematic diagram of the scanning operation of the "first-generation" CT machines. A collimated beam of x rays is passed through the patient's head in a direction transverse to the longitudinal axis. The emerging beam flux on the opposite side of the patient is constantly monitored in a scintillation detector. The x-ray source and detector move together, perpendicular to the beam direction, and roughly 160 distinct measurements of total attenuation of the x-ray beam are made at evenly spaced points along the scan path. The configuration of x-ray beam source and detector is then rotated through a small angle, usually 1°, and the procedure is repeated. The acquisition of absorption information by scanning is continued until an angle of 180° has been swept.

The procedure is called *tomography* (the Greek root *tomos* means to cut or to section) because only those structures lying in the narrow anatomical slice traversed by the beam are imaged. The tightly collimated beam results in imaging that is essentially scatter free and is efficient enough to make applying the procedure practical.

Fundamental to the procedure is the mathematical discovery that a two-dimensional function is determined by its *projections* in all directions. A sampling of projections at angles uniformly distributed about the origin can provide an approximate reconstruction of the function. How much detail can be reconstructed is straightforwardly dependent on the number of angles sampled and the sampling coarseness at each angle. If beam absorption is measured at 160 distinct points along each scanning path and a $1^\circ$ increment in angle is used, nearly 29,000 distinct pieces of x-ray absorption data are acquired. These are employed to reconstruct a two-dimensional map of x-ray absorption as a function of position, presented as a $160 \times 160$ matrix of uniform square-picture elements.

The reconstruction of images from the scanning data is performed by means of a small digital computer. The time required for reconstructing the picture is of the same order of magnitude as that for acquiring the data. Some of the mathematical reconstruction algorithms permit reconstruction to begin as soon as the first projection data come in. These algorithms clearly provide a considerable saving in time by allowing the mathematical reconstruction to take place during the scan operation.

The mathematical algorithms fall into two general classes, the iterative and the analytic. In the *iterative* methods, an initial guess about the two-dimensional pattern of x-ray absorption is made. The projection data predicted by this guess are then calculated, and these predictions are compared with the measured results. Discrepancies between the measured values and the model predictions are employed in a continuous iterative improvement of the model array.

Figure 12.12 shows the scheme by which the model projections are generated and by which the discrepancies between model and measurement are used to best improve the model at each iteration. Each reconstructed picture element is represented by an average attenuation coefficient $\mu_{ij}$, where the subscripts $i$ and $j$ specify the position of the picture element in the image. The relative degree to which each element can remove x-ray flux from the ray at the $k$th beam position at scan angle $\theta$ is expressed by the four-label quantity $W_{ij}^{\theta k}$. These quantities are essentially determined by the geometrical overlap between the finite-width x-ray beam at scan position $\theta k$ and the square-picture element at position $ij$. Clearly, the overwhelming majority of the more than $8 \times 10^8$ quantities $W_{ij}^{\theta k}$ are zero, because in most cases the ray $\theta k$ does not pass through the element $ij$ at all. The model array $\mu_{ij}$ determines the model projection data at each iteration according to

$$I^{\theta k} = I_0 \exp\left( -\sum_{ij} W_{ij}^{\theta k} \mu_{ij} \right) \tag{12.14}$$

$$P^{\theta k} = \ln\left( \frac{I_0}{I^{\theta k}} \right) = \sum_{ij} W_{ij}^{\theta k} \mu_{ij}$$

where $I_0$ is the constant intensity of the input beam and $I^{\theta k}$ is the intensity transmitted of position $k$ at angle $\theta$. The quantities $P^{\theta k}$, conventionally called the projection data for the position $k$ at angle $\theta$, are calculated in the manner shown in order that the observed measurements be converted into quantities that are simple linear combinations of the unknown quantities $\mu_{ij}$.

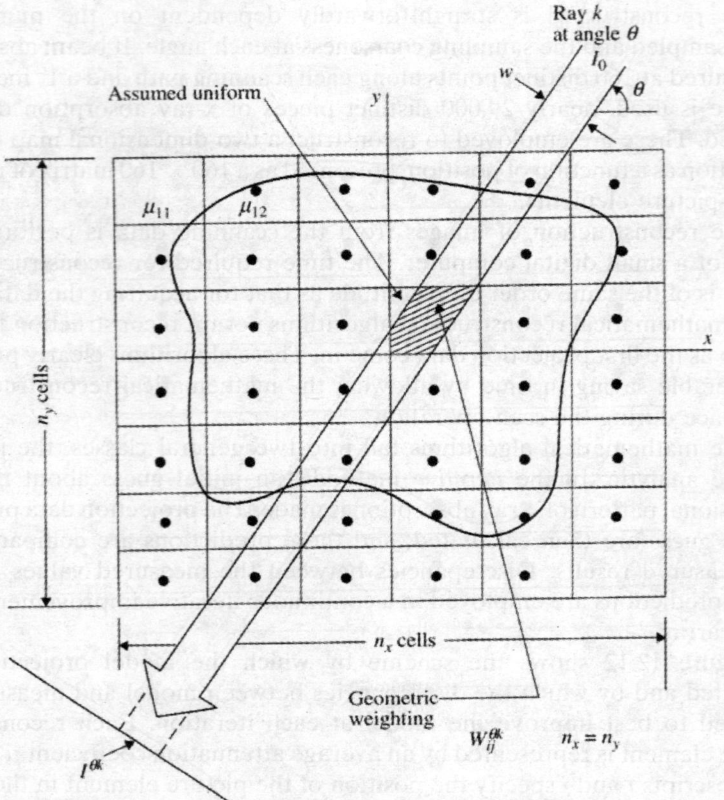


**Figure 12.12** The basic parameters of computerized image reconstruction from projections. Shown are the picture element cells $\mu_{ij}$, a typical projection ray $I^{\theta k}$, and their geometrical overlap $W_{ij}^{\theta k}$. [From Hall (1978).]

Just as the weights $W_{ij}^{\theta k}$ determine which picture elements are involved in the generation of the model projections, they also determine the manner in which the model array is changed at each iteration. In the simplest iterative reconstruction techniques, the discrepancy between the measured and model values of $P^{\theta k}$ is attributed equally to all the elements $ij$ traversed by the ray $\theta k$, and each model-picture element is changed, according to the geometrical weights $W_{ij}^{\theta k}$, to make the model value and the measured value for the scan line under consideration come into agreement. In actual practice, many timesaving variations of this fundamental idea have been successfully tried. Regardless of the exact way in which the model array is modified, the rays $\theta k$ are cyclically iterated until the model values and the measurements of all ray projections are in adequate agreement.

*Analytic* methods differ from iterative methods in a very important way. In analytic methods, the image is reconstructed directly from the projection data without any recourse to comparison between the measured data and the

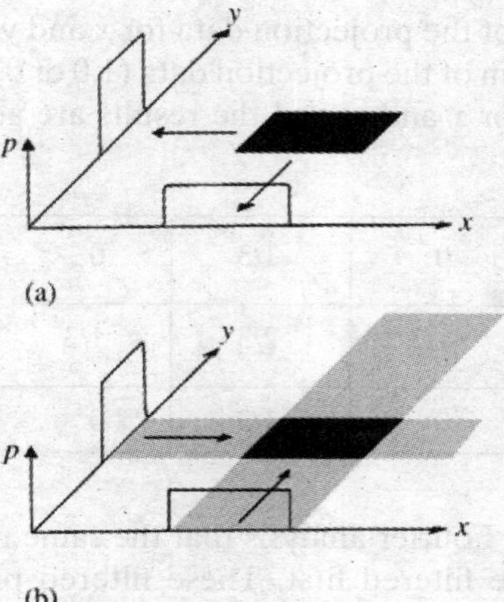


**Figure 12.13 Back projection** (a) Projections of this object in the two directions normal to the $x$ and $y$ axes are measured. (b) These projection data are projected back into the image plane. The area of intersection receives their summed intensities. It is apparent that the back-projected distribution is already a crude representation of the imaged object. [From Brooks and Di Chiro (1975).]

reconstructed model. Fundamental to analytic methods is the concept of *back projection*.

Figure 12.13 illustrates back projection for the case of projections at two angles separated by 90°. As shown, a back-projected image is made by projecting the scan data $P^{\theta k}$ back onto the image plane such that the projection value measured for a given ray is applied to all the points in the image plane that lie on that ray.

The total back-projected image is made by summing the contributions from all the scan angles $\theta$. The summing is carried out by using the same geometrical weights defined in the preceding paragraph. The back-projected image is already a crude reconstruction of the imaged object. More important, the exact relationship between the back-projected image and the desired actual array of attenuation is well understood; the latter can be calculated from the former via Fourier analysis. The back-projected image is Fourier transformed into the frequency domain and filtered with a filter proportional to spatial frequency up to some frequency cutoff. The result is then transformed back into Cartesian coordinates.

**EXAMPLE 12.5** Assume that the object in Figure 12.13(a) occupies the center square of a 3 × 3 square array. Assume that it has a density of 1.0 and that all other squares have a density of zero. Sketch the resulting curves for $p(x)$ and $p(y)$, the projection data for the directions normal to the $x$ and $y$ axes. Sketch the square array shown in Figure 12.13(b), and assign a density for each square in the resulting back projection.

**ANSWER** The sums of the projection data for $x$ and $y$ are equal, as shown in Figure 12.13(a). The sum of the projection data (1.0 or 0) is divided evenly over each block (1/3 or 0) for $x$ and $y$, and the results are added to yield the back projection shown.

| | | |
|---|---|---|
| 0 | 1/3 | 0 |
| 1/3 | 2/3 | 1/3 |
| 0 | 1/3 | 0 |

It can be shown by Fourier analysis that the same result is obtained when the projection data are filtered first. These filtered projections are used to construct the final back-projected image. The filtering operations can also be done in Cartesian space by means of analytic algorithms called *convolution techniques* (Bracewell, 1999).

The first-generation machines used a single pencil beam and a single detector in a translate–rotate scan. Each translation took about 5 s followed by a rotation of 1°, then 1 s delay for the machine to stop vibrating, followed by another translation of the x-ray tube and detector. To rotate over the full 180° took about 20 min. Because x-rays cannot be focused, the x-ray beam was limited to the dimensions of the detector by "coning," using a leaded box in front of the x-ray tube with a hole scaled to the dimension of the detector.

The second generation used an array of 100 or more detectors spaced every 5 mm and the x-ray tube output shaped as a fan beam. The detectors and the x-ray tube rotated together, and there was no need to translate the assembly to cover the field. For the same number of photons detected, the multiple detectors reduced the scan time by a factor of 100 or more. The time to collect information for one slice was less than 10 s. Because a patient could hold his breath for 10 s, it was now possible to take CT images of the chest, but heart motion was a limiting factor in many applications.

The next improvement aligned the third-generation CT machine gantry with several hundred stationary detectors and rotated the x-ray tube. Improvements of the computers, higher output x-ray tubes reduced the scan time to 2 s or less and the slice thickness to around 2 mm. Cables connected the rotating tube to the power supply so that a scan series consisted of a number of winds and unwinds of the cables to make the exposures. For example, the tube would rotate once to make an exposure, the patient table would translate 1 cm, the tube would rotate in the opposite direction while making the next exposure, the table would translate 1 cm, etc. A series of 10 or 15 exposures would permit a study of, say, the liver or abdomen. By using power supplies that rotated with the x-ray tube and by using slip rings to carry power to the assembly, it was not necessary to rotate–reverse–rotate, etc. in order to wind/unwind the x-ray tube cables, and the scan process could proceed with a series of rotate the tube assembly, translate the table, rotate, etc., to complete the exposures for the study.

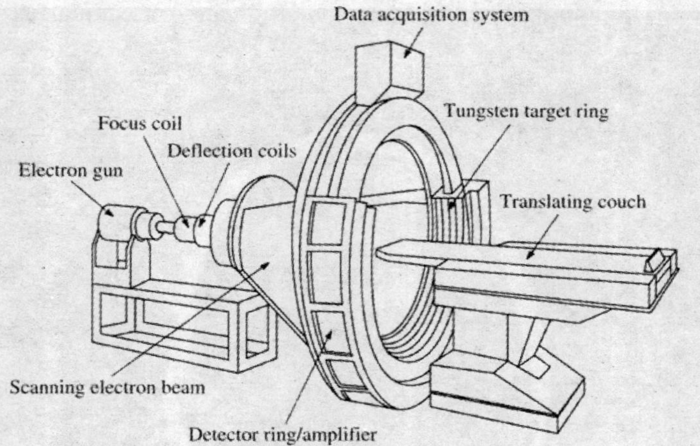


**Figure 12.14** IMATRON electron beam CT system. (Courtesy of Doug Boyd, IMATRON Corp.)

The most recent improvement is to move the table in a smooth, stepless motion while the tube assembly rotates continuously. This helical or spiral scanning method obtains image data faster than five images/s. Another improvement uses paired detectors so that two cuts 1 cm apart are made simultaneously. These fast image acquisition systems make possible CT angiography of the heart, i.e., dynamic studies of the blood vessels of a beating heart. A practical limitation of any of these systems is the difficulty of rotating a 200 kg mass at several rpm while maintaining precision of the position of the source to within a fraction of a millimeter.

Figure 12.14 shows one novel machine, which avoids the practical problem of accelerating the mass of the x-ray tube and power supplies by building the machine in the form of a "demountable" x-ray tube. Here, the electron beam strikes a circular anode almost 2 m diameter, the patient is within the circle, and the ring of detectors is the same as the fourth-generation machines. Such machines take CT angiographic images faster than 30 images/s.

Figure 12.15 shows that the resolution of the third- and fourth-generation machines can be as high as $512 \times 512$ pixels. In some applications, the operator can set the machine to lower values when high resolution is not required and so reduce patient exposure. The early machines used scintillation detectors based on the technology of images for nuclear medicine. In order to pack many detectors into the small space required for high resolution, new detectors were developed. One type uses an "egg crate" assembly of pressurized xenon gas ion chambers. Several hundred cylinder equivalents are arranged in an arc, each feeding an amplifier. The dimensions of each cylinder and the gas pressure are such that the x-ray absorption of the mass of xenon gas along the length of the cylinder is sufficient for detection at reasonable exposure rates (about 10% stopping power). Solid-state detector technology has improved so that small scintillators can be coupled to arrays

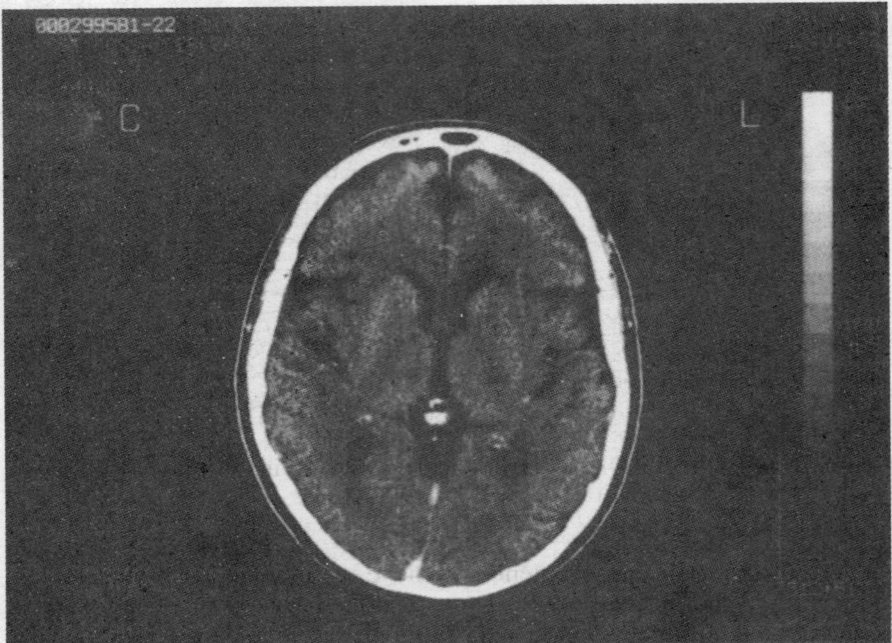


**Figure 12.15 A 512 x 512 pixel CT image of the brain** Note that the increased number of pixels yields improved images. (Photo Courtesy of Philips Medical Systems.)

of photodiodes and still have excellent absorption. Newer detectors convert the x radiation directly into electric signals to multiple integrated-circuit amplifiers.

The linear attenuation coefficient of the x-ray beam of the patient tissue can be expressed in dB/cm. However, this term is dependent on beam energy and is often inconvenient to use. Of greater interest to the diagnostician is the relative attenuation corrected for beam energy and other effects. Tissue attenuation can be characterized by values from −1000 H (air) through 0 H (water) to +1000 H (bone). The units are expressed as H units, or Hounsfield units, and are compensated for beam and other effects. Abnormal tissue, bone density, and body fluids are often found by noting deviations of the attenuation in H units.

Figure 12.16 shows that images are presented at the computer console. The operator controls the window width and level (WWL), brightness, and contrast with a wedge showing H units versus gray levels. Patient information and machine settings are also displayed. The patient table moves a preset distance between scans so that several planes or "cuts" can be imaged. The physician can observe the appearance of objects in several different cuts to get an idea of their shape. Computer programs have also been developed that take the information from several cuts and display that information as a

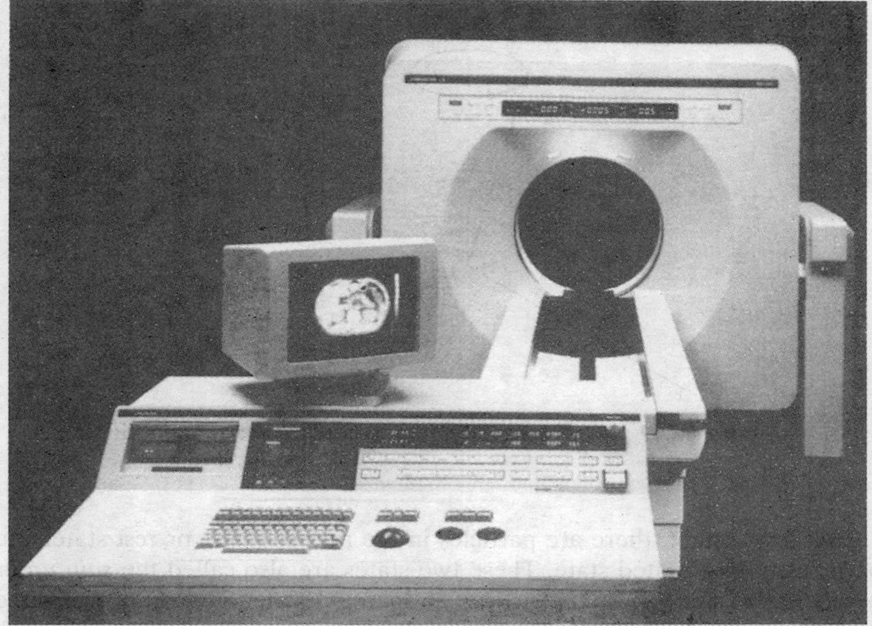

**Figure 12.16** **Control console and gantry assembly of a CT system** (Photo courtesy of Philips Medical Systems.)

three-dimensional image object. For example, the images of cranial bones in several planes can be processed to generate a synthetic image of a complete skull. A duplicate monitor is used in a film camera assembly to photograph the CT images of several cuts and WWLs. Several images are recorded on a single film for the patient record. Physicians often examine CT images at the same time as other type of images, because objects that are obscure in one type of system may be obvious in others.

## 12.8 MAGNETIC RESONANCE IMAGING

Spinning charged particles have a magnetic moment and, when placed in an external magnetic field, tend to align with the field. The usual state would be for the field of the charged particles to align itself N to S, where N refers to the north pole of the particle's field and S refers to the south pole of the external field. However, it is possible for the particles to be oriented N to N and have the property that a slight perturbation causes the particle to flip back to the lower-energy state, N to S, and thereby return energy to the system. The N-to-N state is a high-energy state; it corresponds to an ionized state (or other excited state) of other particles (Block, 2006).

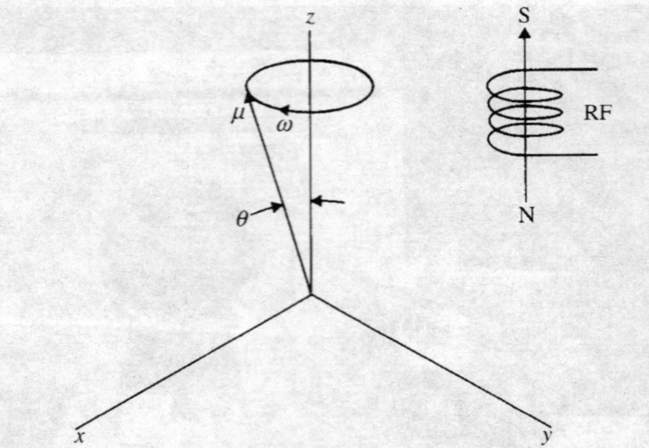


**Figure 12.17 Precession of charged particles in a magnetic field**

At any instant, there are particles in the normal state, or rest state, and particles in the excited state. These two states are also called the *spin up* or parallel state and the *spin down* or antiparallel state. The ratio of excited particles to particles at rest is a function of the energy difference between the states and of the temperature. The quantum energy difference is $\Delta E = hf$, where $h$ is Planck's constant and $f$ is the frequency. The ratio of the populations of normal to excited particles is $N_n/N_e = e^{hfkT}$, where $k$ is Boltzmann's constant and $T$ is the temperature. Actually, the axes of the spinning particles do not remain fixed in the magnetic field but rather precess, or wobble just as a spinning top does in a gravitational field (see Figure 12.17). The precessional frequency can be found from the Larmor relationship, $\omega = \gamma B$, where $\omega$ is $2\pi$ times the precessional frequency, $B$ is the magnetic field, and $\gamma$ is a property of the particle called the *gyromagnetic* ratio. Resonance—the absorption of energy—occurs when radio-frequency energy is applied at the Larmor frequency and causes particles to change state and become excited.

The particles exist in three-dimensional space, and we can assume that the external magnetic field is along the $z$ axis. Precession also occurs around the $z$ axis. If a pulse of radio-frequency (RF) energy at the precessional or Larmor frequency is applied to the system, the particles absorb energy and the precessional axes rotate. They could rotate just 90° or to the point where they precisely reverse direction of alignment (a full 180°). Because the RF energy and the pulse width determine this angular shift, the pulses are called simply 90° or 180° RF pulses. After the pulse, the particles return to the equilibrium ratio at rates determined by thermal coupling to the lattice and by the exchange of magnetic energy between excited and nonexcited particles. The two types of energy decay are called *spin-lattice decay* (with time constant $T_1$) and *spin–spin decay* (with time constant $T_2$). These time constants are quite long, ranging from several milliseconds to seconds, and they depend on the type of particles and the surrounding material. By varying the time between the RF pulses, their type (90° or 180°), and the placement of receiver coils, it is possible to determine the values of $T_1$ and $T_2$.

The patient axis is the $y$ axis. The patient is placed in the constant magnetic field and then the field is perturbed to produce a small magnetic gradient along the $y$ axis. There will be only one small section or slice at a particular magnetic field value. The surrounding RF coils are then pulsed at the frequency corresponding to the Larmor frequency of the particle being studied, usually the hydrogen nucleus. Because the resonant frequency is sharply defined, only those particles within this slice will be excited. The magnetic field is then quickly perturbed across the patient, along the $x$ axis, and the relaxation decay frequency will vary along the $x$ axis as a function of the magnetic field. The selectivity of the radio receiver will separate signals as if they were scan lines orthogonal to both gradient fields. A more elegant receiver, a spectrum analyzer, produces multichannel signals as functions of frequency to feed to the computer. The magnetic field can be either rotated slightly by introducing perturbations in the $z$ axis or can simply produce a single gradient in the $z$ axis to produce additional sets of scan lines. The similarity to CT systems is obvious, and the multiple line signals are processed in the same way.

Because of the reactance of the large magnetic coils, gradient coils are used to incrementally perturb the field, i.e., produce the small magnetic gradient that is the key to MRI imaging. In addition, magnetic shunts may be used to adjust the primary magnetic field. These produce mechanical noises as they drop in place. The cleverness of the system is impressive: Produce an axial magnetic gradient so that only one plane is excited at the Larmor frequency, then rotate this field (a second gradient coil) to produce and tune the receiver to scan lines across the slice following the exciting pulse of RF energy; rotate the gradient field to scan additional sets of lines; receive the signals in a spectrum analyzer (each channel detects the signal from a single line in the plane); and repeat several hundred times to reduce the noise and process signals as done in CT systems to produce the images.

Because of the time relationships of $T_1$ and $T_2$ recovery signals to the initial RF exciting pulse, these may be enhanced by various pulse gate recovery schemes or pulse code systems. By observing the time differences of these signals, the receiver can be gated to accumulate signals of particular time relationships to enhance particular features of the images.

The spinning charged particles could be spinning electrons, either single or unpaired, or charged nuclei—in particular the simplest nucleus, the proton of ionized (in solution) hydrogen. The ratio of excited particles to particles at rest and other properties of particular nuclei determine the sensitivity to nuclear magnetic resonance sensing methods: the nuclear magnetic resonance (NMR) sensitivity. This is a measure of the ease of obtaining useful signals. Table 12.1 characterizes some of the common biological elements.

The nuclear magnetic resonance effects of each of these elements can be measured when a sample is placed in the apparatus with a uniform magnetic field and the excitation frequency is varied. To image a cross section of tissue—in particular, living tissue of a patient—a gradient field is used. For example, if

**Table 12.1 Nuclear Magnetic Resonance Frequencies of Common Biological Elements**

| Element | Percent of Body Weight | Isotope | Relative Sensitivity | NMR Frequency, MHz/T |
|---|---|---|---|---|
| Hydrogen | 10 | $^{1}H$ | 1.0 | 42.57 |
| Carbon | 18 | $^{13}C$ | $1.6 \times 10^{-2}$ | 10.70 |
| Nitrogen | 3.4 | $^{14}N$ | $1.0 \times 10^{-3}$ | 3.08 |
| Sodium | 0.18 | $^{23}Na$ | $9.3 \times 10^{-2}$ | 11.26 |
| Phosphorous | 1.2 | $^{31}P$ | $6.6 \times 10^{-2}$ | 17.24 |

the field were varied about 1.0 T, the NMR frequency of hydrogen would vary about the 42.57 MHz value tissue section, hydrogen would be present in various densities throughout the sample, and a band of returned frequencies would be detected. Fourier analysis is used to determine the amplitude distribution of the returned frequencies, and one "pass" of the back projection (similar to that of a computerized tomographic image) is determined. Unlike CT, the entire scanner does not have to be rotated; the direction of the magnetic gradient is rotated slightly, and the process is repeated to get the next back projection. The back-projection signals are analyzed by the computer to generate an image of the density distribution of hydrogen in that plane or "cut." The cut thickness is determined by carefully restricting the field of the RF antenna of the transmitted signal and the return signal. When the NMR signals are used to produce an image in this way, the technique is called *magnetic resonance imaging*.

Unlike CT, MRI uses no ionizing radiation, and no measurable biological after-effects have been seen. Magnetic resonance imaging appears to be safe, so repeated images of delicate tissue can be made without harm or concern for exposure. By varying the sequence code of the 90° or 180° pulse train, the displayed contrast can be intensified for materials of slightly different $T_1$ and $T_2$ values.

The magnetic field can be quite strong—on the order of 2.0 T or above. Because most ferromagnetic materials saturate close to that level, superconducting coils are used when very strong fields are required. An alternative is to use either a conventional permanent magnet or a resistive-coil electromagnet when the field is 1.0 T or less. A lower magnetic field means that the Larmor frequency is also reduced and that the lower frequencies degrade the intensity of the received signal and the resolution of the final image. However, resistive-magnet MRI machines are suitable for many imaging applications.

The positioning of the patient in the gantry of the MRI machine is similar to the patient's positioning in a CT machine. The MRI gantry is deeper to accommodate the magnet over dimensions that will ensure uniformity of the field and to provide RF shielding for the receiving coils. Magnetic

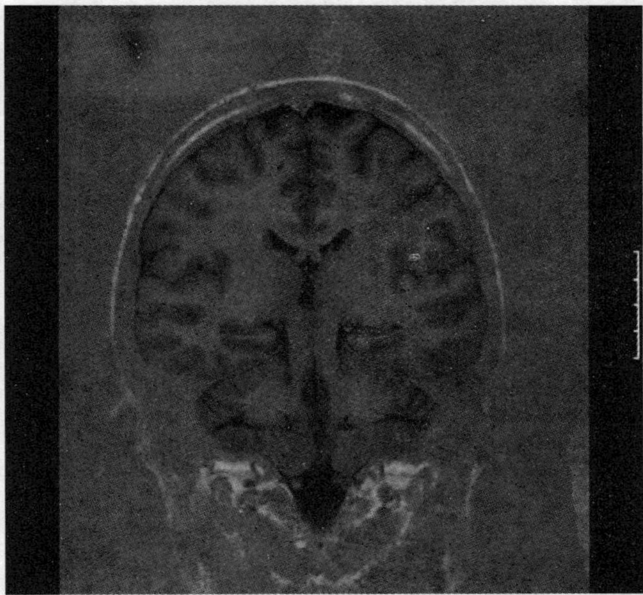

**Figure 12.18 MRI image of the head** Sets of images may be acquired for 1 mm-section thickness at 2 mm apart for diagnosis of the entire volume of the brain. (Photo courtesy of Siemens Medical.)

resonance imaging scans require up to several minutes, but, as Figure 12.18 and Figure 12.19 show, they are similar in general appearance to the tomographic slices or sections of CT images. Both machines can make a number of slices to determine the level of the anatomical object or anomaly. The diagnostician can examine films of several slices from both CT and MRI machines to obtain the necessary information.

Structural MRI scans display only differences in tissue type. Functional MRI (fMRI) displays changes in blood oxygenation levels. Cognitive activity changes metabolism in regions of the brain, which then increase blood flow and increase oxyhemoglobin, which differs in its magnetic properties from deoxyhemoglobin.

Diffusion-weighted imaging (DWI) uses a pulsed field gradient to measure the diffusion of water to diagnose vascular strokes in the brain. Diffusion tensor imaging (DTI) varies the magnetic field in 6 directions to measure direction of diffusion of water to image white matter tracts in investigations of neural networks.

With dynamic contrast enhanced MRI (DCE-MRI), sites acquire a serial set of images before and after the injection of a paramagnetic contrast agent such as gadolinium. The gadolinium changes the local magnetic field, which changes the Larmor frequency, which changes the contrast. This rapid acquisition of images allows an analysis of the variation of the MR signal intensity, before and after contrast enhancement, over time; recorded for each image

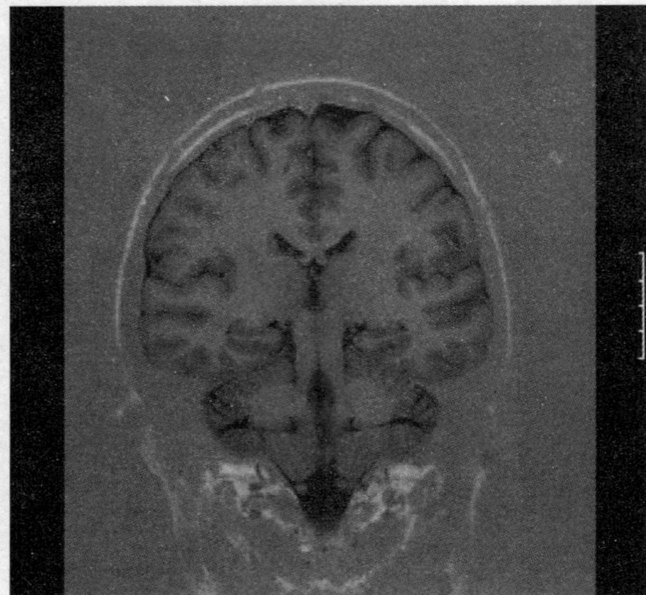

**Figure 12.19** MRI image of the brain. Compare with Figure 12.15. The MRI image shows differences due to hydrogen concentration rather than tissue density, making the bony part of the skull transparent and having a different contrast pattern than the CT image. (Image courtesy of Siemens Medical Systems.)

voxel. As the contrast agent enters the tissue, it increases the MR signal intensity from the tissue by a degree that depends on the local concentration. When the contrast agent leaves the tissue, the MR signal intensity decreases toward the baseline value. Using an appropriate pharmacokinetic model, the difference between the two sets of values can be analyzed to determine blood flow, permeability, and tissue volume fractions for each voxel within ROI.

## 12.9 NUCLEAR MEDICINE

Nuclear medicine enlists radioactive material for the diagnosis of disease and for assessment of the patient. Thus, it differs from radiography in that the source of gamma rays is not external but rather *within* the patient. It also differs in a second very important way: The radioactivity can be attached to materials that are biochemically active in the patient. Therefore, nuclear medicine is said to image *organ function* as opposed to simple organ morphology. The basic imaging situation in nuclear medicine, then, is the measurement of a distribution of radioactivity inside the body of the patient. These distributions can be either static or changing in time (Williams, 2006; Wagner *et al.*, 1995).

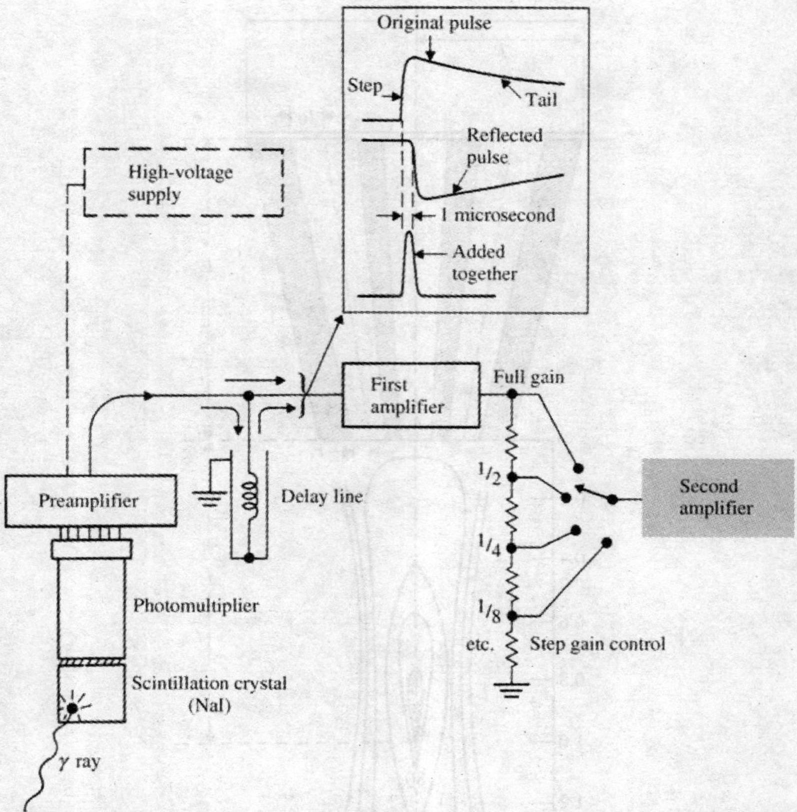


**Figure 12.20** Basic implementation of a NaI scintillation detector, showing the scintillator, light-sensitive photomultiplier tube, and support electronics. (From H. N. Wagner, Jr., ed., *Principles of Nuclear Medicine*. Philadelphia: Saunders, 1968. Used with permission of W. B. Saunders Co.)

Common to nearly all instruments employed in nuclear-medicine imaging is the *sodium iodide detector*, shown in Figure 12.20. The detector consists of three main components: (1) the crystal itself, which scintillates with blue light in linear proportion to the energy a gamma ray loses in it; a photomultiplier tube, which converts this light into a proportional electric signal; and (2) the support electronics, which amplify and shape this electric signal into a usable form. The simplest nuclear-medicine procedures do not involve images at all but consist simply of placing such a detector near the surface of the patient's skin and counting the gamma-ray flux.

The first nuclear-medicine imaging device involved the operator taking such a simple detector and moving it in rectilinear paths relative to the patient, in much the same way as we put together an aerial map of the earth. Any process that involves this rectilinear motion of the detector is called *scanning*.

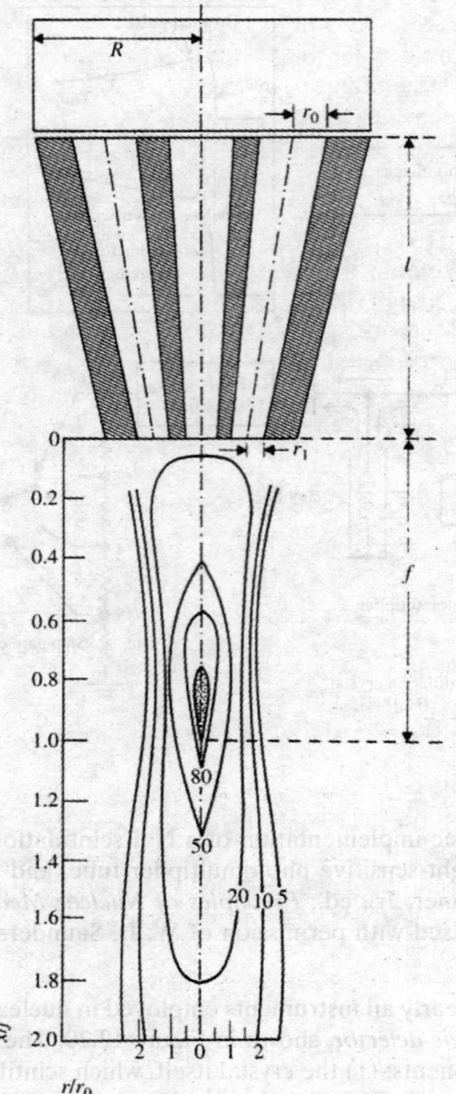


**Figure 12.21** Cross section of a focusing collimator used in nuclear-medicine rectilinear scanning. The contour lines below correspond to contours of similar sensitivity to a point source of radiation, expressed as a percentage of the radiation at the focal point. (From G. J. Hine, ed., *Instrumentation in Nuclear Medicine*. New York: Academic, 1967.)

Figure 12.21 shows how the sodium iodide detector must be *collimated* in a scanning procedure in order to restrict its field of view, both along its longitudinal axis and transverse to it. The extension of the transverse field of view is the primary determinant of mage resolution in a nuclear-medicine scan. If we know the approximate strength of the source, we can combine this information about strength with the basic resolution-element size determined by the collimator to calculate the scan speed necessary to provide the statistical accuracy desired in the image.

For example, consider the nuclear-medicine bone scan, in which an agent that has high metabolic turnover in the skeleton is used to locate sites of the bones involved with cancers originating elsewhere. A typical dose of such an agent is 15 mCi (Ci is the symbol for the standard unit of radioactivity, the curie; $1\ \text{Ci} = 3.7 \times 10^{10}$ nuclear decays/s). The total activity is distributed broadly over the skeleton. This wide distribution, combined with the isotropic distribution of the gamma rays and the absorption of many of those gamma rays in the patient's own tissue, yields a maximal count rate at the body surface of about 1000 cts/s. Typical dimensions of the pixel are $0.5\ \text{cm} \times 0.5\ \text{cm}$. If we demand a statistical fluctuation of 10% (100 cts) in this pixel for the position of greatest count rate, the speed is easily determined; counts per pixel = count rate/(horizontal speed × vertical dimension of pixel). Horizontal speed (cm/min) = count rate/(counts per pixel × vertical dimension of pixel):

$$\frac{1000\ \text{ct}}{\text{s}}\ \frac{60\ \text{s}}{\text{min}}\ \frac{0.25\ \text{cm}^2}{100\ \text{cts}}\ \frac{1}{0.5\ \text{cm}} = \frac{300\ \text{cm}}{\text{min}}$$

In the basic stand-alone nuclear-medicine scanning instrument, a *pulse-height analyzer*, selects events that have the proper gamma-ray energy. These events are used to gate a light source that scans across a film in the same rectilinear fashion in which the detector scans across the patient. The images are smoothed by integrating the rate of detector count in a simple rate-meter circuit. Alternatively, events selected by the pulse-height analyzer may be scaled digitally as a function of position of the detector. The spatial frequency of storage of scaled information is determined by the desire to have two to three picture elements within the basic resolution dimension defined by the detector collimator. The resulting image can be seen on a computer image display shown on a storage oscilloscope or collected on film. Figure 12.22 gives examples of rectilinear scans that were acquired by these two methods.

A second type of nuclear-medicine imaging instrument, introduced about 10 years after the rectilinear scanner, has since become the workhorse of the typical nuclear-medicine laboratory. This is the so-called *gamma camera*, sometimes called the *Anger camera* after its original developer. The gamma camera is a stationary imaging system that is simultaneously sensitive to all the radioactivity in a large field of view. It does not depend on motion of the detector to piece together an image.

Figure 12.23 shows a simplified cross section of such an imaging system. The radiation detector is a single sodium iodide crystal 30 to 40 cm in diameter and 1.2 cm thick. This detector is viewed simultaneously by an array of photomultiplier tubes arranged in a hexagonal pattern at the rear of the detector. When a gamma ray enters the sodium iodide crystal, the resulting scintillation light spreads through the crystal, and each photomultiplier tube

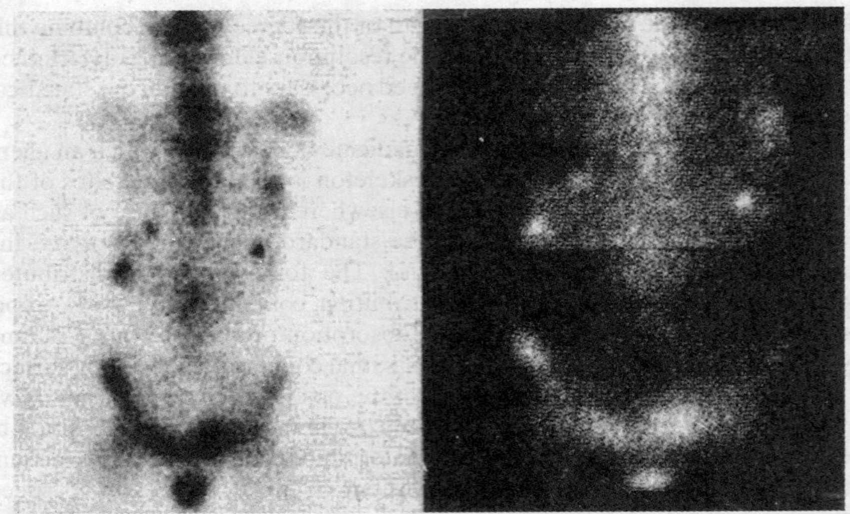

**Figure 12.22** Images of a patient's skeleton were obtained by a rectilinear scanner, in which a technetium-labeled phosphate compound reveals regions of abnormally high metabolism. The conventional analog image is on the left, and the digitized version is on the right.

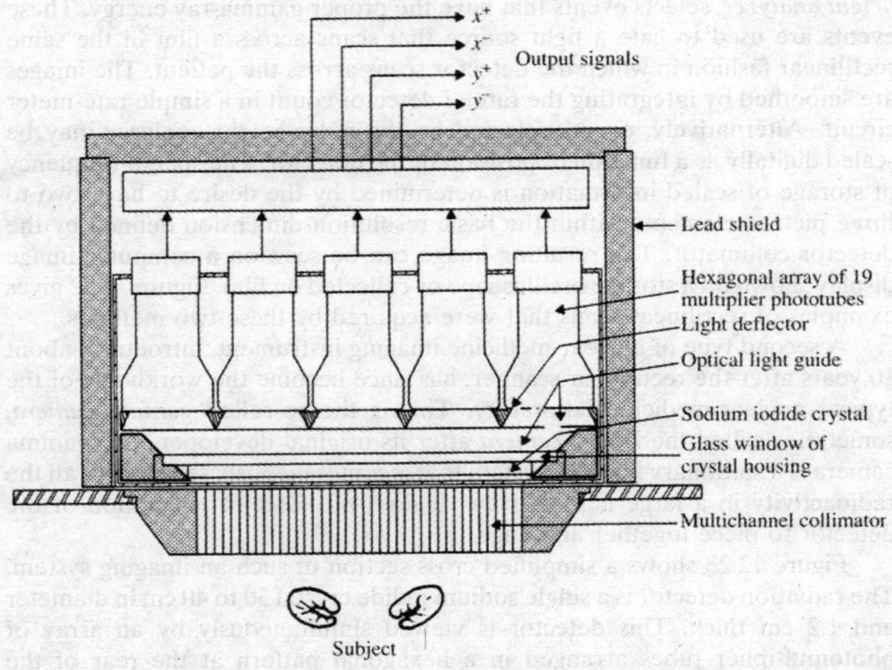


**Figure 12.23** **Cross-sectional view of a gamma camera** (From G. J. Hine, ed., *Instrumentation in Nuclear Medicine*. New York: Academic, 1967.)

receives some portion of the total light. The fraction of the total light seen by each tube depends on the proximity of that tube to the original point of entry of the gamma ray.

The fundamental principle of operation of the gamma camera is that the relative fraction of the total light seen by each tube uniquely determines the position of the original point of entry of the gamma ray. Voltages corresponding to the $x$ and $y$ coordinates of the gamma-ray event are reconstructed from the signals of several photomultiplier tubes in an analog electronic circuit. In a modern instrument, this circuit employs operational amplifiers the gain of which reflects the position of the given photomultiplier tube in the array. The center of the sodium iodide detector is conventionally assigned the position $x = 0$ and $y = 0$.

For example, a photomultiplier tube positioned far from the center in the conventional $+x$ direction but centered in the $y$ direction would have amplifier gains such that the signal from that tube would provide a $+x$ signal disproportionately large relative to the $-x$ signal but would provide equal contribution to the total $+y$ and $-y$ signals. The image can be recorded in both analog and digital form. In the analog form, the $+x$, $-x$, $+y$, and $-y$ signals are used as deflection voltages on the plates of an oscilloscope.

Events that satisfy an energy-discrimination condition briefly unblank the oscilloscope and expose a film on which the composite image is formed. Alternatively, the signals can be digitized, and the resulting digitized $x$ and $y$ coordinates used to determine a computer address corresponding to the position of the event. A digital image is built up by incrementing the appropriate computer address at each event.

Figure 12.24 shows gamma-camera images acquired via these two methods. The most important advantages of the gamma camera, compared to the

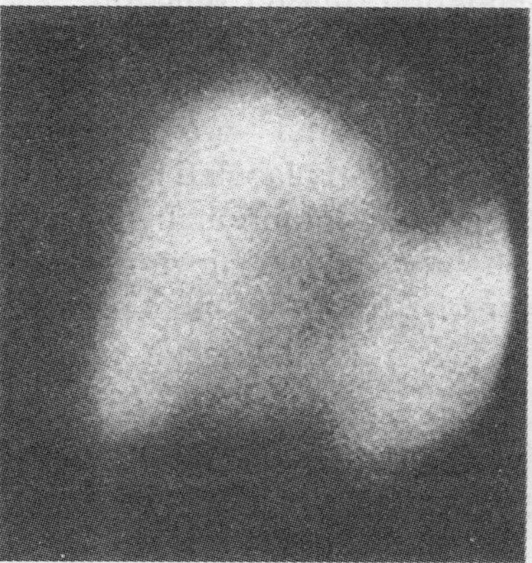

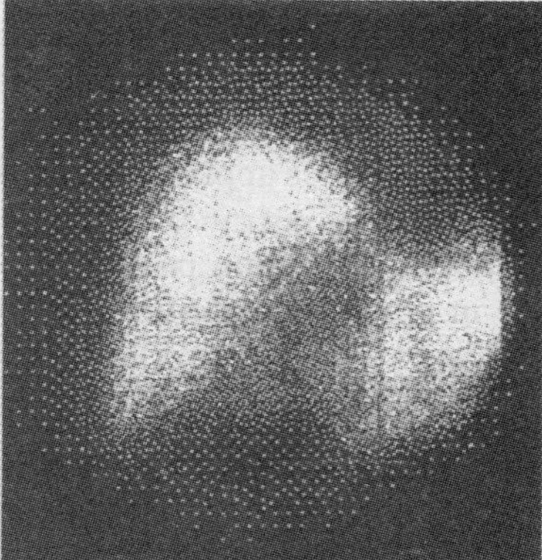

**Figure 12.24** Gamma-camera images of an anterior view of the right lobe of a patient's liver. A colloid labeled with radioactive technetium was swept from the blood stream by normal liver tissue. Left: conventional analog image. Right: digitized version of the same data.

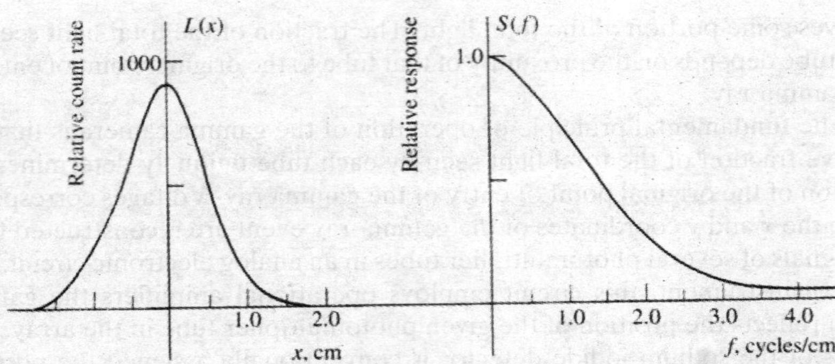


**Figure 12.25** Line-spread response function obtained in a gamma camera under computer control, together with the corresponding modulation transfer function.

rectilinear scanner, are its capability of measuring changes in the distribution of radioactivity as a function of time and the increased use of the emitted photons. Gamma cameras interfaced to computer systems can acquire data at frame rates in excess of 30 frames/s. In fact, even higher frame rates would be conceivable if it were not for safety rules limiting exposure of the patient to radiation.

Because nuclear-medicine images typically have a fundamental resolution distance that is roughly 1% of the image dimension and are composed of only $10^5$ to $10^6$ photons, they are simple to investigate quantitatively and provide a convenient way of studying the basic imaging concepts listed earlier in this chapter. Figure 12.25 shows the measurement of the response of a gamma camera to a line source of radioactivity. The line-spread function of the camera was easily generated by summing over one dimension of the digital image acquired in a nuclear-medicine computer. This line-response function was then Fourier transformed to generate the modulation transfer function.

Figure 12.2 dramatizes the relationship between quality of image and number of photons. It shows images of a so-called thyroid phantom, a small Lucite tank that—when filled with radioactive material—provides a distribution of radionuclides approximating that of a similarly labeled human thyroid. Resolution is demonstrated by the defects of holes intentionally placed in the radioactivity distribution pattern. Each phantom image shown represents an increase in number of photons by a factor of 2 from the one before it.

## 12.10 SINGLE-PHOTON EMISSION COMPUTED TOMOGRAPHY

Single-photon emission computed tomography (SPECT) uses a large-area scintillation assembly similar to that of an Anger camera and rotates it around the patient. Many of the isotopes used in nuclear medicine produce a single photon or gamma ray in the useful range of energies. The collimator is often designed to collect radiation from parallel rays (the collimator is usually focused at infinity), and the collection of signals is used in an image-reconstruction process analogous to methods used in computed tomography (see Figure 12.16). Several planes or slices of activity are reconstructed at the same time. These multiple slices of isotope activity allow the system to show depth information in the volume of interest by constructing several cross-sectional views in addition to the head-on, or planar, view offered by a conventional nuclear camera. The method can also resolve the activity to a smaller volume than conventional Anger camera images. In order to achieve the greater image resolution, the acceptance angle of each hole of the collimator must be restricted, and the collection time must be considerably longer than that of the Anger camera. Single-photon emission computed tomography systems must compensate for variations in attenuation of the patient. As a result, these systems are not used for conducting dynamic studies but only for imaging near-static structures, such as tumors and subtle bone disease. By obtaining three-dimensional information and increased resolution, it is possible to see certain anomalies that are not so clear in conventional x-ray and other nuclear images.

## 12.11 POSITRON EMISSION TOMOGRAPHY

Certain isotopes produce positrons that react with electrons to emit two photons at 511 keV in opposite directions. Positron emission tomography (PET) takes advantage of this property to determine the source of the radiation. If one path is shorter, then the opposite path is longer, and the average signal level is the same without regard to patient attenuation or point of origin. These isotopes have two means of decay, which result in the annihilation of an electron. In one case, the nucleus can capture an orbital electron that combines with one positive charge; alternatively, the nucleus can emit the positive charge as a positron that travels a short distance to combine with an external electron. The combination of the negative and positive particles annihilates the charges and masses of each, energy and momentum are conserved, and two 511 keV gamma rays are emitted in opposite directions.

Positrons emitted by the nucleus have kinetic energy, so they travel a few millimeters before the annihilation emission event. The travel distance and interaction effects blur the dimensions of the region of origin when it is detected. The broadening effect shown in Table 12.2 is the width of the pulse measured at the 10% level. The dimensions of a useful picture element would be about twice these values because of other spreading effects, such as system bandwidth optical effects.

The property of simultaneous emission of two gamma rays in opposite directions gives PET the ability to locate the region of origin. Instead of the multihole collimator found in most gamma cameras, two imaging detectors capable of determining *x*–*y* position are used. Each *x*–*y* pair is accepted if the two scintillation effects are coincident and have energy levels (pulse heights) close to the expected value of 511 keV.

**Table 12.2 Characteristics of Five Isotopes for PET**

| Isotope | Maximal Kinetic Energy | Half-life | Broadening |
|---|---|---|---|
| $^{10}F$ | 640 keV | 110 min | 1.1 mm |
| $^{11}C$ | 960 keV | 20.4 min | 1.9 mm |
| $^{13}N$ | 1.2 MeV | 10.0 min | 3.0 mm |
| $^{60}Ga$ | 1.9 MeV | 62.3 min | 5.9 mm |
| $^{82}Rb$ | 3.4 MeV | 1.3 min | 13.2 mm |

In the simplest PET camera, two modified Anger cameras are placed on opposite sides of the patient [Figure 12.26(a)]. The modification removes the multihole collimator and adds the coincidence and computing circuits. Removing the collimator increases the collection angle and reduces the collection time, which are limitations of SPECT. The camera is rotated slowly around the patient to obtain the additional views needed for reconstruction and to obtain better images. Images can be built up faster when additional pairs of detectors are used. Figure 12.26(b) shows the three pairs of cameras used in the hexagonal-ring camera. Incremental lateral translation and rotation improve the images by compensating for inhomogeneities and gaps of detection. Very elegant cameras can be constructed by using a circular ring of many detectors that surround the patient [Figure 12.26(c)]. The ring detector does not have to be rotated; image positions are resolved by computer analysis of the signals. As in all radionuclide imagers, the level of the radioactivity places a noise bound on the images. Obviously, compromises must be made in the amount of radionuclide administered: It must be large enough to obtain a good image in the time required and small enough to minimize patient exposure to radiation.

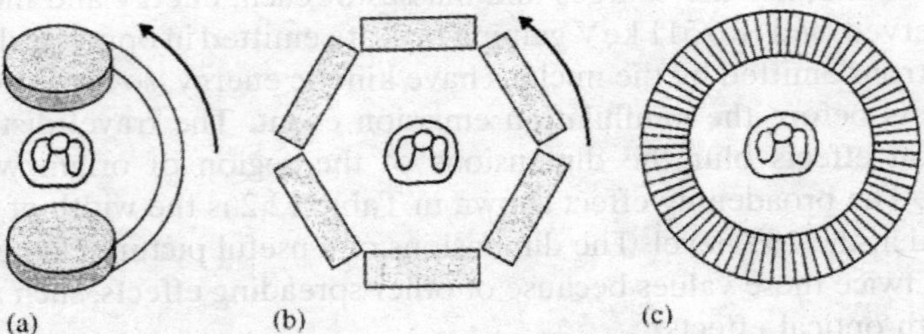


**Figure 12.26 Evolution of the circular-ring PET camera** (a) The paired and (b) the hexagonal ring cameras rotate around the patient. (c) The circular ring assembly does not rotate but may move slightly—just enough to fill in the gaps between the detectors. The solid-state detectors of the ring camera are integrated with the collimator and are similar in construction to detectors used in CT machines.

The advantages of PET over conventional nuclear imaging include the clarity of the cross-sectional views and the availability of positron emitters that can be compounded as metabolites. It is possible to map metabolic activity in the brain by using tagged compounds to observe uptake and clearance.

The measured quantity in PET imaging is the concentration, in tissue, of the positron emitter. To obtain the actual concentration, it is necessary to calibrate and measure the performance of the machine. Because knowing the actual concentration (in μCi/ml) in the patient may not be so important as knowing the fraction taken up in a particular region, the PET camera can be used to measure the tissue concentration in arbitrary units. A short time after the imaging procedure, a sample of the patient's blood may be placed in a well counter (a scintillation counter) to obtain a reference value. Comparison of the tissue and blood activity yields the ratio of isotope uptake. For example, the local cerebral blood volume and the distribution of activity are measured this way. Because the brain adjusts uptake as a function of the use of various metabolites, brain activity can be measured. A rapid sequence of brain images shows the response of the brain to various stimuli and pinpoints areas of abnormal activity.

As different parts of the brain respond to different stimuli, the PET image shows this activity (Figure 12.27). Normal brains generate one image of brain activity, but abnormal functioning, tumors, seizure, and other anomalies may also be clearly visible in the map of activity. The PET image of the brain shows the patient's responses to noise, illumination, changes in mental concentration, and other activities. One method of introducing a suitable isotope for brain

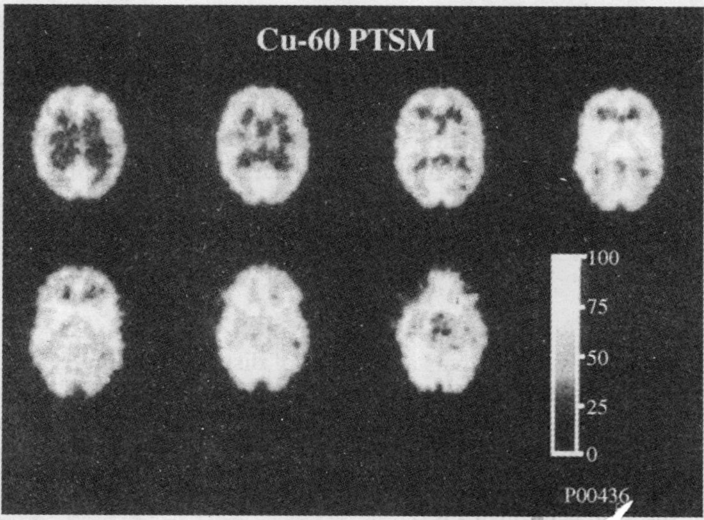


**Figure 12.27 PET image** The trapping of $^{60}$Cu-PTSM (a thiosemicarbazone) reflects regional blood flow, modulated by a nonunity extraction into the tissue. (Photo courtesy of Dr. R. J. Nickles, University of Wisconsin.)

imaging is for the patient to breathe air containing CO made with $^{11}$C. Such short-lived positron-emitting isotopes do not occur in nature but can be created in a small cyclotron. This is done by introducing into the nucleus a proton that, in turn, emits an alpha particle or neutron. For certain elements, the nucleus becomes unstable and emits a positron in a short time. For example, $^{11}$C is prepared in a small cyclotron and has a half-life of 20.4 min. The short half-life means that the isotope must be prepared near the point of use. The radionuclide decays rapidly, exhibits high activity during the time necessary to obtain images, and clears the patient in a short time. Clearance is a function of both the radioactive decay and the biological excretion of the material.

## 12.12 ULTRASONOGRAPHY

We know from old war movies that pulses of sound waves are used to detect submarines. Because wavelength $\lambda$, frequency $f$, and velocity $u$ are related ($u = f\lambda$), it is easy to show that wavelengths in the audible spectrum are only a small fraction of the length of a submarine. A phase change of less than one cycle (360°) would result in a maximum error of position equal to the wavelength: $\lambda = u/f$. To find the error of position of a detected submarine, substitute the velocity of sound in water (1480 m/s), and let $f = 1$ kHz and $\lambda = 1.48$ m. This precision would be adequate for detecting submarines but not for, say, visualizing a human fetus. To obtain precision of 1.48 mm, the frequency of the pulse would have to be increased to 1.0 MHz in the ultrasonic range.

Sound and ultrasound follow rules of propagation and reflection similar to those that govern electric signals. A transmission line must be terminated in its characteristic impedance to avoid reflections. The acoustic impedance $Z$ is a fundamental property of matter and is related to the density $\rho$ and the velocity of sound $u$ : $Z = \rho u$. The fraction of energy $R$ reflected at the normal interface of two different tissue types is and the impedances are those of the tissues on either side of the interface (Kripfgans, 2006).

$$R = \left(\frac{Z_2 - Z_1}{Z_2 + Z_1}\right)^2$$

Acoustic signals diminish as a function of distance, geometry, and attenuation. In free space, the signals decrease as a result of the inverse square law because the energy per unit area is a function of the total area of the imaginary sphere at distance $r$. The signals also decrease as a result of attenuation by the medium. When $\alpha$ is the coefficient of attenuation and $I_0$ is the incident signal intensity, the signal intensity is

$$I = \frac{I_0 e^{-\alpha r}}{r^2}$$

**Table 12.3 Acoustic Properties of Some Tissues at 1.0 MHz**

| Tissue | $u$, m/s | $Z$, g/(cm²·s) | HVL, cm | | $R$ at Interface |
|---|---|---|---|---|---|
| Water | 1496 | $1.49 \times 10^5$ | 4100 | Air/water | 0.999 |
| Fat | 1476 | $1.37 \times 10^5$ | 3.8 | Water/fat | 0.042 |
| Muscle | 1568 | $1.66 \times 10^5$ | 2.5 | Water/muscle | 0.054 |
| Brain | 1521 | $1.58 \times 10^5$ | 2.5 | Water/brain | 0.029 |
| Bone | 3360 | $6.20 \times 10^5$ | 0.23 | Water/bone | 0.614 |
| Air | 331 | 4.13 | 1.1 | Tissue/air | 0.999 |

When $\alpha$ is large compared to $r$, the exponential term dominates, and it is convenient to define the thickness of material where the attenuation of the medium decreases the signal by half (the half-value layer or HVL) independently of the geometrical effects. Table 12.3 lists the HVL for water and some tissues. Note that water is not very *lossy* and that the signal decreases 50% for 41 m of water. However, a 50% decrease occurs through only 2.5 cm of muscle. Most biological tissues have high coefficients of attenuation and low HVLs. Attenuation increases with frequency.

Ultrasound transducers use the piezoelectric properties of ceramics such as barium titanate or similar materials. When stressed, these materials produce a voltage across their electrodes. Similarly, when a voltage pulse is applied, the ceramic deforms. If the applied pulse is short, the ceramic element "rings" at its mechanical resonant frequency. With appropriate electronic circuits, the ceramic can be pulsed to transmit a short burst of ultrasonic energy as a miniature loudspeaker and then switched to act as a microphone to receive signals reflected from the interfaces of various tissue types. The gain of the receiver can be varied as a function of time between pulses to compensate for the high attenuation of the tissues. Ultrasonic energy at the levels used for medical imaging appears to cause no harm to tissue, unlike the ionizing radiation of x rays.

The time delay between the transmitted pulse and its echo is a measure of the depth of the tissue interface. Fine structures of tissues (blood vessels, muscle sheaths, and connective tissue) produce extra echoes within "uniform" tissue structures. At each change of tissue type, a reflection results. Figure 12.28 shows how the interfaces of bodily structures produce the echoes that reveal their locations. This type of simple ultrasonic scanner, the A-mode device, was an early device used to measure the displacement of the brain midline. An A-mode device shows echo intensity as an $x$–$y$ plot. The transducer is placed against the skull and the display gives the echo time of the brain midline (proportional to depth). The transducer is then moved to the other side of the skull and the procedure repeated. The images of normal patients are symmetric so that the brain midline should appear in the same position in the two images. A tumor or large blood clot could move the cerebral hemispheres to shift the midline. This type of simple device is now seldom used and has been

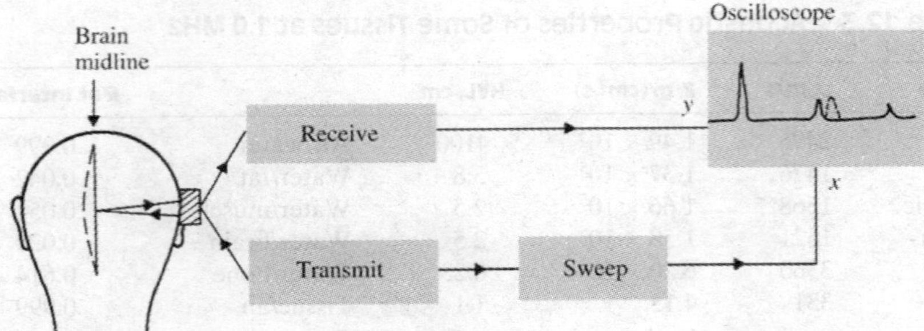


**Figure 12.28** A-mode scan of the brain midline

replaced by more elegant systems that show structures that are far more detailed and also show the brain midline.

**EXAMPLE 12.6** For Figure 12.28, estimate the sweep speed required for a $10 \times 10$ cm display. Estimate the maximal rate of repetition.

**ANSWER** For Fig. 12.26, the round trip acoustic distance is about 0.02 m. Acoustic velocity of water is 1500 m/s. Time $t = d/u = 0.02/1500 = 13.3\ \mu\text{s}$. Choose a sweep speed of 2 μs/cm or 20 μs across the 10 cm display. Maximum repetition rate is $1/(20\ \mu\text{s}) = 50\ \text{kHz}$.

If the strength of the echo signal is used to modulate the intensity of the display against the echo-return time, with zero time at the top of the display and with the appropriate image storage circuits, the image can be shown as moving to the right. This technique presents the position of tissues as a function of time as a time-motion (TM) scan. Figure 12.29 shows the motion of the mitral valve of the heart over three cardiac cycles.

Computer image storage displays or long persistence phosphor display screens can be intensity modulated as the position of the transducer is varied. The display will show the two-dimensional shape of objects. For older systems, the position and direction of the transducer are coupled to the display circuits by a system of pulleys and potentiometers. Newer systems use mechanical scanning or phased arrays within the transducer assembly and display the two-dimensional image relative to the fixed position of the transducer assembly. A computer stores the echo signals for display as a sector. Some sophisticated systems correlate sectors taken from a number of directions and display them as a single image, much improved in quality over an image taken from only one direction. Sector images and most two-dimensional images are called *B-mode images* (see Figure 12.30).

Frequencies from 1.0 MHz to 15 MHz are used for most medical ultrasonography. The operating frequency is chosen to meet the imaging task. Higher

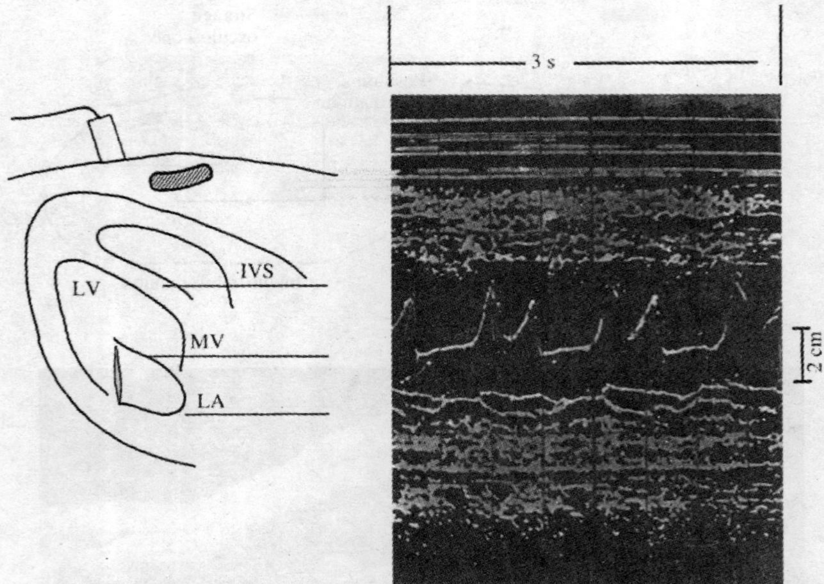


**Figure 12.29 Time-motion ultrasound scan of the mitral valve of the heart** The central trace follows the motions of the mitral valve (MV) over a 3 s period, encompassing three cardiac cycles. The other traces correspond to other relatively static structures, such as the interventricular septum (IVS) and the walls of the left atrium (LA).

frequencies will improve resolution, but increased HVL limits the depth of penetration. However, for special purposes (e.g., ophthalmic and neonatal imaging) where the objects are small, the operating frequency may be increased to 15 MHz or higher and the resolution will permit the observation of very small structures or anomalies.

During endobronchial ultrasound (EBUS), a bronchoscope with the ultrasound transducer at the tip is inserted into the windpipe. Images show whether lung cancer has spread into the windpipe or to the lymph nodes on either side.

Figure 12.31 shows four ultrasonic transducers. The two larger devices use three transducers spinning in fluid-filled enclosures [Figure 12.32(a)]. The midsized device and the smaller, ophthalmic transducer use phased arrays, which can be steered by adjusting the timing of the pulses applied to sets of several ceramic elements. If all elements of the transducer are pulsed at the same instant, the ultrasonic energy will be projected in the forward direction [Figure 12.32(b)]. If the left side elements are pulsed in a delayed sequence, the energy will be projected toward the right with the angle proportional to the timing delay [Figure 12.32(d)]. By adjustment of the timing delay, the beam

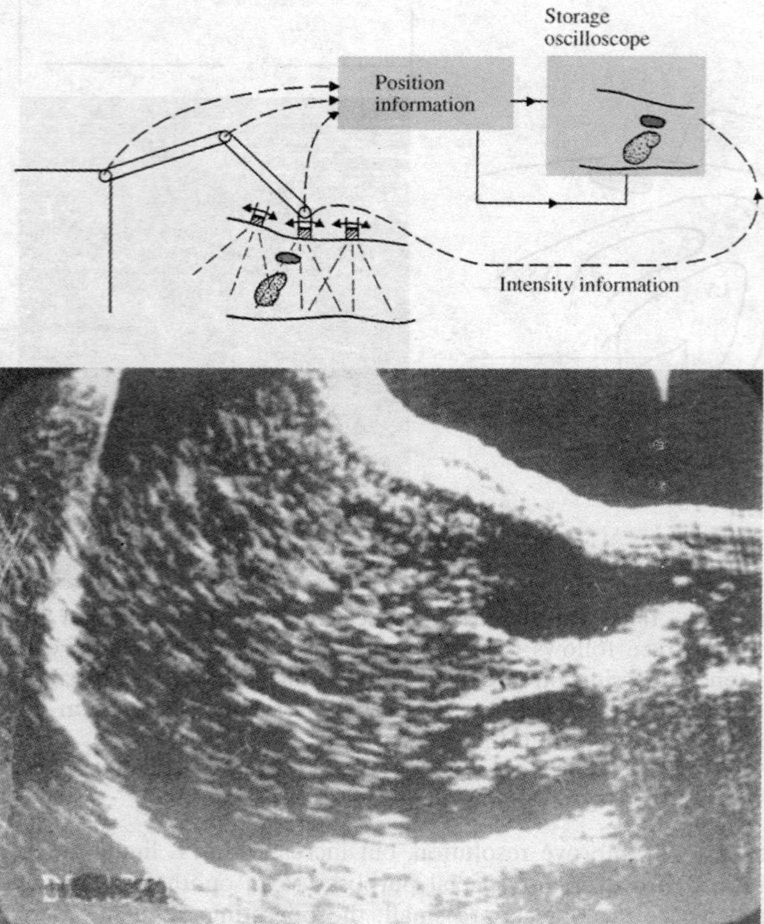


**Figure 12.30** (a) B-mode ultrasonic imaging shows the two-dimensional shape and reflectivity of objects by using multiple-scan paths. (b) This B-mode ultrasonic image, which corresponds to (a), shows the skin of the belly at the top right, the liver at the left center, the gall bladder at the right above center, and the kidney at the right below center. The bright areas within the kidney are the collecting ducts.

may be scanned from side to side. With either the spinning or phased array transducer placed against the skin, the image of a sector is displayed. Phased array transducers have been made small enough to be mounted at the ends of probes for insertion into body cavities such as the rectum for imaging the prostate or the vagina for showing the fetus or the condition of the reproductive organs.

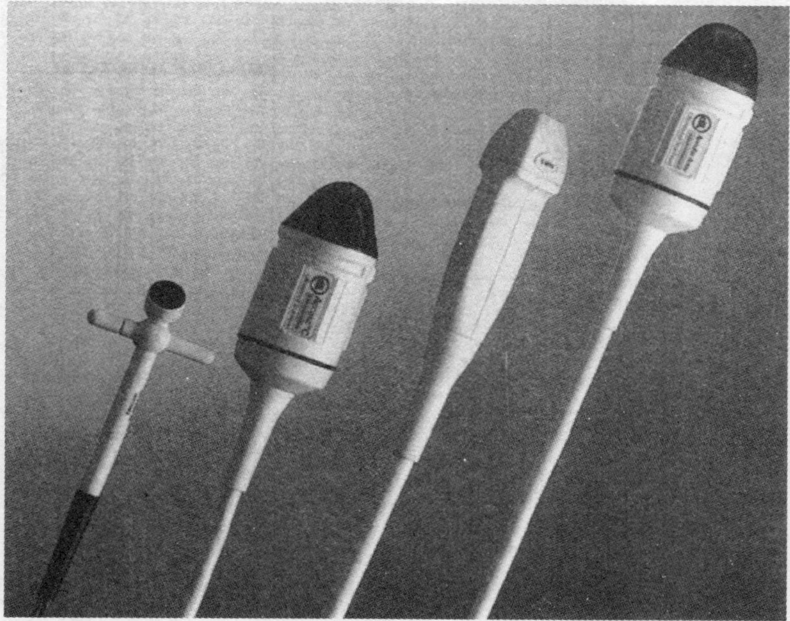

**Figure 12.31** Different types of ultrasonic transducers range in frequency from 12 MHz for ophthalmic devices to 4 MHz for transducers equipped with a spinning head. (Photo courtesy of ATL.)

Even smaller transducers have been made for high-frequency operation. These have been fitted at the tips of catheters and used for examining the characteristics of blood vessels prior to angioplasty. Figure 12.33 shows the appearance of a normal artery taken with a catheter tip transducer. In angioplasty, a balloon is introduced into ischemic or partially closed vessels and then inflated to stretch the walls of the vessel to increase the lumen or diameter and increase blood flow. If the vessel walls are weak, the probe images may show that angioplasty could jeopardize the life of the patient. Following balloon inflation, the probe can be pulled back to determine the dimensions of the stretched walls and verify the integrity of the vessel.

## DUPLEX SCANNERS

Halberg and Thiele (1986) describe the design of a phased array ultrasonic duplex scanner that combines real-time two-dimensional imaging with the pulsed-Doppler method to measure directional blood velocity noninvasively. Figure 12.32(d) shows how a mechanical real-time sector scanner can generate a fan-shaped beam. Figure 12.34 shows the system block diagram. A colored

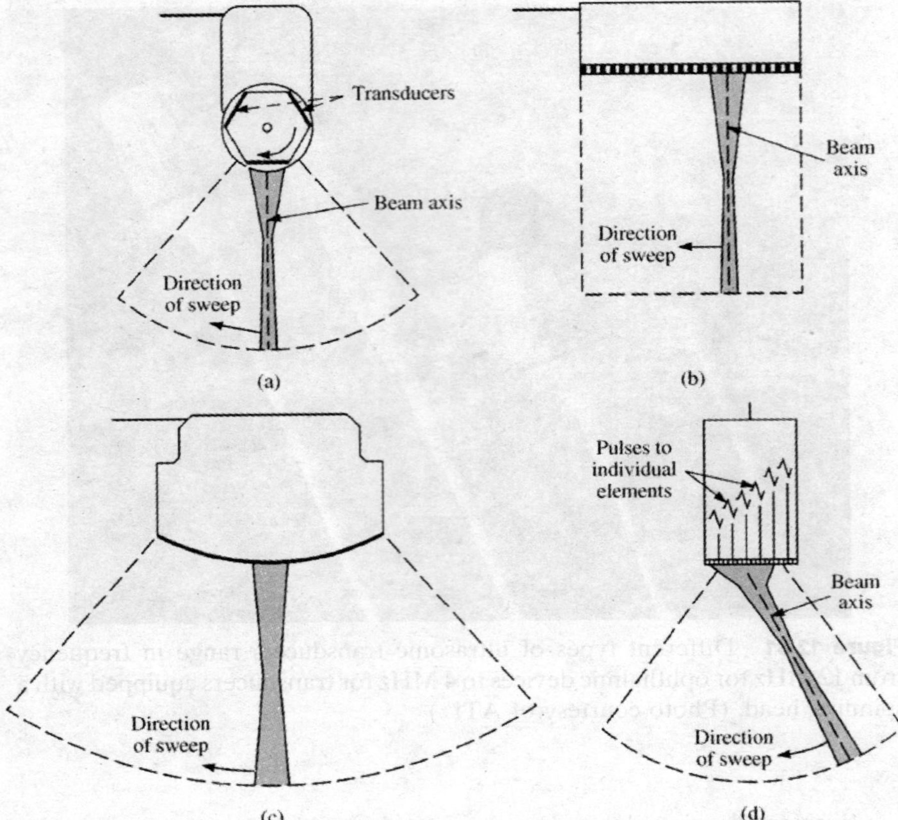


**Figure 12.32 Ultrasound scan heads** (a) Rotating mechanical device. (b) Linear phased array which scans an area of the same width as the scan head. (c) Curved linear array can sweep a sector. (d) Phasing the excitation of the crystals can steer the beam so that a small transducer can sweep a large area.

display from a duplex scanner shows flow into or out of the screen as red or blue against a monochrome background, with the intensity of the color approximating the velocity. This technique is called *color flow imaging* and yields images shown in Figure 12.35.

Because the duplex scanner can distinguish between moving blood and stationary soft plaque, it is useful for diagnosing obstruction in diseased carotid arteries. Pulsed-Doppler techniques are useful in locating and determining in the heart the direction and extent of abnormal flow, valvular abnormalities, shunt lesions such as patent ductus arteriosis, and ventricular and septal defects.

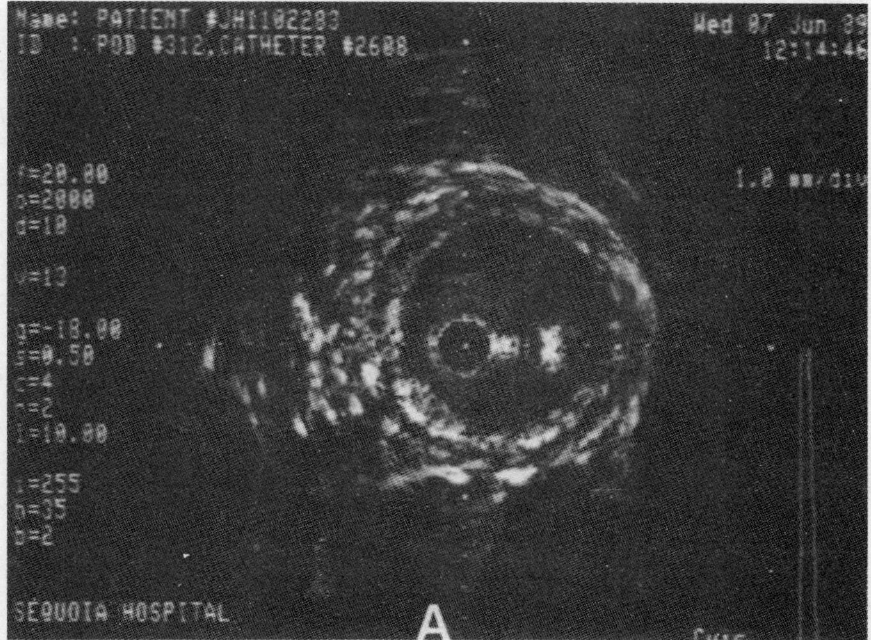


**Figure 12.33** Intravascular ultrasonic image showing the characteristic three-layer appearance of a normal artery. Mild plaque and calcification can be observed at 7 o'clock. (Photo courtesy of Cardiovascular Imaging Systems, Inc.)

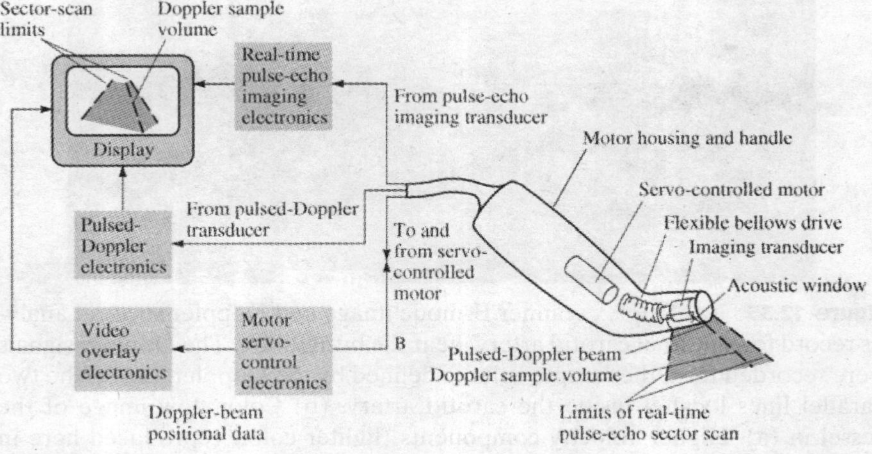


**Figure 12.34** The duplex scanner contains a mechanical real-time sector scanner that generates a fan-shaped two-dimensional pulse-echo image. Signals from a selected range along a selected path are processed by pulsed-Doppler electronics to yield blood velocity. [From Wells (1984).]

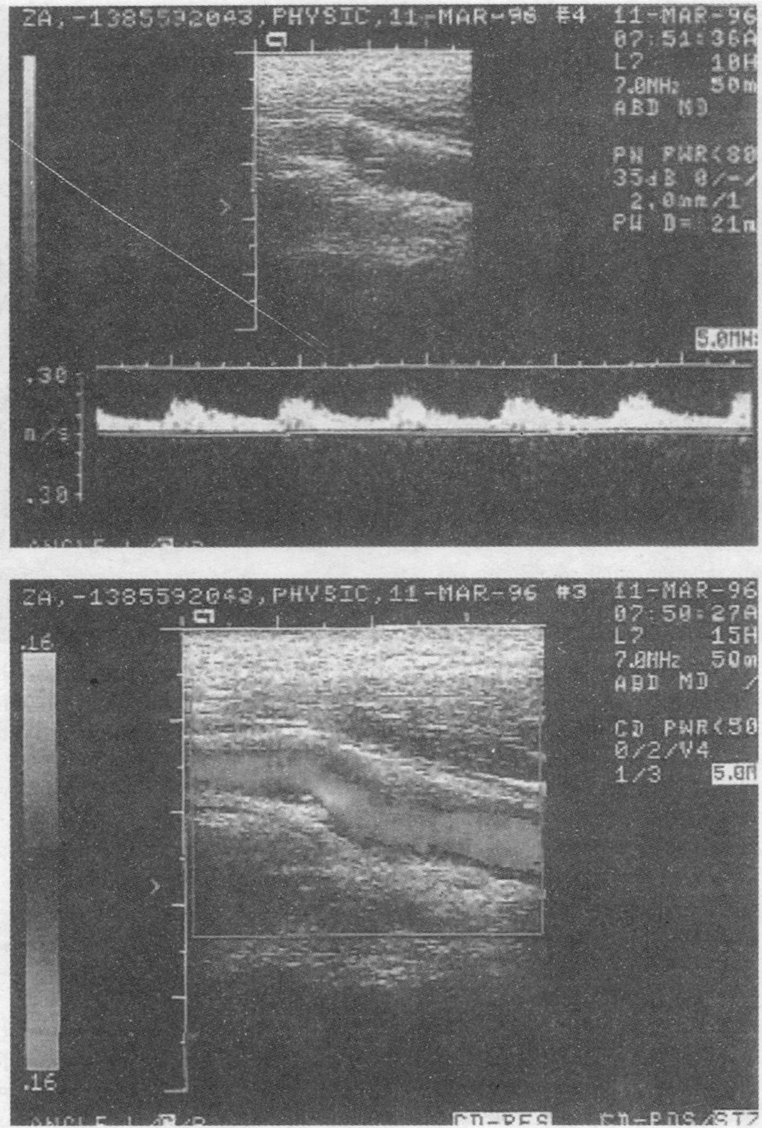


**Figure 12.35** (a) Duplex scanner B-mode image and Doppler spectral analysis record for a normal carotid artery, near the bifurcation. The Doppler signals were recorded from the sample volume defined by the Doppler cursor, the two parallel lines located inside the carotid artery. (b) Color flow image of the vessel in (a). Higher velocity components (lighter color, reproduced here in black and white) are seen where the vessel direction courses more directly toward the transducer.

## 12.13 CONTRAST AGENTS

The images of low contrast structures, blood vessels and anatomic spaces can be enhanced by the injection of a contrast agent. Figure 12.36 shows that for x rays and CT, iodine-based compounds are used as these can be tolerated by the body and expelled quickly. Iodine is a relatively heavy element ($Z = 53$) so that x-ray absorption per atom is high. For MRI, compounds incorporating gadolinium are often used. Gadolinium is unusual in that it is ferromagnetic as a metal and paramagnetic when incorporated in complex organic molecules. Small fat or gas bubbles enclosed in microshells or emulsifiers have different acoustic impedance than most body fluids and will enhance the echo signals.

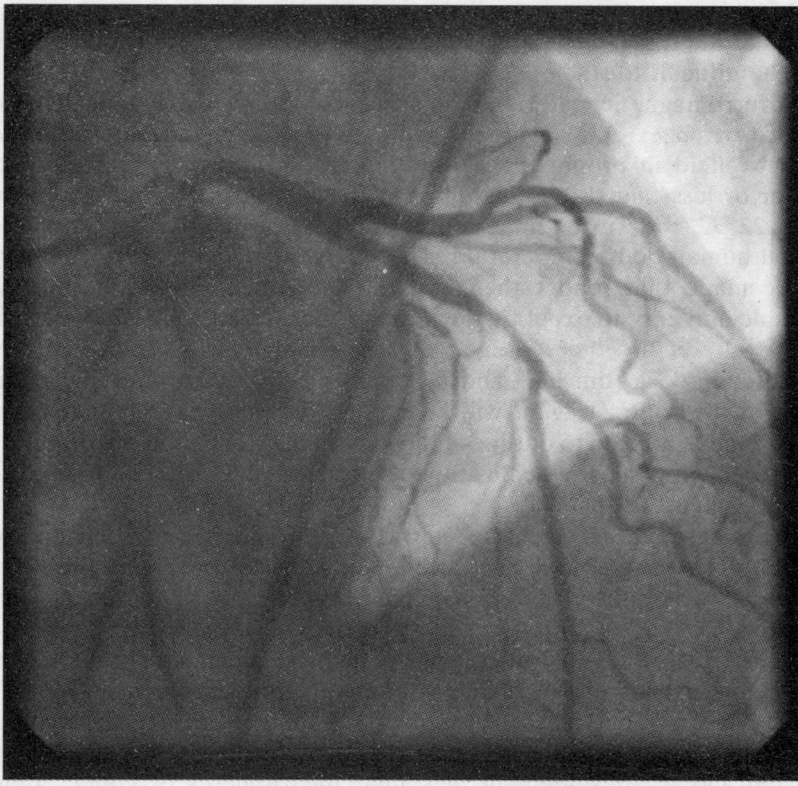


**Figure 12.36** Angiogram of the author taken with iodine-based contrast agent. (Image courtesy of Drs. Hinderaker and Farnham.)

The linear attenuation of x rays was given earlier as $I = I_0 e^{-\alpha x}$, where $\alpha$ is the coefficient of attenuation and $x$ is the thickness of the absorber. The mass attenuation coefficient, $\alpha/\rho$, is found by dividing the linear attenuation coefficient by $\rho$, the mass of the absorber. The mass attenuation coefficient is roughly proportional to $Z^3$, where $Z$ is the atomic number of the absorber. The $Z$ of iodine is 53, and we assume that the average atomic number of blood is less than 5. Iodine contrast agents use complex organic molecules, some having 3 iodine atoms per molecule, usually in the range of 100 to 350 mg/ml. Some iodinated contrast agents are used in angiography and injected into the blood vessels of the heart or other organs to outline the lumens of the blood vessels. Other contrast agents are attached to specialized molecules used as vectors to carry the iodine to, say, the gall bladder or thyroid gland to outline the condition of that organ. As the iodine is expelled by the kidneys, the x-ray image contrast of the urine is increased to permit examination of the ureters, the kidneys, etc. Other iodinated contrast agents increase the contrast of images of the spinal channel and other body cavities, which would otherwise be quite difficult to study.

A ferromagnetic material, such as iron, can show a magnetic field in the absence of an external magnetic field. A paramagnetic material shows a magnetic field in proportion to the external field, the proportion can be greater or less than 1.0. Gadolinium is unusual in that it is ferromagnetic below 22 °C (the Curie temperature) and paramagnetic above it. Since the normal human body temperature is 37 °C, paramagnetic organic molecules can be made that render the high $Z$ (64) element, normally poisonous, tolerable and easy to expel by the kidneys. Because the local magnetic field will be altered by the presence of a paramagnetic substance, the MRI relaxation or decay times, $T_1$ and $T_2$, will also be changed and a high contrast image of the contrast agent will be produced. Such paramagnetic contrast agents can be injected to outline and help visualize lesions in the brain, spine, and associated tissues. Visualization of intracranial lesions due to injuries or tumors is greatly enhanced.

An ideal contrast agent for ultrasound would have impedance quite different from water, blood or nearby tissue in order to increase the visibility of the agent. As in the case for other contrast agents, the material must be well tolerated by the body and readily excreted. Early contrast agents were emulsified oils, which had to be used in high concentrations to be effective. Streams of small air bubbles were not tolerated or the bubbles accreted to form ineffective larger bubbles. The discovery of fullerenes, very large spherical carbon molecules capable of enclosing small volumes, suggested further research and the development of similar microspheres of human albumin enclosing a minuscule volume of air. Further work substituted octafluoropropane gas for the air. The fluorine compound is less soluble in water so that the useful lifetime of the albumin–microsphere–octafluoropropane is several minutes. Such contrast agents, also called *gas microbubbles*, injected into the bloodstream permit the ready visualization of heart structures not easily seen without the contrast agent such as the coronary valves, the apex, and the shape of the ejected fraction of the blood.

## PROBLEMS

**12.1** How much time does it take to transmit a single television frame over telephone lines that have a bandwidth of 3 kHz?

**12.2** A computer monitor uses a noninterlaced scheme with a 4:3 aspect ratio (the height is 3/4 of the width) frame rate of 67 frames/s, 480 visible scan lines, 640 pixels visible/line, 10% retrace time for each vertical and horizontal scan. Find the minimum bandwidth required. Find the bandwidth if the system were redesigned for high resolution and changed to 1024 total scan lines with 920 lines visible and with 1280 pixels visible per line (10% retrace time). How would the bandwidth be affected if the systems were designed for interlaced scanning and the frame rate was 1/2 the field rate (equal to the original frame rate)?

**12.3** A square $8 \times 8$ checkerboard is to be imaged using a raster scan system. The board is centered in this square image. When it is rotated 45° with respect to the image axes, its corners are just touching the centers of the image boundaries. Describe the horizontal and vertical characteristics of this raster scan and the total cycles/image required to detect all the checkerboard squares.

**12.4** Calculate $N_e$ for $S(f) = 1/(1 + 2f)$, where $f$ is in cycles per millimeter.

**12.5** Three elements of an optical system have $N_e = 1$, 2, and 4 cycles/mm. Calculate the system $N_e$.

**12.6** A new imaging system was tested for spatial frequency response, and it was observed that the amplitude response was constant from 0 to 10 lp/mm and then fell linearly to zero response at 20 lp/mm. How would this system compare to one having a noise-equivalent bandwidth of 15 lp/mm?

**12.7** Suppose we make our measurements in the plane of the patient and are required to see the smallest pixel of about 0.25 mm (about 2 line pairs/mm). If the contrast of the object is about 10%, the QDE of the image detector is 50%, the *RL* is about 3%, the image rate is 10/s, and the total exposure time is 10 min, what is the approximate total incident exposure? This level of exposure could be seen in an interventional radiographic procedure.

**12.8** For all other variables fixed, including probability of detection, plot the dimension $d$ of an object versus contrast $C$ for an x-ray image.

**12.9** When an x-ray machine is set for a normal film of the abdomen, around 100 kV, the energy distribution of the beam is such that 4% of the beam can penetrate and exit the patient. If we want to see objects 0.5 mm in diameter that can modulate the beam 50%, what level of incident exposure in R is required? What if the size of the object were 0.2 mm and the modulation (contrast) was 10%?

**12.10** Radiation requirements are based on the statistical independence of the x-ray photons producing an image. If the SNR required is, say, 100, then

10,000 photons are required, on average, per pixel. If the image is to be digitized to 10 bits, 1024 levels, why is it necessary to have so many photons per pixel?

**12.11** The Hounsfield units are a measure of amplitude resolution in computed tomography. If we need to resolve to 1.0% of amplitude, what does this mean in terms of radiation requirements when compared to conventional radiography (3 to 5% amplitude resolution)? What is the effect of taking thinner slices in CT in terms of surface (of the patient) incident exposure?

**12.12** For the ray $\theta k$ shown in Figure 12.12, estimate and list the value for each nonzero $W_{ij}^{\theta k}$. For ease of calculating, assume that a complete overlap of beam and pixel corresponds to a $W_{ij}^{\theta k} = 1.0$.

**12.13** Our measurement for the ray shown in Figure 12.12 yields $I_0/I^{\theta k} = 2.0$. Calculate our best guess for $\mu_{ij}$ using the $W_{ij}^{\theta k}$ values from Problem 12.12.

**12.14** A patient is placed in the strong magnetic field of an MRI imager. The field is 2.0 T, and the blood velocity (blood is an electric conductor) is 10 cm/s. What is the induced voltage gradient across a blood vessel? Could this be harmful?

**12.15** In block-diagram form, show the design of a nuclear-medicine pulse-height analyzer. For each random pulse entering it that has an energy between two limits, it should give only one count. Note that for energies greater than both limits, the output pulse of the detector amplifier passes through both limits twice (rising and falling wave).

**12.16** For the gamma camera, describe the *x*- and *y*-signal contribution from a photomultiplier that is located in the lower left of the detector array.

**12.17** A gamma camera has a line-source response function of $k\exp(-2|x|)$, where $k$ is a constant and $x$ is in centimeters. Calculate the transfer function $S(f)$ of the system.

**12.18** Draw a block diagram for an A-scan ultrasonic signal amplifier that corrects for ultrasonic attenuation with distance.

**12.19** Why are ultrasound images of bone structures distorted? Why don't we observe a similar effect with air cavities?

**12.20** In Problem 12.07, if the geometry of the imaging system were such that the patient's skin was 70 cm from the x-ray source and the input of the detector, an image intensifier tube, was 100 cm from the source, how would this affect the exposure to the skin of the patient (assuming that the image features were measured at the image intensifier)?

**12.21** Three measurements are made of the output of a medical x-ray machine using an ion chamber and electrometer (calibrated in mR) located 100 cm away from the focal spot (source) of the x-ray tube and several thin sheets of aluminum placed at the collimator. The machine was set to 80 kVp, 600 mA, and 0.1 s. The output of the machine was 380 mR (0.0 mm Al), 200 mR (3.0 mm Al), and 163 mR (4.0 mm Al). Find the HVL and output in mR/(mA·s).

**12.22** X-ray tube current is set by adjusting filament current. Assume a constant filament resistance, mean filament temperature of 2000 K, and filament work function of 2.2 eV. What precision is required of the filament control circuit to keep the emission current to within 5% of its set value?

**12.23** A microbubble ultrasound contrast agent is injected as a bolus (an injection of sufficient volume and speed of injection to displace all of the blood in a blood vessel for a short distance). By the time the injected material reaches the heart, it has been diluted by the blood to around 5% of the volume. Assume that the impedance is the volume average, the impedance of the contrast agent is 100 and that of blood is the same as that of water. What is the fraction of ultrasound energy reflected at the boundary of normal and infused blood?

**12.24** The 100 ml ion chamber of an automatic exposure control is exposed to 1 mR. The R is defined as 1 esu/ml conducted per R of exposure, 1 esu = $3.33 \times 10^{-10}$ C. How much charge is conducted by the chamber? What is the voltage change on the 1000 pF integrating capacitor?

## REFERENCES

Block, W. F., "Magnetic resonance imaging." In J. G. Webster (ed.), *Encyclopedia of Medical Devices and Instrumentation*, 2nd ed., New York: Wiley, 2006, Vol. 4, pp. 283–298.

Bracewell, R. N., *The Fourier Transform and Its Applications*, 3rd ed., New York: McGraw-Hill, 1999.

Brooks, R. A., and G. Di Chiro, "Theory of image reconstruction in computed tomography." *Radiology*, 1975, 117, 561–572.

Brooks, R. A., and G. Di Chiro, "Principles of computer-assisted tomography (CAT) in radiographic and radioisotopic imaging." *Phys. Med. Biol*, 1976, 21, 689–732.

Christensen, D. A., *Ultrasound Bioinstrumentation*. New York: Wiley, 1988.

Kripfgans, O., "Ultrasonic imaging." In J. G. Webster (ed.), *Encyclopedia of Medical Devices and Instrumentation*, 2nd ed., New York: Wiley, 2006, Vol. 6, pp. 453–473.

Halberg, L. I., and K. E. Thiele, "Extraction of blood flow information using Doppler-shifted ultrasound." *Hewlett-Packard J.*, 1986, 37(6), 35–40.

Hall, E. L., *Computer Picture Processing and Recognition*. New York: Academic, 1978.

Hine, G. S., (ed.), *Instrumentation in Nuclear Medicine*. New York: Academic, 1967.

Johns, H. E., and J. R. Cunningham, *The Physics of Radiology*, 5th ed. Springfield, IL: Charles C. Thomas, 1990.

Phelps, M. E., J. C. Mazziota, and H. R. Schelbert (eds.), *Positron Emission Tomography and Autoradiography*. New York: Raven, 1986.

Tornai, M, "X-ray equipment design." In J. G. Webster (ed.), *Encyclopedia of Medical Devices and Instrumentation*. 2nd ed., New York: Wiley, 2006, Vol. 6, pp. 550–560.

Wagner, H. N., Jr., Z. Szabo, and J. W. Buchanan (eds.), *Principles of Nuclear Medicine*. 2nd. ed., Philadelphia: Saunders, 1995.

Wells, P. N. T., "Medical ultrasonics." *IEEE Spectrum*, 1984, 21(12), 44–51.

Williams, L. E., "Nuclear medicine instrumentation." In J. G. Webster (ed.), *Encyclopedia of Medical Devices and Instrumentation*. 2nd ed., New York: Wiley, 2006, Vol. 5, pp. 90–106.

# 13

# THERAPEUTIC AND PROSTHETIC DEVICES

Michael R. Neuman

As noted in earlier chapters of this book, a major use of medical electronic instrumentation is in diagnostic medicine. Most instruments sense various physiological signals, carry out some processing of these signals, and display or record them. There is, however, a class of medical electronic devices that are useful therapeutically and as prostheses. Electric stimulators of one form or another represent an important subgroup in this area. Also available are other devices, such as incubators, ventilators, heart–lung machines, artificial kidneys, diathermy devices, and electrosurgical instruments. In this chapter we examine some of these devices and look briefly at their principles of operation.

## 13.1 CARDIAC PACEMAKERS AND OTHER ELECTRIC STIMULATORS

A wide variety of electric stimulators is used in patient care and research. They range from very low-current, low-duty-cycle stimulators, such as the cardiac pacemaker, to high-current single-pulse stimulators, such as defibrillators. In this section, we examine the pacemaker in detail and look at other applications of electric stimulators.

### CARDIAC PACEMAKERS

The cardiac pacemaker is an electric stimulator that produces periodic electric pulses that are conducted to electrodes normally located within the lining of the heart (the endocardium). The stimulus thus conducted to the heart causes it to contract; this effect can be used prosthetically in disease states in which the heart is not stimulated at a proper rate on its own. The principal pathologic conditions in which cardiac pacemakers are applied are known collectively as *heart block*. These are reviewed by Murray (2006) and Schaldach (1992); Webster (1995) reviews pacemaker design details.

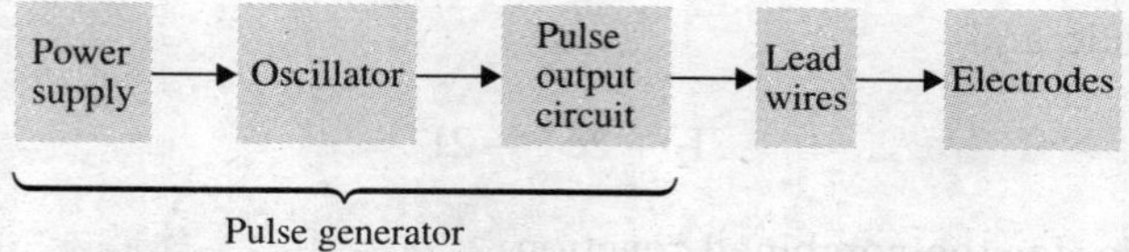


**Figure 13.1** **Block diagram of an asynchronous cardiac pacemaker**

An *asynchronous* pacemaker is one that is free running. Its electric stimulus appears at a uniform rate regardless of what is going on in the heart or the rest of the body. It therefore gives a fixed heart rate. It was the first type of pacemaker that was developed in the mid-twentieth century (Greatbatch, 2000).

Figure 13.1 is a block diagram of an asynchronous pacemaker. The power supply is necessary to supply energy to the pacemaker circuit. Primary battery sources are used.

The oscillator establishes the pulse rate for the pacemaker; this, in turn, controls the pulse output circuit that provides the stimulating pulse to the heart. This pulse is conducted along lead wires to the cardiac electrodes.

Each of these blocks is important in the construction of the pacemaker, and each must be made highly reliable, because faulty operation of this device can cost a patient's life.

Another component of the overall construction of the pacemaker that is not included in Figure 13.1 is the package itself. Not only must the package of an implanted pacemaker be compatible and well tolerated by the body, but it must also provide the necessary protection to the circuit components in order to ensure their reliable operation. The body is a corrosive environment, so the package must be designed to operate well in this environment, while occupying minimal volume and mass.

Today, cardiac pacemakers are contained in hermetically sealed metal packages. Titanium and stainless steel are frequently used for the package. Special electron beam or laser welding techniques have been developed to seal these packages without damaging the electronic circuit or the power source. These metal packages take up less volume and are more reliable than the earlier, polymer-based packages.

Although simple, asynchronous pacemakers such as that shown in Figure 13.1 are seldom used anymore, we can learn about pacemakers in general by examining each of the blocks in more detail.

***Power Supply*** The usual power supply for implantable pacemakers is a battery made up of primary cells. Customary practice in the early 1970s was to change the pacemaker generator every two years due to limitations of the batteries used at that time. It was not until the lithium iodide battery was introduced into use in pacemakers that the lifetime of the cardiac pacemaker was significantly increased (Greatbatch *et al.*, 1971). The fundamental lithium iodide cell involves the reactions

$$\mathrm{Li} \rightarrow \mathrm{Li}^{+} + \mathrm{e}^{-} \qquad (13.1)$$

at the cathode and

$$I_2 + 2e^- \rightarrow 2I^- \tag{13.2}$$

at the anode, for the combined reaction

$$2Li + I_2 \rightarrow 2LiI \tag{13.3}$$

This cell has an open-circuit voltage of 2.8 V and is much more reliable than the batteries that had been used before. Its major limitation is its relatively high source resistance. Essentially all of presently applied pacemakers utilize various forms of lithium batteries as their power source.

***Timing Circuit*** The asynchronous pacemaker represents the simplest kind of pacemaker because it provides a train of stimulus pulses at a constant rate regardless of the functioning of the heart. A free-running oscillator is all that is required for the timing pulse in such a system. More advanced pacemakers, such as are used today, still have timing circuits to determine when a stimulus should be applied to the heart, but complex logic circuits, quartz crystal control, and even a microprocessor replace the simple, free-running oscillator. An overview of the function of some of these systems will be presented later in this chapter.

***Output Circuit*** The pulse output circuit of the pacemaker generator produces the actual electric stimulus that is applied to the heart. At each trigger from the timing circuit, the output circuit generates an electric stimulus pulse that has been optimized for stimulating the myocardium through the electrode system that is being applied with the generator. Constant-voltage or constant-current amplitude pulses are the two usual types of stimuli produced by the output circuit. Constant-voltage amplitude pulses are typically in the range of 5.0 to 5.5 V with a duration of 500 to 600 μs. Constant-current amplitude pulses are typically in the range of 8 to 10 mA with pulse durations ranging from 1.0 to 1.2 ms. Rates for asynchronous pacemakers range from 70 to 90 beats/min, whereas pacemakers that are not fixed rate typically achieve rates ranging from 60 to 150 beats/min.

## LEAD WIRES AND ELECTRODES

Because, in most pacemaker designs, the generator is located at some position remote from the heart itself, there must be an appropriate conduit to carry the electric stimuli to the heart and to apply them in the appropriate place. The lead wires, in addition to being good electrical conductors, must be mechanically strong. Their distal ends must not only withstand the constant motion of the beating heart, but as the individual in whom the pacemaker is implanted moves about, these lead wires have to be able to withstand the stress of being flexed in various positions. A second requirement of the lead-wire system is that it must be well insulated. If this is not the case, wherever faults in the insulation occur, there is effectively another stimulating electrode that, in addition to possibly stimulating the tissue in its vicinity, shunts important stimulating current away from its intended point of application on the heart.

To meet these requirements, the lead wires presently used consist of interwound helical coils of spring-wire alloy molded in a silicone-rubber or polyurethane cylinder. The helical coiling of the wire minimizes stresses applied to it, and the multiple strands serve as insurance against failure of the pacemaker following rupture of a single wire. The soft compliant silicone-rubber or polyurethane encapsulation maintains flexibility of the lead-wire assembly and provides electrical insulation and biological compatibility.

Cardiac pacemakers are either of the *unipolar* or the *bipolar* type. In a unipolar device, a single electrode is in contact with the heart, and negative-going pulses are connected to it from the generator. A large indifferent electrode is located somewhere else in the body, usually mounted on the generator, to complete the circuit. In the bipolar system, two electrodes are placed within the heart, and the stimulus is applied across these electrodes. Both systems of electrodes require approximately the same stimulus for efficient cardiac pacing, as long as negative-going pulses are applied in the unipolar system.

There are clinically applied pacemakers utilizing each system. The electrodes themselves are normally pressed against the inside surface of the heart (endocardial or intraluminal electrodes). It is possible to introduce the electrodes into the heart through a shoulder or neck vein so that it is not necessary to expose the heart surgically during the implantation process.

As with the lead wires, the materials of which electrodes are made are important. The electrodes must be able to stand up to the repeated stress they may encounter as a result of the mechanical activity of the heart, and they must remain in place to provide effective pacing. They must also be made of materials that do not dissolve during long-term implantation, cause undue irritation to the heart tissue adjacent to them, or undergo electrolytic reactions when the stimulus is applied. To avoid any junctional electrolytic corrosion problems, these electrodes are often made of the same materials as the lead wires. Electrodes should also be made of materials that minimize biological interaction such as dense fibrous capsule formation around the electrode. Significant capsule formation can increase the threshold required for stimulation.

Several materials are used for pacemaker electrodes and lead wires. These include platinum and alloys of platinum with other materials: various formulations of stainless steel, carbon, and titanium; and specialized alloys such as Elgiloy (40% cobalt, 20% chromium, 15% iron, 15% nickel, 7% molybdenum, 2% manganese, and traces of carbon and beryllium, originally developed for wrist watch main springs that could endure repeated winding and unwinding without fatigue) and MP35N (35% nickel, 35% cobalt, 20% chromium, 10% molybdenum, and a trace of iron). In early pacemakers, a common type of failure was associated with breakage of the lead wire. Today, thanks to technological advances such as those just described, this problem has been

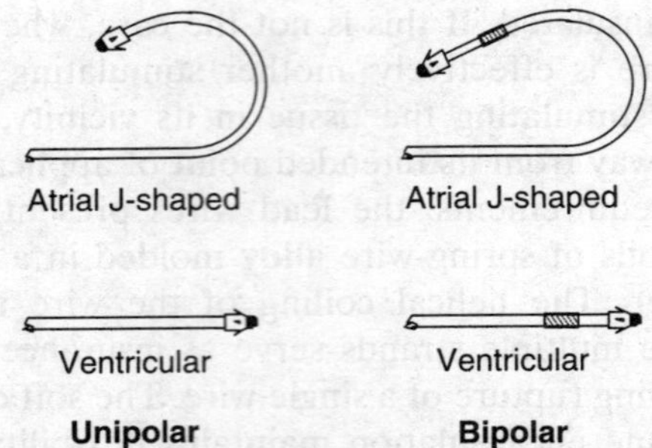


**Figure 13.2** Unipolar and bipolar implementations of both J-shaped and nonpreshaped leads. All models have distal cathode. Bipolar designs typically have a ring anode proximal 10 to 15 mm on the lead. [From Webster (1995).].

greatly reduced, and lead wires and electrodes usually remain in place when the generator circuit and batteries are replaced.

Figure 13.2 shows the basic structure of typical unipolar intraluminal electrodes where the current travels from the tip to the pacemaker can. The ventricular lead passes through the tricuspid valve and the plastic wings embed in the right ventricle while the conducting bands around the circumference of the solid intraluminal probe contact the endocardium (internal surface of the heart wall) and electrically stimulate it. The atrial lead is J-shaped to contact the atrial wall. For the bipolar leads, the current travels between the tip and the ring.

## SYNCHRONOUS PACEMAKERS

Often patients require cardiac pacing only intermittently, because they can establish a normal cardiac rhythm between periods of block. For these patients, it is not necessary to stimulate the ventricles continuously; in some cases, continuous stimulation can even result in serious complications. For example, if an artificial stimulus falls in the repolarization period following a spontaneous ventricular contraction, ventricular tachycardia or fibrillation can result. Thus it is important in these cases that the artificial pacemaker not compete with the heart's normal pacing action. Such a situation can be achieved with an asynchronous pacemaker by making the rate sufficiently high that the heart does not have a chance to beat on its own between pacemaker stimuli. A better solution, however, involves the use of synchronous pacemakers.

There are two general forms of synchronous pacemakers: the demand pacemaker and the atrial-synchronous pacemaker. Figure 13.3 shows the *demand* pacemaker. It consists of a timing circuit, an output circuit, and electrodes, just like those of the asynchronous pacemaker, but it has a feedback loop as well. The timing circuit is set to run at a fixed rate, usually 60 to 80 beats/min. After each stimulus, the timing circuit resets itself, waits the appropriate interval to provide the next stimulus, and then generates the next pulse.

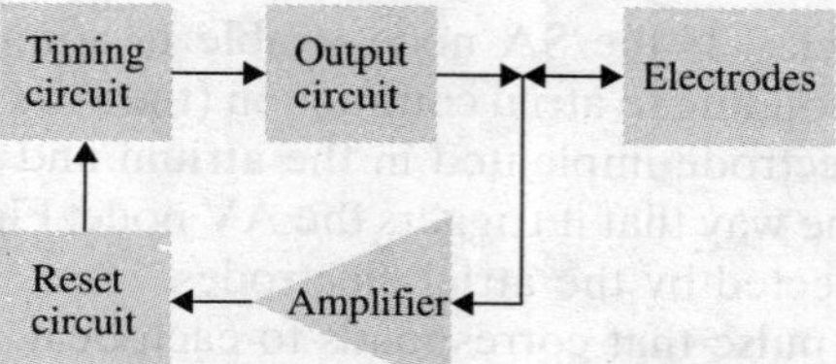


**Figure 13.3 A demand-type synchronous pacemaker** Electrodes serve as a means of both applying the stimulus pulse and detecting the electric signal from spontaneously occurring ventricular contractions that are used to inhibit the pacemaker's timing circuit.

However, if during this interval a natural beat occurs in the ventricle, the feedback circuit detects the QRS complex of the ECG signal from the electrodes and amplifies it. This signal is then used to reset the timing circuit. It awaits its assigned interval before producing the next stimulus. If the heart beats again before this stimulus is produced, the timing circuit is again reset and the process repeats itself. Thus we see that, when the heart's conduction system is operating normally and the heart has a natural rate that is greater than the rate set for the timing circuit, the pacemaker remains in a standby mode, and the heart operates under its own pacing control. In this way the heart can respond to changing demands of the organism by changing its rate in the usual manner. If, on the other hand, temporary heart block occurs, the pacemaker takes over and stimulates the heart at the fixed rate of the timing circuit.

The *atrial-synchronous* pacemaker is a more complicated circuit, as shown in Figure 13.4. In this case, the pacemaker is designed to replace the blocked conduction system of the heart. The heart's physiological pacemaker, located at the SA node, initiates the cardiac cycle by stimulating the atria to contract and then providing a stimulus to the AV node, which, after appropriate delay,

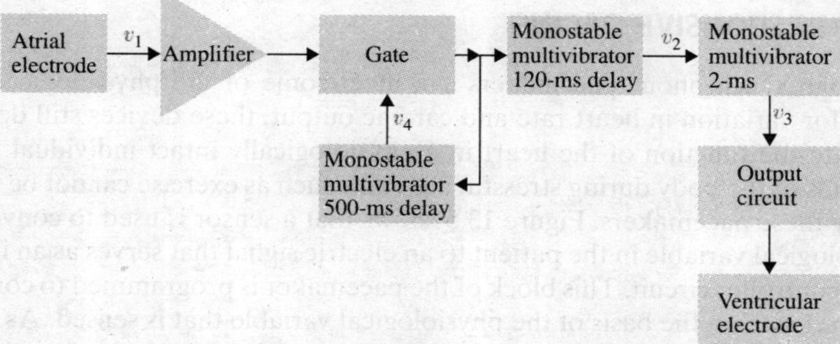


**Figure 13.4** An atrial-synchronous cardiac pacemaker, which detects electric signals corresponding to the contraction of the atria and uses appropriate delays to activate a stimulus pulse to the ventricles.

stimulates the ventricles. If the SA node is able to stimulate the atria, the electric signal corresponding to atrial contraction (the P wave of the ECG) can be detected by an electrode implanted in the atrium and used to trigger the pacemaker in the same way that it triggers the AV node. Figure 13.4 shows the voltage $v_1$ that is detected by the atrial electrodes.

This voltage is a pulse that corresponds to each beat. The atrial signal is then amplified and passed through a gate to a monostable multivibrator giving a pulse $v_2$ of 120 ms duration, the approximate delay of the AV node. Another monostable multivibrator giving a pulse duration of 500 ms is also triggered by the atrial pulse. It produces $v_4$, which causes the gate to block any signals from the atrial electrodes for a period of 500 ms following contraction. This eliminates any artifact caused by the ventricular contraction from stimulating additional ventricular contractions. Thus the pacemaker is refractory to any additional stimulation for 500 ms following atrial contractions.

The falling edge of the 120 ms-duration pulse, $v_2$, is used to trigger a monostable multivibrator of 2 ms duration. Thus the pulse $v_2$ acts as a delay, allowing the ventricular stimulus pulse $v_3$ to be produced 120 ms following atrial contraction. Then $v_3$ controls an output circuit that applies the stimulus to appropriate ventricular electrodes.

Often atrial-synchronous pacemakers have provisions to run at a fixed rate in case the atrial stimulus is lost. This is achieved by combining the demand-pacemaker system with the atrial-stimulus pacemaker system so that an atrial stimulus disables a fixed-rate timing circuit. If the stimulus is absent, the fixed-rate timing circuit takes over and controls the output circuit in the same way as in the asynchronous pacemaker.

The pacing systems shown in Figures 13.3 and 13.4 are represented as having individual circuit blocks. As with the fixed-rate pacemaker, the blocks in these diagrams illustrate the functions carried out by the pacemaker system. These functions are now carried out by microprocessor systems within the pacemaker. Thus it is not possible to find individual components that make up a specific block in an actual device.

## RATE-RESPONSIVE PACING

Although synchronous pacemakers can meet some of the physiological demand for variation in heart rate and cardiac output, these devices still do not replicate the function of the heart in a physiologically intact individual. The demands of the body during stressful activities such as exercise cannot be fully met by these pacemakers. Figure 13.5 shows that a sensor is used to convert a physiological variable in the patient to an electric signal that serves as an input to the controller circuit. This block of the pacemaker is programmed to control the heart rate on the basis of the physiological variable that is sensed. As with the demand pacemaker, this controller can determine whether any artificial pacing is required and can keep the pacemaker in a dormant state when the patient's natural pacing system is functional. The remainder of the pacing system is the same as described in this chapter for other generators.

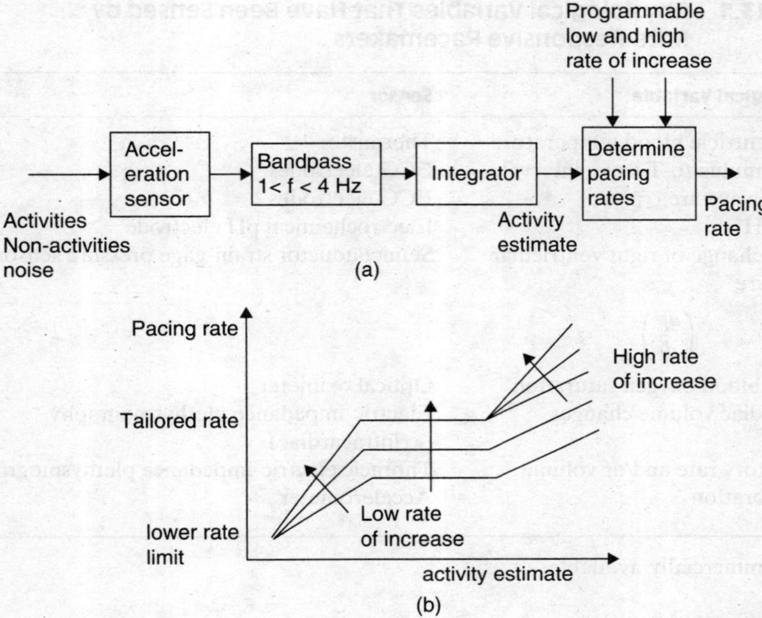


**Figure 13.5** (a) The signal from an acceleration sensor within the rate-responsive pacemaker is bandpass filtered to minimize noise, then rectified and low-pass filtered to yield the activity estimate. (b) The physician selects a programmable curve that has a more sensitive acceleration and/or pacing-rate relationship during low and high levels of activity, with a less sensitive intermediate slope to maintain stability during ordinary workloads. [From Webster (1995).].

The sensor can be located within the pacemaker itself, or it can be located at some other point within the body. In the latter case, it is necessary to connect the sensor to the pacemaker by using a lead-wire system.

Many different physiological variables have been used to control rate-responsive pacemakers. Table 13.1 lists some of these variables and, for each, a sensor that can be used to measure that variable in an implanted system. Each of these variables requires a different control algorithm for the control circuit. In some cases, simple proportional control can be used; in other cases, more complex control algorithms are necessary. For example, when the temperature of the venous blood is used as the control variable, derivative control has been found to be important. As a patient begins strenuous exercise, the venous blood temperature begins to decrease because the increased blood flow to the periphery returns cooler blood to the circulation. This decrease lasts for only about a minute, however, and then the venous blood temperature increases, as a result of the increased metabolic activity in the peripheral skeletal muscles, to a temperature that is above the patient's resting body temperature. If it is to perform similarly to the physiologically intact cardiovascular control system,

**Table 13.1 Physiological Variables That Have Been Sensed by Rate-Responsive Pacemakers**

| Physiological Variable | Sensor |
|---|---|
| Right-ventricle blood temperature | Thermistor |
| ECG stimulus-to-T-wave interval | ECG electrodes |
| ECG R-wave area | ECG electrodes |
| Blood pH* | Electrochemical pH electrode |
| Rate of change of right ventricular pressure* $\left(\frac{dp}{dt}\right)$ | Semiconductor strain-gage pressure sensor |
| Venous blood oxygen saturation* | Optical oximeter |
| Intracardiac volume changes | Electric-impedance plethysmography (intracardiac) |
| Respiratory rate and/or volume | Thoracic electric-impedance plethysmography |
| Body vibration | Accelerometer |

*Not commercially available.

the pacemaker must have a controller that can recognize these changes and respond to them with an increase in heart rate.

Although we generally think of cardiac pacemakers as implantable devices, there also are external versions of this electric stimulator. Fixed-rate, asynchronous pacemakers are appropriate for external devices, because controls for various pacing functions (such as rate) are located on the circuit and can be adjusted by the clinical staff. Intracardiac electrodes are used, and they are introduced percutaneously through a peripheral vein. The external pacemaker is used for patients who are expected to require pacing for only a few days while they are in the intensive-care unit or who are awaiting implantation of a permanent pacemaker. Frequently, external pacemakers are used for patients recovering from cardiac surgery to correct temporary conduction disturbances resulting from the surgery. As the patient recovers, normal conduction returns and use of the pacemaker is discontinued.

An external transcutaneous cardiac pacemaker can apply 80 mA pulses through 50 $cm^2$ electrodes on the chest. But this procedure is painful, so it is used only for emergency or temporary situations (Bocka, 1989).

A typical modern pacemaker is quite small compared to earlier versions. The complete package is about the size of a pocket watch and has a special connector to attach the lead-wire-electrode system. Figure 13.6 shows the evolution of the modern pacemaker. The upper left shows an early form of the pacemaker encapsulated in a biocompatible silicone elastomer. The upper right shows a more recent epoxy resin encapsulated pacemaker. The lifetime of these devices was limited by the battery and the packaging materials. The lower left shows a hermetically sealed metal package in a robust package and

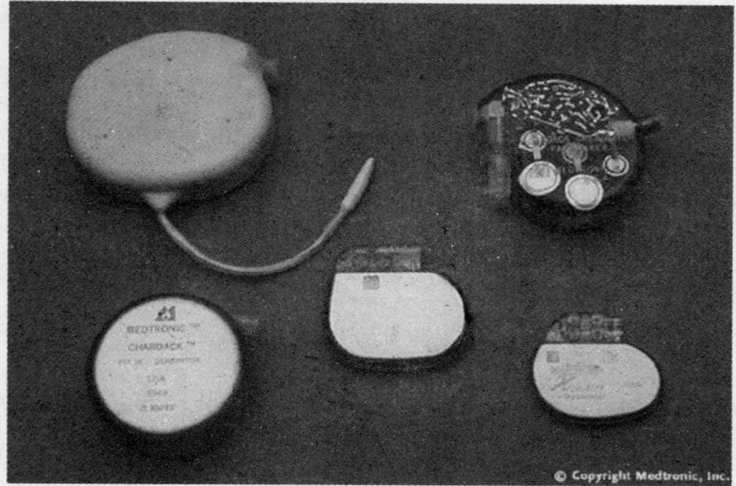


**Figure 13.6** Examples of early pacemakers (top row) and metal encapsulated devices (bottom row). The two units on the bottom right are modern pacemakers that are about the size and mass of a pocket watch. (Photograph courtesy of Medtronic Corp.).

somewhat smaller volume and mass, but the pacemakers were still rather bulky. The advent of lithium batteries and large-scale integrated circuits made it possible for pacemakers to become much lighter and thinner as shown by the remaining two currently used pacemakers in Figure 13.6.

**EXAMPLE 13.1** A cardiac pacemaker delivers 5 V pulses of 2 ms duration to bipolar electrodes, that can be approximated as being a 2 kΩ-resistive load. The mean pulse rate of the pacemaker is 70 per min. The pulses represent 25% of the energy consumed by the pacemaker. The pacemaker is powered by two lithium cells connected in series to give a voltage of 5.6 V. As the designer of this circuit, you are called upon to specify a battery capable of operating the pacemaker for 10 years. What is the minimal acceptable capacity for each cell?

**ANSWER** The energy per stimulus pulse will be

$$E_p = \frac{v^2}{R}T = \frac{(5\,\text{V})^2}{2\,\text{k}\Omega} \times 2\,\text{ms} = 25\,\mu\text{J} \tag{E13.1}$$

The number of pulses in 10 years (including 2 leap years) will be

$$\begin{aligned} N &= 70\,\text{min}^{-1} \times 60\,\text{min/h} \times 24\,\text{h/day} \times 365.25\,\text{day/year} \times 10\,\text{year} \\ &= 3.68 \times 10^8\ \text{pulses} \end{aligned} \tag{E13.2}$$

Thus the total energy will be

$$E_t = NE_p = 3.68 \times 10^8 \times 25\,\mu\text{J} = 9.2\,\text{kJ} \tag{E13.3}$$

The energy supplied by the battery must be four times as great

$$E_b = 4E_t = 36.8\,\text{kJ} \tag{E13.4}$$

If, for the sake of argument (because it would be unwise to draw such a large current from these cells due to polarization and source resistance effects), we draw a current of 1 A from the battery, it would be supplying a power of 5.6 W. The period of time over which this power would have to be supplied to give an energy $E_b$ would then be

$$t = \frac{E_b}{5.6\,\text{W}} = 6.57\,\text{ks} = 1.83\,\text{h} \tag{E13.5}$$

Thus, the battery capacity must be at least 1.83 A·h, or rounding off, 2 A·h to operate this pacemaker.

## BLADDER STIMULATORS

Urinary incontinence and other neurological bladder dysfunctions can, in some cases, be treated by electric stimulation. In the case of incontinence, the sphincter muscles surrounding the urethra are unable to contract sufficiently to occlude the urethra, and increased pressure within the bladder due to coughing, laughing, or neurologically excited excessive contraction of the detrusor muscle of the bladder wall can result in the uncontrollable passage of urine. Several investigators and manufacturers are considering practical ways to control this problem through electric stimulation (Susset, 1973). These involve placing stimulating electrodes in or near the muscles involved in sphincter control of the urethra or on the nerves supplying these muscles. The electrodes stimulate electrically, with pulses of durations of from 0.5 to 5 ms at a repetition rate from 20 to 100 pulses/s, depending on the individual system.

When neural electrodes are used, pulse duration can be shortened to be in the range of 100 to 400 μs. Average stimulating currents (during the pulse) are of the order of 1 mA. Electrodes are frequently placed directly on sphincter muscles, and optimal locations are determined during the implantation surgery by placing a balloon attached to a pressure sensor within the urethra in the region of the sphincters and locating the electrodes such as to give a maximal increase in pressure within the balloon during stimulation.

Noninvasive stimulating electrodes have also been described. In the case of women, such electrodes can be placed on a vaginal pessary that is positioned so as to position the electrodes against the anterior vaginal wall, posterior to the urethra. In men, an anal plug containing electrodes can be used to stimulate the sphincter muscles of the urethra. Although limited studies have shown these devices to be efficacious, they have not been popular with patients.

Some patients need continuous stimulation to avoid incontinence, and the high rate of stimulation calls for a greater power supply over a period of time

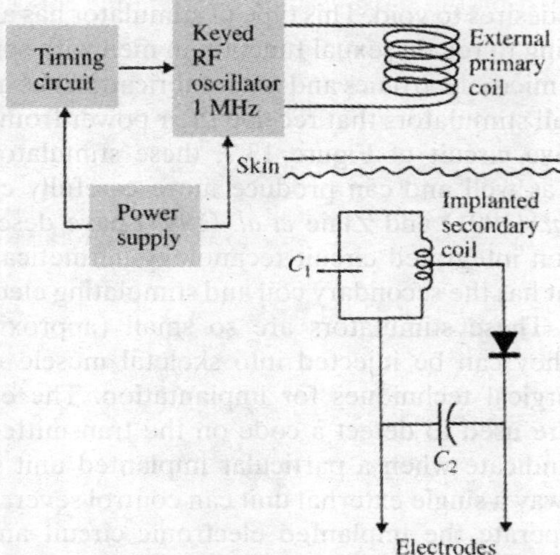


**Figure 13.7 A transcutaneous RF-powered electric stimulator** Note that the implanted circuit of this stimulator is entirely passive and that the amplitude of the pulse supplied to the electrodes is dependent on the coupling coefficient between the internal and external coils.

that is greater than that required for the cardiac pacemaker. For this reason, techniques of transcutaneous stimulation are often used.

One kind of transcutaneous stimulator used in this application is the radio-frequency (RF) unit shown in Figure 13.7. The implanted circuit is entirely passive, with the internal secondary coil located just beneath the skin and coupled to an external primary coil placed over it. The primary coil is driven by a 1 MHz RF oscillator that is keyed by the timing circuit to produce the desired pulses. The power supply for this external circuitry is made up of replaceable or rechargeable batteries. The internal circuit consists of a capacitor $C_1$ to resonate the secondary coil to the oscillator frequency, a diode detector, and a filter capacitor $C_2$ to remove the RF component from the detected pulse waveform. The stimulus is then applied directly to the electrodes. Although the percutaneous transmission of energy is not very efficient, signal amplitudes of several volts can be obtained at the electrodes with primary-to-secondary coil spacings of approximately 1 cm.

Bladder stimulators are also used to help patients who otherwise cannot do so to void. Patients with certain neurological injuries find themselves unable to pass their urine because they cannot contract their detrusor muscle. Stimulators have been developed that can be controlled externally to cause the detrusor muscle to contract. This enables the patient to expel the contents of the bladder at will. To effect complete emptying, such stimulators require multiple electrodes on or within the bladder wall or on the spinal nerves that innervate the bladder. Again the RF percutaneous technique can be used; this time it is necessary only to bring the transmitting unit over the secondary coil when the patient desires to void. This type of stimulator has also been shown to be useful in helping to regain sexual function in men with spinal-cord injuries. Advancement in microelectronics and microfabrication has made it possible to develop very small stimulators that receive their power from external sources. Unlike the passive circuit of Figure 13.7, these stimulators contain active circuit elements as well and can produce more carefully controlled electric pulses. Loeb *et al.* (1991) and Ziaie *et al.* (1993) have described stimulators based upon silicon integrated circuit technology hermetically packaged in a glass cylinder that has the secondary coil and stimulating electrodes integrated into the device. These stimulators are so small (approximately 2 mm in diameter) that they can be injected into skeletal muscle rather than using open incision surgical techniques for implantation. The electronics on the implanted unit are used to detect a code on the transmitted signal from the primary coil to indicate when a particular implanted unit should produce a stimulus. In this way a single external unit can control several implanted units. The power to operate the implanted electronic circuit and to provide the stimulus pulse comes from the signal produced by the external unit.

## MUSCLE STIMULATORS

There have been various applications of electric stimulation to muscle. Stimulators can be used in physical therapy to determine whether muscle groups are able to contract by applying external stimuli to these muscles and observing the results. Stimulators are especially useful in cases in which temporary paralysis can result from atrophy of the muscle caused by disuse, which significantly reduces the mass of the muscle. By periodic direct stimulation of the muscle, the clinician can exercise the muscle, even though the normal neurostimulation is not available. Electric stimulation of muscle can also be used to regain function of paralyzed muscles when the paralysis is a result of neurological injury. It has been demonstrated that patients with spinal-cord injury can regain some crude function of specific skeletal muscles by means of programmed electric stimulation. One such example is an individual whose muscles controlling a hand are completely paralyzed; electric stimulation can enable the person to gain or enhance some ability to grasp. This technique has been used in patients with spinal-cord injuries secondary to traumatic accidents (Peckham, 1987). Fine-wire electrodes are placed in the flexor and extensor muscles controlling finger movement, and these electrodes are stimulated in different sequences to enable the patient to go through various grasping and releasing motions. The patient is able to control the stimulators by moving his or her contralateral shoulder.

Muscle stimulators have also been used to help patients gain function of the lower extremities. Functional electric stimulation (FES) systems have been developed that enable paraplegic patients to stand, walk, and even climb stairs (Marsolais and Kobetic, 1987; Venkatasubramanian *et al.*, 2006). Several electric stimulators are used, and a computer control system determines the timing of the stimulus bursts to the various muscles of the lower extremities.

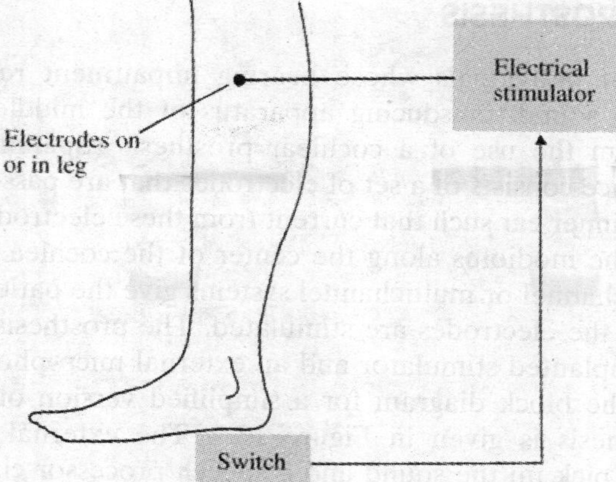


**Figure 13.8** A stimulator system for use on stroke patients suffering from gait problems associated with drop foot.

As with stimulation of the upper extremities, electrodes are placed in the muscle to be stimulated and actually stimulate the nerves that innervate the muscle. Stimulation of these nerves causes the muscle to contract (Nardin *et al.*, 1995).

Another example of a stimulator that is commercially available is one concerned with problems of stroke victims. Often these patients encounter gait problems that are evidenced in a condition known as *drop foot*. In this case, an individual picks up the paralyzed foot to walk but is unable to lift the ball of the foot, so it drags along the ground. The person is thus particularly susceptible to tripping.

The drop foot prosthesis shown in Figure 13.8 can help to minimize this problem. It consists of a switch in the heel of the patient's shoe. The contacts of the switch close when the patient takes weight off his foot. This switch controls a stimulator that continuously stimulates the muscles responsible for lifting the foot. When the individual again places weight on the foot, the switch contacts are opened and the stimulus is stopped. These devices are commercially available but have had only limited acceptance in the United States. In Europe they have been in use for several years.

Stimulus parameters for skeletal-muscle stimulators vary widely according to the type of stimulation, the number of channels, the type of electrode used, and the factor of safety chosen by the designer. Constant-current stimulators are popular in this application, because the charge transferred per stimulus pulse is constant regardless of the electrode load impedance. The pulse currents used range from 2 to 20 mA at pulse durations of 1 ms. These constant-current pulses can produce voltage peaks (Figure 5.23) ranging from 3 to 30 V at the electrodes. Thus, if constant current is to be maintained, the power-supply voltage for the stimulator must exceed this.

## COCHLEAR PROSTHESIS

Profoundly deaf individuals whose hearing impairment results from dysfunction of the sound-transducing apparatus of the middle and inner ear can benefit from the use of a cochlear prosthesis (Spelman, 2006; Clark, 2003). This device consists of a set of electrodes that are passed into the scala tympani of the inner ear such that current from these electrodes can stimulate the nerves of the modiolus along the center of the cochlea. Prostheses that employ single-channel or multichannel systems give the patient the sensation of sound when the electrodes are stimulated. The prosthesis consists of two sections: the implanted stimulator and an external microphone and stimulus control unit. The block diagram for a simplified version of a multichannel cochlear prosthesis is given in Figure 13.9. The external unit includes a microphone to pick up the sound and a speech processor circuit. This block determines what specific characteristics of the sound picked up by the microphone will be used to control the stimulating electrodes. A simple form of such a processor is a set of bandpass filters arranged such that the output signal from these filters represents the sound intensity in a particular passband as a function of time. The signal from each bandpass filter is then used to control the stimulator such that it stimulates a particular set of electrodes in the cochlea.

The stimulus controller block takes the information from the speech processor and uses it to determine when a stimulus pulse should be applied to a particular set of electrodes. In multichannel systems, this block can carry out a multiplexing function as well as a stimulator control function. The output from the stimulus controller circuit drives one or several external coils that are applied to the skin behind the ear directly over a similar coil that is implanted under the skin. The signal and enough power to drive the stimulator are thus transmitted by electric induction via a technique similar to that shown in Figure 13.7.

The input and power supply to the implanted unit come from the internal coil. The stimulator circuit applies an appropriate electric pulse to the electrode pair selected by the stimulus controller.

The electrode array consists of one or more pairs of very small electrodes that are placed on a flexible structure that can assume the spiral shape of the cochlea. Electrodes are positioned such that they face the basilar membrane when the electrode is inserted into the scala tympani. Electrodes have been made from fine wires cast in an elastomer such as silicone or as an array of

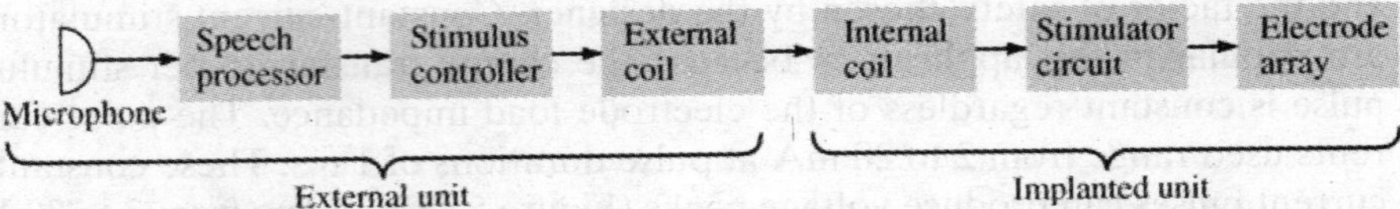


**Figure 13.9** The cochlear prosthesis stimulates an electrode array within the cochlea.

thin-film-deposited electrodes on a flexible polymeric substrate. Needless to say, given the size of the cochlea, these electrodes must be very small.

Although the cochlear prosthesis seems very similar to other types of electric stimulators used for therapeutic purposes, it is unique in one respect that is related to the speech processor and stimulus controller. The sound the patient "hears" is not the same as that heard by the intact ear. Methods of encoding speech into stimulus patterns are evolving, and patients currently have limited recognition of words. Nevertheless, many profoundly deaf patients have benefited from cochlear prostheses, and this technology has moved from the research laboratory to clinical care.

## VISUAL PROSTHESIS

Electrical stimulation of regions of the occipital cortex of the brain and the optic nerve can give the sensation of light to individuals with certain types of blindness. In recent years investigators have begun to explore the potential of developing a visual prosthesis that would take advantage of this fact in creating rudimentary images for blind patients. Early work by Brindley and Lewin (1968) has shown that this is feasible. Research efforts employing stimulation of the occipital cortex of the brain and miniature arrays of stimulating electrodes on the retina have begun, and the neural prosthesis program of the National Institutes of Health in the United States has targeted the development of a visual prosthesis as an important area of research. Although we are far from achieving the potential of this new technology, it represents an exciting challenge for the future of electrical stimulation of tissue (Yanai *et al.*, 2007).

Another form of visual prosthesis that is under development is a system that directly stimulates the retina and the ganglion cells within the retina. This approach can directly map the image on to the retina, but the optic nerve must be intact for the patient to perceive an image. Ultrasmall and high-density electrodes are fabricated using silicon microelectronic technology and surgically implanted in the eye. The visual information is sent to this electrode system via short-range wireless techniques (Chapter 6). Mokwa (2007) presents an example of such a system, and Cohen (2007) reviews the special biologic problems that need to be overcome for retinal and cortical visual prostheses to become practical.

## PAIN SUPPRESSION AND TRANSCUTANEOUS NERVE STIMULATION

Electric stimulation of tissues is sometimes used as a means of suppressing pain. Both battery-powered and transcutaneous RF-powered stimulators have been developed to alleviate severe intractable pain (Simpson, 2003). Such devices have met with varying degrees of success. The amount of paresthesia or anesthesia often depends on the selection of the patient. And in some cases the effectiveness of the stimulation decreases after periods of continuous stimulation. The gate-control theory of pain states that stimulation of certain neurons can have an inhibitory effect on the transmission of pain information from peripheral nerves to the spinal cord. This theory has led to the development of electronic circuits that can stimulate this inhibitory action and can, therefore, be used in the control of pain. Several investigators have studied these stimulators, which are applied to skin surface electrodes, and have found that in many cases (but not all), transcutaneous electric nerve stimulation does reduce perceived pain (Madnani *et al.*, 2006). (Placebo effects were also seen in some cases where stimulators that provided no stimulus were used.)

A wide variety of stimulus waveforms are used with various transcutaneous electrical nerve stimulation (TENS) devices. They range from monophasic rectangular to biphasic spike pulses that are modulated in terms of amplitude, width, or rate. Burst modulation is another popular scheme. Outputs cover a wide range of voltages and currents up to 60 V and 50 mA, and pulse rates range from 2 to 200 pulses/s. Pulse widths also show a wide variation—from 20 to 400 μs. Burst rates are generally around 2 bursts/s. Needless to say, this wide variety of stimulus variables demonstrates the current lack of information on just what the mechanism of TENS is and what the optimal stimulus should be. Nevertheless, many investigators have shown this phenomenon to be helpful to patients suffering from postoperative pain or pain associated with terminal cancer, and the use of TENS devices has been shown to reduce the amount of pain medication required by many patients.

Transcutaneous electrical nerve stimulation stimulators are similar to the asynchronous pacemaker illustrated in Figure 13.1. Electrodes come in various sizes and shapes, but they are in general similar to skin surface electrodes used for monitoring biopotentials (see Chapter 5). A popular form of electrode consists of strips of silicone elastomer made conductive by loading with carbon particles. One electrode is placed on either side of an incision site by means of a conductive adhesive layer, and these electrodes are stimulated in the bipolar mode.

Although this technique is yet not well understood from the standpoint of physiological mechanisms, it offers potential relief to patients suffering from postoperative or intractable pain.

## 13.2 DEFIBRILLATORS AND CARDIOVERTERS

As we learned in Section 4.6, cardiac fibrillation is a condition wherein the individual myocardial cells contract asynchronously with only very local patterns relating the contraction of one cell and that of the next. This serious condition reduces the cardiac output to near zero, and it must be corrected as soon as possible to avoid irreversible brain damage to the patient and death. It is one of the most serious medical emergencies of the cardiac patient. Hence resuscitative measures must be instituted very quickly and definitely within 5 min after the attack.

Electric shock to the heart can be used to reestablish a more normal cardiac rhythm. Electric machines that produce the energy to carry out this function are known as *defibrillators*. The most common type is the rectangular-wave defibrillator. Defibrillation by electric shock is usually carried out by passing current transthoracically, by using large-area electrodes placed against the anterior thorax (Roth, 2006). The physician can achieve defibrillation of the heart with lower levels of current when electrodes are placed directly on the heart, but this can be accomplished only when the heart is exposed in a surgical procedure. Lower energy defibrillation can also be accomplished through endocardial electrodes placed in the heart that are similar to pacemaker electrodes. Such electrodes are used with implantable cardioverter defibrillators that are located subcutaneously with electrodes and lead wires entering the heart through the venous system.

## CAPACITIVE-DISCHARGE DC DEFIBRILLATORS

A short high-amplitude defibrillation pulse can be obtained by using the capacitive-discharge circuit shown in Figure 13.10. In this case, a half-wave rectifier driven by a step-up transformer is used to charge the capacitor $C$. A good rule of thumb is to keep charging time under 10 s.

The clinician discharges the capacitor when the electrodes are firmly in place on the body by starting the timing circuit. The capacitor is discharged through the electrodes and the patient's torso, which represent a primarily resistive load of about 50 Ω that can vary from patient to patient. The process can be repeated if necessary.

When external electrodes are used, energies as high as 400 J may be required. The energy stored in the capacitor is given by the well-known equation

$$E = \frac{Cv^2}{2} \tag{13.4}$$

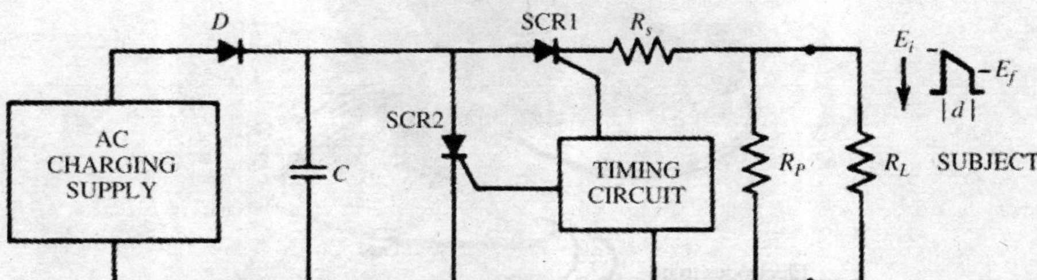


**Figure 13.10** The square and trapezoidal waveform defibrillator may have a battery that drives the ac charging supply. Diode $D$ rectifies the ac to charge capacitor $C$. Series SCR1 is turned on to deliver current to subject $R_L$. The timing circuit calculates the charge delivered, then after duration $d$, shunt SCR2 short circuits the charge. [From Geddes (1984).].

where $C$ is the capacitance and $v$ is the voltage to which the capacitor is charged. Electrolytic capacitors used in defibrillators are about 200 μF and are charged to about 2 kV. This stored energy is not necessarily the same energy that is delivered to the patient. Losses in the discharge circuit and at the electrodes result in an actual delivered energy that is lower.

## AUTOMATIC EXTERNAL DEFIBRILLATOR

Figure 13.11 shows an automatic external defibrillator that can be used by an operator with little training. The electrodes are placed on the body, which ensures that the operator is not exposed to high voltages.

**EXAMPLE 13.2** A simplified form of defibrillator consists of a dc voltage source that charges a capacitor through a series resistor $R_s$ to a voltage sufficiently high to store enough energy to defibrillate a patient through chest electrodes using an energy of 300 J. Assume that the effective resistance between the electrodes on the patient's chest is 100 Ω and that 90% of the energy of the capacitor will be delivered to the patient within 8 ms. (a) What size capacitor should be used? (b) What voltage should the capacitor be charged to initially?

**ANSWER** (a) The energy stored on the capacitor is

$$E = \frac{1}{2}Cv^2 \tag{E13.6}$$

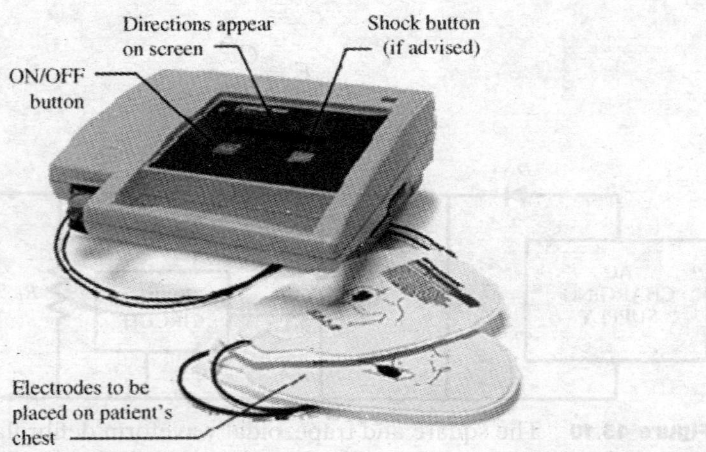


**Figure 13.11** An automatic external defibrillator (AED) visually and vocally instructs the operator to place the conductive adhesive polymer electrodes on the upper and lower chest. It measures the electrocardiogram, and if it detects ventricular fibrillation, it instructs the operator to press the shock button.

where $v$ is the voltage to which $C$ was initially charged. During discharge, the energy dissipated by the load resistance $R_L$ will be

$$E = \frac{v^2}{R_L} \int_0^t e^{-\frac{2t}{R_L C}} dt \tag{E13.7}$$

90% of this energy will be dissipated by

$$e^{-\frac{2t}{R_L C}} = 0.1 \tag{E13.8}$$

or

$$t = R_L C \frac{\ln(0.1)}{2} \tag{E13.9}$$

Because $t$ is required to be 8 ms

$$C = -\frac{2t}{R_L[\ln(0.1)]} = \frac{-2 \times 8 \times 10^{-3}\ \text{s}}{100\ \Omega \times [-2.3]} = 69.6\ \mu\text{F} \tag{E13.10}$$

(b) We can now determine the voltage to which the capacitor should be charged from (E13.6)

$$v = \sqrt{\frac{2E_t}{C}} = \sqrt{\frac{2 \times 300\ \text{J}}{69.6 \times 10^{-6}\ \text{F}}} = 2,940\ \text{V} \tag{E13.11}$$

## CARDIOVERTERS

When an operator applies an electric shock of the magnitude of that from a dc defibrillator to the patient's chest during the T wave of the ECG, there is a strong risk of producing ventricular fibrillation in the patient. Because the most frequent use of defibrillation is to terminate ventricular fibrillation, this problem does not occur; there is no T wave. If, on the other hand, the patient suffers from an atrial arrhythmia, such as atrial tachycardia, fibrillation, or flutter, which in turn causes the ventricles to contract at an elevated rate, dc defibrillation can be used to help the patient revert to a normal sinus rhythm. In such a case, it is indeed possible accidentally to apply the defibrillator output during a T wave (ventricular repolarization) and cause ventricular fibrillation. To avoid this problem, special defibrillators are constructed that have synchronizing circuitry so that the output occurs immediately following an R wave, well before the T wave occurs.

Figure 13.12 is a block diagram of such a defibrillator, which is known as a *cardioverter*. Basically, the device is a combination of the cardiac monitor (Section 6.9) and the defibrillator. Electrocardiography electrodes are placed on the patient in the location that provides the highest R wave with respect to the T wave. The signal from these electrodes passes through a switch that is

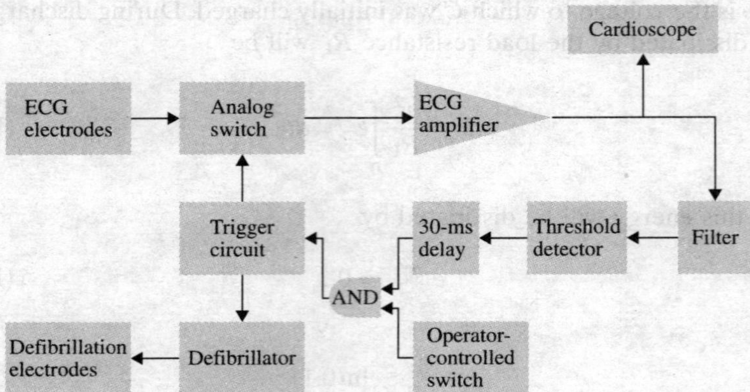


**Figure 13.12** In a cardioverter, the defibrillation pulse must be synchronized with the R wave of the ECG so that it is applied to a patient shortly after the occurrence of the R wave.

normally closed, connecting the electrodes to an appropriate amplifier. The output of the amplifier is displayed on a cardioscope so that the operator can observe the patient's ECG to see, among other things, whether the cardioversion was successful—or, in extreme cases, whether it produced more serious arrhythmias.

The output from the amplifier is also filtered and passed through a threshold detector that detects the R wave. This activates a delay circuit that delays the signal by 30 ms and then activates a trigger circuit that opens the switch connecting the ECG electrodes to the amplifier to protect the amplifier from the ensuing defibrillation pulse. At the same time, it closes a switch that discharges the defibrillator capacitor through the defibrillator electrodes to the patient. This R-wave-controlled switch discharges the defibrillator only once after the operator activates the defibrillator switch. Thus when the operator closes the defibrillator switch, it is discharged immediately after the next QRS complex. After the discharge of the defibrillator, the switch connecting the ECG electrodes to the amplifier is again closed, so that the operator can observe the cardiac rhythm on the cardioscope to determine the effectiveness of the therapy.

## IMPLANTABLE AUTOMATIC DEFIBRILLATORS

It is well known that electrodes placed directly on the myocardium require less energy to defibrillate the heart than do transthoracic electrodes. It is also widely accepted that the earlier defibrillation can be achieved, the better it is for the patient. Thus it was inevitable that implantable automatic defibrillators would be developed (Singer, 1994). These devices, similar in appearance to the implantable pacemaker although somewhat larger, consist of a means of sensing cardiac fibrillation or ventricular tachycardia, a power-supply and an energy-storage component, and electrodes for delivering a stimulus pulse should it be needed. The need for defibrillation is determined by processing the electric signals picked up by the implanted defibrillation electrodes. In some experimental devices, mechanical signals related to ventricular tachycardia and myocardial fibrillation were used to determine the need for a fibrillation pulse.

Energy storage adequate to provide pulses of from 5 to 30 J is necessary in the implantable defibrillator. This is considerably less than the amount of energy required for both the transthoracic defibrillator and those used on the exposed heart. The electrodes used with the implantable defibrillator are larger than those used with a cardiac pacemaker. They are usually located in the ventricular lumen or on the epicardium.

Although the first human implant of an automatic defibrillator occurred in 1980, it was not until 8 years later that commercial devices appeared on the market. Today, the implantable defibrillator is part of the cardiologist's armamentarium for treating cardiac fibrillation and tachyarrhythmias, just as the pacemaker has become a major therapeutic method for treating bradyarrhythmias.

## 13.3 MECHANICAL CARDIOVASCULAR ORTHOTIC AND PROSTHETIC DEVICES

Cardiovascular orthotic prosthetic devices are primarily mechanical in nature, but they are always associated with various pieces of electronic instrumentation that are necessary to control the devices and to monitor their operation.

### CARDIAC-ASSIST DEVICES

It has been the goal of cardiac surgeons and cardiologists to develop mechanical pumps that can be used to aid the failing heart after acute traumatic insults such as myocardial infarction or cardiac surgery. Devices ranging from pumps that can completely replace the heart to a device to reduce the load driven by the heart are being considered. In the latter case, physicians have developed several cardiac-assist devices that are used clinically as a bridge to heart transplant surgery. An aortic-balloon system is an example of one such system that is used clinically. It consists of a long sausage-shaped balloon that can be introduced into the aorta through a femoral artery and connected to an external drive apparatus (Weller and Morrow, 2006).

The operation of this intra-aortic balloon pump is quite simple. Let us consider the balloon as being in the aorta in its inflated state, occupying a major portion of the aortic lumen but still allowing blood to flow past it. At the initiation of the next ventricular contraction, suction is applied to the balloon, causing it to collapse. The blood pumped by the left ventricle enters the aorta and replaces the volume previously occupied by the balloon. This requires only low pressure and demands less effort from the left ventricle. After the contraction, the aortic valve closes, and pressurized $CO_2$ is applied to the balloon, causing it to expand. $CO_2$ is used because it is more soluble in blood than air is. Thus, if the balloon or its supply tubing should leak or rupture, there is less risk of fatal gas embolism.

As the balloon expands, it forces the blood surrounding it out of the aorta and into the rest of the body. Hence the balloon does much of the work normally done by the left ventricle and causes the blood to circulate to the periphery. The process is repeated after the next ventricular contraction.

This device must rely on a sophisticated system of electronic controls to detect ventricular contractions either from a pressure sensor at the arch of the aorta or, more commonly, from the ECG. The signal must then go through appropriate delay circuits to control the suction and pressurized $CO_2$ supplied to the balloon. Appropriate sensors must also be included in the system to ensure that alarms are sounded if any leaks occur.

**EXAMPLE 13.3** An intra-aortic balloon pump device is being applied to a patient in cardiovascular shock. The patient's blood pressure is 80/60, and his heart rate is 85 beats per min. The patient's cardiac output has been determined to be 2.5 liters/min. Once the balloon cardiac-assist device has been started, the patient's systolic blood pressure at the heart drops to 65 mm Hg; the heart rate and cardiac output remain the same. After several hours on the balloon, the systolic pressure is back to 80 mm Hg, the heart rate has dropped to 78 beats/min, and the cardiac output has risen to 3.4 liters/min. Estimate the work done by the heart per beat and per minute before and after the balloon pump was started, as well as several hours later. If the balloon pumps against an average diastolic pressure of 60 mm Hg, how much work is it doing?

**ANSWER** For purposes of simplifying our analysis, to get an estimate of cardiac work, let us assume that the heart pumps against a constant pressure that is equal to the systolic pressure. The work per beat is then

$$W = \int_0^{V_s} P_s dV = P_s V_s \tag{E13.12}$$

where $P_s$ is the systolic blood pressure and $V_s$ is the stroke volume, which is related to cardiac output CO by

$$V_s = \frac{\text{CO}}{\text{HR}} \tag{E13.13}$$

where HR is the heart rate. Before the balloon is applied,

$$W = 80\,\text{mm Hg} \times \frac{2.5\,\text{liters/min}}{85\,\text{min}^{-1}} = 2.35\,\text{mm Hg liters/beat} \tag{E13.14}$$

The work per minute

$$W = 2.35 \text{ mm Hg liters/beat} \times 85 \text{ beats/min}$$
$$= 200 \text{ mm Hg} \cdot \text{liters/min}. \tag{E13.15}$$

After the balloon has been started,

$$W = 65 \text{ mm Hg} \times \frac{2.5 \text{ liters/min}}{85 \text{ min}^{-1}} = 1.91 \text{ mm Hg liters/beat} \tag{E13.16}$$

or 162.5 mm Hg liters/min. Thus the immediate effect of the assist device is to reduce the work done by the heart without affecting cardiac output. The balloon pump must now do work in pumping the blood after the aortic valve has closed. This work is given by

$$W = 60 \text{ mm Hg} \times \frac{2.5 \text{ liters/min}}{85 \text{ min}^{-1}} = 1.76 \text{ mm Hg liters/beat} \tag{E13.17}$$

or 150 mm Hg liters/min. Note that the sum of this work and that of the heart is greater than the original work of the heart before the balloon was applied.

After the balloon pump has been working for several hours, cardiac output is improved, and the heart can do more work. The work is now

$$W = 80 \text{ mm Hg} \times \frac{3.4 \text{ liters/min}}{78 \text{ min}^{-1}} = 3.49 \text{ mm Hg liters/beat} \tag{E13.18}$$

or 272 mm Hg liters/min. This improvement in cardiac performance is due in part to the increased perfusion of the heart itself during diastole, which results from the augmented diastolic pressure from inflation of the balloon.

## PUMP OXYGENATORS

In cardiac surgery it is often necessary to stop the heart from pumping during certain procedures of the operation. In this case, to keep the patient alive it is necessary to replace the heart's pumping action and also the oxygenation normally provided by the lungs, because they are usually not functioning either. Machines known as *pump oxygenators* have been developed that can carry out these functions (D'Alessandro and Michler, 2006). They consist of pumps for maintaining arterial-blood pressure connected in series with oxygenators that increase the blood $O_2$ content and remove $CO_2$. In surgery, the pump oxygenator is usually connected between the superior and inferior venae cavae or between the right atrium and a femoral artery, as shown in Figure 13.13. In some cases a femoral-artery-to-femoral-vein-bypass technique is used to keep all cannulae away from the heart.

Various types of pumps can be used. Roller pumps and multiple-finger pumps are often employed, because the pump itself does not come in contact with the blood. Disposable tubing that is pinched between the propagating rollers or fingers can be used to contain the blood. Pulsatile pumps—consisting of a chamber subjected to the reciprocating motion of a piston, membrane, or

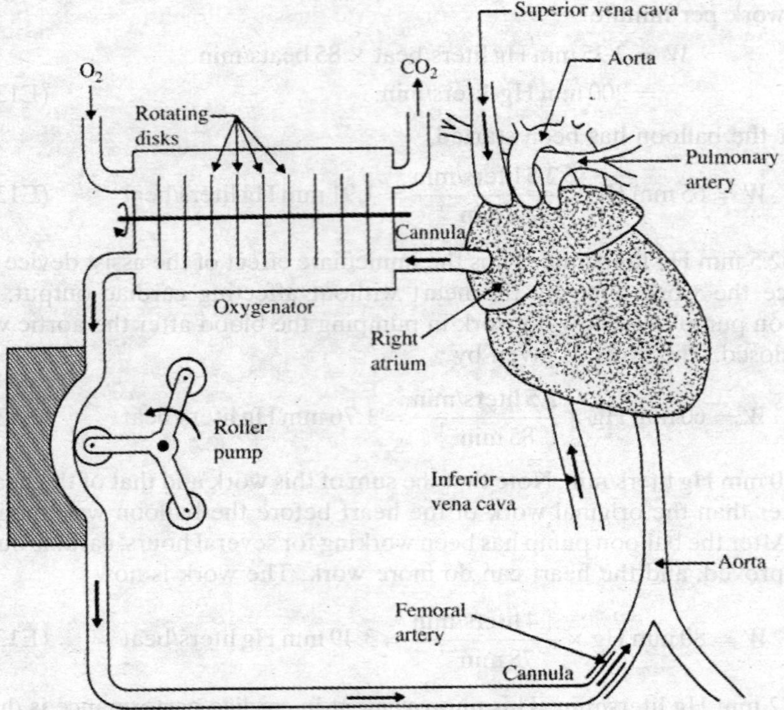


**Figure 13.13 Connection of a pump oxygenator to bypass the heart** A disk-type oxygenator is used with a roller pump. Venous blood is taken from a cannula in the right atrium, and oxygenated blood is returned through a cannula in the femoral artery.

bladder—are also used, with appropriate check valves to direct the flow. Such pumps more closely follow the normal action of the heart and produce a pulsatile blood pressure.

Two general types of oxygenators are used with these prosthetic devices. One is the *film* type, in which a large-surface-area film of blood is drawn into contact with a nearly 100% $O_2$ atmosphere by rotating disks (Figure 13.13). The second type is the *membrane* oxygenator, in which blood flows through fine tubes of a membrane permeable to gas. This device has a large exchange-surface area to allow the gas transfer to take place.

Studies have shown the membrane oxygenator to have less deleterious effects on the blood than film and other direct types of oxygenators. The membrane separates the liquid blood phase from the gaseous oxygen phase, whereas in direct oxygenators such as that shown in Figure 13.13, blood and oxygen are in direct contact. This can denature some of the protein components of the blood, which can lead to formation of clots and emboli in the patient.

Pump oxygenator systems are also applied in newborn intensive care. Infants who have severe lung disease that cannot be treated any other way have been put on pump oxygenators for several days to allow the diseased lung to "rest." The lungs recover in a significant number of these infants, who can then be removed from the pump oxygenator. This therapy, which is based on the extracorporeal membrane oxygenator (ECMO), has been demonstrated to be effective for seriously ill term infants, but the same approach has not shown any therapeutic efficacy in adults.

### TOTAL ARTIFICIAL HEART

Blood pumps have been miniaturized and constructed of such materials that they can replace the natural hearts of patients. They are implanted in the thoracic cavity and operate via pneumatic and electric connections to an external drive apparatus (Zapanta, 2006). Such devices were the subject of many popular press reports during the period in which they were studied in human subjects. The most notable of the devices were the Jarvic 7 and the AbioCor. They have been used as both a temporary and a permanent heart replacement in humans, but neither has become routine clinical devices. Total heart replacements enabling patients to live for up to 620 days after surgery have been reported. Technical and biological problems, however, continue to plague these devices, and their use has been halted pending further improvement. Ventricular assist devices are available for temporary use (McCarthy, 1995).

Electronic instrumentation is essential when pumps or pump oxygenators are used. It is necessary to monitor the hemodynamics of the patient during the procedure. In addition, the ECG, aortic, and central-venous pressure waveforms must be carefully watched. The pump oxygenator itself must also be monitored. The degree of oxygenation of the blood, as well as its pressure, must be recorded. In addition, it is necessary to protect the patient from leaks in the system that could cause $O_2$ to enter the blood vessels or result in the serious loss of blood.

## 13.4 HEMODIALYSIS

One of the most important prosthetic devices in modern medicine is the artificial kidney, which is periodically connected to the circulatory systems of uremic patients to remove metabolic waste products from their blood. A general scheme for the operation of this device is shown in Figure 13.14.

There are two basic units in a hemodialysis system: the exchanger and the dialysate delivery system. The exchanger consists of the dialysis chamber itself, which is a compartment containing the patient's blood and a compartment containing the dialysate. These two compartments are separated by a semipermeable membrane that allows the waste components in the blood to diffuse through to the dialysate, which carries them away.

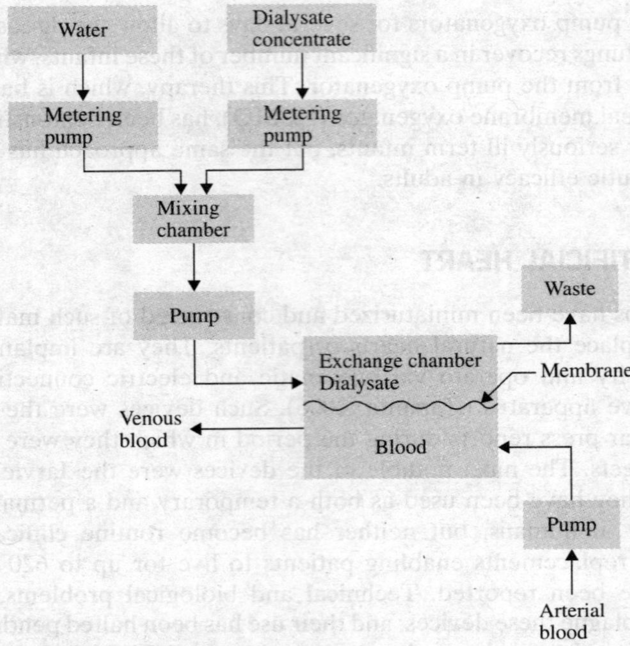


**Figure 13.14 An artificial kidney** The dialysate delivery system in this unit mixes dialysate from a concentrate before pumping it through the exchange chamber.

There are three basic types of exchangers in use. The *coil dialyzer* consists of a tube made of the semipermeable membrane material wound into a coil, in such a way that the dialysate can be circulated between individual turns of it. This is the most commonly used type of dialyzer. It has the limitation that the coil must be fairly long to provide a large effective surface area for mass transport, and it thus imposes a relatively high resistance to the flow of blood. For this reason, and to maintain effective blood flow, it is necessary to put a pump in series with the arterial-blood supply to increase the pressure. However, the increased pressure improves the ultrafiltration rate of the membrane. It is important in this unit that the dialysate also be forcibly circulated to ensure rapid mixing. Because fresh dialysate must be available to the surface of the membrane throughout the coil, a pump is necessary for the dialysate as well.

The second type of exchanger used in artificial-kidney systems is the *parallel-plate dialyzer*. It is constructed similarly to a multilayer parallel-plate capacitor, with the plates made of semipermeable-membrane material. Blood is circulated between alternate pairs of plates, and the dialysate is circulated between the other plates. Each plate thus serves as a membrane between dialysate and blood. The blood flows in thin sheets to maximize the surface-to-volume ratio for the dialyzer.

The third type of exchange apparatus is the *hollow-fiber kidney*. This consists of from 10,000 to 15,000 hollow fibers, with an internal diameter of approximately 0.2 mm and a length of approximately 150 mm, connected in parallel. The blood flows in the lumen of the fibers while the dialysate surrounds them. The walls of the fibers serve as the semipermeable membrane. The dialysate is pumped through the space surrounding the fibers to achieve the most efficient exchange.

The remainder of the artificial kidney consists of the dialysate-delivery system. The dialysate is made up of water with various solutes added. Either it is prepared in a batch and pumped through the dialysis chamber, or (in applications in which large amounts of dialysate are used) a concentrated solution of the solutes is made and automatically mixed with pure water to achieve the correct concentration (Figure 13.14). Metering pumps administer the correct amount of dialysate concentrate and water into a mixing chamber to produce the dialysate, which is then pumped through a dialysis chamber, where it picks up the metabolic waste products. It is then discarded.

As in the case of the cardiovascular prostheses, described in Section 13.3, the hemodialysis apparatus does not require any electronic instrumentation to function. However, in using this device with patients, the clinician finds that several pieces of electronic instrumentation greatly aid in its application and operation. Because only a membrane separates the patient's blood from the dialysate, it is important that any leaks in the membrane be detected immediately before serious losses of blood occur. In some cases, in fact, dialysate can leak into the patient's circulatory system. The blood is usually at a higher pressure than the dialysate, so loss of blood is the hazard of major concern. The dialysate is a clear liquid, and the presence of blood in it can be detected as a colorimetric or optical density change; thus optical systems are used to detect leaks. In addition, instruments monitor the pressure in the blood compartment to detect rapidly any abnormalities, such as major leaks or clotting phenomena, which might change the pressure.

The gross concentration of electrolytes of the dialysate is also monitored by electronic instrumentation. Because the solute is made up of electrolytes, the overall concentration of these in the dialysate is determined by impedance techniques. Thus, by measuring the conductivity of the dialysate in the mixing chamber, instruments can detect any major abnormalities in concentration before the dialysate enters the dialysis chamber.

Another problem common to both hemodialysis units and the pump oxygenator is that air bubbles cannot be tolerated in the blood that reenters the patient: This produces air emboli that may be life threatening. Thus it is important that some type of bubble detector be included in the path of the blood before it reenters the body. If bubbles are detected, the blood pump is turned off until the technician operating the dialyzer solves the problem.

**EXAMPLE 13.4** The electric conductivity $\sigma$ (S/cm) of an electrolytic solution such as dialysate can be approximated by

$$\sigma = \sum_i N_i q_i \mu_i \tag{E13.19}$$

where $N_i$ = number of ions of $i$ per cm$^3$, $q_i$ = charge on ions of $i$, $\mu_i$ = mobility of ions of $i$ in solution, cm$^2$/V·s.

The equation is summed for all ionic species present in the solution. Assume that the dialysate is made up of 0.9 g equivalents of cations having a single electronic charge per ion and a mean mobility of 0.623 cm$^2$/(V·s) and that the same amount of oppositely charged anions having a mobility of 0.986 cm$^2$/(V·s). Determine the conductivity of the dialysate solution. How much it will change if 0.05 g equivalents of an anion are added to the solution?

**ANSWER** The conductivity of the solution as given by (E13.19) will be

$$\sigma = 0.9 \times 6.023 \times 10^{23}\ \text{liter}^{-1} \times 10^{-3}\ \text{liter/cm}^3 \times 1.6 \times 10^{-19}\ \text{C}(0.623 + 0.986)\ \text{cm}^2/(\text{V}\cdot\text{s}) = 139.6\ \text{S/cm} \qquad \text{(E13.20)}$$

If we increase the concentration of ions in the dialysate by 0.05 g equivalents, the first term on the right-hand side of (E13.20) becomes 0.95, and the result will be increased by a factor of 0.95/0.9 or 1.056. The conductivity becomes $\sigma = 147.4$ S/cm.

Thus, an electronic circuit to detect ionic changes in the dialysate roughly 5% would have to be sensitive to a conductivity change of that amount.

## 13.5 LITHOTRIPSY

Kidney stones can cause great discomfort to the patient as they are passed through the urinary tract, and their presence may eventually lead to loss of function of the affected kidney. An open incision surgical technique known as *lithotomy* can be used to remove the stone, and this procedure includes all the risks, complications, discomfort, and disability of major surgery. *Lithotripsy* refers to noninvasive or minimally invasive surgical techniques for removing kidney stones without these risks and complications. The technique involves disintegration of the stone *in vivo* so that it can pass through the urinary tract in the form of small particles the passage of which does not result in severe discomfort or disability (Weizer and Preminger, 2006).

In percutaneous lithotripsy, a probe is guided under x-ray fluoroscopy through a small incision into the location of the kidney stone. Either mechanical shock waves are produced at the tip of the probe by a controlled electric discharge (spark), or the probe contains an ultrasonic transducer that produces ultrasonic waves. Each of these forms of energy is used to break up the kidney stone so that it can be withdrawn in pieces through the probe guide element or can be allowed to pass through the urinary tract.

Extracorporeal shock-wave lithotripsy is an entirely noninvasive method that can be used to break up kidney stones. Figure 13.15 shows the basic structure of a shock-wave lithotripter. Many mechanical shock waves are

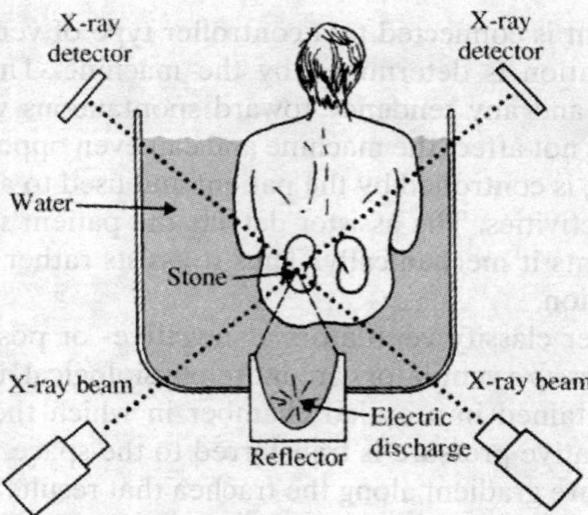


**Figure 13.15** In extracorporeal shock-wave lithotripsy, a biplane x-ray apparatus is used to make sure the stone is at the focal point of spark-generated shock waves from the ellipsoidal reflector.

produced at one focus of an ellipsoidal reflector such that these waves converge to another focal point several centimeters away from the reflector. The reflector and the patient are submerged in demineralized, degassed water in such a way that the patient can be moved until the stone is located at the focal point of the shock wave. This positioning of the patient is critical, and a biplane x-ray system is used to establish the position of the stone at the focal point as well as to monitor its disintegration. A high-voltage pulse (approximately 20 kV) is applied to the spark gap, and the discharge produces a shock wave that is propagated through the water to the focal point. The patient is placed on a gantry support that can be precisely positioned as the operator observes the stone on the biplane x-ray monitors. Once the patient is appropriately positioned, multiple-shock waves are generated by multiple discharges across the spark gap. Up to 2000 shock waves may be necessary to reduce a kidney stone to 1 to 2 mm fragments that can pass through the urinary tract.

With this treatment, most patients are able to resume full activity within two days. This is considerably less time than surgical treatment by lithotomy would entail. Although the apparatus is complex and expensive to purchase and operate, the overall savings for the patient and the health-delivery system are clear.

## 13.6 VENTILATORS

An important factor in respiratory therapy is being able to assist patients in ventilating their lungs. Various mechanical devices have been developed over the years to carry out this function. These devices, known as *ventilators* or *respirators*, can be separated into two general categories: the *controller* and the *assister* (Cairo, and Pilbeam, 1999).

When a patient is connected to a controller type of ventilator, his or her respiratory ventilation is determined by the machine. The device sets the ventilatory cycle, and any tendency toward spontaneous ventilation on the patient's part does not affect the machine and can even oppose it. The assister, on the other hand, is controlled by the patient and used to augment his or her own ventilation activities. The assister detects the patient's attempt at ventilation and augments it mechanically. Thus it assists rather than controls the patient in ventilation.

We can further classify ventilators as negative- or positive-pressure devices. *Negative-pressure* ventilators are more physiological, in that the body of the patient is contained in a sealed chamber in which the pressure can be reduced. This negative pressure is transferred to the space within the thorax, producing a pressure gradient along the trachea that results in air entering the lungs. Pressure is then returned to atmospheric, allowing the lungs to recoil to their original shape and to expel some of their air. *Positive-pressure* ventilators, on the other hand, blow air into the lungs by increasing the pressure in the trachea. This causes the lungs to expand due to internal pressure and then to recoil naturally, expelling a portion of the air once the positive pressure is removed. Even though negative pressure ventilators are more physiological, they are by necessity large and limit access to the patient for therapy. For these reasons, they are seldom used clinically today.

Ventilators can be time cycled, volume cycled, or pressure cycled. Negative-pressure ventilators are usually time cycled. This means that the negative pressure is applied to the body for a given period of time and then released for another given period of time before the process is repeated. Modern time cycled ventilators are electronically controlled. Microprocessors are used to establish the cycling or the rate of ventilation, as well as the ratio between inspiration and expiration times or volumes. These electronic circuits activate solenoid valves that regulate the airflow.

In the *volume-controlled* ventilator, the progression of the cycles of the ventilator is controlled by the volume of air administered to the patient. Thus, if a machine is set to cycle on a given volume, it does not cycle until that volume of air has been administered to the patient. It also has a pressure-override valve, so that if, while the machine is in the process of administering the set volume, the pressure exceeds a predetermined maximal value, the ventilator will cycle whether or not the appropriate volume has been administered. This is an important safety consideration, because uncontrolled pressures could cause serious damage. In the *pressure-cycled* ventilator, air is administered to the patient until the pressure reaches a predetermined limit, at which time the ventilator switches to its expiratory portion of the cycle, and the process is repeated.

For some patients with sleep disorders, as they fall asleep, the muscles in the airways relax and permit the airway to close. After about 30 s, their oxygen level decreases to the level where it wakes them up. This cycle repeats all night long, resulting in loss of sleep. Figure 13.16 shows a continuous-positive-airway-pressure apparatus that keeps the airway open to improve sleep.

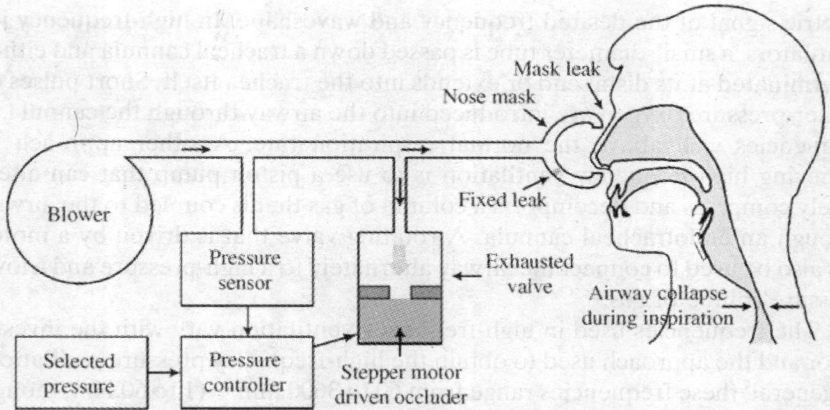


**Figure 13.16** A continuous-positive-airway-pressure (CPAP) apparatus blows air through the nose to prevent airway collapse during sleep. During expiration, the pressure sensor senses the increased pressure and raises the arrow-shaped occluder to make expiration easier.

The arrow-shaped occluder is down during inspiration to increase airway pressure and up during expiration to make expiration easier.

## HIGH-FREQUENCY VENTILATORS

A technique for ventilating patients at frequencies much higher than the normal respiration rate has been investigated and has seen limited clinical use. Not only are the inspiration–expiration frequencies higher than normal, but the actual volume of air moved per "breath" is on the order of the anatomical dead space of the pulmonary system. Because the anatomical dead space constitutes the volume of the conducting airway, the upper airway, trachea, and bronchial tree, high-frequency ventilation is unusual from the standpoint of volume as well as frequency (Hamilton, 1988).

The physiological mechanisms of gas transport in high-frequency ventilation constitute various combinations of volume transport and molecular diffusion (Chang, 1984). Even though it is unlikely that a molecule of oxygen entering the airway would enter the alveoli at normal breathing frequencies and tidal volumes equivalent to the volumes used in high-frequency ventilation, when this process is carried out at high frequencies, increased mixing occurs in the airway. This can be the result of turbulence, asymmetric velocity profiles, and molecular diffusion that occur at the elevated frequencies. The net effect is that the mixed gases in the airway do in fact reach the alveoli, making it possible for the alveoli to be effectively ventilated.

High-frequency ventilation principles can be put into practice in several different ways. The easiest method is to generate the high-frequency pressure waves by means of a large, low-frequency loud speaker that is driven by an electric signal of the desired frequency and waveshape. In high-frequency jet ventilators, a small-diameter tube is passed down a tracheal cannula and either is terminated at its distal end or extends into the trachea itself. Short pulses of higher-pressure oxygen are introduced into the airway through the cannula at frequencies well above the normal respiration rate. Another approach to achieving high-frequency ventilation is to use a piston pump that can alternately compress and decompress a column of gas that is coupled to the airway through an endotracheal cannula. A rotating valve that is driven by a motor can also be used to connect the airway alternately to a high-pressure and a low-pressure source of gas.

The frequencies used in high-frequency ventilation vary with the investigator and the approach used to obtain the high-frequency pressure oscillation. In general, these frequencies range from 60 to 3600 $min^{-1}$ (1 to 60 Hz), though frequencies in the vicinity of 900 $min^{-1}$ (15 Hz) are popular. Inspiration-to-expiration ratios can usually be varied from 1:1 to 1:4, and waveshapes ranging from sinusoidal to rectangular can be achieved. Like conventional ventilators, high-frequency ventilators are usually electronically controlled.

## 13.7 INFANT INCUBATORS

The care of premature newborns often requires that they be in an environment in which temperature is elevated and controlled, because they are unable to regulate their own temperatures. When infants are kept in a chamber maintained within a specific temperature range, $O_2$ requirements are minimized. This is especially important for premature newborns, who are more susceptible to respiratory problems than full-term infants, because of developmental limitations and because their lungs may be unable to supply enough oxygen to meet elevated demands. By minimizing oxygen demands to maintain body temperature, more oxygen is available for growth. Such controlled-temperature environments are maintained in infant incubators.

Temperature-controlled air is passed through the chamber in which the baby is located to maintain it at a set temperature. The temperature is controlled in modern units by means of the proportional control system shown in Figure 13.17. The temperature in the air-supply line varies a thermistor resistance that is compared with a fixed resistance that corresponds to the set temperature. If the temperature of the air entering the infant's chamber is lower than the set temperature, power is applied to the heater to correct for this difference. In the proportional-controller system, the amount of power applied to the heater is proportional to the difference between the actual air temperature and the set point. This means that the amount of power decreases as the temperature approaches the set point, an important feature in effecting more precise control and minimizing overshoot of the set point.

The control system shown in Figure 13.17 uses the thermistor in a bridge circuit, with the set-point resistance as another arm of the bridge. The bridge

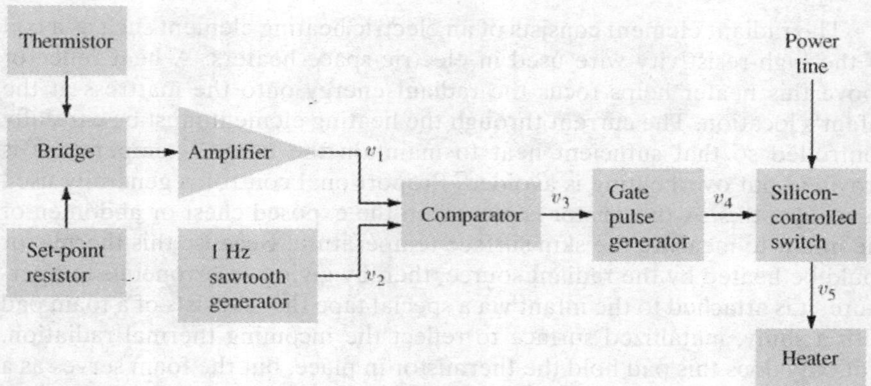


**Figure 13.17** Block diagram of a proportional temperature controller used to maintain the temperature of air inside an infant incubator.

output is amplified, giving the voltage $v_1$ at the output, which is proportional to the difference in temperature between the thermistor and the set point.

Some incubators, instead of controlling the air temperature directly, use the skin temperature of the infant as a control parameter. The thermistor is placed against the skin of the infant over the liver so that it gives a reading representative of the infant's core temperature. The controller is set to maintain the infant's skin at a given temperature. If the infant is cooler than the set point, the air entering the chamber of the incubator is heated an amount proportional to the difference between the set temperature and the baby's actual temperature.

Incubators also have a simple alarm system to alert the clinical staff if there is any dangerous overheating of the device. The system embodies a temperature-controlled switch that carries power to an audible alarm when, if ever, the temperature exceeds the safe limit. Often there is a buzzer connected in series with a switch that is activated by a bimetallic strip. This keeps the system simple and reliable. In some cases, this circuit also immediately reduces power to the heater to stop the overheating.

Infants lose a large percentage of their body heat by radiation. In some clinical situations, the intensive care of term and preterm infants requires that large portions of their skin surface be exposed to enable the clinical staff to observe the infant's condition, carry out special procedures, and attach various therapeutic and monitoring devices. It may be inconvenient to have such infants in an incubator where body temperature is maintained by means of heated air and convection. Accordingly, incubators consisting of radiant warmers have been developed. The infant is placed on a mattress under a radiant heating element. Low walls surround the mattress so that there is no risk of the infant falling off the device, but the remainder of the area surrounding the infant is open to allow access to the patient. This is in contrast to the warm-air convection incubator, where the infant must be accessed through arm ports.

The radiant element consists of an electric heating element such as a coil of the high-resistivity wire used in electric space heaters. A heat reflector above this heater helps focus the radiant energy onto the mattress at the infant's location. The current through the heating element must be carefully controlled so that sufficient heat to maintain the infant's temperature is provided but overheating is avoided. Proportional control is generally used to achieve this. A thermistor is placed on the exposed chest or abdomen of the infant to measure the skin surface temperature. Because this thermistor could be heated by the radiant source, thereby giving an erroneous temperature, it is attached to the infant via a special tape that consists of a foam pad with a shiny, metallized surface to reflect the incoming thermal radiation. Not only does this pad hold the thermistor in place, but the foam serves as a thermal insulator, and the reflecting surface minimizes the direct effect of radiation on the thermistor.

Premature and, in some cases, full-term infants often develop respiratory distress or other anomalies. These infants can stop breathing and such apnea is life threatening. A tap on the incubator wall or a slap on the foot or other physical stimulation is usually all such infants need to remind them to take another breath. Thus it is important to detect when apnea has persisted for a given period of time and to alert clinical personnel so that they can immediately attend to the infant. Various types of apnea monitors have been developed to carry out this function. They detect ventilation by one of the following methods (Chapter 9): transthoracic impedance or movement of the baby's abdominal and/or chest wall. An alarm is sounded when respiratory activity ceases for periods of greater than a preset time, in the range of 15 to 30 s.

## 13.8 DRUG DELIVERY DEVICES

One of the principal activities of clinical medicine is the pharmacologic treatment of diseases. Traditionally, this has been carried out by administering drugs and other materials in individual doses by the oral, subcutaneous, intramuscular, or intravenous route. In some cases, however, these methods of administration are not satisfactory, because drug levels vary from one administration to the next. For drugs the therapeutic levels of which are close to their toxic levels, this type of administration results in either toxic side effects or suboptimal therapy. Methods of using physical devices to administer drugs continuously within a narrow therapeutic range have been developed to overcome these problems.

### DRUG INFUSION PUMPS

Controlled infusion of fluids and drugs is a well-established technique in the hospital. Intravenous (IV) therapy from a gravity-fed fluid reservoir is extensively used in cases ranging from the treatment of severe infections to intensive care in the operating room and postoperatively. These fluids are frequently routed by gravity feed through some type of constriction that controls the total amount of fluid administered. Although this method is widely used in hospitals and is relatively inexpensive, it is limited in that careful control of the amount of fluid or drug administered is not possible. In those cases where precise control is necessary, some type of volumetric controller or a complete pumping system must be used (Ozcelir, 2006).

In the case of a volumetric controller, the amount of fluid administered through a gravity-feed system is carefully regulated. Most clinical intravenous fluid administration sets include a drip chamber where the fluid passes through a fixed-diameter capillary tube and forms drops that drip from the tube into the chamber when they reach a certain volume. The clinician adjusts the flow rate to produce a certain number of drops per unit of time. A simple controller can achieve the same function by photoelectrically observing each drop as it interrupts a light beam passing from a light-emitting diode source to a photodetector such as a phototransistor. A device containing the light source and light detector can be clamped on the drip chamber of a conventional IV administration set and used to control a valve located between the fluid reservoir and the drip chamber. The clinician determines the number of drops required per unit time and sets the controller to deliver drops at the required rate.

Another approach is to use a peristalsis pump such as a roller pump (see Figure 13.13) to allow only a certain amount of fluid to pass from a gravity-fed reservoir to the patient. The inside diameter of the tubing and the propagation velocity of the peristalsis wave determine the amount of fluid administered.

There are other methods that can be used to meter the amount of fluid administered. All these systems require some type of electronic control to maintain steady infusion at a fixed, predetermined rate. Though earlier systems utilized a dc motor to drive a piston pump at a rate determined by a gear system, stepping motors are used today, and the angular velocity is controlled by digital electronics. Figure 13.18 shows a system to provide a series of pulses to the stepping motor at a precise frequency so that it drives the metering pump to supply the fluid at the desired rate. The pulse rate required for the desired infusion rate is set by the operator, who adjusts the rate-setting control. The advantage of using a stepping motor and this system is that the motor advances by a known amount for each applied pulse. Thus, by precisely controlling the number of pulses applied to the stepping motor, it is

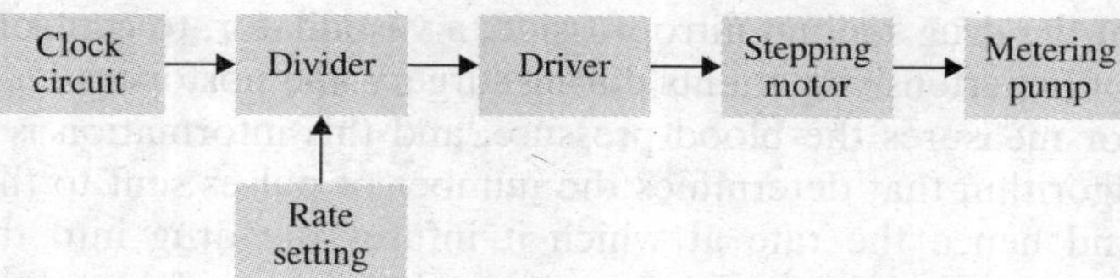


**Figure 13.18** **Block diagram of the electronic control system for a fluid or drug delivery pump**

possible to control precisely its angular displacement. By precisely controlling the rate at which pulses are applied to the motor, it is possible to control its angular velocity. This degree of control is not possible with open-loop analog motors.

**EXAMPLE 13.5** A roller drug infusion pump is driven by a stepper motor that advances the shaft and rollers 1.8° per step. The rollers are on arms that have a radius of 4 cm, and the tube that they compress has an inner diameter of 5 mm. What pulse rate must be supplied to the stepper motor for the drug to be infused into the patient at a rate of 0.5 ml/min?

**ANSWER** The circumference of the circle traversed by the rollers will be

$$l_c = 2\pi r = 2\pi \times 4\,\text{cm} = 25.13\,\text{cm} \tag{E13.21}$$

In one step the rollers will advance by

$$\Delta l = \frac{1.8}{360}(25.13\,\text{cm}) = 0.126\,\text{cm} \tag{E13.22}$$

The cross-sectional area of the tube in the pump is

$$A = \frac{\pi(0.5\,\text{cm})^2}{4} = 0.196\,\text{cm}^2 \tag{E13.23}$$

So for each step the pump delivers

$$V = 0.196\,\text{cm}^2 \times 0.126\,\text{cm} = 0.0247\,\text{cm}^3 \tag{E13.24}$$

of drug. To deliver 0.5 cm$^3$ of drug per minute, the stepper motor should receive

$$p = \frac{0.5\,\text{cm}^3/\text{min}}{0.0247\,\text{cm}^3} = 20.21\,\text{pulses/min} \tag{E13.25}$$

Infusion systems can be used in two general ways. For an open-loop device, the operator sets the desired infusion rate, and the fluid or drug is delivered at that rate until the setting is changed. The closed-loop system involves operating the pump in such a way as to keep a physiological variable as close as possible to a desired value. An example of such a system is the use of controlled infusion of the drug sodium nitroprusside, a vasodilator, to control the blood pressure of hypertensive patients during surgery and postoperatively. A pressure sensor measures the blood pressure, and this information is fed into a control algorithm that determines the number of pulses sent to the stepping motor—and hence the rate at which it infuses the drug into the patient. Investigators have shown that the automatic control of blood pressure in this way is more efficacious than the manual control of blood pressure via the same chemical agent.

## AMBULATORY AND IMPLANTABLE INFUSION SYSTEMS

Miniature infusion pumps have been developed for patients with special therapeutic needs. Insulin pumps that are small enough to be worn by a patient are routinely used to help diabetic patients control their blood glucose. These insulin-delivery systems are currently run open loop, because there is no reliable, continuously operating glucose sensor available for such a system. The patient controls the rate of infusion, after taking into account his or her activity level, meals, and occasional self-administered serum glucose tests.

Miniature pumps that are only slightly larger than an implantable cardiac pacemaker have been developed for implantable drug delivery. These pumps apply a known pressure to a reservoir of the drug, and there is a high-resistance connection between the pump and the site where the drug is to be infused, which is usually a vein. This high-resistance connection is generally a long, thin capillary tube that is wound around the periphery of the pump. The constant pressure in the reservoir and the fixed resistance of the tube maintain a steady but slow rate of infusion of the drug into the venous circulation. Implantable pumps, therefore, utilize a concentrated form of the agent to be infused. Nevertheless, it is periodically necessary to refill the reservoir. This is done percutaneously by means of a needle that can enter the reservoir and refill it without any of the drug leaking into the surrounding tissues. This technique is no more uncomfortable to the patient than receiving an injection.

Implantable pumps have also been used for delivering drugs to a specific tissue. This technique has been found useful in cancer chemotherapy, because systemic administration of the cytotoxic agents used would have far more serious side effects than the patient experiences when the agent is administered locally.

Implantable closed-loop drug delivery systems are of great interest for biomedical therapy because with the appropriate control algorithm they should be able to imitate the normal behavior of organs that are malfunctioning. The classic example of a closed-loop drug delivery system is the artificial pancreas. This device consists of an implantable pump of the type described in previous paragraphs. This pump, as shown in Figure 13.19, has a reservoir containing insulin and a control valve that determines the flow rate of insulin into the surrounding tissue from which it is picked up by the circulation. The valve in turn is controlled by an electronic control system that performs the

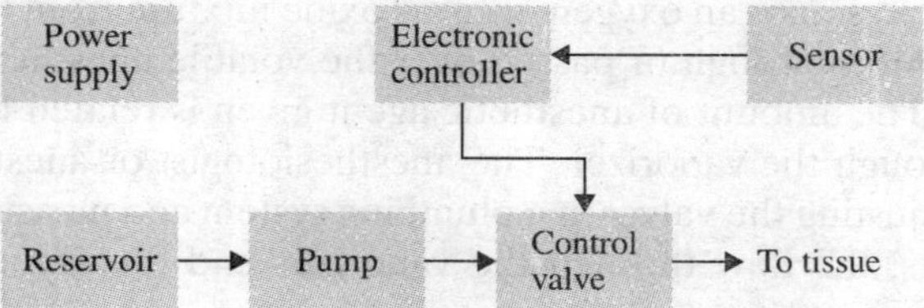


**Figure 13.19** A block diagram of an implantable artificial pancreas showing the major components of the system.

control algorithm for the device. A glucose sensor determines the body's glucose level and serves as the input device for the control system. Elevated glucose levels cause the pump to dispense increased amounts of insulin, while reduced glucose levels have the opposite effect. Most of these components have been developed in implantable form, and miniature closed-loop insulin delivery systems should be quite feasible with the exception of one component: the sensor. Although various investigators have developed glucose sensors that function in vitro, reliable miniature *in vivo* sensors capable of measurements for many years are not available. Without this crucial component, the implantable artificial pancreas is constrained to being a dream for the future.

Long-term drug delivery from passive devices has been demonstrated and utilized in some products. The basic principle has been described and reduced to practice by Langer (1995) and consists of a polymer matrix in which the drug is dispersed that is implanted in tissue. The drug slowly leaches from this material and is taken up by the capillaries in the surrounding tissue whereupon it is dispersed throughout the body by the cardiovascular system. By choosing appropriate materials and forming them in a specific shape, the drug can be leached out to give a desired level in the body appropriate for the therapeutic situation. An example of such a device is a thin polymer cylinder that can be injected beneath the skin and slowly leaches the hormone progesterone to provide contraceptive protection lasting several months in women. Even though these devices do not require electronic control systems, and they must operate open loop, they have several clinical advantages due to their simplicity.

## ANESTHESIA MACHINES

A special case of a controlled drug delivery system is the anesthesia machine (Ehrenwerth and Eisenkraft, 1993). This device enables anesthesiologists and anesthetists to administer volatile anesthetic agents to patients in the operating room through their lungs. There are three sections to the typical anesthesia machine. The first is the gas supply and delivery system. Here oxygen and nitrous oxide from central hospital sources or small storage cylinders on the anesthesia machine are mixed in the desired proportions. Flow meters indicate the amount of each gas that is delivered, and the operator can adjust the flow rate to get the desired ratio and total volume.

The second section of the anesthesia machine is the vaporizer. In this section, pure oxygen or an oxygen–nitrous oxide mixture from the gas delivery system is bubbled through or passed over the volatile anesthetic agent in the liquid phase. The amount of anesthetic agent given is related to the flow rate of the gas through the vaporizer. The anesthesiologist or anesthetist controls this rate by adjusting the valves in a plumbing system and measuring, by means of flow meters, the flow through the vaporizer and the amount of gas that bypasses it.

The final section of the anesthesia machine is the patient breathing circuit. This section is responsible for delivery of the anesthesia-producing gases to the patient and removal of expired gases coming from the patient. This portion of the system is a closed circuit. That is, the gas administered to the patient is introduced via a one-way (check) valve through one section of tubing, and the expired gas passes through a different section of tubing, again via a one-way valve. Thus the expired gas is separated from the inspiratory line. The expired gas is passed through a carbon dioxide absorber to remove the carbon dioxide and is reintroduced into the inspiratory line. A reservoir bag is connected in the circuit to provide low-pressure gas storage and to enable the anesthesiologist or anesthetist to assist in ventilating the patient when necessary. Expiratory gas can also be removed from the patient breathing circuit and passed through a scavenging system to remove the anesthetic agent before the gas is vented to the atmosphere. The patient breathing circuit can be connected to a ventilator for those patients who need assistance in ventilation.

## 13.9 SURGICAL INSTRUMENTS

There are many devices that can be classified as surgical instruments; to consider all of them would require several volumes. There are, however, electric and electronic devices that are important in the surgical care of patients, in addition to those used for monitoring patients in the operating and recovery rooms. In the next two sections, we examine two of these: the electrosurgical unit and the laser.

### ELECTROSURGICAL UNIT

Electric devices to assist in surgical procedures by providing cutting and hemostasis (stopping bleeding) are widely applied in the operating room. These devices are also known as *electrocautery apparatuses*. They can be used to incise tissue, to destroy tissue through desiccation, and to stop bleeding by causing coagulation of blood. The process involves the application of an RF arc between a probe and tissue to cause localized heating and damage to that tissue.

The basic electrosurgical unit is shown in Figure 13.20(a) (Pearce, 2006). The high-frequency power needed to produce the arc comes from a high-power, high-frequency generator. The power to operate the generator comes from a power supply, the output of which may in some cases be modulated to produce a waveform more appropriate for particular actions. In this case, a modulator circuit controls the output of the generator. The application of high-frequency power from the generator is ultimately controlled by the surgeon through a control circuit, which determines when power is applied to the electrodes to carry out a particular action. Often the output of energy from the high-frequency generator needs to be at various levels for various jobs. For this reason, a coupling circuit is inserted between the generator output and the electrodes to control this energy transfer.

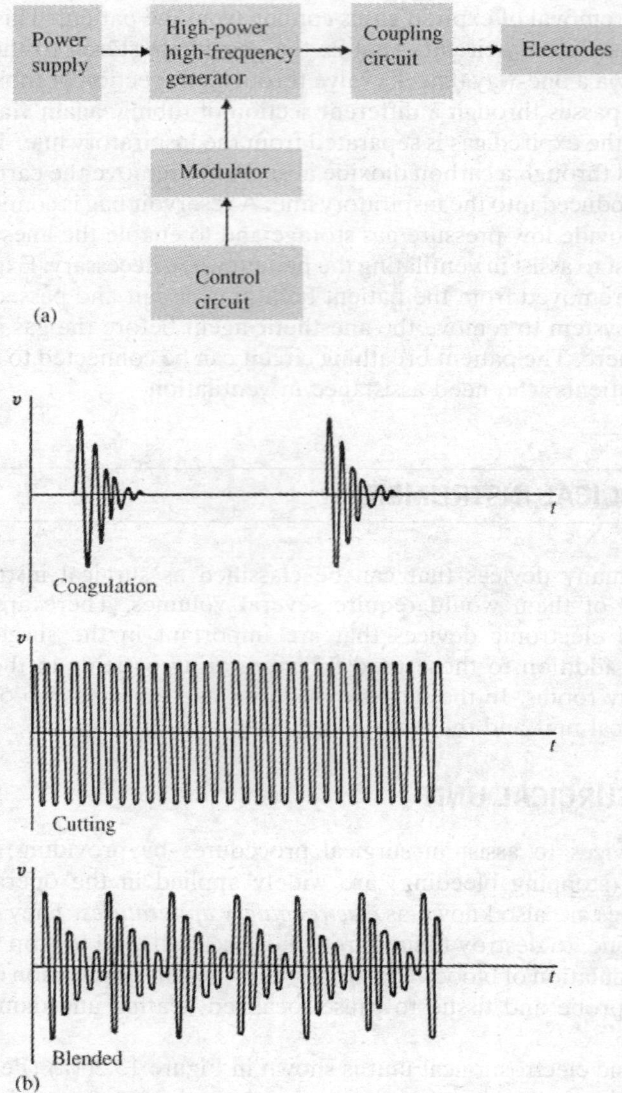


**Figure 13.20** (a) Block diagram for an electrosurgical unit. High-power, high-frequency oscillating currents are generated and coupled to electrodes to incise and coagulate tissue. (b) Three different electric voltage waveforms available at the output of electrosurgical units for carrying out different functions.

The electric waveforms generated by the electrosurgical unit differ for its different modes of action. To bring about desiccation and coagulation, the device uses damped sinusoidal pulses, as shown in Figure 13.20(b). The RF sine waves have a nominal frequency of 250 to 2000 kHz and are usually pulsed at a rate of 120 per second. Open-circuit voltages range from 300 to 2000 V, and power into a 500 Ω load ranges from 80 to 200 W. The magnitude of both voltage and power depends on the particular application.

Cutting is achieved with a CW RF source, as shown in Figure 13.20(b). Often units cannot produce truly continuous waves, as shown in Figure 13.20(b), and some amplitude modulation is present. Cutting is done at higher frequency, voltage, and power, because the intense heat at the spark destroys tissue rather than just desiccating it, as is the case with coagulation. Frequencies range from 500 kHz to 2.5 MHz, with open-circuit voltages as high as 9 kV. Power levels range from 100 to 750 W, depending on the application.

The cutting current usually results in bleeding at the site of incision, and the surgeon frequently requires "bloodless" cutting. Electrosurgical units can achieve this by combining the two waveforms, as shown in Figure 13.20(b). The frequency of this *blended* waveform is generally the same as the frequency for the cutting current. For best results, surgeons prefer to operate at a higher voltage and power when they want bloodless cutting than when they want cutting alone.

Many different designs for electrosurgical units have evolved over the years. Modern units generate their RF waveforms by means of solid-state electronic circuits. Older units were based on vacuum tube circuits and even utilized a spark gap to generate the waveforms shown in Figure 13.20(b).

A block diagram of a typical electrosurgical unit is shown in Figure 13.21. The RF oscillator provides the basic high-frequency signal, which is amplified and modulated to produce the coagulation, cutting, and blended waveforms. A function generator produces the modulation waveforms according to the mode selected by the operator. The RF power output is turned on and off by means of a control circuit connected either to a hand switch on the active electrode or to a foot switch that can be operated by the surgeon. An output circuit couples the power generator to the active and dispersive electrodes. The entire unit derives its power from a power-supply circuit that is driven by the power lines.

Electrodes used with electrosurgical units come in various sizes and shapes, depending on the manufacturer and the application. The active electrode is a scalpel-like probe that is shaped for the function for which it is intended. The

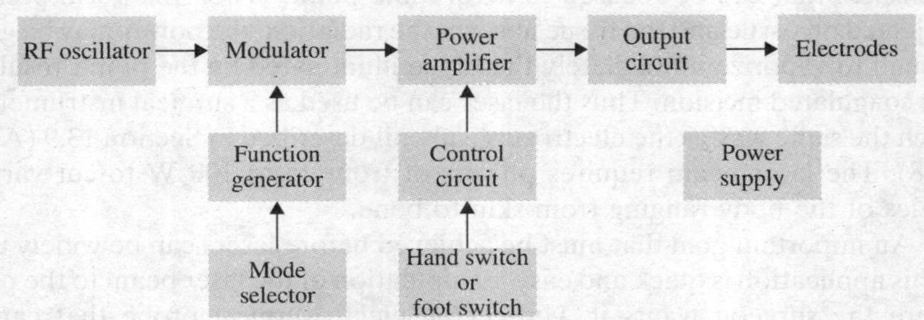


**Figure 13.21 Block diagram of a typical electrosurgical unit**

simplest form consists of a probe that appears to be similar to a test probe used with an electronic instrument such as a multimeter or an oscilloscope. A pointed metallic probe fits into an insulating handle and is held by the surgeon as one would hold a pencil. The finger switch located on the handle is momentarily depressed when the surgeon wants to apply power to the probe.

Whereas the purpose of the active probe is to apply energy to the local tissue at the tip of the probe and thereby to effect coagulation, cutting, or both, the dispersive electrode has a different function. It must complete the RF circuit to the patient without having current densities high enough to damage tissue. The simplest dispersive electrode is a large, reusable metal plate placed under the buttocks or back of the patient. Most procedures use a 70 $cm^2$ disposable conductive adhesive polymer dispersive electrode placed on the thigh. Another type has a gel-soaked sponge backed by metal foil and surrounded by foam and pressure-sensitive adhesive. Another capacitive type has a thin Mylar insulator backed by foil and its entire face coated with pressure-sensitive adhesive. It is important that this electrode make good contact with the patient over its entire surface so that "hot spots" do not develop.

### RADIO-FREQUENCY CATHETER ABLATION

Extra-conductive accessory pathways between the cardiac atria and ventricles may permit excitation to travel in circles and cause tachycardia. These extra pathway sites can be mapped by inserting a collapsed 64-electrode catheter into the heart chamber and expanding it into a basket to measure conduction times. Then a catheter is introduced to the sites and RF current at about 500 kHz heats the pathways to 50 °C to destroy (ablate) the conductive pathways. A temperature sensor at the electrode tip may be used to control the temperature (Huang, 1995).

## 13.10 THERAPEUTIC APPLICATIONS OF THE LASER

As we saw in Section 2.13, the laser makes available coherent light at high intensities that can be focused to a very fine point. When this focal point is projected on tissue and the tissue absorbs the radiation, the power may be great enough to vaporize immediately the tissue illuminated by the point, resulting in a coagulated incision. Thus the laser can be used as a surgical instrument in much the same way as the electrosurgical unit described in Section 13.9 (Auth, 1988). The laser beam requires powers of from 25 to 100 W to cut various tissues of the body ranging from skin to bone.

An important goal that must be achieved before lasers can be widely used in this application is quick and easy manipulation of the laser beam to the point where the surgeon wants it. Unlike the electrosurgical probe that can be connected to its generator by a flexible insulated lead wire, the laser must be coupled to its point of application through a system of mirrors and a lens. The powers required are high enough to make the laser too large to be manipulated by itself, so this coupling scheme becomes important but cumbersome.

The laser has some important applications in other aspects of medicine (Judy, 2000). Because it can be used in the control of bleeding through photocoagulation and heating, the laser has been applied through a fiber-optic endoscope in the coagulation of bleeding gastric ulcers. In some cases, the power is sufficiently great to stop bleeding in experimentally induced lesions in dogs.

In ophthalmology, the laser has found an important therapeutic application. Laser photocoagulators are able to repair detached retinas much more quickly than conventional photocoagulators, thereby minimizing the risk of damage to the retina due to movement of the eyes. Such systems are now commercially available and are in use at many institutions. Lasers have also been investigated as diagnostic and therapeutic instruments in many centers. This work ranges from dentistry to oncology (the study and treatment of tumors). Laser radiation is even being investigated in the clinical laboratory for analysis of tissue and fluid specimens taken from patients as well as diagnosing malignant tumors *in vivo*.

## PROBLEMS

**13.1** An asynchronous cardiac pacemaker operates at a rate of 70 pulses/min. These pulses are of 2 ms duration and have amplitude 5 V when driving a 500 Ω load.

**a.** What is the total energy supplied to this load over a 10 year period?

**b.** Suppose that 35% of the energy from the power supply goes into the output pulses. What must be the capabilities of the power supply to operate the pacemaker for 10 years?

**c.** Assume that the power supply is two 2.8 V lithium cells. What must the milliampere–hour capacity of each cell be to operate this pacemaker for 10 years?

**d.** Even though a pacemaker such as this would have a 10 year capacity in its power supply, it is found that when it is implanted, the power supply becomes exhausted in a little over 5 years. Can you suggest some of the reasons why this theoretical calculation disagrees with actual practice?

**13.2** An important problem in the clinical application of pacemakers is to determine when a given pacemaker is about to fail. Then surgeons may replace it before there is a failure that puts the patient at extreme risk. Describe a technique that could be used to determine the status of the battery of an implanted pacemaker that cannot be directly contacted with electric probes connected to test instruments. It is possible to place electrodes on the surface of the patient's body to observe signals from the pacemaker. Assume that you can use any of the test equipment available to the medical electronics engineer.

**13.3** There are some limitations on the use of synchronous cardiac pacemakers, especially when the patient is in the vicinity of strong electromagnetic fields, such as those produced by nearby microwave ovens, powerful radio transmitters, and radar stations. Discuss these limitations and describe the mechanisms involved.

**13.4** For the demand type of synchronous pacemaker shown in Figure 13.3, draw an appropriate waveform diagram that describes the operation of this pacemaker with and without spontaneous ventricular beats.

**13.5** How might the atrial-synchronous pacemaker shown in Figure 13.4 be modified to enable it to operate asynchronously in the absence of atrial contractions? Draw a block diagram for the modified circuit, and explain its operation.

**13.6** Compare the power requirements for a bladder stimulator that produces 5 V pulses—each having a duration of 2 ms, at a frequency of 100 pulses/s—with those of the cardiac pacemaker described in Problem 13.1. Do you think the power requirements of this stimulator make battery operation possible?

**13.7** The circuit of the RF-powered bladder stimulator of Figure 13.6 produces pulses of RF energy that have a voltage of 10 V rms as seen across the primary coil. The source impedance of the generator may be considered to be very low. The secondary coil has 1.2 times the number of turns of the primary and is coupled to the primary with a coupling coefficient of 0.5. What is the pulse amplitude seen across the electrodes when the tissue appears as a 500 Ω resistive load? What is the load impedance that the RF oscillator sees?

**13.8** The effective load resistance seen by the electrodes of an electric stimulator used for pain suppression can increase with time following the implantation of the stimulator and the healing of the site. Discuss the way this affects the efficacy of the stimulator. List the precautions that can be taken in the design of the circuit to minimize these problems.

**13.9** It was stated in the text that there is often a discrepancy between the stored energy in a capacitive-discharge cardiac defibrillator and the energy that is actually given to the patient during discharge. Explain what you believe to be reasons for this discrepancy and what can be done to minimize it.

**13.10** Capacitor-discharge cardiac defibrillators can be constructed with relatively small capacitances charged to high voltages or with comparatively large capacitances charged to lower voltages. Contrast the two types of defibrillators. List and discuss the advantages and disadvantages of each.

**13.11** If a capacitive-discharge cardiac defibrillator is discharged on a patient when the electrodes are not firmly in contact with the patient's chest wall, serious complications can develop. Describe what these are from the standpoint of what happens to the patient and the waveform produced by the defibrillator.

**13.12** What precautions should a clinician take when it is necessary to defibrillate a patient who has an implanted pacemaker of either the synchronous or the asynchronous type?

**13.13** The 200 μF capacitor of the defibrillator circuit shown in Figure 13.10 is charged to 2 kV. When the electrodes are attached to the patient, a 50 Ω resistive load is seen

**a.** Calculate the peak current passing through the patient during the discharge under these conditions.

**b.** Calculate the time constant of the discharge.

**13.14** When it is necessary to defibrillate a patient, the clinician must be assured that the defibrillator will operate properly. Therefore, it is necessary for the clinical engineer to have an aggressive program of testing and preventive maintenance of all cardiac defibrillators in the hospital. The key to this program is a method of evaluating the performance of each defibrillator. Design an instrument that is capable of measuring what you believe to be the key parameters of a cardiac defibrillator to assure the clinician that it is operating properly.

**13.15** Instrumentation is needed to control a balloon-type cardiac-assist device. It must detect the R wave of the ECG and use this to control the mechanism for deflation of the balloon, followed by reinflation. Design the necessary instrumentation and control system in block-diagram form.

**13.16** Design an instrumentation system for use with a pump–oxygenator system such as that shown in Figure 13.13. This system should monitor the oxygen saturation and pressure of the blood being reinfused into the body, as well as the pressure of the venous-return blood. Specify the sensors to be used in the instrumentation system, and explain why your choice is the most desirable. Show the electronics in block-diagram form, and include alarm circuitry to detect elevated arterial and venous pressures as well as reduced oxygen saturation.

**13.17** An artificial-kidney system must be protected from leaks across the dialyzing membrane. Design an instrumentation system that can provide this protection, and describe its operation.

**13.18** Sketch the flow and pressure at the mouth versus time for the continuous-positive-airway-pressure apparatus shown in Figure 13.16 during a complete breathing cycle and, explain the waveforms.

**13.19** A capacitive electrosurgical dispersive electrode has a Mylar insulator that is 0.002 in. thick and has an area of 70 $cm^2$. Find the relative dielectric constant for plastic, and calculate the impedance at 500 kHz.

**13.20** A broken lead wire on the back-plate or thigh-plate electrode of an electrosurgical unit can produce serious burns. Can you describe a way to eliminate this problem using an ancillary electronic circuit?

## REFERENCES

Auth, D. C, "Laser scalpel." In J. G. Webster (ed.), *Encyclopedia of Medical Devices and Instrumentation*. New York: Wiley, 1988, pp. 1717–1725.

Bocka, J. J., "External transcutaneous pacemakers." *Ann. Emerg. Med.*, 1989, 18, 1280–1286.

Brindley, G. S., and W. S. Lewin, "The sensations produced by electrical stimulation of the visual cortex." *J. Physiol.,* 1968, 196, 479–493.

Cairo, J., and S. Pilbeam, *Mosby's Respiratory Care Equipment*, 6th Ed., St. Louis: C. V. Mosby, 1999.

Chang, H. K., "Mechanisms of gas transport during ventilation by high-frequency oscillation." *J. Appl. Physiol.*, 1984, 56, 553–563.

Clark, G., *Cochlear Implants: Fundamentals and Applications*. New York: Springer, 2003.

Cameron T., G. E. Loeb, R. A. Peck, J. H. Schulman, P. Strojnik, and P. R. Troyk, "Micromodular implants to provide electrical stimulation of paralyzed muscles and limbs." *IEEE Trans. Biomed. Eng.*, 1997, 44(9), 781–790.

Cohen E. D., "Prosthetic interfaces with the visual system: biological issues." *J. Neural Eng.*, 2007, 4(2), R14–31

D'Alessandro, D., and R. Michler, "Heart-lung machines." In J. G. Webster (ed.), *Encyclopedia of Medical Devices and Instrumentation*. 2nd ed. New York: Wiley, 2006, Vol. 3, pp. 459–462.

Ehrenwerth, J., and J. B. Eisenkraft, *Anesthesia Equipment: Principles and Applications*. St. Louis: Mosby, 1993.

Geddes, L. A., *Cardiovascular Devices and their Applications*. New York: John Wiley & Sons, 1984.

Greatbatch, W., *The Making of the Pacemaker: Celebrating a Lifesaving Invention*, Amherst, NY: Prometheus, 2000.

Greatbatch, W., J. Lee, W. Mathias, M. Eldridge, J. Moser, and A. Schneider, "The solid-state lithium battery." *IEEE Trans. Biomed. Eng.*, 1971, BME-18, 317.

Hamilton, L. H., "Ventilators, high frequency." In J. G. Webster (ed.), *Encyclopedia of Medical Devices and Instrumentation*. New York: Wiley, 1988, pp. 2858–2864.

Huang, S. K. S. (ed.), *Radiofrequency Catheter Ablation of Cardiac Arrhythmias. Basic Concepts and Clinical Applications*. Armonk, NY: Futura, 1995.

Judy, M. M., "Biomedical Lasers." In J. D. Bronzino (ed.), *The Biomedical Engineering Handbook*, 2nd ed., Boca Raton, FL: CRC Press, 2000, pp. 85-1–85-13.

Langer, R., "1994 Whitaker Lecture: polymers for drug delivery and tissue engineering." *Ann. Biomed. Eng.*, 1995, 23, 101–111.

Loeb, G. E., C. J. Zamin, J. H. Schulman, and P. R. Troyk, "Injectable microstimulator for functional electrical stimulation." *Med. Biol. Eng. Comput.*, 1991, 29, NS13–NS19.

Madnani, A., S. Madnani, R. Carr, and J. Wells, "Transcutaneous electrical nerve stimulation (TENS)." In J. G. Webster (ed.), *Encyclopedia of Medical Devices and Instrumentation*, 2nd ed. New York: Wiley, 2006, Vol. 6, pp. 437–452.

Marsolais, E. B., and R. Kobetic, "Functional electrical stimulation for walking in paraplegics." *J. Bone Joint Surg.*, 1987, 69, 728–733.

McCarthy, P. M., "HeartMate implantable left ventricular assist device: bridge to transplantation and future applications." *Ann. Thoracic Surg.*, 1995, 59, S46–51.

Mokwa, W., An implantable microsystem as a vision prosthesis. *Med. Device Technol.*, 2007, 18(6), 20, 22–23.

Murray, A., "Pacemakers." In J. G. Webster (ed.), *Encyclopedia of Medical Devices and Instrumentation*, 2nd ed. New York: Wiley, 2006, Vol. 5, pp. 217–224.

Nardin, M., B. Ziaie, J.Von Arx, A. Coghlan, M. Dokmeci, and K. Najafi,"An inductively powered microstimulator for functional neuromuscular stimulation.". In C. C. Cristalli, J. Amlaner, and M. R. Neuman (eds.), *Biotelemetry XIII: Proc. 13th Int. Symp. Biotelemetry*. Strasbourg: International Society on Biotelemetry, 1995, pp. 99–104.

Ozcelir, S., "Drug infusion systems." In J. G. Webster (ed.), *Encyclopedia of Medical Devices and Instrumentation*, 2nd ed. New York: Wiley, 2006, Vol. 2, pp. 495–508.

Pearce, J. A., *Electrosurgery*. New York: John Wiley, 1986.

Pearce J., "Electrosurgical unit." In J. G. Webster (ed.), *Encyclopedia of Medical Devices and Instrumentation*, 2nd ed. New York: Wiley, 2006, pp. 156–177.

Peckham, P. H., "Functional electrical stimulation: Current status and future prospects of applications to neuromuscular system in spinal cord injury." *Paraplegia*, 1987, 25, 274–288.

Roth, B. J., "Defibrillators." In J. G. Webster (ed.). *Encyclopedia of Medical Devices and Instrumentation*, 2nd ed. New York: Wiley, 2006, Vol. 2, pp. 406–410.

Sawan M., M. M. Hassouna, J. S. Li, F. Duval, and M. M. Elhilali, "Stimulator design and subsequent stimulation parameter optimization for controlling micturition and reducing urethral resistance." *IEEE Trans. Rehab. Eng.*, 1996, 4(1): 39–46.

Schaldach, M., *Electrotherapy of the Heart*. Berlin: Springer, 1992.

Simpson, B. A. (ed.), *Electrical Stimulation and the Relief of Pain*. Amsterdam: Elsevier, 2003.

Singer, I. (ed.). *Implantable Cardioverter-Defibrillator*. Mt. Kisco, New York: Futura Publishing, 1994.

Spelman, F. A., "Cochlear prosthesis." In J. G. Webster (ed.), *Encyclopedia of Medical Devices and Instrumentation*, 2nd ed. New York: Wiley, 2006, Vol. 2, pp. 133–141.

Susset, J. G., "The electrical drive of the urinary bladder and sphincter." In W. S. Fields and L. A. Leavitt (eds.) *Neural Organization and Its Relevance to Prosthetics*. New York: Intercontinental, 1973, pp. 319–342.

Venkatasubramanian, G., R. Jung, and J. D. Sweeny, "Functional electrical stimulation." In J. G. Webster (ed.), *Encyclopedia of Medical Devices and Instrumentation*, 2nd ed. New York: Wiley, 2006, Vol. 3, pp. 347–366.

Webster, J. G. (ed.). *Design of Cardiac Pacemakers*. Piscataway, NJ: IEEE Press, 1995.

Weizer, A. Z., and G. M. Preminger, "Lithotripsy." In J. G. Webster (ed.), *Encyclopedia of Medical Devices and Instrumentation*, 2nd ed. New York: Wiley, 2006, Vol. 4, pp. 258–266.

Weller, P., and D. Morrow, "Intraaortic balloon pump." In J. G. Webster (ed.), *Encyclopedia of Medical Devices and Instrumentation*, 2nd ed. New York: Wiley, 2006, Vol. 4, pp. 162–171.

Yanai, D., J. D. Weiland, M. Mahadevappa, R. J. Greenberg, I. Fine, and M. S. Humayun, "Visual performance using a retinal prosthesis in three subjects with retinitis pigmentosa." *Am. J. Ophthalmol.,* 2007, 143(5) 820–827.

Zapanta, C. M., "Heart, artificial." In J. G. Webster (ed.), *Encyclopedia of Medical Devices and Instrumentation*, 2nd ed. New York: Wiley, 2006, Vol. 3, pp. 449–459.

Ziaie, B., M. Nardin, J. Von Arx, and K. Najafi, "A single channel implantable microstimulator for functional neuromuscular stimulation (FNS)." *Proc. 7th Int. Conf. Solid State Sensors Actuators*, 1993, Yokohama, Japan, pp. 450–453.

# 14

# ELECTRICAL SAFETY

Walter H. Olson

Medical technology has substantially improved health care in all medical specialties and has reduced morbidity and mortality for critically ill patients. Nevertheless, the increased complexity of medical devices and their utilization in more procedures result in about 10,000 device-related patient injuries in the United States each year. Most of these injuries are attributable to improper use of a device as a result of inadequate training and lack of experience. Medical personnel rarely read user manuals until a problem has occurred. Furthermore, medical devices eventually fail, so engineers must develop fail-safe designs.

The safe design and the safe use of medical instrumentation are broad subjects that involve nearly all medical procedures, every conceivable form of energy, and the familiar concept that everything that *can* go wrong eventually *will* go wrong. Medical procedures usually expose the patient to more hazards than the typical home or workplace, because in medical environments the skin and mucous membranes are frequently penetrated or altered, and because there are many sources of potentially hazardous substances and energy forms that could injure either the patient or the medical staff. These sources include fire, air, earth, water, chemicals, drugs, microorganisms, vermin, waste, sound, electricity, natural and unnatural disasters, surroundings, gravity, mechanical stress, and people responsible for acts of omission and commission, not to mention radiation from x rays, ultrasound, magnets, ultraviolet light, microwaves, and lasers (Dyro, 2006). Although this chapter focuses on electrical safety, it is important to recognize that there are also many other aspects of medical instrumentation safety (Charney *et al.*, 1990, Fagerhaugh *et al.*, 1987, Geddes, 1995).

In the 1980s, many minimum performance standards were written for most medical devices. Issues for the 1990s include inappropriate use of electrical connectors, sterilization efficacy, medical waste, and laser safety.

In this final chapter we focus on electrical safety and discuss the physiological effects of electric current, shock hazards, methods of protection, electrical safety standards, and electrical-safety testing procedures. Our objectives are to understand the possible hazards and to learn how safety features can be incorporated into the design of medical instruments we have studied in previous chapters.

## 14.1 PHYSIOLOGICAL EFFECTS OF ELECTRICITY

For a physiological effect to occur, the body must become part of an electric circuit. Current must enter the body at one point and leave at some other point. The magnitude of the current is equal to the applied voltage divided by the sum of the series impedances of the body tissues and the two interfaces at the entry points. The largest impedance is often the skin resistance at the contact surface. Three phenomena can occur when electric current flows through biological tissue: (1) electric stimulation of excitable tissue (nerve and muscle), (2) resistive heating of tissue, and (3) electrochemical burns and tissue damage for direct current and very high voltages.

Let us now discuss the psychophysical and physiological effects that occur in humans as the magnitude of applied electric current progressively increases. The chart in Figure 14.1 shows the approximate range of currents needed to produce each effect when 60 Hz current is applied for 1 to 3 s via AWG No. 8 copper wires that a 70 kg human holds in each hand. Then, in the section that follows, we will examine the effect of each of these conditions (weight of the individual and so on).

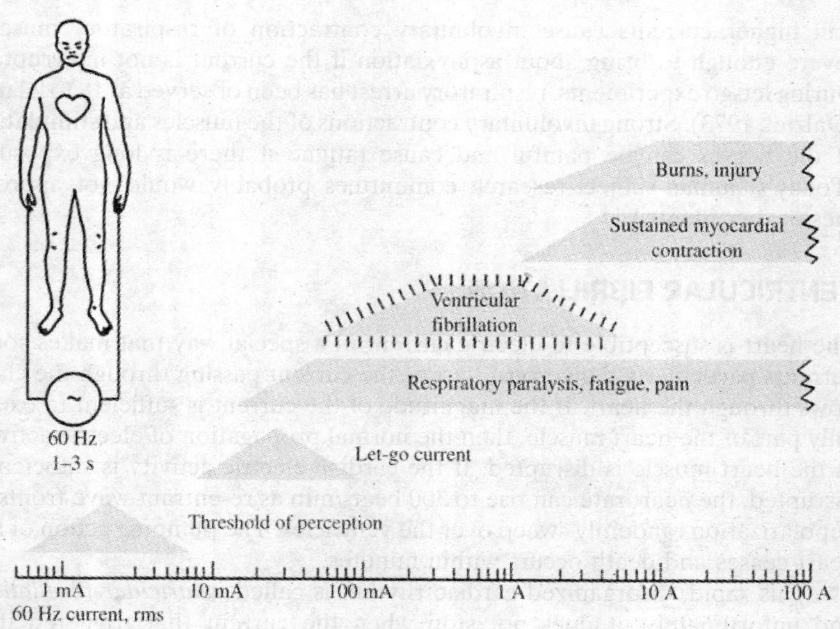


**Figure 14.1 Physiological effects of electricity** Threshold or estimated mean values are given for each effect in a 70 kg human for a 1 to 3 s exposure to 60 Hz current applied via copper wires grasped by the hands.

## THRESHOLD OF PERCEPTION

For the conditions just stated, when the local current density is large enough to excite nerve endings in the skin, the subject feels a tingling sensation. Current at the *threshold of perception* is the minimal current that an individual can detect. This threshold varies considerably among individuals and with the measurement conditions. When someone with moistened hands grasps small copper wires, the lowest thresholds are about 0.5 mA at 60 Hz. Thresholds for dc current range from 2 to 10 mA, and slight warming of the skin is perceived.

## LET-GO CURRENT

For higher levels of current, nerves and muscles are vigorously stimulated, and pain and fatigue eventually result. Involuntary contractions of muscles or reflex withdrawals by a subject experiencing any current above threshold may cause secondary physical injuries, such as might result from falling off a ladder. As the current increases further, the involuntary contractions of the muscles can prevent the subject from voluntarily withdrawing. The *let-go current* is defined as the maximal current at which the subject can withdraw voluntarily. The minimal threshold for the let-go current is 6 mA.

## RESPIRATORY PARALYSIS, PAIN, AND FATIGUE

Still higher currents cause involuntary contraction of respiratory muscles severe enough to bring about asphyxiation if the current is not interrupted. During let-go experiments, respiratory arrest has been observed at 18 to 22 mA (Dalziel, 1973). Strong involuntary contractions of the muscles and stimulation of the nerves can be painful and cause fatigue if there is long exposure. (Today's human-subject-research committees probably would not approve these experiments.)

## VENTRICULAR FIBRILLATION

The heart is susceptible to electric current in a special way that makes some currents particularly dangerous. Part of the current passing through the chest flows through the heart. If the magnitude of the current is sufficient to excite only part of the heart muscle, then the normal propagation of electric activity in the heart muscle is disrupted. If the cardiac electric activity is sufficiently disrupted, the heart rate can rise to 300 beats/min as re-entrant wave fronts of depolarization randomly sweep over the ventricles. The pumping action of the heart ceases and death occurs within minutes.

This rapid, disorganized cardiac rhythm is called *ventricular fibrillation*, and unfortunately, it does not stop when the current that triggered it is removed. Ventricular fibrillation is the major cause of death due to electric shock. The threshold for ventricular fibrillation for an average-sized human varies from about 75 to 400 mA. Normal rhythmic activity returns only if a brief high-current pulse from a defibrillator is applied to depolarize all the cells of the heart muscle simultaneously. After all the cells relax together, a normal rhythm usually returns. In the United States, approximately 1000 deaths per year occur in accidents that involve cord-connected appliances.

### SUSTAINED MYOCARDIAL CONTRACTION

When the current is high enough, the entire heart muscle contracts. Although the heart stops beating while the current is applied, a normal rhythm ensues when the current is interrupted, just as in defibrillation. Data from ac-defibrillation experiments on animals show that minimal currents for complete myocardial contraction range from 1 to 6 A. No irreversible damage to the heart tissue is known to result from brief applications of these currents (Roy *et al.*, 1984).

### BURNS AND PHYSICAL INJURY

Very little is known about the effects of currents in excess of 10 A, particularly for currents of short duration. Resistive heating causes burns, usually on the skin at the entry points, because skin resistance is high. Voltages greater than 240 V can puncture the skin. The brain and other nervous tissue lose all functional excitability when high currents pass through them. Furthermore, excessive currents may stimulate muscular contractions that are strong enough to pull the muscle attachment away from the bone (Lee *et al.*, 1992).

## 14.2 IMPORTANT SUSCEPTIBILITY PARAMETERS

The physiological effects previously described are for an average 70 kg human and for 60 Hz current applied for 1 to 3 s to moistened hands grasping a No. 8 copper wire. The current needed to produce each effect depends on all these conditions, as explained below. Safety considerations dictate thinking in terms of minimal rather than average values for each condition.

### THRESHOLD AND LET-GO VARIABILITY

Figure 14.2 shows the variability of the threshold of perception and the let-go current for men and women (Dalziel, 1973). On this plot of percentile rank versus rms current in milliamperes, the data are close to the straight lines shown, so a Gaussian distribution may be assumed. For men, the mean value for the threshold of perception is 1.1 mA; for women, the estimated mean is 0.7 mA. The minimal threshold of perception is 500 μA. When the current was applied to ECG gel electrodes, the threshold of perception averages only 83 μA with a range of 30 to 200 μA (Tan and Johnson, 1990). Recent data for surface electrical stimulation of skeletal muscle showed that sensory threshold

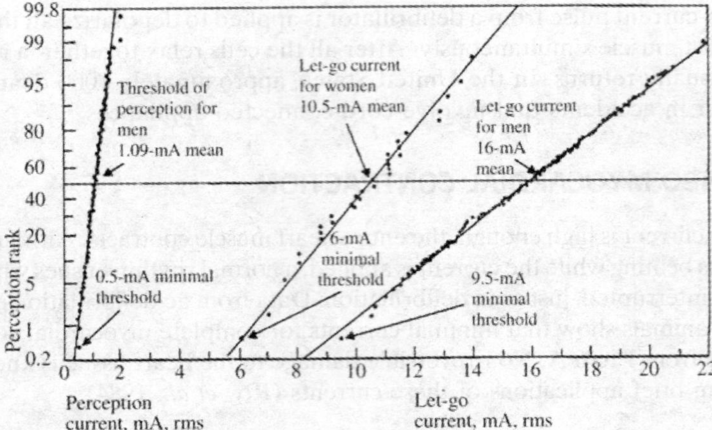


**Figure 14.2 Distributions of perception thresholds and let-go currents** These data depend on surface area of contact (moistened hand grasping AWG No. 8 copper wire). (Replotted from C. F. Dalziel, "Electric Shock," *Advances in Biomedical Engineering*, edited by J. H. U. Brown and J. F. Dickson III, 1973, 3, 223–248.)

was 43% ($p < 0.001$) lower in women and supramotor threshold was 17% ($p < 0.01$) less for women (Maffiuletti *et al.*, 2008).

Let-go currents also appear to follow Gaussian distributions, with mean let-go currents of 16 mA for men and 10.5 mA for women. The minimal threshold let-go current is 9.5 mA for men and 6 mA for women. Note that the range of variability for let-go current is much greater than the range for threshold-of-perception current.

## FREQUENCY

Figure 14.3 shows a plot of let-go current versus frequency of the current. Unfortunately, the minimal let-go currents occur for commercial power-line frequencies of 50 to 60 Hz. For frequencies below 10 Hz, let-go currents rise, probably because the muscles can partially relax during part of each cycle. And at frequencies above several hundred hertz, the let-go currents rise again.

## DURATION

To estimate the ventricular fibrillation (VF) risk of electromuscular incapacitation devices (EMDs), it is important to understand the excitation behavior of myocardial cells. Geddes and Baker (1989) presented the cell membrane excitation model by a lumped parallel *RC* circuit that represents the resistance and capacitance of the cell membrane. This model determines the cell excitation thresholds that exceed about 20 mV for varying rectangular pulse durations *d* by assigning the rheobase currents $I_r$ (for very long pulse durations) and cell

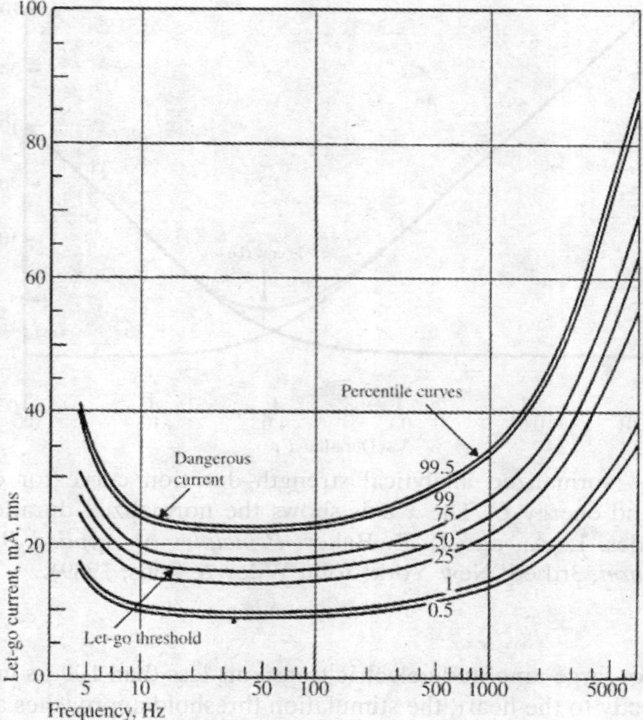


**Figure 14.3 Let-go current versus frequency** Percentile values indicate variability of let-go current among individuals. Let-go currents for women are about two-thirds the values for men. (Reproduced, with permission, from C. F. Dalziel, "Electric Shock," *Advances in Biomedical Engineering*, edited by J. H. U. Brown and J. F. Dickson III, 1973, 3, 223–248.)

membrane time constant $\tau = RC$. Figure 14.4 shows that for short durations the stimulation current threshold $I_d$ is inversely related to the pulse duration $d$ by the well-known strength–duration equation

$$I_d = \frac{I_r}{1 - e^{-d/\tau}} \tag{14.1}$$

**EXAMPLE 14.1** A cardiac pacemaker company wants to minimize pacing duration $d$ while keeping current at 3 times $I_r$. Assume cardiac membrane $\tau = 2$ ms, and calculate $d$.

**ANSWER** Use (14.1): $0.33 = 1 - e^{-d/0.002}$, $0.67 = e^{-d/0.002}$, $\ln 0.67 = -d/0.002 = -0.4$, $d = 0.8$ ms.

A single electric stimulus pulse can induce VF if it is delivered during the vulnerable period of cardiac repolarization that corresponds to the T wave on

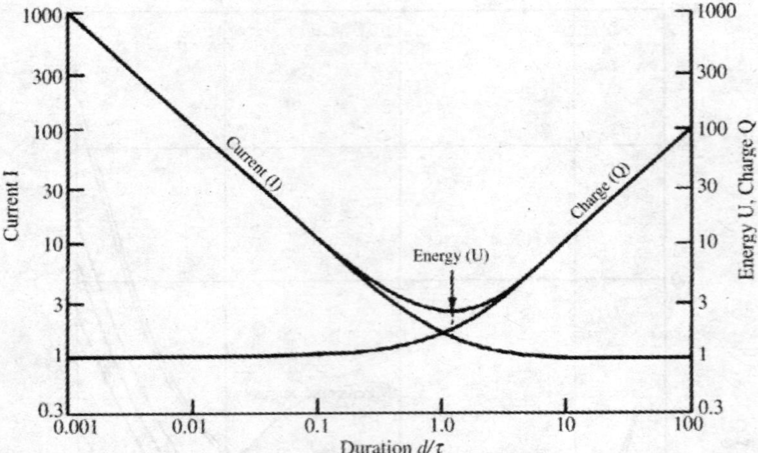


**Figure 14.4** Normalized analytical strength–duration curve for current $I$, charge $Q$, and energy $U$. The $x$ axis shows the normalized duration of $d/\tau$. (From Geddes, L. A., and L. E. Baker, *Principles of Applied Biomedical Instrumentation*, 3rd ed. New York: John Wiley & Sons, 1989).

the ECG. For large-amplitude electric transients less than 100 μs in duration applied directly to the heart, the stimulation threshold approaches a constant charge transfer density of $3.5\ \mu C \cdot cm^{-2}$. For normal hearts, the ratio of the fibrillation stimulation threshold to the single-beat stimulation threshold is 20:1 to 30:1 for electrodes on the heart and 10:1 to 15:1 for chest surface electrodes (Geddes *et al.*, 1986). For 60 Hz current applied to the extremities, the fibrillation threshold increases sharply for shocks that last less than about 1 s, as shown in Figure 14.5. Shocks must last long enough to take place during the vulnerable period that occurs during the T wave in each cardiac cycle (Reilly, 1998). For the 100 μs pulses of electric fences (IEC, 2006) and Tasers, Figure 14.4 shows that much higher currents are required for excitation.

## BODY WEIGHT

Several studies using animals of various sizes have shown that the fibrillation threshold increases with body weight. Fibrillating current increases from 50 mA rms for 6 kg dogs to 130 mA rms for 24 kg dogs. These findings deserve more study, because they are used to extrapolate fibrillating currents for humans.

## POINTS OF ENTRY

When current is applied at two points on the surface of the body, only a small fraction of the total current flows through the heart, as shown in Figure 14.6(a). These large, externally applied currents are called *macroshocks*.

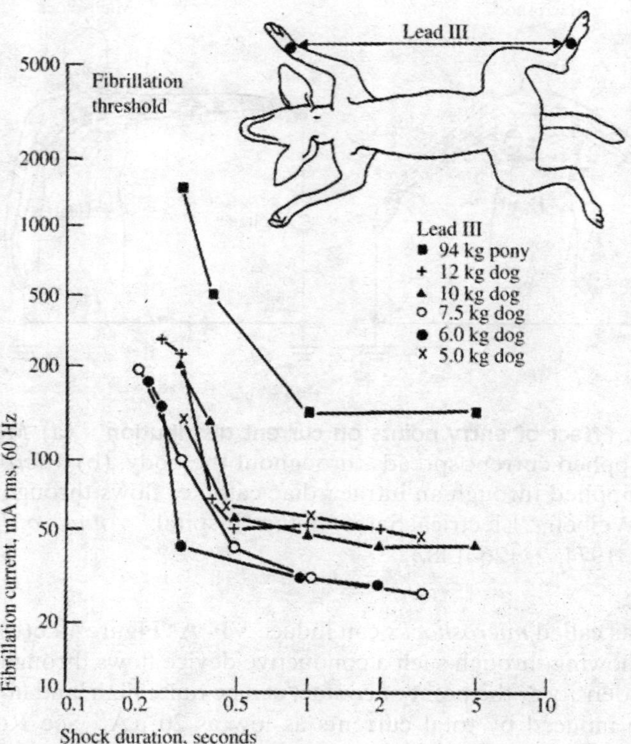


**Figure 14.5** Fibrillation current versus shock duration. Thresholds for VF in animals for 60 Hz ac current. Duration of current (0.2 to 5 s) and weight of animal body were varied. (From L. A. Geddes, *IEEE Trans. Biomed. Eng.*, 1973, 20, 465–468. Copyright 1973 by the Institute of Electrical and Electronics Engineers. Reproduced with permission.)

The magnitude of current needed to fibrillate the heart is far greater when the current is applied on the surface of the body than it would be if the current were applied directly to the heart. The importance of the location of the two macroshock entry points is often overlooked. If the two points are both on the same extremity, the risk of fibrillation is small, even for high currents. For dogs, the current needed for fibrillation is greater for ECG lead I (LA–RA) electrodes than for ECG leads II and III (LL–RA and LL–LA) (Geddes, 1973). The protection afforded by the skin resistance (15 kΩ to 1 MΩ for 1 $cm^2$) is eliminated by many medical procedures that require insertion of conductive devices into natural openings, skin incisions, skin abrasion, or electrode gel.

If the skin resistance is bypassed, less voltage is required to produce sufficient current for each physiological effect.

Patients are particularly vulnerable to electric shock when invasive devices are placed in direct contact with cardiac muscle. If a device provides a conductive path to the heart that is insulated except at the heart, then very

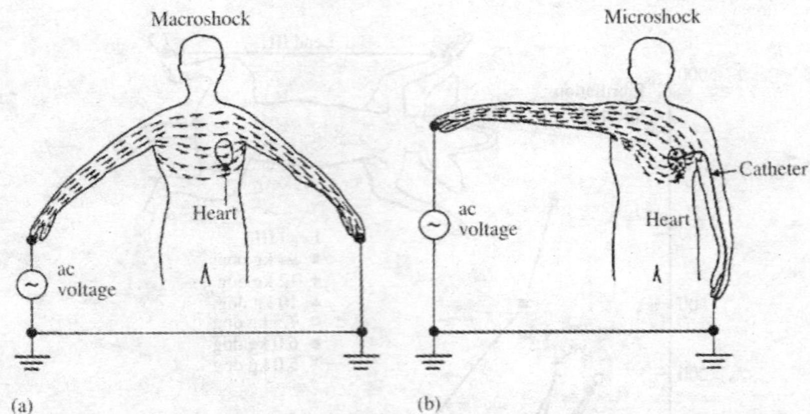


**Figure 14.6 Effect of entry points on current distribution** (a) *Macroshock:* Externally applied current spreads throughout the body. (b) *Microshock:* All the current applied through an intracardiac catheter flows through the heart. (From F. J. Weibell, "Electrical Safety in the Hospital," *Annals of Biomedical Engineering*, 1974, 2, 126–148.)

small currents called *microshocks* can induce VF. As Figure 14.6(b) shows, all the current flowing through such a conductive device flows through the heart. The current density at the point of contact can be quite high, and fibrillation in dogs can be induced by total currents as low as 20 μA. [See Roy (1980).] Application of 60 Hz ac for 5 s test periods to a ventricular pacing catheter during implantable cardioverter–defibrillator implant testing in 40 patients showed intermittent capture with a minimum current of 20 μA, continuous capture with hemodynamic collapse with a minimum current of 32 μA and VF persisting after ac termination with a minimum current of 49 μA (Figure 14.7) (Swerdlow *et al.*, 1999.) The other connection can be at any point on the body. The widely accepted safety limit to prevent microshocks is 10 μA.

## 14.3 DISTRIBUTION OF ELECTRIC POWER

Electric power is needed in health-care facilities not only for the operation of medical instruments but also for lighting, maintenance appliances, patient conveniences (such as television, hair curlers, and electric toothbrushes), clocks, nurse call buttons, and an endless list of other electric devices. A first step in providing electrical safety is to control the availability of electric power and the grounds in the patients' environment. This section is concerned with methods for safe distribution of power in health-care facilities. Then, in the sections that follow, we will discuss various macroshock and microshock hazards (Klein, 1996).

A simplified diagram of an electric-power-distribution system is shown in Figure 14.8. High voltage (4800 V) enters the building—usually via

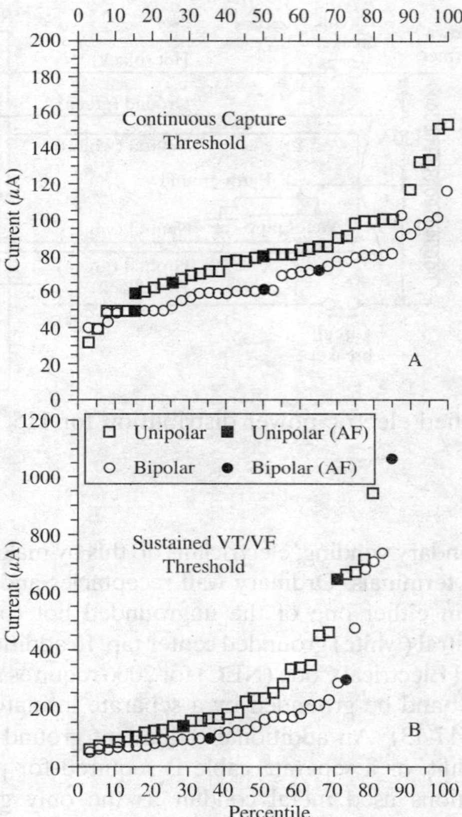


**Figure 14.7** Percentile plot of thresholds for continuous capture and VF (or sustained VT). Cumulative percent of patients is shown on abscissa and root-mean-square ac current (in μA) on ordinate. Squares denote unipolar data; circles denote bipolar data. Solid symbols identify data from patients in whom the only clinical arrhythmia was atrial fibrillation (AF). (*Top*) Thresholds for continuous capture. Current strength of 50 μA caused continuous capture in five patients (12%) with unipolar ac and in nine (22%) with bipolar ($P = 0.49$). (*Bottom*) Thresholds for sustained VT/VF. These plots do not reach 100% because sustained-VT/VF thresholds exceeded maximum output of stimulator in six patients (15%) with bipolar ac and eight (20%) with unipolar ac. [From Swerdlow, C. D., W. H. Olson, M. E. O' Connor, D. M. Gallik, R. A. Malkin, M. Laks, "Cardiovascular collapse caused by electrocardiographically silent 60-Hz intracardiac leakage current – Implications for electrical safety." *Circulation.*, 1999, 99, 2559–2564.]

underground cables. The secondary of a step-down transformer develops 240 V. This secondary has a grounded center tap to provide two 120 V circuits between ground and each side of the secondary winding. Some heavy-duty devices (such as air conditioners, electric dryers, and x-ray machines) that require 240 V are placed

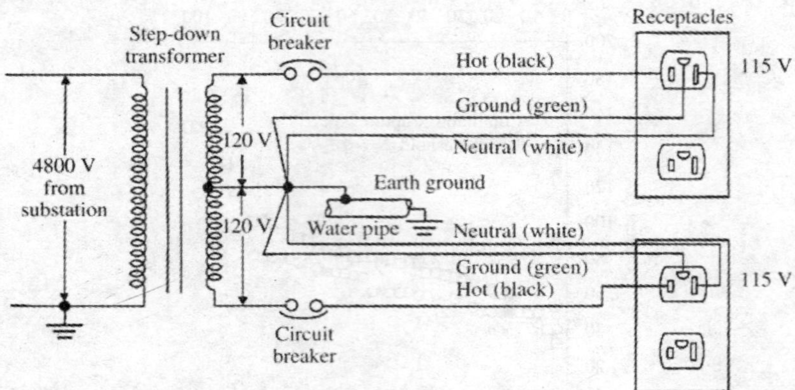


**Figure 14.8** Simplified electric-power distribution for 115 V circuits. Power frequency is 60 Hz.

across the entire secondary winding; electricians do this by making connections to the two ungrounded terminals. Ordinary wall receptacles and lights operate on 120 V, obtained from either one of the ungrounded hot (black) transformer terminals and the neutral (white) grounded center tap. In addition, for health-care facilities, the National Electrical Code (NEC) for 2006 requires that all receptacles be "Hospital Grade" and be grounded by a separate insulated (green) copper conductor (Article 517-13). An additional redundant ground path through the metal raceway, conduit, or a separate cable is required for patient-care areas. Some older installations used metal conduit as the only ground conductor. Conduit grounds are generally unsatisfactory, because corrosion and loose conduit connections make them unreliable.

## PATIENTS' ELECTRICAL ENVIRONMENT

Of course, a shock hazard exists between the two conductors supplying either a 240 V or a 120 V appliance. Because the neutral wire on a 120 V circuit is connected to ground, a connection between the hot conductor and *any* grounded object poses a shock hazard. Microshocks can occur if sufficient potentials exist between exposed conductive surfaces in the patients' environment. The following maximal potentials permitted between any two exposed conductive surfaces in the vicinity of the patient are specified by the 2006 NEC, Article 517-15:

1. General-care areas, 500 mV under normal operation
2. Critical-care areas, 40 mV under normal operation

In general-care areas, patients have only incidental contact with electric devices. For critical-care areas, hospital patients are intentionally exposed to electric devices, and insulation of externalized cardiac conductors from conductive surfaces is required. In critical-care areas, all exposed conductive surfaces in the vicinity of the patient must be grounded at a single patient-grounding point (Section 14.8). Also, periodic testing for continuity between the patient ground and all grounded surfaces is required.

Each patient-bed location in general-care areas must have at least four single or two duplex receptacles. Each receptacle must be grounded. At least two branch circuits with separate automatic overcurrent devices must supply the location of each patient bed. For critical-care areas, at least six single or three duplex receptacles are required for each location of a patient bed. Two branch circuits are also required, at least one being an individual branch circuit from a single panelboard. A patient-equipment grounding point (Section 14.8) is permitted for critical-care areas. For details, see NEC 70–2006, Article 517-19.

## ISOLATED-POWER SYSTEMS

Even installing a good separate grounding system for each patient cannot prevent possibly hazardous voltages that can result from ground faults. A *ground fault* is a short circuit between the hot conductor and ground that injects large currents into the grounding system. These high-current ground faults are rare, and usually the circuit breakers open quickly. If the center tap of the step-down transformer were not grounded, then very little current could flow, even if a short circuit to ground developed. So long as both power conductors are isolated from ground, a single ground fault will not allow the large currents that cause hazardous potentials between conductive surfaces.

Isolation of both conductors from ground is commonly achieved with an *isolation transformer*. A typical isolated-power system is shown in Figure 14.9. In an isolated system such as this, if a single ground fault from either conductor

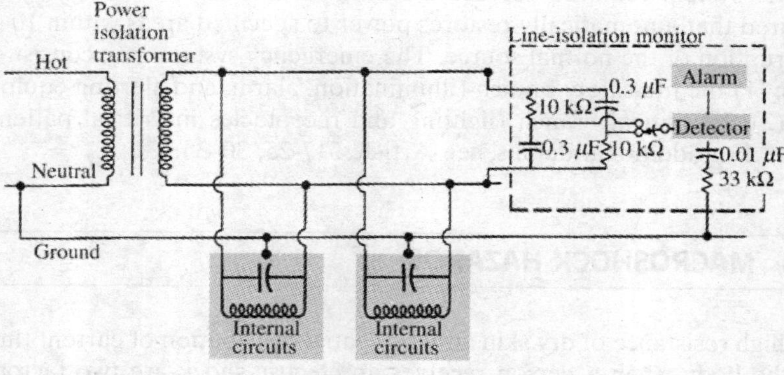


**Figure 14.9** Power-isolation-transformer system with a line-isolation monitor to detect ground faults.

to ground occurs, the system simply reverts to a normal grounded system. A second fault from the other conductor to ground is then required to get large currents in the grounds.

A continually operating *line-isolation monitor* (LIM) (also called a *dynamic ground detector*) must be used with isolation transformers to detect the occurrence of the first fault from either conductor to ground. This monitor alternately measures the total possible resistive and capacitive leakage current *(total hazard current)* that would flow through a low impedance *if it were connected* between either isolated conductor and ground. When the total hazard current exceeds 3.7 to 5.0 mA for normal line voltage, a red light and an audible alarm are activated. The LIM itself has a monitor hazard current of 1 mA. This makes the allowed fault total hazard current for all appliances served by the transformer somewhat less than 5 mA.

The kinds of corrective action that should be taken when the alarm goes off must be explained to medical personnel so that they do not overreact. The periodic switching in some line-isolation monitors produces transients that can interfere with monitoring of low-level physiological signals (ECG and EEG) and give erroneous heart rates. Or it can trigger synchronized defibrillators and aortic-balloon assist pumps during the wrong phase of the patient's heart cycle. Some LIMs avoid these problems by using continuous two-channel circuitry instead of measuring the total hazard current by switching between each line and ground.

Isolated-power systems were originally introduced to prevent sparks from coming into contact with flammable anesthetics such as ether. The NEC requires isolated-power systems only in those operating rooms and other locations where flammable anesthetics are used or stored.

### EMERGENCY-POWER SYSTEMS

Article 517 of the 2006 National Electrical Code specifies the emergency electric system required for heath-care facilities. An emergency system is required that automatically restores power to specified areas within 10 s after interruption of the normal source. The emergency system may consist of two parts: (1) the life-safety branch (illumination, alarm, and alerting equipment) and (2) the critical branch (lighting and receptacles in critical patient-care areas). For additional details, see Article 517-25, 30–35.

## 14.4 MACROSHOCK HAZARDS

The high resistance of dry skin and the spatial distribution of current throughout the body when a person receives an electric shock are two factors that reduce the danger of VF. Furthermore, electric equipment is designed to minimize the possibility of humans coming into contact with dangerous voltages.

## SKIN AND BODY RESISTANCE

The resistance of the skin limits the current that can flow through a person's body when that person comes into contact with a source of voltage. The resistance of the skin varies widely with the amount of water and natural oil present. It is inversely proportional to the area of contact.

Most of the resistance of the skin is in the outer, horny layer of the epidermis. For 1 $cm^2$ of electric contact with dry, intact skin, resistance may range from 15 kΩ to almost 1 MΩ, depending on the part of the body and the moisture or sweat present. If skin is wet or broken, resistance drops to as low as 1% of the value for dry skin. By contrast, the internal resistance of the body is about 200 Ω for each limb and about 100 Ω for the trunk. Thus internal body resistance between any two limbs is about 500 Ω. These values are probably higher for obese patients, because the specific resistivity of fat is high. Actually, the distribution of current in various tissues in the body is poorly understood.

Any medical procedure that reduces or eliminates the resistance of the skin increases possible current flow and makes the patient more vulnerable to macroshocks. For example, biopotential electrode gel reduces skin resistance. Electronic thermometers placed in the mouth or rectum also bypass the skin resistance, as do intravenous catheters containing fluid that can act as a conductor. Thus patients in a medical-care facility are much more susceptible to macroshock than the general population.

## ELECTRIC FAULTS IN EQUIPMENT

All electric devices are of course designed to minimize exposure of humans to hazardous voltages. However, many devices have a metal chassis and cabinet that medical personnel and patients may touch. If the chassis and cabinet are not grounded, as shown in Figure 14.10(a), then an insulation failure or shorted component between the black hot power lead and the chassis results in a 115 V potential between the chassis and any grounded object. If a person simultaneously touches the chassis and any grounded object, a macroshock results.

The chassis and cabinet can be grounded via a third green wire in the power cord and electric system, as shown in Figure 14.10(b). This ground wire is connected to the neutral wire and ground at the power-distribution panel. Then, when a fault occurs between the hot conductor and the chassis, the current flows safely to ground on the green conductor. If the ground-wire resistance is very low, the voltage between the chassis and other grounded objects is negligible. If enough current flows through the ground wire to open the circuit breaker, this will call people's attention to the fault.

Note that direct faults between the hot conductor (or any high voltage in the device) and ground are not common. Little or no current flows through the ground conductor during normal operation of electric devices. The ground conductor is not needed for protection against macroshock until a hazardous

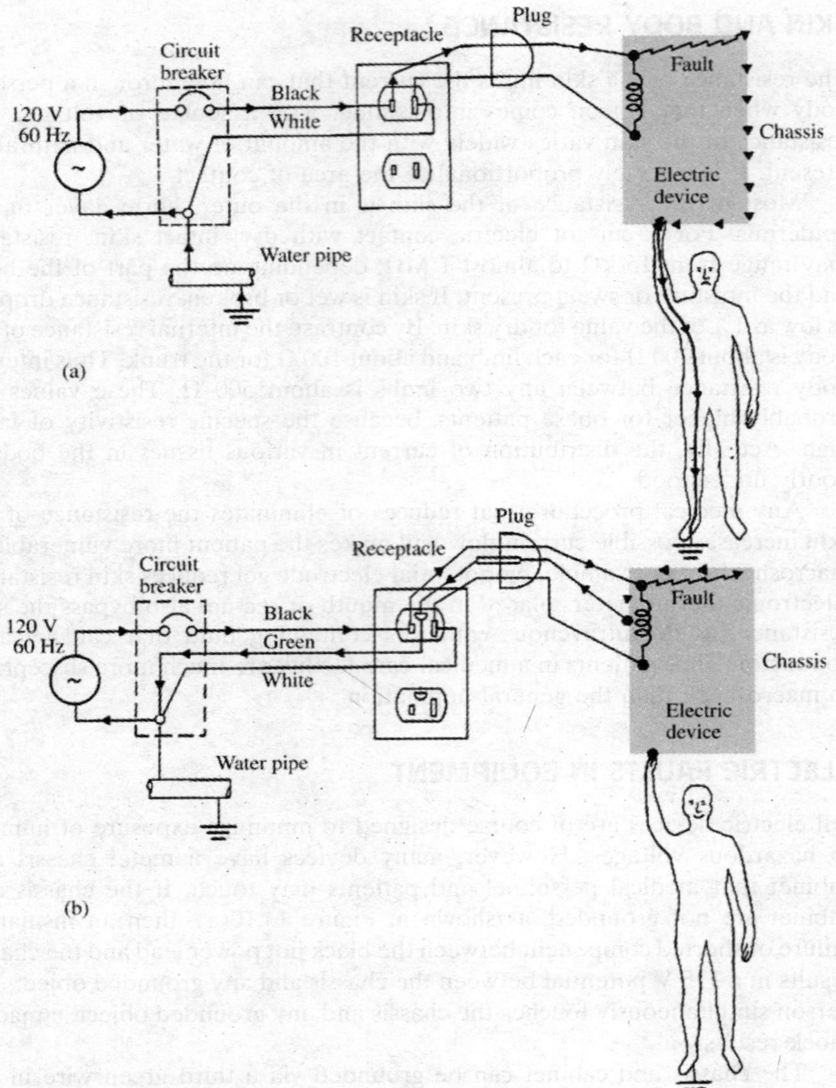


**Figure 14.10** Macroshock due to a ground fault from hot line to equipment cases for (a) ungrounded cases and (b) grounded chassis.

fault develops. Thus a broken ground wire or a poor connection of a receptacle ground is not detected during normal operation of the device. For this reason, continuity of the ground wire in the device and the receptacle must be tested periodically.

Faults inside electric devices may result from failures of insulation, shorted components, or mechanical failures that cause shorts. Power cords are particularly susceptible to strain and physical abuse, as are plugs and receptacles. Ironically, it is possible for a device's chassis and cabinet to become hot because a ground wire is in the power cord. If the ground wire is open anywhere between the power cord and ground, then a frayed cord could permit contact between the hot conductor and the broken ground wire leading to the chassis. Often, macroshock accidents result from carelessness and failure to correct known deficiencies in the power-distribution system and in electric devices.

Fluids—such as blood, urine, intravenous solutions, and even baby formulas—can conduct enough electricity to cause temporary short circuits if they are accidentally spilled into normally safe equipment. This hazard is particularly acute in hospital areas that are subject to wet conditions, such as hemodialysis and physical therapy areas. The cabinets of many electric devices have holes and vents for cooling that provide access for spilled conductive fluids. The mechanical design of devices should protect patient electric connections from this hazard.

## 14.5 MICROSHOCK HAZARDS

Microshock accidents in patients who have direct electric connections to the heart are usually caused by circumstances unrelated to macroshock hazards. Microshocks generally result from *leakage currents* in line-operated equipment or from differences in voltage between grounded conductive surfaces due to large currents in the grounding system. The microshock current can flow either into or out of the electric connection to the heart.

### LEAKAGE CURRENTS

Small currents (usually on the order of microamperes) that inevitably flow between any adjacent insulated conductors that are at different potentials are called *leakage currents*. Although most of the leakage current in line-operated equipment flows through the stray capacitance between the two conductors, some resistive leakage current flows through insulation, dust, and moisture.

The most important source of leakage currents is the currents that flow from all conductors in the electric device to lead wires connected either to the chassis or to the patient. Leakage current flowing to the chassis flows safely to ground if a low-resistance ground wire is available, as shown in Figure 14.11(a). If the ground wire is broken, then the chassis potential rises above ground, and a patient who touches the chassis *and* has a grounded electric connection to the heart may receive a microshock [Figure 14.11(b)]. If there is a connection from the chassis to the patient's heart *and* a connection to ground anywhere on the body, this could also cause a microshock [Figure 14.11(c)].

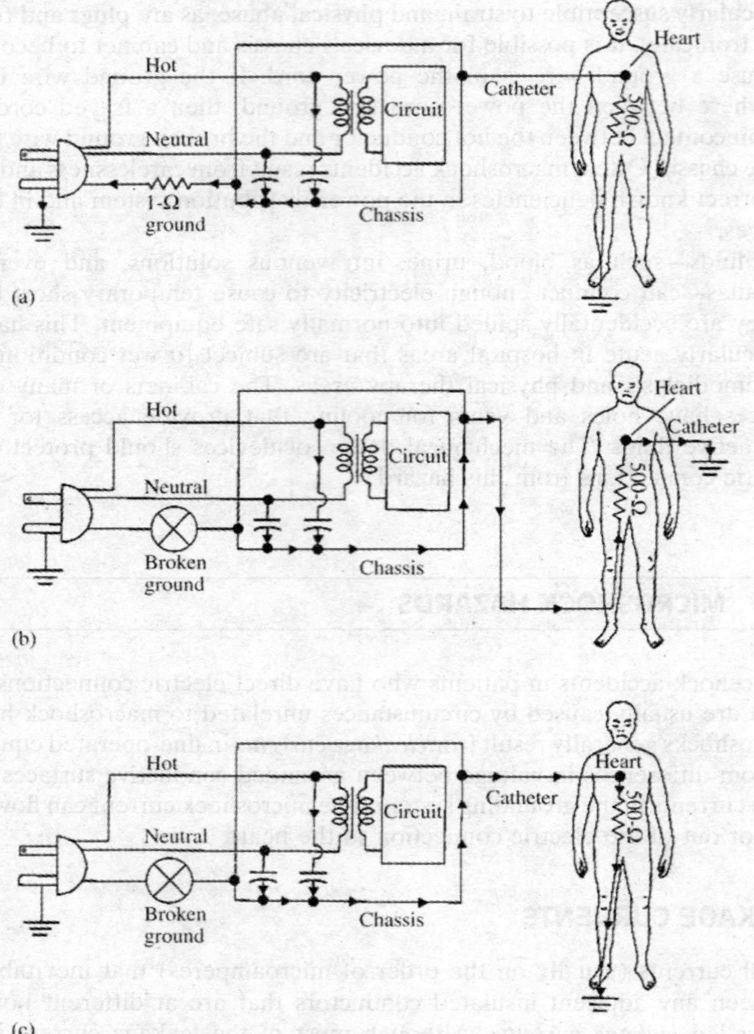


**Figure 14.11 Microshock leakage-current pathways** Assume 100 μA of leakage current from the power line to the instrument chassis, (a) intact ground; 99.8 μA flows through the ground, (b) broken ground; 100 μA flows through the heart, (c) broken ground; and 100 μA flows through the heart in the opposite direction.

## CONDUCTIVE SURFACES

The source that produces the microshock current need not be leakage current from line-operated equipment. Small potentials between any two conductive surfaces near the patient can cause a microshock if either surface makes contact with the heart and the other surface contacts any other part of the body. An example is given later in this section.

## CONDUCTIVE PATHS TO THE HEART

Specific types of electric connections to the heart can be identified. The following clinical devices make patients susceptible to microshock.

1. Epicardial or endocardial electrodes of externalized temporary cardiac pacemakers
2. Electrodes for intracardiac electrogram (EGM) measuring and stimulation devices
3. Liquid-filled catheters placed in the heart to
   a. Measure blood pressure
   b. Withdraw blood samples
   c. Inject substances such as dye or drugs into the heart

It should be emphasized that a patient is in danger of microshock only when there is some electric connection to the heart. The internal resistance of liquid-filled catheters is much greater (50 kΩ to 1 MΩ) than the resistance of metallic conductors in pacemaker and EGM electrode leads. Internal resistance of the body to microshock is about 300 Ω, and the resistance of the skin can be quite variable.

In dogs, the surface area of the intracardiac electrode is an important determinant of minimal fibrillating current (Roy *et al.*, 1980). Figure 14.12 shows that as catheter electrodes get smaller, so does the total current needed to fibrillate. This means that current density at the tip of the intracardiac electrode is the important microshock parameter. Smaller catheter electrodes may have larger internal resistance.

**EXAMPLE 14.2** From Figure 14.1, find the current required for arm-to-arm VF. Assume that all this current passes through the area of the heart (about $10 \times 10$ cm). Calculate the current density through the heart. How does this compare with the lowest value current density from Figure 14.12?

**ANSWER** Figure 14.1 shows minimal current for VF by macroshock of 75 mA. For $10 \times 10$ cm cross-sectional area, the current density $J = 75{,}000\ \mu\text{A}/10{,}000\ \text{mm}^2 = 7.5\ \mu\text{A}/\text{mm}^2$. Figure 14.12 shows for 90 mm$^2$ a current for VF of 1000 μA, or $J = 1000\ \mu\text{A}/90\ \text{mm}^2 = 11.1\ \mu\text{A}/\text{mm}^2$. This comparison supports the view that macroshock and microshock cause VF by the same mechanism.

***Microshock via Ground Potential Differences*** An example of microshock illustrates the need for a single reference ground point of each patient in

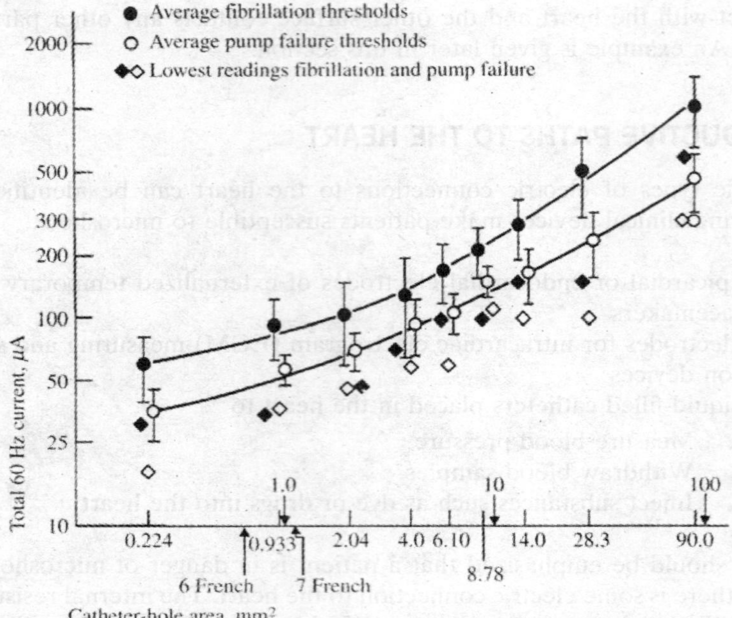


**Figure 14.12** Thresholds of VF and pump failure versus catheter area in dogs. (From O. Z. Roy, J. R. Scott, and G. C. Park, "Ventricular Fibrillation and Pump Failure Thresholds Versus Electrode Area," *IEEE Transactions on Biomedical Engineering*, 1976, 23, 45–48. Reprinted with permission.)

critical-care areas and the need for a 40 mV limit on the difference in potential between conductive surfaces in these areas.

Figure 14.13 shows a patient in the intensive-care unit (ICU) who is connected to an ECG monitor that grounds the right-leg electrode to reduce 60 Hz interference. In addition, the patient's left-ventricular blood pressure is being monitored by an intracardiac saline-filled catheter connected to a metallic pressure sensor that is also grounded. Assume that these two monitors are connected to grounded three-wire wall receptacles on separate circuits that can come from a central power-distribution panel many meters away. A microshock can occur when any device with a ground fault that does not open the circuit breaker is operated on *either* circuit.

Figure 14.13(a) shows the scheme of this hazard; Figure 14.13(b) shows an equivalent circuit. Suppose that a faulty electric floor polisher, which is dusty and damp, allows 5 A to flow to the distribution panel on the ground wire. The floor polisher functions properly, so the fault is not noticed by the operator. The ground wire could easily have a 0.1 Ω resistance, so 500 mV could appear across the patient between the ECG-monitor ground and the pressure-monitor ground. If the resistance of the patient's body and of the liquid-filled catheter is less than 50 kΩ, a current in excess of the 10 μA safe limit could flow. Of course, more current would flow if the ground

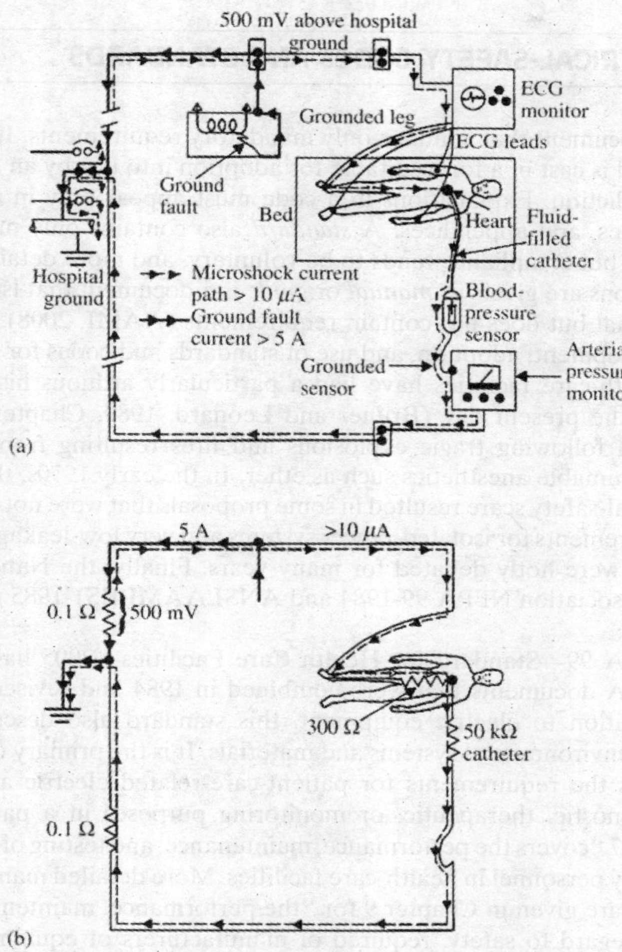


**Figure 14.13** (a) Large ground-fault current raises the potential of *one* ground connection to the patient. The microshock current can then flow out through a catheter connected to a different ground. (b) Equivalent circuit. Only power-system grounds are shown.

resistance or fault current were higher or if the catheter resistance were lower. If a grounded pacing catheter were to be used instead of the liquid-filled catheter in this example, then much smaller differences in ground potential would exceed the safe limit.

Most low-voltage hazards can be avoided if the grounds of all devices used in the vicinity of each patient are connected to a single patient-grounding point. This also prevents faults at one patient's bedside from affecting the safety of other patients. Modern pressure sensors and ECG monitors provide electrical isolation for all patient leads.

## 14.6 ELECTRICAL-SAFETY CODES AND STANDARDS

A *code* is a document that contains only mandatory requirements. It uses the word *shall* and is cast in a form suitable for adoption into law by an authority that has jurisdiction. Explanations in a code must appear only in fine-print notes, footnotes, and appendices. A *standard* also contains only mandatory requirements, but compliance tends to be voluntary, and more detailed notes and explanations are given. A *manual* or *guide* is a document that is informative and tutorial but does not contain requirements (AAMI, 2008).

The development, adoption, and use of standards and codes for electrical safety in health-care facilities have had a particularly arduous history that continues to the present day (Bruner and Leonard, 1989, Chapter 9). The process began following tragic explosions and fires resulting from electric ignition of flammable anesthetics such as ether. In the early 1970s, the microshock electrical-safety scare resulted in some proposals that were not practical. Implicit requirements for isolated-power systems and very low-leakage current requirements were hotly debated for many years. Finally, the National Fire Protection Association NFPA 99-1984 and ANSI/AAMI ES1-1985 standards were adopted.

The NFPA 99—Standard for Health Care Facilities—2005 has evolved from 12 NFPA documents that were combined in 1984 and revised every 3 years. In addition to electric equipment, this standard also describes gas, vacuum, and environmental systems and materials. It is the primary document that describes the requirements for patient-care-related electric appliances used for diagnostic, therapeutic, or monitoring purposes in a patient-care area. Chapter 7 "covers the performance, maintenance, and testing of electrical equipment" by personnel in health-care facilities. More detailed manufacturer requirements are given in Chapter 9 for "the performance, maintenance, and testing with regard to safety, required of manufacturers of equipment used within health-care facilities." Annex 2 concerns "the safe use of high-frequency (100 kHz to microwave frequencies) electricity in health-care facilities.

The National Electrical Code—2006, Article 517—Health Care Facilities is published by the NFPA and is widely adopted and enforced by state, county, and municipal authorities having jurisdiction. Requirements vary for general-care areas, critical-care areas, and wet locations. The major sections are I. General; II. Wiring and Protection; III. Essential Electrical System; IV. Inhalation Anesthetizing Locations; V. X-Ray Installations; VI. Communications, Signaling Systems, Data Systems, Fire-Alarm Systems, and Systems Less than 120 Volts, Nominal; and VII. Isolated Power Systems.

The Association for the Advancement of Medical Instrumentation (AAMI) developed an American National Standard on "Safe Current Limits for Electromedical Apparatus," ANSI/AAMI ESI—1993. This standard concerns limits on chassis and patient-lead leakage currents, which are fixed from dc to 1 kHz and increase from 1 kHz to 100 kHz. For single-fault conditions

**Table 14.1 Limits on Leakage Current for Electric Appliances**

| Electric Appliance | Chassis Leakage, μA | Patient-Lead Leakage, μA |
|---|---|---|
| Appliances not intended to contact patients | 100 | Not applicable |
| Appliances not intended to contact patients and single fault | 500 | Not applicable |
| Appliances with *nonisolated* patient leads | 100 | 10 |
| Appliances with *nonisolated* leads and single fault | 300 | 100 |
| Appliances with *isolated* patient leads | 100 | 10 |
| Appliances with *isolated* leads and single fault | 300 | 50 |

See Section 14.12 for specific test conditions and requirements.

only the patient-lead leakage current was relaxed from 10 μA to 50 μA and the chassis leakage current was relaxed from 100 μA to 300 μA. These changes were hotly challenged by the American Heart Association committee on electrocardiography (Laks *et al.*, 1994; Laks *et al.*, 1996). Laks said this change "constitutes experimentation on humans without their consent to determine the safe range of such currents."

The International Electrotechnical Commission (IEC) 60601-1 (2006) standard has been adopted by all other standards organizations, including the limit on leakage current for medical electric devices. This conformity to a widely supported international standard is endorsed by the Health Industry Manufacturers Association (HEMA), the National Electrical Manufacturers Association (NEMA), and the U.S. Food and Drug Administration (FDA). The IEC 60601-1 standard allows a "patient auxiliary current" up to 100 μA at not less than 0.1 Hz to permit amplifier bias currents and impedance plethysmography if the current is not intended to produce a physiological effect.

The present limits on leakage currents for the IEC 60601-1 2005 standard are shown in Table 14.1.

## 14.7 BASIC APPROACHES TO PROTECTION AGAINST SHOCK

There are two fundamental methods of protecting patients against shock. First, the patient can be completely isolated and insulated from all grounded objects and all sources of electric current. Second, all conductive surfaces within reach of the patient can be maintained at the same potential, which is not necessarily ground potential. Neither of these approaches can be fully achieved in most practical environments, so some combination of the two methods must usually suffice.

Not only must all hospital patients be protected from macroshocks, but all visitors and staff must be protected as well. Patients with reduced skin resistance (perhaps coupled to electrodes), invasive connections (such as intravenous catheters), or exposure to wet conditions (as happens during dialysis) need extra protection. The small numbers of patients with accessible electric connections to the heart need additional protection from microshock currents. Many of the specific methods of protection described here can be used in combination to provide redundant safeguards. It is also necessary to consider cost–benefit ratios with respect to both the purchase cost of safety equipment and the periodic maintenance costs of such equipment.

## 14.8 PROTECTION: POWER DISTRIBUTION

### GROUNDING SYSTEM

Low-resistance grounds that can carry currents up to circuit-breaker ratings are clearly essential for protecting patients against both macroshock and microshock, even when an isolated-power system is used. Figure 14.10 shows the importance of adequate grounds for protection against macroshock. Grounding is equally significant in preventing microshock (see Figure 14.11). A grounding system protects patients by keeping all conductive surfaces and receptacle grounds in the patient's environment at the same potential. It also protects the patient from ground faults at other locations.

The grounding system has a *patient-equipment grounding point*, a *reference grounding point*, and connections, as shown in Figure 14.14. The patient-equipment grounding point is connected individually to all receptacle grounds, metal beds, metal door and window frames, water pipes, and any other conductive surface. These connections should not exceed 0.15 Ω. The difference in potential between receptacle grounds and conductive surfaces should not exceed 40 mV. Each patient-equipment grounding point must be connected individually to a reference grounding point that is in turn connected to the building service ground.

### ISOLATED POWER-DISTRIBUTION SYSTEM

Unfortunately, even a good equipotential grounding system cannot eliminate voltages produced between grounds by large ground faults that cause large ground currents. However, these ground faults are rare in high-quality and properly maintained equipment. The isolation transformers discussed in Section 14.3 and shown in Figure 14.9 prevent this unlikely hazard. The isolated power system also reduces leakage current somewhat, but not below the 10 μA safe limit. There is usually enough capacitance between the transformer secondary circuit and ground to preclude protection against microshocks with isolation transformers. Isolated power systems provide considerable protection against macroshocks,

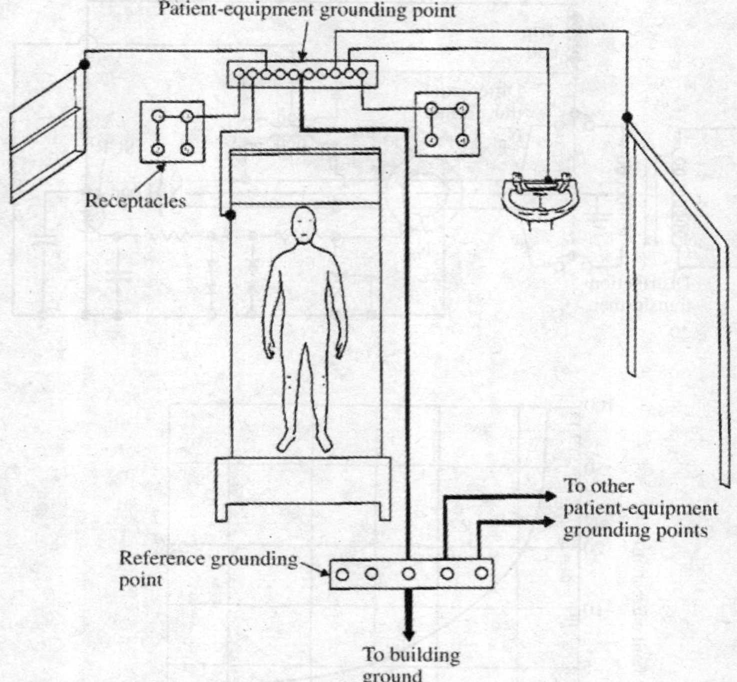


**Figure 14.14 Grounding system** All the receptacle grounds and conductive surfaces in the vicinity of the patient are connected to the patient-equipment grounding point. Each patient-equipment grounding point is connected to the reference grounding point that makes a single connection to the building ground.

particularly in areas subject to wet conditions. Isolated power systems are only necessary in locations where flammable anesthetics are used. The additional protection against microshocks provided by isolation transformers does not generally justify the high cost of these systems.

## GROUND-FAULT CIRCUIT INTERRUPTERS (GFCI)

Ground-fault circuit interrupters disconnect the source of electric power when a ground fault greater than about 6 mA occurs. In electric equipment that has negligible leakage current, the current in the hot conductor is equal to the current in the neutral conductor. The GFCI senses the difference between these two currents and interrupts power when this difference, which must be flowing to ground somewhere, exceeds the fixed rating. The devices make no distinction among paths the current takes to ground: That path may be via the ground wire or through a person to ground (Figure 14.10).

Most GFCIs use a differential transformer and solid-state circuitry, as shown in Figure 14.15(a). The trip time for the GFCI varies inversely with the

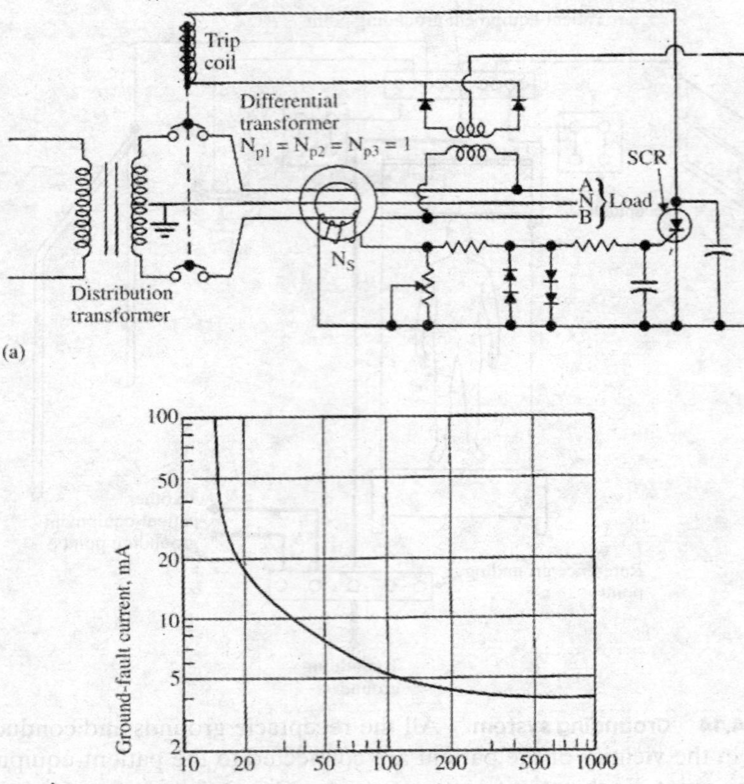


**Figure 14.15 Ground-fault circuit interrupters** (a) Schematic diagram of a solid-state (three-wire, two-pole, 6 mA) GFCI. (b) Ground-fault current versus trip time for a GFCI. [Part (a) is from C. F. Dalziel, "Electric Shock," in *Advances in Biomedical Engineering*, edited by J. H. U. Brown and J. F. Dickson III, 1973, 3: 223–248.]

magnitude of the ground-fault current, as shown in Figure 14.15(b). The GFCI is used with conventional three-wire grounded power-distribution systems. When power is interrupted by a GFCI, the manual reset button on the GFCI must be pushed to restore power. Most GFCIs have a momentary pushbutton that creates a safe ground fault to test the interrupter.

**EXAMPLE 14.3** Most GFCIs have a momentary push button that creates a safe ground fault to test the interrupter. On Figure 14.15, *design* the modifications to permit this test.

**ANSWER** Add from B to earth ground a resistor in series with a momentary push-button switch so current flows outside the magnetic core. $R = V/I = 120\ \text{V}/12\ \text{mA} = 10\ \text{k}\Omega$.

The 2006 National Electrical Code requires that there be GFCIs in circuits serving bathrooms, garages, outdoor receptacles, swimming pools, and construction sites (Articles 210-8,680-5). NFPA 99 requires the use of GFCIs in wet locations, particularly hydrotherapy areas, where continuity of power is not essential.

Ground-fault circuit interrupters are not sensitive enough to interrupt microshock levels of leakage current, so they are primarily macroshock-protection devices. They can, however, prevent some microshocks by interrupting the source of large ground-fault currents that cause differences in potential in grounding systems.

However, circuits in patient-care areas generally should not include GFCIs, because the loss of power to life-support equipment due to GFCIs is probably more hazardous to the patient than most small ground faults would be. Where brief power interruptions can be tolerated, the low cost of GFCIs ($10) make them an attractive alternative to isolated power-distribution systems ($2000).

## 14.9 PROTECTION: EQUIPMENT DESIGN

### RELIABLE GROUNDING FOR EQUIPMENT

The importance of an effective grounding system for equipment has already been illustrated (Figure 14.10). Most failures of equipment grounds occur either at the ground contact of the receptacle or in the plug and cable leading to the line-powered equipment. Hospital-grade receptacles and plugs and "Hard Service" (SO, ST, or STO) or "Junior Hard Service" (SJO, SJT, or SJTO) power cords must be used in all patient areas. Molded plugs should be avoided, because surveys have shown that 40% to 85% of these plugs develop invisible breaks within 1 to 10 years of hospital service. Strain-relief devices are recommended both where the cord enters the equipment and at the connection between cord and plug. A convenient cord-storage compartment or device reduces cord damage. Equipment grounds are often deliberately interrupted by improper use of the common three-prong-to-two-prong adapter (*cheater adapter*).

### REDUCTION OF LEAKAGE CURRENT

Reduction of leakage current in the chassis of equipment and in patient leads is an important goal for designers of all line-powered instruments. Special low-leakage power cords are available (<1.0 μA/m). Leakage current inside the chassis can be reduced by using layouts and insulating materials that minimize the capacitance between all hot conductors and the chassis. Particular attention must be given to maximizing the impedance from patient leads to hot conductors and from patient leads to chassis ground. Most modern equipment meets the leakage-current limits given in Section 14.6. Old equipment with higher leakage should not be used with patients susceptible to microshocks unless proper grounding is ensured.

## DOUBLE-INSULATED EQUIPMENT

The objective of grounding is to eliminate hazardous potentials by interconnecting all conductive surfaces. An equally effective approach is to use a separate layer of insulation to prevent contact of any person with the chassis or any exposed conductive surface. Primary insulation is the normal functional insulation between energized conductors and the chassis. A separate secondary layer of insulation between the chassis and the outer case protects personnel even if a ground fault to the chassis occurs. The outer case, if it is made of insulating material, may serve as the secondary insulation. All switch levers and control shafts must be double insulated (for example, plastic knobs may have recessed screws). Double insulation generally reduces leakage current. For medical instruments, both layers of insulation should remain effective, even when conductive fluid is spilled. Double insulation protects against both macroshock and microshock.

## OPERATION AT LOW VOLTAGES

Most solid-state electronic diagnostic equipment can be powered by low-voltage batteries ($<10$ V) or low-voltage isolation transformers. Macroshock is avoided if the voltage is low enough to be safe even when the device is applied directly to wet skin. Low-voltage ac-powered equipment can still cause microshock if the current is applied directly to the heart. However, low-voltage ac equipment is generally safer than high-voltage ac equipment. See Section 164 in Article 517 of the 2006 National Electrical Code for requirements for low-voltage equipment used in inhalation-anesthetizing locations.

## ELECTRICAL ISOLATION

Isolation amplifiers are devices that break the ohmic continuity of electric signals between the input and output of the amplifier. This isolation includes different supply-voltage sources and different grounds on each side of the isolation barrier. Isolation amplifiers usually consist of an instrumentation amplifier at the input followed by a unity-gain isolation stage. Figure 14.16(a) shows a general model for an isolation amplifier that has a triangular operational amplifier symbol split by a perfect isolation barrier (dashed line). The very high impedance across the barrier is modeled by the isolation capacitance and resistance. The isolation voltage $v_{ISO}$ is the potential that can exist between the input common and the output common (note the different ground symbols) and is rated from 1 to 10 kV without breakdown. The rejection of this voltage by the amplifier is specified by the isolation-mode rejection ratio (IMRR). The desired input voltage $v_{SIG}$, the input common-mode voltage $v_{CM}$,

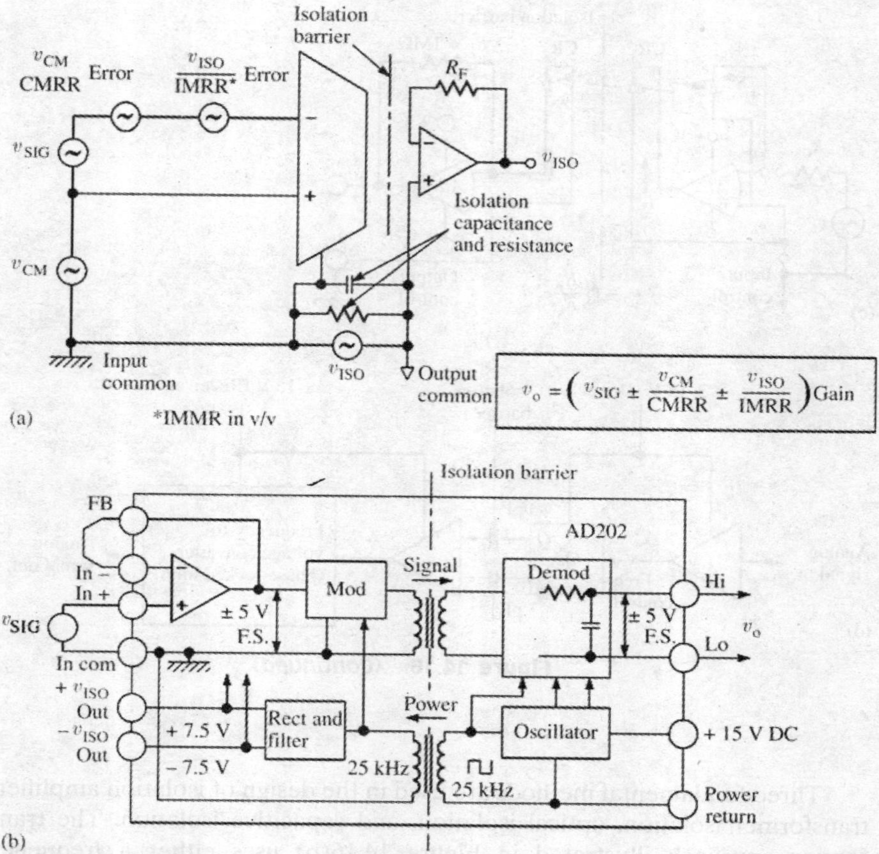


**Figure 14.16 Electrical isolation of patient leads to biopotential amplifiers** (a) General model for an isolation amplifier. (b) Transformer isolation amplifier (courtesy of Analog Devices, Inc., AD202). (c) Simplified equivalent circuit for an optical isolator (copyright 1989 Burr-Brown Corporation. Reprinted in whole or in part with the permission of Burr-Brown Corporation. Burr Brown ISO100). (d) Capacitively coupled isolation amplifier (Horowitz and Hill, *Art of Electronics*, Cambridge Univ. Press, 1989, Burr Brown ISO106).

and the common-mode rejection ratio (CMRR) are the same as for a non-isolated amplifier. Typical maximal ratings for $v_{CM}$ are only $\pm 10$ V. The input common may be connected to the source in applications that break ground loops or may be floated to make possible simpler, two-wire connections to the source and reference of the common-mode signal across the isolation barrier to the output common. The three main features of an isolation amplifier are high ohmic isolation between input and output (>10 MΩ), high isolation-mode voltage (>1000 V), and high common-mode rejection (>100 dB).

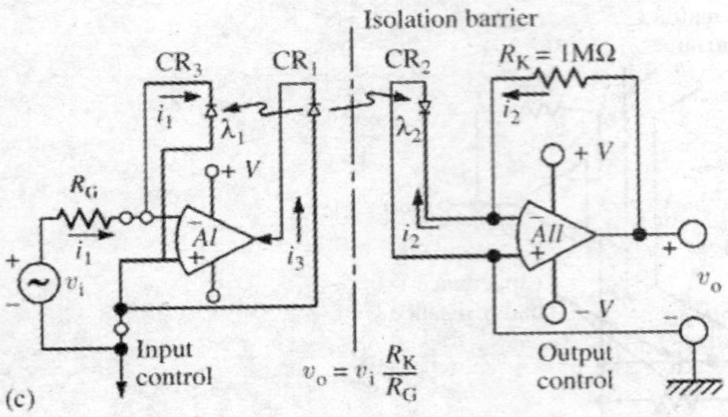


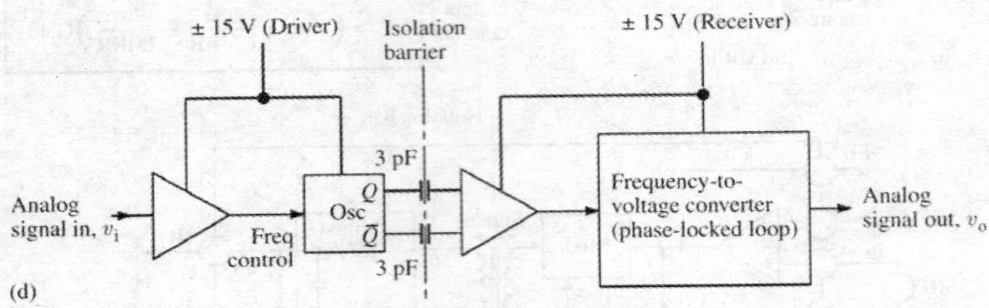


**Figure 14.16** *(Continued)*

Three fundamental methods are used in the design of isolation amplifiers: transformer isolation, optical isolation, and capacitive isolation. The transformer approach illustrated in Figure 14.16(b) uses either a frequency-modulated or a pulse-width-modulated carrier signal with small signal bandwidths up to 30 kHz to carry the signal. It uses an internal dc-to-dc converter composed of a 25 kHz oscillator, transformer, rectifier, and filter to supply isolated power. The optical method uses an LED on the source side and a photodiode on the output side. No modulator–demodulator is needed, because the signal all the way to dc is transmitted optically. A matched photodiode on the source side is used with feedback to improve linearity. Increased light from the forward-biased LED $CR_1$ causes increased reverse leakage current through $CR_2$ and $CR_3$ (see Figure 2.22). The simplified circuit in Figure 14.16(c) operates only for one polarity of input signal. The capacitive method, shown in Figure 14.16(d), uses digital encoding of the input voltage and frequency modulation to send the signal across a differential ceramic capacitive barrier. There is no feedback, though a power supply is needed on both sides of the barrier. The peak isolation voltage can be as high as 8 kV, and bandwidth up to 70 kHz is available.

**EXAMPLE 14.4** For the isolation barrier in Figure 14.16, calculate the capacitance to limit the 60 Hz, 120 V current to 10 μA.

**ANSWER** $Z = 120\,\text{V}/10\,\mu\text{A} = 12\,\text{M}\Omega$, $C = 1/(\omega|Z|) = 1/(2\pi 60 \times 12\,\text{M}\Omega) = 221\,\text{pF}$.

## ISOLATED HEART CONNECTIONS

Undoubtedly the best way to minimize the hazards of microshock is to isolate or eliminate electric connections to the heart. Fully insulated connectors for external cardiac pacemakers powered by batteries have greatly reduced this hazard. Modern blood-pressure sensors are designed with triple insulation between the column of liquid, the sensor case, and the electric connections (Figure 2.5). Catheters with conductive walls have been developed that provide electric contact all along that part of the catheter that is inside the patient, so that microshock current is distributed throughout the body, not concentrated at the heart. Conductivity of the catheter wall does not affect measurements of pressure made with liquid-filled catheters. Catheters that contain sensors in the tip for measuring blood pressure and flow should have low leakage currents.

# 14.10 ELECTRICAL-SAFETY ANALYZERS

Commercially available instruments called *electrical-safety analyzers* are useful for testing both medical-facility power systems and medical appliances (Anonymous, 1988). These analyzers range in complexity from simple conversion boxes used with any volt–ohm meter to computerized automatic measurement systems with bar code readers that generate written reports of test results. The features to consider are accuracy, ease of use, testing time, and cost. The analyzers also reduce errors caused by incorrect test setups and reduce the risk of shock to the person performing tests such as applying line voltage to patient leads to test isolation. Automated methods for measuring leakage current for medical equipment have been developed (Hu *et al.*, 2005).

# 14.11 TESTING THE ELECTRIC SYSTEM

When we test systems of electric distribution and line-powered equipment, we must consider the safety of both the patients and the personnel conducting the tests. We shall briefly describe and comment on only the common tests.

## TESTS OF RECEPTACLES

Receptacles should be tested for proper wiring, adequate line voltage, low ground resistance, and mechanical tension. The common three-light receptacle

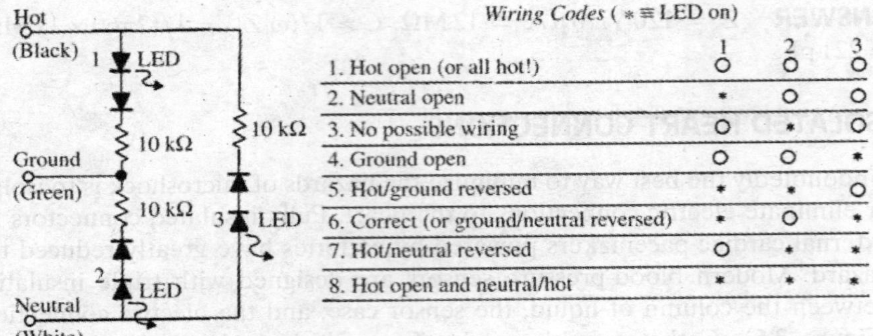


*Wiring Codes* ( * ≡ LED on)

| | 1 | 2 | 3 |
|---|---|---|---|
| 1. Hot open (or all hot!) | O | O | O |
| 2. Neutral open | * | O | O |
| 3. No possible wiring | O | * | O |
| 4. Ground open | O | O | * |
| 5. Hot/ground reversed | * | * | O |
| 6. Correct (or ground/neutral reversed) | * | O | * |
| 7. Hot/neutral reversed | O | * | * |
| 8. Hot open and neutral/hot | * | * | * |

**Figure 14.17 Three-LED receptacle tester** Ordinary silicon diodes prevent damaging reverse-LED currents, and resistors limit current. The LEDs are ON for line voltages from about 20 V rms to greater than 240 V rms, so these devices should not be used to measure line voltage.

testers shown in Figure 14.17 are deficient in several respects. These devices were designed to check only the wiring, but even so, they can indicate only 8 ($2^3$) of 64 ($4^3$) possible states for an outlet. The three lights have only two states ($2^3$), whereas each of the three outlet contacts has four states ($4^3$)—hot, neutral, ground, and open.

These testers give an OK reading when the ground and neutral wires are transposed and when the green and white wires are hot and the black wire is grounded. (Opening of the circuit breaker would probably call attention to the latter miswiring and to several others as well.)

Ground resistance can be measured by passing up to 1 A through the ground wire and measuring the voltage between ground and neutral. Anyone doing these ground-wire tests should take care not to incur the microshock hazards described in Section 14.5 (and shown in Figure 14.13). The resistance of neutral wiring can be tested similarly, by passing the current through the neutral conductor. Ground or neutral resistance should not exceed 0.2 Ω. The minimal mechanical retaining force for each of the three contacts is about 115 g (4 oz).

## TESTS OF THE GROUNDING SYSTEM IN PATIENT-CARE AREAS

The NFPA 99 requires both voltage and impedance measurements with different limits for new and existing construction. The voltage between a reference grounding point (see Figure 14.14) and exposed conductive surfaces should not exceed 20 mV for new construction. For existing construction, the limit is 500 mV for general-care areas and 40 mV for critical-care areas. The impedance between the reference grounding point and receptacle grounding contacts must be less than 0.1 Ω for new construction and less than 0.2 Ω for existing construction.

## TESTS OF ISOLATED-POWER SYSTEMS

Isolated-power systems should have equipotential grounding that is similar to that of unisolated systems (Figure 14.14). The line-isolation monitor (Figure 14.9) should trigger a visible (red) and an audible alarm when the total hazard current (resistive and capacitive leakage currents and LIM current) reaches a threshold of 5 mA under normal line-voltage conditions. The LIM should not trigger the alarm for a fault-hazard current of less than 3.7 mA. For complete specifications, see the latest NFPA 99 standard.

## 14.12 TESTS OF ELECTRIC APPLIANCES

### GROUND-PIN-TO-CHASSIS RESISTANCE

The resistance between the ground pin of the plug and the equipment chassis and exposed metal objects should not exceed 0.15 Ω during the life of the appliance (Figure 14.18).

During the measurement of resistance, the power cord must be flexed at its connection to the attachment plug and at its strain relief where it enters the appliance.

### CHASSIS LEAKAGE CURRENT

Leakage current emanating from the chassis, as measured in Figure 14.19(a), should not exceed 500 μA for appliances with single fault not intended to contact patients and should not exceed 300 μA for appliances that are intended for use in the patient care vicinity. These are limits on rms current for sinusoids from dc to 1 kHz, and they should be obtained with a current-measuring device of 1000 Ω or less. Figure 14.19(b) shows a suitable circuit. The limits on leakage current apply whether the polarity of the power line is correct or reversed,

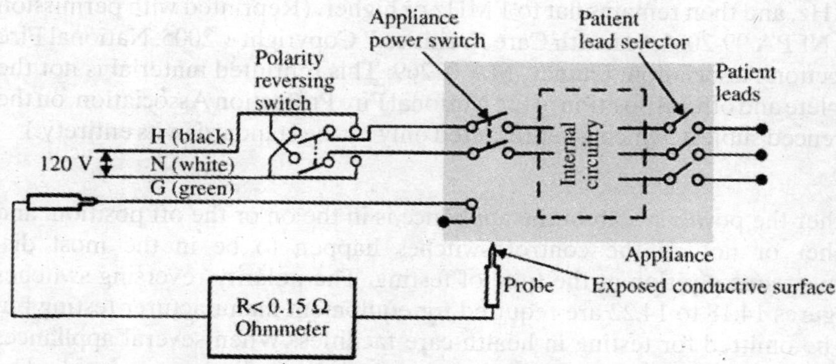


**Figure 14.18** Ground-pin-to-chassis resistance test

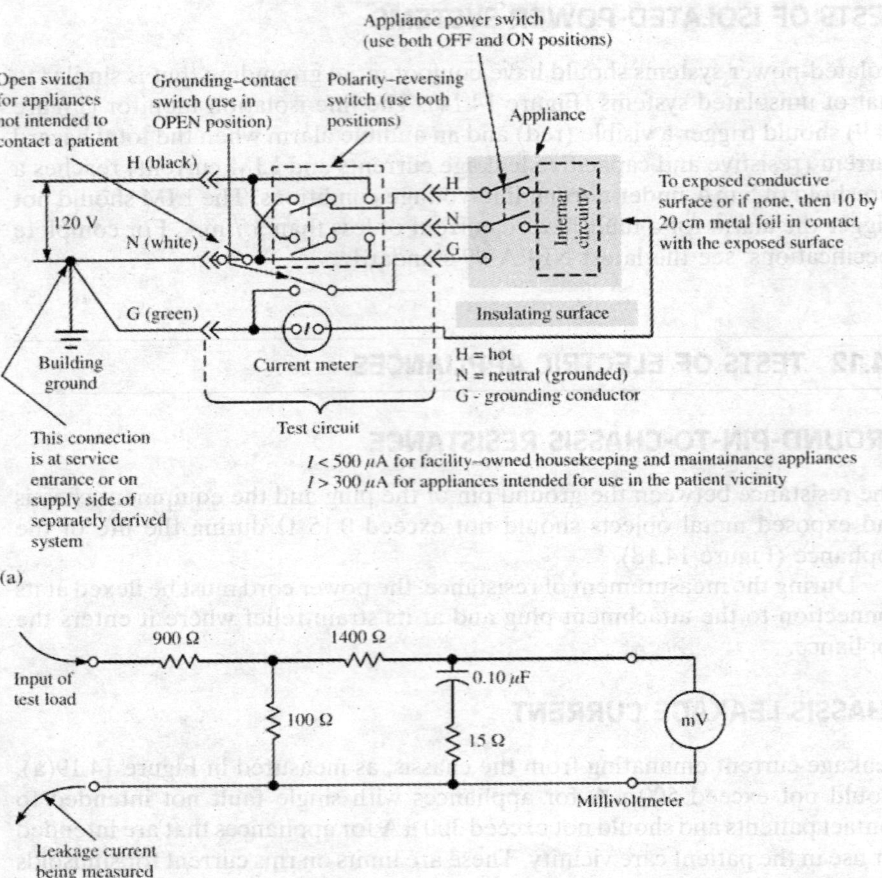


**Figure 14.19** (a) Chassis leakage-current test. (b) Current-meter circuit to be used for measuring leakage current. It has an input impedance of 1 kΩ and a frequency characteristic that is flat to 1 kHz, drops at the rate of 20 dB/decade to 100 kHz, and then remains flat to 1 MHz or higher. (Reprinted with permission from NFPA 99-2005, "Health Care Facilities," Copyright ©2005, National Fire Protection Association, Quincy, MA 02269. This reprinted material is not the complete and official position of the National Fire Protection Association, on the referenced subject, which is represented only by the standard in its entirety.)

whether the power switch of the appliance is in the on or the off position, and whether or not all the control switches happen to be in the most disadvantageous position at the time of testing. The polarity-reversing switches in Figures 14.18 to 14.22 are required for equipment manufacturer testing but may be omitted for testing in health-care facilities. When several appliances are mounted together in one rack or cart, and all the appliances are supplied by one power cord, the complete rack or cart must be tested as one appliance.

## LEAKAGE CURRENT IN PATIENT LEADS

Leakage current in patient leads is particularly important because these leads are the most common low-impedance patient contacts. Limits on leakage current in patient leads should be 50 μA. Isolated patient leads must have leakage current that is less than 10 μA. Only *isolated* patient leads should be connected to catheters or electrodes that make contact with the heart. Leakage current between individual or interconnected patient leads and ground should be measured with the patient leads active, as shown in Figure 14.20.

In addition, leakage current between any pair of leads or between any single lead and all the other patient leads should be measured, as indicated in Figure 14.21.

Finally, the leakage current that would flow through patient leads to ground if line voltage were to appear on the patient should be tested. This leakage current is called *isolation current* or *risk current*. Application of power-line voltage and frequency to the isolated patient leads should produce an isolation current to ground that is less than 50 μA (Figure 14.22).

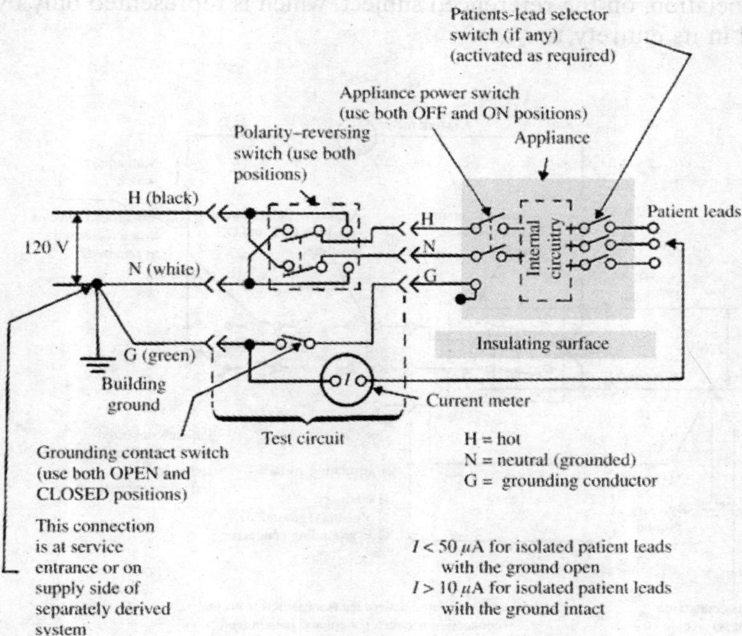


**Figure 14.20** Test for leakage current from patient leads to ground. (Reprinted with permission from NFPA 99-2005, "Health Care Facilities," Copyright © 2005, National Fire Protection Association, Quincy, MA 02269. This reprinted material is not the complete and official position of the National Fire Protection Association, on the referenced subject, which is represented only by the standard in its entirety.)

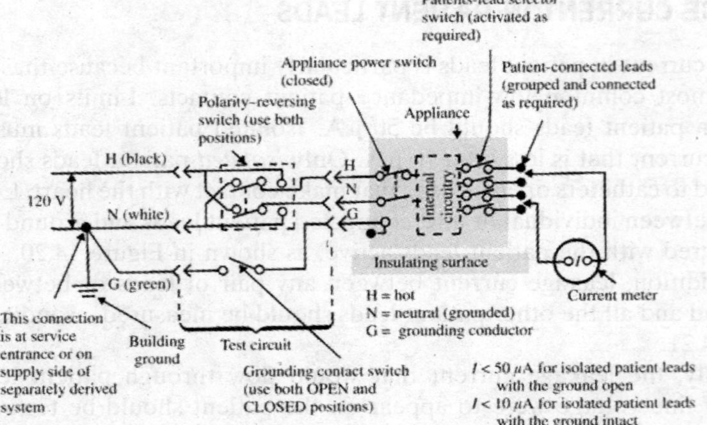


**Figure 14.21** Test for leakage current between patient leads (Reprinted with permission from NFPA 99-2005, "Health Care Facilities," Copyright ©2005, National Fire Protection Association, Quincy, MA 02269. This reprinted material is not the complete and official position of the National Fire Protection Association, on the referenced subject, which is represented only by the standard in its entirety.)

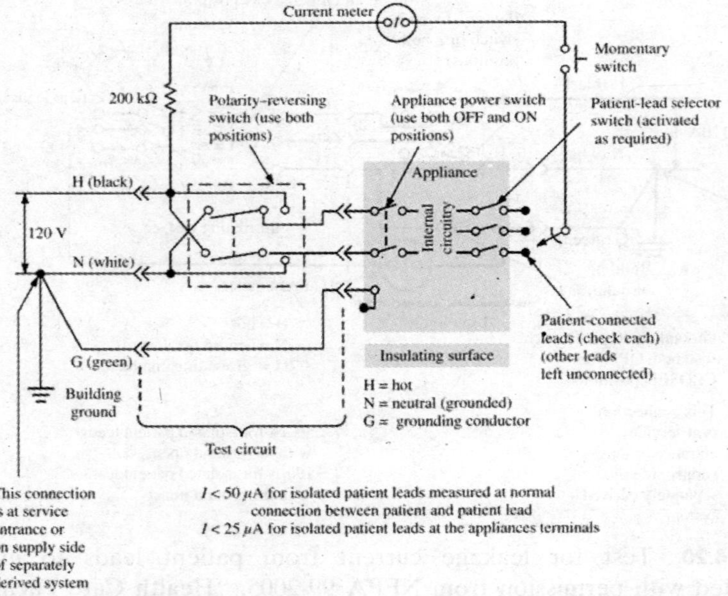


**Figure 14.22** Test for ac isolation current. (Reprinted with permission from NFPA 99-2005, "Health Care Facilities," Copyright © 2005, National Fire Protection Association, Quincy, MA 02269. This reprinted material is not the complete and official position of the National Fire Protection Association, on the referenced subject, which is represented only by the standard in its entirety.)

## CONCLUSION

Adequate electrical safety in health-care facilities can be achieved at moderate cost by combining a good power-distribution system, careful selection of well-designed equipment, periodic testing of power systems and equipment, and a modest training program for medical personnel. Fortunately, the electrical-safety scare of the early 1970s has led to increased knowledge and greater safety for both patients and medical personnel.

## PROBLEMS

**14.1** Assume that the cell membranes of a very large number of cells in parallel can be modeled by a 1 Ω resistor in parallel with a 100 μF capacitor. Determine the rms sinusoidal current versus frequency necessary to depolarize the cells. Assume that the peak potential of the cell membrane must be raised 20 mV above its resting potential to exceed threshold. Plot your results together with those shown in Figure 14.3, and compare.

**14.2** From your knowledge of cardiac electrophysiology (Section 4.6), explain what rhythm would result from an intense 100 ms shock that occurred during (a) the P wave, (b) the R wave, (c) the T wave, and (d) diastole. From these results, explain the shape of the curves shown in Figure 14.5.

**14.3** Resketch Figure 14.6(b) for the case in which a catheter made of conductive plastic is used.

**14.4** If the secondary earth ground in Figure 14.8 were not connected, would this prevent electrocution under no-fault conditions? What would be the result in case of a primary-to-secondary fault in the transformer?

**14.5** The LIM in Figure 14.9 has a monitor hazard current that is too high. Redesign it to achieve a lower monitor hazard current of 25 μA by changing the value of a *single* passive component shown and adjusting the detector threshold.

**14.6** Design the simplest line-isolation monitor that would be capable of detecting a *single* fault from either line to ground.

**14.7** Some authors hypothesize that it is current density flowing through the cell membrane that raises the resting potential of the cell to exceed threshold. Replot Figure 14.12 to show the average current density of the fibrillation threshold versus area of the catheter. Is the foregoing hypothesis correct? Explain any discrepancies.

**14.8** Calculate the maximal safe capacitance between a liquid-filled catheter and dc-isolated pressure-sensor leads for a 120 V, 60 Hz fault in the sensor leads.

**14.9** Compute the resistivity of the liquid necessary for safe operation of a liquid-filled catheter that is 1 m long and has a radius of 1.13 mm. Use the data given in Roy *et al.* (1980) (shown in Figure 14.12). Assume that the patient is grounded and that a 120 V fault develops at the sensor.

**14.10** Draw a complete equivalent circuit, and compute the rms current through the patient's heart for the following situation. The patient's hand touches a faulty metal lamp that is 120 V rms above ground. A saline-filled catheter ($R = 50\,\text{k}\Omega$) for measuring blood pressure is connected to the patient's heart. Some of the pressure-sensor strain-gage wiring is grounded, and the sensor is somewhat isolated electrically. However, there is 20 MΩ of leakage resistance in the insulation between the ground and the saline in the sensor. There is also 100 pF of capacitance between the ground and the saline. Assume that the skin resistance of the patient is 1 MΩ. Is there a microshock hazard?

**14.11** Show how a single electric instrument can be the path for microshock current flowing both to and from the patient, at the same time. Use complete diagrams, and do a sample calculation.

**14.12** Devise your own hospital-patient microshock situation. Give complete details, including a diagram and equivalent circuit. Describe all tests, and give the standards for test results necessary to ensure the safety of the patient.

**14.13** Figure 14.15 is designed for two-phase operation. Redesign it (draw a circuit diagram) for one-phase operation.

**14.14** Design a tester for an electric receptacle that will indicate as many states as possible, including those not detected by the common three-LED receptacle testers (Figure 14.17).

**14.15** A power engineer receives a lethal macroshock while standing in water and simultaneously touching the ungrounded metal casing on a high-voltage, 60 Hz power transformer. Assume that the resistance of the skin on the engineer's hand is 100 kΩ and that the resistance of the skin on the engineer's feet is negligible. A capacitance of 25 nF is measured between the transformer casing and the high-voltage conductors. Find the minimal value of the high voltage, assuming that 75 mA is the minimal fibrillating macroshock. Draw an equivalent circuit.

**14.16** In Figure 14.16(c), the diodes are forward-biased for only *one* polarity of $v_i$. Redesign the circuit such that it works for *both* polarities of $v_i$. Consider the op-amp summer as a possibility.

**14.17** Figure 14.1 shows us that 60 Hz arm-to-arm current of 100 mA rms causes VF. Assume $I_r$ in (14.1) is 60 Hz peak current of 141 mA and that $\tau = 3\,\text{ms}$. Calculate $I_d$ for a Taser that has $d = 100\,\mu\text{s}$.

## REFERENCES

AAMI, *AAMI Electrical Safety Manual, 2008, A Comprehensive Guide to Electrical Safety Standards for Healthcare Facilities.* Arlington, VA: Association for the Advancement of Medical Instrumentation, 2008.

AAMI, *American National Standard, Safe Current Limits for Electromedical Apparatus.* (ANSI/AAMIES1–1993). Arlington, VA: Association for the Advancement of Medical Instrumentation, 1993.

Anonymous, "Electrical safety analyzers." *Health Devices*, 1988, 17, 283–309; "Update." *Health Devices*, 1989, 18, 411–413.

Bruner, J. M. R., and P. F. Leonard, *Electrical Safety and the Patient*. Chicago: Year Book Medical Publishers, 1989.

Charney, and W., J. Schirmer, *Essentials of Modern Hospital Safety*. Chelsea, MI: Lewis Publishing, 1990.

Dalziel, C. F., "Electric shock." In J. H. U. Brown and J. F. Dickson III (eds.), *Advances in Biomedical Engineering*, 1973, 3, 223–248.

Dyro, J. F., "Safety program, hospital." In J. G. Webster (ed.), *Encyclopedia of Medical Devices and Instrumentation*, 2nd ed. New York: Wiley, 2006, Vol. 6, pp. 109–122.

*The National Electrical Code 2006 Handbook*, Quincy, MA: National Fire Protection Association, 2006.

Fagerhaugh, S. Y., A. Strauss, B. Suczek, and C. L. Wiener, *Hazards in Hospital Care: Ensuring Patient Safety*. San Francisco, CA: Jossey-Bass, 1987.

Geddes, L. A., *Handbook of Electrical Hazards and Accidents*. Boca Raton, FL: CRC Press, 1995.

Geddes, L. A., J. D. Bourland, and G. Ford, "The mechanism underlying sudden death from electric shock." *Med. Instrum.*, 1986, 20, 303–315.

Geddes, L. A., and L. E. Baker, *Principles of Applied Biomedical Instrumentation*, 3rd ed. New York: Wiley, 1989.

Hu, Y., L. Y. Pang, X. B. Xie, X. H. Li, and K. D. K. Luk, "Automated leakage current measurement for medical equipment safety." *Proceedings of IEEE Engineering in Medicine and Biology*, 2005, 440–442.

IEC 60601-1 2006 *Household and similar electrical appliances—Safety—Part 2-76: Particular requirements for electric fence energizers*, (IEC 60335-2-76, Edition 2.1).

Klein, B. R., *Health Care Facilities Handbook*, 5th ed. Quincy, MA: National Fire Protection Association, 1996.

Laks, M., R. Arzbaecher, J. Bailey, A. Berson, S. Briller, and D. Geselowitz, "Will relaxing safe current limits for electromedical equipment increase hazards to patients? " *Circulation*, 1994, 89, 909–910.

Laks, M., R. Arzbaecher, J. Bailey, D. Geselowitz, and A. Berson, "Recommendations for safe current limits for electrocardiographs." *Circulation*, 1996, 93, 837–839.

Lee, R. C., E. G. Cravalho, and J. F. Burke, *Electrical Trauma: The Pathophysiology, Manifestations and Clinical Management*. Cambridge, England: Cambridge University Press, 1992.

Maffiuletti, N. A., A. J. Herrero, M. Jubeau, F. M. Impellizzeri, M. Bizzini, "Differences in electrical stimulation thresholds between men and women." *Ann. Neurol.*, 2008, 63, 507–512.

NFPA No. 99-2005, *Standard for Health Care Facilities.* Quincy, MA: National Fire Protection Association, 2005.

Reilly, J. P., *Applied Bioelectricity: From Electrical Stimulation to Electropathology*. New York: Springer, 1998.

Roy, O. Z., "Summary of cardiac fibrillation thresholds for 60 Hz currents and voltages applied directly to the heart." *Med. Biol. Eng. Comput.*, 1980, 18, 657–659.

Roy, O. Z., A. J. Mortimer, B. J. Trollope, and E. J. Villeneuve, "Effects of short-duration transients on cardiac rhythm." *Med. Biol. Eng. Comput.*, 1984, 22, 225–228.

Roy, O. Z., J. R. Scott, and G. C. Park, "60 Hz ventricular fibrillation and pump failure thresholds versus electrode area." *IEEE Trans. Biomed. Eng.*, 1976, 23, 45–48.

Staewen, W. S., "Electrical safety reconsidered—the new AAMI electrical safety standard." *Biomed. Instrum. Tech.*, 1994, 28, 131–132.

Swerdlow, C. D., W. H. Olson, M. E. O'Connor, D. M. Gallik, R. A. Malkin, and M. Laks, "Cardiovascular collapse caused by electrocardiographically silent 60-Hz intracardiac leakage current—implications for electrical safety." *Circulation*, 1999, 99, 2559–2564.

Tan, K. S., and D. L. Johnson, "Threshold of sensation for 60 Hz leakage current: Results of a survey." *Biomed. Instrum. Tech.*, 1990, 24, 207–211.

# APPENDIX

## APPENDIX A.1

### Physical Constants

| | |
|---|---|
| $g = 9.8\ \text{m/s}^2$ | Acceleration due to gravity |
| $c = 3 \times 10^8\ \text{m/s}$ | Velocity of light |
| $\sigma = 5.67 \times 10^{-12}\ \text{W/(cm}^2 \cdot \text{K}^4)$ | Stefan–Boltzmann constant |
| $k = 1.38 \times 10^{-23}\ \text{J/K}$ | Boltzmann's constant |
| $h = 6.63 \times 10^{-34}\ \text{J} \cdot \text{s}$ | Planck's constant |
| $R = 8.31\ \text{J/(mol} \cdot \text{K)}$ | Gas constant |
| $F = 96{,}500$ C/equivalent | Faraday's constant (Equivalent = mole/valence) |
| $q = -1.602 \times 10^{-19}\ \text{C}$ | Charge on the electron |
| $\varepsilon_0 = 8.8 \times 10^{-12}\ \text{F/m}$ | Dielectric constant of free space |
| $N = 6.02 \times 10^{23}$ molecules/mol | Avogadro's number |

## APPENDIX A.2

### International System of Units (SI) Prefixes (Thompson and Taylor, 2008)

| Multiplication Factor | Prefix | Symbol |
|---|---|---|
| $10^{24}$ | yotta | Y |
| $10^{21}$ | zetta | Z |
| $10^{18}$ | exa | E |
| $10^{15}$ | peta | P |
| $10^{12}$ | tera | T |
| $10^{9}$ | giga | G |
| $10^{6}$ | mega | M |
| $10^{3}$ | kilo | k |
| $10^{-1}$ | deci | d |
| $10^{-2}$ | centi | c |

| Multiplication Factor | Prefix | Symbol |
|---|---|---|
| $10^{-3}$ | milli | m |
| $10^{-6}$ | micro | μ |
| $10^{-9}$ | nano | n |
| $10^{-12}$ | pico | p |
| $10^{-15}$ | femto | f |
| $10^{-18}$ | atto | a |
| $10^{-21}$ | zepto | z |
| $10^{-24}$ | yocto | y |

# APPENDIX A.3

## International System of Units (Thompson and Taylor, 2008)

| To Convert from | To | Multiply by |
|---|---|---|
| degree | radian (rad) | 0.0175 |
| inch | meter (m) | 0.0254 |
| gallon | liter (l) | 3.79 |
| cycles per second | hertz (Hz) | 1.0 |
| minute | second (s) | 60 |
| hour | minute (min) | 60 |
| day | hour (h) | 24 |
| pound | kilogram (kg) | 0.454 |
| 0.012 kg of carbon-12 | mole (mol) | 1.0 |
| pound-force | newton (N) | 4.45 |
| degree Rankine | Kelvin (K) | $t_K = t_R^o/1.8$ |
| calorie | joule (J) | 4.186 |
| British thermal unit | joule (J) | 1055 |
| horsepower | watt (W) | 745 |
| cm $H_2O$ | pascal (Pa) | 98.1 |
| mm Hg (torr) | pascal (Pa) | 133.3 |
| psi | pascal (Pa) | 6895 |
| atmosphere | pascal (Pa) | 101325 |
| poise | pascal·second (Pa·s) | 0.1 |
| | volt (V) | |
| | ampere (A) | |
| | ohm (Ω) | |
| mho | Siemens (S) | 1.0 |
| gauss | tesla (T) | 0.0001 |
| maxwell | weber (Wb) | $10^{-8}$ |
| | farad (F) | |
| | decibel (dB) | |
| | candela (cd) | |
| roentgen (R) | coulomb per kilogram (C/kg) | 0.000258 |
| rad | gray (Gy) | 0.01 |
| curie (Ci) | becquerel (Bq) | $3.7 \times 10^{10}$ |

## REFERENCES

Thompson, A., and Taylor, B. N., Guide for the Use of the International System of Units (SI). NIST Special Publication 811. Gaithersburg, MD: National Institute of Standards and Technology, 2008. http://physics.nist.gov/cuu/pdf/sp811.pdf

# APPENDIX A.4

**Abbreviations**

| Abbreviation | Term |
|---|---|
| AAMI | Association for the Advancement of Medical Instrumentation |
| AAP | Axon action potential |
| ac | Alternating current |
| ACA | Automatic Clinical Analyzer |
| ADC | Analog-to-digital converter |
| AF | Audio frequency |
| AIDS | Acquired immune deficiency syndrome |
| AM | Amplitude modulation |
| ANSI | American National Standards Institute |
| ATP | Analytical test pack |
| ATR | Attenuated total reflection |
| AV | Atrioventricular |
| AWG | American wire gage |
| CAD | Computer-aided design |
| CC | Closing capacity |
| CCD | Charge-coupled device |
| CMRR | Common-mode rejection ratio |
| CNS | Central nervous system |
| CPAP | Continuous positive airway pressure |
| CPU | Central processing unit |
| CSF | Cerebrospinal fluid |
| CV | Closing volume |
| cv | Coefficient of variation |
| CVP | Central venous pressure |
| CW | Continuous wave |
| *D* | *d/dt* |
| DAC | Digital-to-analog converter |
| dc | Direct current |
| DNA | Deoxyribonucleic acid |
| DPG | Diphosphoglycerate |
| EBR | Electron beam recording |
| ECG | Electrocardiogram |
| ECMO | Extracorporeal membrane oxygenator |
| ECO | Engineering change order |
| ECoG | Electrocorticogram |

| Abbreviation | Term |
|---|---|
| EEG | Electroencephalogram |
| EGM | Myocardial electrogram |
| EIA | Electronics industries association |
| ELISA | Enzyme-linked immunosorbent assay |
| emf | Electromotive force |
| EMG | Electromyogram |
| ENG | Electroneurogram |
| EOG | Electro-oculogram |
| EPROM | Erasable programmable read-only memory |
| ERG | Electroretinogram |
| ERP | Early-receptor potential |
| ERV | Expiratory reserve volume |
| FDA | Food and Drug Administration |
| FEF | Forced expiratory flow |
| FET | Field-effect transistor |
| FEV | Forced expiratory volume |
| FM | Frequency modulation |
| FRC | Functional residual capacity |
| FVC | Forced vital capacity |
| GC | Gas chromatograph |
| GFCI | Ground-fault circuit interrupter |
| GLC | Gas-liquid chromatograph |
| GM | Geometric mean |
| GSR | Galvanic skin response |
| GRIN | Graded index |
| HCT | Hematocrit |
| Hb | Hemoglobin |
| HPTS | Hydroxypyrene trisulfonic acid |
| IC | Inspiratory capacity |
| IC | Integrated circuit |
| ICU | Intensive-care unit |
| ID | Inside diameter |
| IMFET | Immunologically sensitive field-effect transistor |
| IR | Infrared |
| ISE | Ion-sensitive electrode |
| ISFET | Ion-sensitive field-effect transistor |
| IV | Intravenous |
| $j$ | $+\sqrt{-1}$ |
| LED | Light-emitting diode |
| LIM | Line isolation monitor |
| lps | Liters per second |
| LRP | Late-receptor potential |
| MBC | Maximal breathing capacity |
| MCH | Mean corpuscular hemoglobin |
| MCHC | Mean corpuscular hemoglobin concentration |
| MCV | Mean corpuscular volume |
| MEFV | Maximal expiratory flow volume |

(*Continued*)

| Abbreviation | Term |
|---|---|
| MEG | Magnetoencephalogram |
| MMF | Maximal midexpiratory flow |
| MOSFET | Metal-oxide-semiconductor field-effect transistor |
| MRI | Magnetic resonance imaging |
| MTBF | Mean time between failures |
| MTF | Modulation transfer function |
| NDIR | Nondispersive infrared analysis |
| NEC | National Electric Code |
| NEMA | National Electrical Manufacturers Association |
| NEP | Noise-equivalent power |
| NFPA | National Fire Protection Association |
| NIST | National Institute of Standards and Technology |
| NREM | Nonrapid eye movement |
| OD | Outside diameter |
| ODC | Oxyhemoglobin dissociation curve |
| PA | Pulmonary artery |
| PCTA | Percutaneous translumenal coronary angioplasty |
| PEEP | Positive end expiratory pressure |
| PEF | Peak expiratory flow |
| PEP | Pre-ejection period |
| PFT | Pulmonary function tests |
| PIM | Patient interface module |
| PM | Photomultiplier |
| p-p | Peak-to-peak |
| PROM | Programmable read-only memory |
| PSP | Postsynaptic potential |
| PT | Phototransistor |
| PVC | Premature ventricular contraction |
| PVC | Polyvinyl chloride |
| RAM | Random-access memory |
| RAS | Reticular activating system |
| RBC | Red blood cell |
| RDW | Erythrocyte volume distribution width |
| REM | Rapid eye movement |
| RF | Radiofrequency |
| RIA | Radioimmunoassay |
| rms | Root-mean-square |
| ROM | Read-only memory |
| RV | Residual volume |
| SA | Sinoatrial |
| SCR | Silicon-controlled rectifier |
| SEC | Secondary-electron conduction |
| SEM | Standard error of the mean |
| SHR | Signal-to-hysteresis ratio |
| SMA | Sequential multiple analyzer |
| SMU | Single motor unit |
| SNR | Signal-to-noise ratio |
| SQUID | Superconducting quantum interference device |

| Abbreviation | Term |
|---|---|
| SVP | Surge-voltage protection |
| TBP | Total-body plethysmograph |
| TCD | Thermal-conductivity detector |
| TLC | Total lung capacity |
| TLC | Thin-layer chromatograph |
| TV | Television |
| TVC | Timed vital capacity |
| UL | Underwriters' Laboratory |
| VC | Vital capacity |
| VCVS | Voltage-controlled voltage source |
| VLSI | Very large scale integration |
| WBC | White blood cell |
| WPW | Wolff–Parkinson–White |
| YAG | Yttrium aluminum garnet |

# APPENDIX A.5

## Chemical Elements

| Element and Symbol | Atomic Number | Atomic weight (C = 12) | Element and Symbol | Atomic Number | Atomic weight (C = 12) |
|---|---|---|---|---|---|
| Actinium (Ac) | 89 | | Mercury (Hg) | 80 | 200.59 |
| Aluminum (Al) | 13 | 26.9815 | Molybdenum (Mo) | 42 | 95.94 |
| Americium (Am) | 95 | | Neodymium (Nd) | 60 | 144.24 |
| Antimony (Sb) | 51 | 121.75 | Neon (Ne) | 10 | 20.179 |
| Argon (Ar) | 18 | 39.948 | Neptunium (Np) | 93 | 237.0482 |
| Arsenic (As) | 33 | 74.9216 | Nickel (Ni) | 28 | 58.71 |
| Astatine (At) | 85 | | Niobium (Nb) | 41 | 92.9064 |
| Barium (Ba) | 56 | 137.34 | Nitrogen (N) | 7 | 14.0067 |
| Berkelium (Bk) | 97 | | Nobelium (No) | 102 | |
| Beryllium (Be) | 4 | 9.01218 | Osmium (Os) | 76 | 190.2 |
| Bismuth (Bi) | 83 | 208.9806 | Oxygen (O) | 8 | 15.9994 |
| Boron (B) | 5 | 10.81 | Palladium (Pd) | 46 | 106.4 |
| Bromine (Br) | 35 | 79.904 | Phosphorus (P) | 15 | 30.9738 |
| Cadmium (Cd) | 48 | 112.40 | Platinum (Pt) | 78 | 195.09 |
| Calcium (Ca) | 20 | 40.08 | Plutonium (Pu) | 94 | |
| Californium (Cf) | 98 | | Polonium (Po) | 84 | |
| Carbon (C) | 6 | 12.011 | Potassium (K) | 19 | 39.102 |
| Cerium (Ce) | 58 | 140.12 | Praseodymium (Pr) | 59 | 140.9077 |
| Cesium (Cs) | 55 | 132.9055 | Promethium (Pm) | 61 | |
| Chlorine (Cl) | 17 | 35.453 | Protactinium (Pa) | 91 | 231.0359 |
| Chromium (Cr) | 24 | 51.996 | Radium (Ra) | 88 | 226.0254 |
| Cobalt (Co) | 27 | 58.9332 | Radon (Rn) | 86 | |

(*Continued*)

| Element and Symbol | Atomic Number | Atomic weight (C = 12) | Element and Symbol | Atomic Number | Atomic weight (C = 12) |
|---|---|---|---|---|---|
| Columbium (Cb) | (see niobium) | | Rhenium (Re) | 75 | 186.2 |
| Copper (Cu) | 29 | 63.546 | Rhodium (Rh) | 45 | 102.9055 |
| Curium (Cm) | 96 | | Rubidium (Rb) | 37 | 85.4678 |
| Dysprosium (Dy) | 66 | 162.50 | Ruthenium (Ru) | 44 | 101.07 |
| Einsteinium (Es) | 99 | | Samarium (Sm) | 62 | 150.4 |
| Erbium (Er) | 68 | 167.26 | Scandium (Sc) | 21 | 44.9559 |
| Europium (Eu) | 63 | 151.96 | Selenium (Se) | 34 | 78.96 |
| Fermium (Fm) | 100 | | Silicon (Si) | 14 | 28.086 |
| Fluorine (F) | 9 | 18.9984 | Silver (Ag) | 47 | 107.868 |
| Francium (Fr) | 87 | | Sodium (Na) | 11 | 22.9898 |
| Gadolinium (Gd) | 64 | 157.25 | Strontium (Sr) | 38 | 87.62 |
| Gallium (Ga) | 31 | 69.72 | Sulfur (S) | 16 | 32.06 |
| Germanium (Ge) | 32 | 72.59 | Tantalum (Ta) | 73 | 180.9479 |
| Gold (Au) | 79 | 196.9665 | Technetium (Tc) | 43 | 98.9062 |
| Hafnium (Hf) | 72 | 178.49 | Tellurium (Te) | 52 | 127.60 |
| Helium (He) | 2 | 4.0026 | Terbium (Tb) | 65 | 158.9254 |
| Holmium (Ho) | 67 | 164.9303 | Thallium (Tl) | 81 | 204.37 |
| Hydrogen (H) | 1 | 1.0080 | Thorium (Th) | 90 | 232.0381 |
| Indium (In) | 49 | 114.82 | Thulium (Tm) | 69 | 168.9342 |
| Iodine (I) | 53 | 126.9045 | Tin (Sn) | 50 | 118.69 |
| Indium (Ir) | 77 | 192.22 | Titanium (Ti) | 22 | 47.90 |
| Iron (Fe) | 26 | 55.847 | Tungsten (W) | 74 | 183.85 |
| Krypton (Kr) | 36 | 83.80 | Uranium (U) | 92 | 238.029 |
| Lanthanum (La) | 57 | 138.9055 | Vanadium (V) | 23 | 50.9414 |
| Lawrencium (Lr) | 103 | | Wolfram (W) | (See tungsten.) | |
| Lead (Pb) | 82 | 207.2 | Xenon (Xe) | 54 | 131.30 |
| Lithium (Li) | 3 | 6.941 | Ytterbium (Yb) | 70 | 173.04 |
| Lutetium (Lu) | 71 | 174.97 | Yttrium (Y) | 39 | 88.9059 |
| Magnesium (Mg) | 12 | 24.305 | Zinc (Zn) | 30 | 65.37 |
| Manganese (Mn) | 25 | 54.9380 | Zirconium (Zr) | 40 | 91.22 |
| Mendelevium Md) | 101 | | | | |

# INDEX

**T**